NOTES ON CANINE INTERNAL

NOTES ON CANINE INTERNAL MEDICINE

Fourth Edition

Victoria L. Black,
MA, VetMB, FHEA, DipECVIM-CA, MRCVS
Senior Clinician in Small Animal Medicine
EBVS® European Specialist in Small Animal Internal Medicine
RCVS Specialist in Small Animal Medicine
Langford Vets, Bristol Veterinary School
Bristol, UK

Kathryn F. Murphy,
BVSc, DSAM, PGCertHE, DipECVIM-CA, FRCVS
EBVS® European Specialist in Small Animal Internal Medicine,
RCVS Specialist in Small Animal Medicine
Rowe Referrals, Bristol
VetCT
UK

Jessie Rose Payne,
BVetMed, MVetMed, PhD, DipACVIM (Cardiology), MRCVS
Senior Clinician in Cardiology
ACVIM Specialist in Veterinary Cardiology
RCVS Specialist in Veterinary Cardiology
Langford Vets, Bristol Veterinary School
Bristol, UK

Edward J. Hall,
MA, VetMB, PhD, DipECVIM-CA, FRCVS
Emeritus Professor of Small Animal Internal Medicine
EBVS® European Specialist in Small Animal Internal Medicine
RCVS Specialist in Small Animal Medicine (Gastroenterology)
University of Bristol
Bristol, UK

WILEY Blackwell

Edition History
Wright Imprint by IOP Publishing Limited
(1e, 1983; 2e, 1986)
Blackwell Science Ltd (3e, 2003)

Registered Offices
John Wiley & Sons, Inc., 111 River Street, Hoboken, NJ 07030, USA
John Wiley & Sons Ltd, The Atrium, Southern Gate, Chichester, West Sussex, PO19 8SQ, UK

Editorial Office
9600 Garsington Road, Oxford, OX4 2DQ, UK

For details of our global editorial offices, customer services, and more information about Wiley products visit us at www.wiley.com.

Wiley also publishes its books in a variety of electronic formats and by print-on-demand. Some content that appears in standard print versions of this book may not be available in other formats.

Library of Congress Cataloging-in-Publication Data

Names: Hall, E. J. (Ed J.) author. | Black, Victoria L., 1985- author. |
  Murphy, K. F. (Kate F.), author. | Payne, Jessie Rose, 1985- author.
Title: Notes on canine internal medicine / Victoria L. Black, Kathryn F.
  Murphy, Jessie Rose Payne, Edward J. Hall.
Other titles: Canine internal medicine
Description: Fourth edition. | Hoboken, NJ : Wiley-Blackwell, 2022. |
  Hall's name appears first in third edition.
Identifiers: LCCN 2022000939 (print) | LCCN 2022000940 (ebook) | ISBN
  9781119744771 (paperback) |
  ISBN 9781119744788 (adobe pdf) |
  ISBN 9781119744795 (epub)
Subjects: MESH: Dog Diseases | Handbook
Classification: LCC SF991 (print) | LCC SF991 (ebook) | NLM SF 991 | DDC
  636.7/0896–dc23/eng/20220209
LC record available at https://lccn.loc.gov/2022000939
LC ebook record available at https://lccn.loc.gov/2022000940

Cover Design: Wiley
Cover Images: Courtesy of Edward J. Hall, Jessie Rose Payne, Kathryn F. Murphy, and Victoria L. Black

Set in 9/11.5pt Sabon by Straive, Pondicherry, India
Printed in Singapore
M112334_080422

We all recognise the patience and support of our respective families during the production of this book. However, individually we wish to dedicate it specifically to:

All the vets and vet students I have met with a curious approach to our patients – your enthusiasm continues to inspire and motivate.

Victoria L. Black

Those who inspired me to know more as a student and resident (particularly Ed!) and my colleagues, clients and patients who continue to encourage me to learn more.

Kathryn F. Murphy

My patients, who make each day different from the last and continue to inspire me to learn every day.

Jessie Rose Payne

All the Medicine Residents and colleagues (particularly Kate and Vicki!) I have worked with, who have pushed me to learn more.

Edward J. Hall

CONTENTS

Section 5
Organ Systems   247

"When you hear hoofbeats, look for horses — not zebras."[*]

In 1983, in the first edition of Notes on Canine Internal Medicine, Peter Darke provided a revolutionary new and simplified diagnostic approach to internal medicine problem solving. It was not long before his book was to be found in the pocket of every veterinary undergraduate in the UK, as well as being an important first source of information for practitioners. The second and third editions built on this success. However, it is now nearly 20 years since the third and last edition and, in that time, our knowledge of canine internal medicine and our ability to investigate and treat cases has grown almost exponentially. Standard internal medicine texts now often fill two large volumes, detailing the underlying pathophysiology that is essential to understand diseases fully. However, there remains a need for a concise text to aid students and busy practitioners.

Whilst we acknowledge the importance of pathophysiology in internal medicine, in first opinion practice knowing the three most likely differential diagnoses for a problem is of more use than knowing ten obscure and unlikely ones despite potentially similar pathophysiological mechanisms. Thus, in this book, we have provided separate lists of the 'common causes' of medical problems, and the 'uncommon causes'. Our personal experiences and geographical location inevitably bias our opinions on what are the most common causes of any specific problem but please note that these two lists are in alphabetical order and not order of prevalence. We are also not indicating the relative incidence of specific problems seen in first opinion practice, although practitioners will already know that dermatological and GI problems are most common. Our opinions on what are the best approaches to a specific problem are based on the scientific evidence, where it is available, and on our personal experience.

This edition follows a similar pattern to the third edition, with sections on presenting complaints, physical findings, and laboratory abnormalities. We have added a new section on imaging patterns, and again finish with a section covering diseases of the major organ systems. The authorship has been expanded to ensure we have the expertise to cover all areas of internal medicine, including Peter Darke's own discipline of cardiology. We have also included information on behavioural, dermatological and ophthalmological problems focused on where these are manifestations of systemic disease. We do not believe in a totally algorithmic approach as used in some texts and have highlighted key clinical clues which, when using the results of history-taking, physical examination, laboratory tests and imaging findings, should guide the clinician's investigation in the right direction and avoid unnecessary testing.

As noted in the first edition, the recognition that not everything in internal medicine is black and white is part of its challenge; and not every patient 'reads the textbook'. We still believe in the advice of the first edition that '*basic, careful history-taking and thorough and, if necessary, repeated clinical examination are fundamental procedures that may yield a diagnosis in a complicated or unresolved case*'. One should always remember that there is always one more question to be asked, or one more investigation to be performed on problem cases, and one should never be afraid to go back to the beginning and start again.

V.L.B, K.F.M., J.R.P. and E.J.H.
2022

---

[*] Source uncertain; https://quoteinvestigator.com/2017/11/26/zebras/

ACKNOWLEDGEMENTS

The initial inspiration for this book was Peter Darke's and we are honoured to write this new edition. The book retains its original title to emphasise its aim to be easily accessible notes for the veterinary practitioner and student to assist their diagnostic investigations of medically ill dogs.

USING THIS BOOK

SECTION 1

Presenting complaints
- In this section, the common presenting complaints are listed alphabetically according to a stylised format.
- Each problem is defined, and the expected clinical signs listed although not every case will show every sign.
- Causes for the problem are divided into 'common' and 'uncommon' to guide the reader, but are only the opinion of the authors, and may vary in different geographical locations.
- For each problem a logical diagnostic approach is suggested; any numbering indicates a suggested order for the investigations:
  - Clinical clues in the history.
  - Potential findings in the clinical examination.
  - Laboratory findings that aid the diagnosis.
  - Key results from imaging.
  - Special tests that may confirm the diagnosis.

SECTION 2

Physical problems

In this section, significant findings from the physical examination are listed alphabetically.
- Each problem is defined.
- Common and uncommon causes, listed alphabetically, are suggested for each problem.
- Related clinical signs are listed.
- For each problem a logical diagnostic approach is suggested.
- Key findings to look for in the history and physical examination are noted; not all will be present in every case.
- Laboratory findings that aid the diagnosis are noted.
- Key results of imaging are noted.
- Special tests that may confirm the diagnosis are listed.

SECTION 3

Laboratory abnormalities
In this section laboratory abnormalities of haematology, serum biochemistry and urinalysis are listed alphabetically.

- The abnormality is defined.
- Causes are listed alphabetically, and the likely degree of severity is suggested.
- The diagnostic interpretation for the abnormality is given.
- Adjunctive tests that may help support or confirm the diagnosis are given.

SECTION 4

Imaging patterns

Differential diagnoses for specific plain radiographic and ultrasonographic patterns and appearances are listed. Relevant further imaging modalities (contrast radiography, cross-sectional imaging, i.e. CT and MRI) are suggested.

SECTION 5

Organ systems

The relevant clinical presentations and physical, laboratory and imaging abnormalities (identified in Sections 1–4, respectively) are given for each major internal organ system. Then the diagnostic approach and the methods of investigation of each organ system are briefly explained. Finally, the more common diseases of each system are covered alphabetically. For each, its aetiology, predisposition, historical clues, clinical signs, laboratory test results, treatment and monitoring, sequelae and prognosis are given in note form.

COMMONLY USED ABBREVIATIONS

Commonly used scientific and medical abbreviations listed here are used throughout the book without further expansion. All other abbreviations are spelled out in each section, and are listed at the end of the book with the Index.

ACTH	adrenocorticotrophic hormone
ALP (SAP)	(serum) alkaline phosphatase
ALT	alanine aminotransferase
BID	twice daily (q12h)
CBC	complete blood count
ECG	electrocardiogram
EDTA	ethylenediaminetetra-acetic acid
ELISA	enzyme-linked immunosorbent assay
HCT	haematocrit
IgA	immunoglobulin A
IM	intramuscular
IV	intravenous
NPO	*nil per os* (nothing by mouth)
NSAID	non-steroidal anti-inflammatory drug
PCR	polymerase chain reaction
PCV	packed cell volume
PO	*per os*
QID	four times daily (q6h)
q.v.	*quod vide* (see related material)
RBC	red blood cell
SC	subcutaneous
SID	once daily (q24h)
T4	thyroxine
TID	three times daily (q8h)
WBC	white blood cell

SECTION 1
PRESENTING COMPLAINTS

In this section, the common presenting complaints are listed alphabetically according to a stylised format.

- Each problem is defined, and the expected clinical signs listed, although not every case will show every sign.
- Causes for the problem are divided into 'common' and 'uncommon' to guide the reader, but are only the opinion of the authors, and may vary in different geographical locations.
- For each problem a logical diagnostic approach is suggested; any numbering indicates a suggested order for the investigations:
  - Clinical clues in the history.
  - Potential findings in the clinical examination.
  - Laboratory findings that aid the diagnosis.
  - Key results from imaging.
  - Special tests that may confirm the diagnosis

PRESENTING COMPLAINTS

1.1 ABORTION

DEFINITION

The spontaneous expulsion of one or more fetuses before the end of full-term pregnancy, i.e. when the fetus is incapable of independent life.

RELATED CLINICAL SIGNS

- Abdominal pain
- Abnormal vulval discharge
- Fever
- Lethargy/depression
- Premature whelping is reported with live or dead pups or no live pups at term

COMMON CAUSES

Infectious
- Bacterial
  - *Brucella canis* in endemic countries; not endemic in UK
  - *Streptococcus* infection
- Viral: Canine herpesvirus-1 (CHV-1)

Non-infectious
- Congenital defects: various lethal defects
- Genetic causes: various lethal defects
- Maternal factors:
  - Illness
    - Diabetes mellitus (DM)
    - Eclampsia
    - Pregnancy toxaemia
  - Drugs
    - Corticosteroids
    - Griseofulvin
    - Itraconazole
    - Phenylephrine
    - Prolactin inhibitors
    - Prostaglandins
    - Progesterone-receptor blockers
  - Toxins: insecticides, plant toxins
- Trauma
- Hypoluteinization (low progesterone)
- Advanced age
- Traumatic: dystocia

UNCOMMON CAUSES

Infectious
- Bacterial
  - *Escherichia coli*
  - *Campylobacter*
  - *Leptospira*
  - *Salmonella*
- Fungal
- Protozoal
  - *Leishmania*
  - *Neospora*
  - *Toxoplasma*
- Viral
  - Bluetongue virus
  - Canine adenovirus 1
  - Canine distemper virus
  - Canine parvovirus 1 (minute virus)

DIAGNOSTIC APPROACH

Clinical clues
Predisposition
- Advanced age
- Previous history of abortion
  - Assess for hypoluteinization by checking progesterone concentrations

History
- Abnormal vulval discharge
- Bitch whelps early with live or dead pups or no pups at term

Clinical examination
Visual inspection
- Often unremarkable

Notes on Canine Internal Medicine, Fourth Edition. Victoria L. Black, Kathryn F. Murphy, Jessie Rose Payne, and Edward J. Hall.

PRESENTING COMPLAINTS

Physical examination
- Abdominal contractions and expulsion of fetus(es) in later pregnancy
- Vulval discharge: purulent, haemorrhagic, green, black, malodorous

Laboratory findings
Haematology
- May be normal
- HCT often low in pregnancy due to decreased plasma volume, e.g. 30–35% compared to 45–55%
- Mild mature neutrophilia common in pregnancy, may sometimes be more pronounced changes or bands

Serum biochemistry
- May be normal

Urinalysis
- May show evidence of inflammation with free catch or catheter samples

Imaging
Plain radiographs
- May show evidence of dystocia

Ultrasound
- May show evidence of fetal death

Special tests
- Examination of fetus post mortem
- Virus isolation/bacterial culture/PCR of fetus/placenta/vaginal secretions/milk

Tests of dam
- Serology ± PCR of dam for CHV-1, *B. canis*
- Serum progesterone to assess if sufficient to maintain pregnancy: should be > 2 ng/ml (6 nmol/l); if less than these values for > 48 hours suggests hypoluteinization but can be seen due to fetal death
- Thyroid hormone analysis: total T4/thyroid-stimulating hormone (TSH)

1.2 ALOPECIA

DEFINITION

Absence of hair from areas of skin that normally carry hairs, due either to a failure of production or to an increased loss of hair. Hypotrichosis refers to thinning of hair. Hair loss may be focal or diffuse, and symmetrical or non-symmetrical.

RELATED CLINICAL SIGNS

- Endocrinopathies are likely to cause concurrent systemic signs such as changes in drinking, eating, exercise tolerance and body weight
- Loss or absence of hair
- Self-traumatic lesions if pruritic skin disease

COMMON CAUSES

Primary follicular disease
Inherited abnormalities of follicular structure, ranging from absence of follicles that normally produce hair of a particular colour to complete absence of follicles, are uncommon except in specific breeds.

Secondary follicular disease
- Bacterial folliculitis/superficial pyoderma
- Demodectic mange
- Hyperadrenocorticism (HAC)
  - Iatrogenic
  - Pituitary- or adrenal-dependent
- Hypothyroidism
- Interdigital pyoderma
- *Malassezia* infection
- Seasonal flank alopecia (cyclic follicular dysplasia)

Self-trauma when pruritic
- Atopy
- Fleas and flea-allergic dermatitis
- Pyotraumatic dermatitis ('hot spot')
- Sarcoptic mange
- Secondary bacterial pyoderma

UNCOMMON CAUSES

Primary follicular disease
- Alopecia areata
- Alopecia mucinosa/follicular mucinosis: Shar pei
- (Auto)immune skin disease
  - Dermatomyositis
  - Erythema multiforme
  - Exfoliative cutaneous lupus erythematosus (ECLE)
  - Systemic lupus erythematosus
  - Pemphigus foliaceous
  - Sebaceous adenitis
- Catagen arrest: Weimaraners
- Colour mutant/dilution
- Congenital hypotrichosis/alopecia
- Follicular dysplasia
  - Black hair follicular dysplasia
  - Breed-specific follicular dysplasia
    - Loss of primary but retention of secondary hairs changing coat to reddish-brown: Siberian Husky and Alaskan Malamute
    - Flank and saddle region involved initially in red or black dogs: Dobermann
    - Flank and saddle hair loss: Airedale terrier, Boxer, English bulldog, Staffordshire terrier
    - Hair loss around face and over dorsum; cyclic initially but eventually permanent: Curly-coated Retriever, Irish Water spaniel, Portuguese Water dog
  - Medullary trichomalacia: German shepherd
  - Pili torti
  - Trichorrhexis nodosa
- Follicular lipidosis: Rottweiler
- Hairless breeds
- Pattern baldness
  - Caudal thigh: Greyhounds
  - Neck, trunk and thighs: Portuguese Water dog, American Water spaniel
  - Pinnal: Dachshund
  - Ventral and caudal: Boston Terrier, Chihuahua, Dachshund, Manchester Terrier, Whippet
- Pressure/traction alopecia: focal hair loss over bony prominences and sites of friction by collars, harnesses and coats
- Pseudopelade
- Subcorneal pustular dermatosis
- Trichoptilosis: Golden retriever

Secondary follicular disease
- Adrenal sex hormone imbalance/adrenal hyperplasia syndrome (alopecia X)
- Anagen defluvium
  - Cancer chemotherapy – greatest risk with curly- or wire-haired coats
  - Endocrinopathies
  - Infection
- Cicatricial (scar-related)
- Cold agglutinin disease
- Contact dermatitis
- Cutaneous vasculitis
- Dermatomyositis
- Dermatophytosis
- Epitheliotropic lymphoma including mycosis fungoides
- Follicular arrest
  - Post-clipping
  - Protein/calorie malnutrition
- Hepatocutaneous sydrome: more typically causes painful footpad hyperkeratosis
- Hyperoestrogenism
  - Adrenal gland disease
  - Excessive oestrogen administration (for urinary incontinence)
  - Excessive phytoestrogen ingestion (e.g. flaxseed)
  - Inadvertent exposure to human transdermal hormone replacement product
  - Ovarian remnant follicular cyst formation or malignant transformation
  - Testicular Sertoli cell tumour
- Hypo-oestrogenism
- Hyposomatotropism (pituitary dwarf)
- Hypotestosteronism
- Leishmaniosis
- Nutritional
  - Biotin deficiency
  - Vitamin A or E deficiency
- Radiation therapy
- Systemic lupus erythematosus (SLE)
- Telogen effluvium
  - Injection reaction
    - Epidural
    - Post-vaccinal
  - Post-partum
  - Pregnancy
  - "Stress"
- Thallium poisoning
- Vitamin A deficiency
- Zinc-responsive dermatosis

Self-mutilation
- Acral lick/flank sucking/neurodermatitis
- Cheyletiella
- Food allergy
- Lice
- *Trombicula* (Harvest mite)

DIAGNOSTIC APPROACH

1 Identification of infectious agents by sello-tape strips, skin scrapes, hair plucks, bacterial and fungal cultures, and empirical treatment trials.
2 The presence or absence of pruritus narrows the differential diagnosis.
   If pruritic:
   - After ruling out infectious causes, trial therapy for bacterial pyoderma, fleas and possibly also for *Sarcoptes*, is acceptable
   - Intradermal skin testing is performed to identify atopic reactions
   - If all negative, an exclusion food trial is indicated
   If non-pruritic:
   - Consider endocrinopathy or breed-related problem
   - Skin biopsy is indicated if no cause is obvious

Clinical clues
- Pattern of hair loss and sites of self-mutilation can be informative
   q.v. Clinical examination
- Broken hairs on trichogram and ulcerated skin suggest self-trauma due to pruritus
- Concurrent systemic signs of polyuria/polydipsia (PU/PD), exercise intolerance, polyphagia or weight gain are suggestive of an endocrinopathy
- Non-symmetrical alopecia is suggestive of self-trauma or infection
- Presence of fleas or 'flea dirt' is diagnostic
- Repeated scratching and rubbing indicate pruritic causes
- Seasonality is suggestive of atopy, ectoparasites or seasonal flank alopecia
- Symmetrical alopecia is suggestive of an endocrinopathy
- Bilaterally symmetrical alopecia starting on the trunk is considered the hallmark of an

endocrinopathy, but pruritic skin disease can also appear symmetrical.
- Evidence of pruritus:
  - Positive scratch reflex
  - Broken hairs, not hair loss

Predisposition
Breed predisposition may suggest primary follicular diseases:
- Canine hairless breeds: American Hairless Terrier, Argentine Pila, Chinese Crested, Mexican Hairless (Xoloitzcuintli), Peruvian Inca Orchid
- Colour-mutant alopecia: blue/fawn/red Dobermann, blue Chow Chow, blue Dachshund, blue Great Dane, blue Whippet, fawn Irish setter
- Follicular dysplasia: Curly-coated Retriever, Irish Water Spaniel, Portuguese Water dog
- Dermatomyositis: Collies

History
- Colour-mutant alopecia develops in young adults
- Congenital or hereditary hypotrichosis is usually evident from an early age
- Slow onset and bilateral truncal alopecia is suggestive of endocrinopathy
- Testicular mass, pendulous prepuce and attractiveness to other male dogs is suggestive of functional Sertoli cell tumour
- Other clinical signs (e.g. PU/PD, weight change) suggest a possible endocrinopathy

Clinical examination
Visual inspection
- Broken hairs if pruritic, otherwise hairs are absent
- Lesions secondary to self-trauma: erythema, excoriation, lichenification, hyperpigmentation
- Presence of fleas or 'flea dirt'
- Pustules, erythema, scaling in pyoderma

Physical examination
- Thickened skin in hypothyroidism
- Thinned skin in HAC
- Distribution of self-mutilation
  - Dorso-lumbar with flea-allergic dermatitis
  - Ear margins and elbows with sarcoptic mange

- Face, feet and ventrum with atopy
- Feet and ventrum with contact allergy
- Face, ears and feet with food allergy
- Face, ears, feet or multifocal with demodecosis
- Face, feet, mucocutaneous junctions with autoimmune skin disease
- Distribution of hair loss
  - Focal
    - Alopecia areata
    - Cicatricial
    - Demodecosis
    - Dermatophytosis
    - Injection reaction
    - Pattern baldness
    - Superficial pyoderma/bacterial folliculitis
  - Multifocal or diffuse but patchy
    - Colour dilution
    - Demodecosis
    - Dermatomyositis
    - Dermatophytosis
    - Epitheliotropic lymphosarcoma
    - Follicular dysplasia
    - Superficial pyoderma/bacterial folliculitis
  - Symmetrical, generalised, diffuse
    - Demodecosis
    - Dermatophytosis
    - Endocrinopathies
    - Superficial pyoderma/bacterial folliculitis
    - Telogen effluvium
    - Hair loss from the caudal trunk and thighs
    - Flea allergic dermatosis
    - Follicular dysplasia
    - Hyperoestrogenism
    - Pattern baldness of Greyhounds
  - Hair loss from the pinnae
    - Atopy
    - Cold agglutinin disease
    - Dermatophytosis
    - Demodectic mange

- Otitis externa
- Pemphigus erythematosus
- Pemphigus foliaceus
- Pinnal pattern baldness
- Sarcoptic mange
- Subcorneal pustular dermatosis
- Hair loss from the feet
  - Atopy
  - Contact dermatitis
  - Demodectic mange
  - Pemphigus diseases
  - Interdigital pyoderma
  - Thallium poisoning

Laboratory findings

Haematology and serum biochemistry
- Unremarkable unless underlying endocrinopathy, e.g. hypercholesterolaemia in hypothyroidism, increased ALP activity in HAC

Dermatological investigations
- Bacterial and fungal cultures
- Hair plucks – *Demodex*, ringworm
- Hypercholesterolaemia and increased ALP in HAC
- Sellotape strips cytology: *Malassezia*
- Skin scrapes: *Sarcoptes*, *Demodex*

Imaging
- Usually unnecessary and unremarkable unless systemic signs (e.g. endocrinopathy)

Special tests
- Dynamic cortisol testing for HAC
- Exclusion diet trial
- Intradermal skin tests
- Sarcoptic mange antibody
- Therapeutic trial for sarcoptic mange
- Skin biopsy
- Thyroid function tests

1.3 ALTERED BEHAVIOUR

DEFINITION

A change in response to or interaction with the environment. Abnormal behaviour can be observed as a spectrum of consciousness (*q.v.* section 1.4) ranging from reduced response to even noxious stimuli to manic behaviour and hyperactivity. Animals may also demonstrate changes in sleep-wake cycles, social relationships, repetitive activities, or spatial disorientation.

Behavioural disorders and medical disorders causing behaviour change present a significant challenge due to the considerable overlap in presentations. Behavioural disorders can be considered *after* medical disorders have been excluded and are more common in younger animals presenting with increased reactivity or vigilance.

RELATED CLINICAL SIGNS

- Aggression
- Dullness and reduced responsiveness, *q.v.* section 1.4
- Excessive grooming
- Hyperactivity (excessive pacing, circling, altered sleep patterns)
- Inappropriate elimination
- Repetitive behaviours (fly catching, overgrooming, tail chasing, flank sucking)

COMMON CAUSES

Pain
- Ear disease
- Neuropathic
- Orthopaedic

Intracranial disorders
- Cognitive dysfunction
- Hydrocephalus
- Idiopathic epilepsy
- Inflammatory (meningoencephalitis of unknown origin)
- Neoplasia

Metabolic disorders
- Hepatic encephalopathy (portosystemic shunts, chronic hepatitis, acute hepatic failure)
- Hyperadrenocorticism
- Hypertension
- Hypothyroidism
- Toxins

Intestinal disorders
- Idiopathic chronic inflammatory enteropathy (CIE)/inflammatory bowel disease (IBD)
- Neoplasia

Urinary tract disorders
- Atopy
- Dermatological disorders
- Ectopic ureters
- Parasitic infection
- Urinary tract infection
- Urolithiasis

UNCOMMON CAUSES

Metabolic disorders
- Hyperthyroidism
- Phaeochromocytoma

Intracranial disorders
- Infectious disease, e.g. *Cryptococcus*, distemper, *Toxoplasma*, *Neospora*
- Storage disease

Dermatological disorders
- Bacterial hypersensitivity

Ocular disorders causing pain or impairing vision
- Cataracts
- Progressive retinal atrophy
- Uveitis

DIAGNOSTIC APPROACH

Thorough screening for medical disorders should be considered in young animals, or in patients with acute onset change. Environment, social interactions, exercise routine, and training history may influence likelihood of behavioural disorders.

Clinical clues
Predisposition
- Cognitive dysfunction and orthopaedic pain: older dogs
- Portosystemic shunt (PSS): young dogs and some breeds are predisposed (e.g. Yorkshire terriers, Miniature schnauzers, Pugs, Irish Wolfhounds)

- Some repetitive behaviours have breed associations:
  - Flank sucking: Dobermanns
  - Fly catching: CKCS
  - Hind-end checking: Miniature Schnauzers
  - Self-mutilation: Springer spaniels
  - Tail chasing: German shepherds
- Neuropathies can be heritable disorders, e.g. sensory neuropathy in Border collies

History
- Assess for risk of toxin exposure if acute onset change
- Circumstance of occurrence may increase suspicion of
  - pain disorders after rest or after exercise
  - metabolic disease, e.g. after eating may increase suspicion of a PSS

Clinical examination
Visual inspection
- Behaviour during consultation, or during circumstance of typical occurrence: video recordings of abnormal behaviour are encouraged
- Haircoat changes are suggestive of endocrine disorders
- In young dogs, examine for
  - disproportionate stunting, e.g. congenital hypothyroidism
  - domed cranium ± open fontanelle in hydrocephalus
  - stature, e.g. small size in EPI, PSS

Physical examination
Thorough examination for source of pain, with specific attention to musculoskeletal system
- Neurological and ophthalmic examination
- Rectal examination in cases of inappropriate elimination to assess for rectal, urethral, and prostatic disorders

Laboratory findings
Haematology
- May reveal microcytosis ± hypochromasia in PSS
- Mild, normocytic, normochromic, poorly-regenerative anaemia in hypothyroidism

Serum biochemistry
- Evidence of hepatic dysfunction (e.g. decreased albumin, cholesterol, urea, glucose, increased ammonia), including increased bile acids; increased liver enzyme activities not typical in PSS but detected in other hepatopathies
- Enteropathy may present with panhypoproteinaemia (hypoalbuminaemia and hypoglobulinaemia) ± low serum cholesterol
- Hypercholesterolaemia in hypothyroidism

Imaging
Plain radiographs
- In cases with excessive grooming may detect underlying musculoskeletal disease including degenerative joint disease or neoplasia

Ultrasound
- Abnormal vessel ± renomegaly may be observed in PSS
- Adrenal gland size in cases suspicious for hyperadrenocorticism
- Intestinal wall layering for enteropathy
- Liver size and echotexture when suspicious of hepatic dysfunction

Special tests
- Cobalamin and folate in cases with a suspicion of enteropathy, particularly relevant to cases of fly catching, inappropriate elimination, or pica
- Computed tomography (CT) angiogram to assess for PSS if not detected on ultrasound examination
- Low-dose dexamethasone suppression LDDS test (± ACTH stimulation test) to assess for hyperadrenocorticism
- Liver biopsy for hepatopathy
- Total thyroxine and TSH to assess for hypothyroidism
- Treatment trials
  - Non-steroidal anti-inflammatory drug (NSAID) or other analgesic trial for suspected pain
  - Antiepileptic therapy where partial seizures are a consideration
  - Exclusion diet trial where atopy or enteropathy is suspected

1.4 ALTERED CONSCIOUSNESS

DEFINITION

Consciousness is the state of arousal and ability to respond to the external environment. Diminished consciousness can be graded based upon lack of responsiveness to increasingly stimulatory external events. State of consciousness is an important component of the modified Glasgow Coma Scale (MGCS), useful prognostically and for monitoring purposes.

Consciousness is primarily determined by the ascending reticular activating system, an important set of neurons found within the brainstem. Disorders of the brainstem can result in dysfunction of these neurons, with a consequent reduced state of arousal of the individual. Diffuse forebrain dysfunction (cerebral disorders) may also result in diminished consciousness in some circumstances (*q.v.* modified Glasgow Coma Scale in section 5.8).

RELATED CLINICAL SIGNS

Grades of dysfunction
Depressed or obtunded
- Reduced responsiveness to external visual or auditory stimuli
  - Associated with brainstem, diffuse forebrain disorders, or systemic disease
  - Can have intermittent periods of more normal mentation

Stuporous
- Semi-comatose, responsive only to repeated noxious stimuli
  - Typically associated with brainstem disorders, including brain herniation

Comatose
- Unresponsive to repeated noxious stimuli
  - Typically associated with brainstem disorders, including brain herniation

Delirious
- Hyperactive with excessive or abnormal responses to external stimuli
  - Typically associated with forebrain disease

COMMON CAUSES

Congenital
- Hydrocephalus
- PSS

Inflammatory
- Meningoencephalitis of unknown origin (MUO)

Infectious
- Bacterial empyema, e.g. extension of otitis media
- Lungworm (*Angiostrongylus vasorum*)

Iatrogenic
- Head trauma
- Toxins or drugs, e.g. sedation or anaesthesia, hallucinogens

Metabolic
- Electrolyte disturbances, especially changes in osmolarity due to too-rapid correction of sodium disturbances
- Hepatic encephalopathy
- Hypoglycaemia
- Severe systemic disease, e.g. sepsis, congestive heart failure, etc.

Neoplastic
- Primary central nervous system (CNS) tumours: meningioma, glioma, lymphoma

Vascular
- Thromboembolic or haemorrhagic stroke

UNCOMMON CAUSES

Congenital
- Storage disease: signs may develop as dog ages

Infectious
- Distemper
- Protozoal: *Toxoplasma, Neospora*
- Rabies

Iatrogenic

- Complication of cerebrospinal fluid (CSF) sampling in dogs with increased intracranial pressure

Vascular

- Hyperviscosity, e.g. hyperglobulinaemia, hyperlipidaemia, primary erythrocytosis

DIAGNOSTIC APPROACH

Clinical clues

Predisposition

- Congenital disorders maybe suspected in young dogs, especially those with conformational changes
  - Disproportionate stunting, e.g. congenital hypothyroidism (*q.v.* section 1.45)
  - Domed cranium ± open fontanelle in hydrocephalus
  - Small stature in PSS
- Small purebred middle-aged dogs are predisposed to meningoencephalitis of unknown origin (e.g. Maltese terrier, Pug, West Highland White terrier [WHWT])

History

- Anti-parasitic prophylaxis may indicate lesser risk of *Angiostrongylus* infection
- Lifestyle may increase index of suspicion for infectious disease, e.g. raw-fed may increase suspicion of toxoplasmosis or exposure to toxins or risk of trauma

Clinical examination

Visual inspection

- Interaction with the environment, increasing external stimuli (to include visual and auditory tests)

Physical examination

- Assess for signs of systemic disease in cases of obtundation; mentation changes may be secondary to this, or, in multisystemic disease, may detect abnormalities on examination
- Heart rate and blood pressure (BP): a patient with bradycardia (pulse rate < 60 beats/minute) and hypertension (systolic BP > 160 mmHg) is at risk of increased intracranial pressure (Cushing's reflex)

Neurological examination

- Cranial nerve assessment is particularly important in stuporous and comatose animals given the high suspicion of a brainstem disorder
- Focus on assessment of forebrain (mentation, proprioception, menace response and response to nasal stimulation) and brainstem (proprioception and cranial nerves) functions
- MUO typically presents with a multifocal lesion localisation, whereas metabolic disease typically results in symmetrical deficits localising to the forebrain

Ophthalmic examination

- Papilloedema (optic disc swelling) is suggestive of increased intracranial pressure

Laboratory findings

Haematology

- Assess for signs of severe systemic disease (e.g. marked leukocyte changes supportive of an inflammatory focus)
- Increased PCV in primary erythrocytosis (typically > 68%)
- May reveal microcytosis ± hypochromasia in PSS

Serum biochemistry

- Evidence of hepatic dysfunction (low albumin, cholesterol, urea, glucose, increased ammonia) and increased bile acids
- Increased liver enzyme activities are not typical in PSS but are detected in other hepatopathies
- Hypoglycaemia
- Sodium concentrations: review previous results in hospitalised animals to assess for changes in sodium indicating too-rapid correction of marked hypernatraemia

Imaging

NB: Cross-sectional imaging (MRI) is often indicated for primary CNS diseases

Plain radiographs

- Screening in cases with a high suspicion of multisystemic disorders (e.g. assessing for neoplasia)

- Skull radiographs may be useful in cases of head trauma, but rarely in hydrocephalus

Ultrasound
- Assess for liver size and echotexture when suspicious of hepatic dysfunction. Renomegaly may also be observed in PSS.
- Screening in cases with a high suspicion of multisystemic disorders (e.g. assessing for neoplasia)

Special tests
- Assessment of haemostasis (platelet count, buccal mucosal bleeding time, prothrombin time [PT] and activated partial thromboplastin time [aPTT], thromboelastography) to assess for risk of hypo- or hypercoagulability where vascular disorder is suspected
- Baermann's technique, AngioDetect® or faecal smear to identify *Angiostrongylus* infection
- CSF analysis – cytology and biochemistry, PCR for *Toxoplasma* and *Neospora*
- EEG (electroencephalography) or BAER (brainstem auditory evoked response)
- MRI
- Response to mannitol or hypertonic saline in patients with suspected increased intracranial pressure

1.5 ANOREXIA/HYPOREXIA/INAPPETENCE

DEFINITION

A decline in food intake through loss of appetite whilst still physically able to eat
- Anorexia indicates a complete lack of food intake
- Dysorexia is a diminished, disordered or unnatural appetite (*q.v.* section 1.36)
- Hyporexia is a significant reduction in food intake
- Inappetence implies a decline in food intake through either a loss of appetite or a selective appetite
- Pseudo-anorexia is a condition where a dog wants to eat but is unwilling or physically unable to do so because of orthopaedic or neuromuscular dysfunction or pain associated with eating

RELATED CLINICAL SIGNS

- Pseudo-anorexia: the dog may try to eat but stop quickly because of pain or difficulty swallowing
- True anorexia: the dog will not attempt to eat, or may turn away as if nauseated

COMMON CAUSES

Anorexia/inappetence
- Diabetic ketoacidosis
- Drugs: many
- Fever
- Gastrointestinal (GI) disease
- Hepatic disease
- Hypercalcaemia
- Infectious/inflammatory diseases
- Neoplasia
- Pain
- Pancreatitis
- Uraemia

Pseudoanorexia
- Dental disease
  - Abscessed tooth root
  - Fractured tooth
- Oesophagitis
- Retrobulbar abscess/periorbital cellulitis
- Unpalatable diet

UNCOMMON CAUSES

True anorexia
- Anosmia, *q.v.* section 1.6
- Cardiac failure
- Drugs

- Hypoadrenocorticism
- Sialoadenitis
- Severe respiratory disease
  - Advanced neoplasia (primary or metastatic)
  - Diaphragmatic rupture
  - Pneumonia
  - Pleural effusion
- Neurological disease
  - Cerebral oedema
  - Hydrocephalus
  - Hypothalamic disease
    - Congenital cystic lesions
    - Infection/inflammation
    - Neoplasia
    - Trauma
- Psychological (food aversion)
  - Anxiety
  - Hospitalisation
  - Loss of companion
  - Social stress

Pseudo-anorexia

- Blindness
- Cranial nerve deficits
- Craniomandibular osteopathy
- Jaw fracture
- Oropharyngeal inflammation/ulceration
- Oropharyngeal neoplasia
- Osteomyelitis of jaw
- Temporal myositis
- Temporomandibular joint (TMJ) disease
  - Jaw locking
  - TMJ dysplasia or dislocation
- Tetanus
- Trigeminal neuritis/neuropraxia

DIAGNOSTIC APPROACH

Anorexia/hyporexia are common, non-specific findings with many potential causes.
1 Rule out dietary causes, drug administration, stressors.
2 Determine from history and direct observation whether the dog wants to eat or not and whether it is physically able to.
3 Pseudo-anorexia will be caused by a cranial nerve deficit or a lesion in the mouth, pharynx or oesophagus.
4 Examination of the mouth may require sedation or anaesthesia, and imaging of the skull.
5 Complete physical examination and relevant lab tests and imaging for causes of true anorexia.

Clinical clues
Predisposition
- Craniomandibular osteopathy in WHWT

History
- Coughing or other respiratory signs
- Does dog attempt to eat and then drop or regurgitate food, or does it avoid food?
- Nausea (e.g. signs of lip-smacking, retching, etc.) in metabolic or GI disease
- PU/PD in liver and renal disease
- Seizures if intracranial disease
- Stressful event leading to food aversion
- Traumatic event if jaw fracture
- Vomiting and/or diarrhoea with GI disease and hypoadrenocorticism
- Weight loss in excess of what is expected from not eating suggests increased energy usage, e.g. metabolic disease, neoplasia, etc.

Clinical examination
Visual inspection
- Depression
- Drooling saliva
- Dyspnoea if cardiac failure
- Open mouth if trigeminal neuropraxia or jaw locking
- Unilateral exophthalmos if retrobulbar abscess

Physical examination
- Abdominal masses palpable
- Abnormal lung and heart sounds
- Halitosis if oral disease
- Pain or resistance on opening mouth if myositis, foreign body (FB) or retrobulbar abscess
- *Risus sardonicus*, erect ears, muscle stiffness and spasms in tetanus

- Temporal muscle atrophy with myositis
- Trismus with myositis or TMJ disorder

Laboratory findings
Variable, often within normal limits (WNL)

Haematology
- Inflammatory leukogram with infection or inflammatory diseases

Biochemistry
- Azotaemia
  - Plus isosthenuria in renal failure
  - Pre-renal (hypersthenuria) in dehydration due to hypodipsia

- Hypercalcaemia most frequently associated with malignancy, especially lymphosarcoma and anal sac adenocarcinoma; primary hyperparathyroidism is rare
- Hyponatraemia / hyperkalaemia in hypoadrenocorticism
- Increased liver enzyme activities, bile acids ± bilirubin in hepatic diseases

Special tests
- Complete neurological examination
- Multiple depending on suspected condition

1.6 ANOSMIA

DEFINITION

The loss of the sense of smell. The most common reason for presentation is when an owner of a hunting dog perceives their dog has lost the ability to find game, or a detection dog is unable to find the substance it has been trained to seek. Even then, other signs of nasal disease are more likely to prompt presentation.

RELATED CLINICAL SIGNS

- Epistaxis, nasal discharge, sneezing
- Facial deformity
- Temporal muscle atrophy
- Xerostomia

COMMON CAUSES

- Diseases of the nasal cavity
  - Lymphoplasmacytic rhinitis
  - Neoplasia
  - Sino-nasal aspergillosis

UNCOMMON CAUSES

- Distemper
- Forebrain disease
- Sensory decline with age

- Sensory overload (temporary)
- Skull fracture(s)
- Trigeminal neuritis
- Traumatic/destructive lesions of the cribriform plate
  - Fungal infection
  - Neoplasia

DIAGNOSTIC APPROACH

It is difficult to assess olfaction but cranial nerve assessment, in particular nasal sensation, should be undertaken unless there is obvious nasal disease.

Clinical clues
Predisposition
- Sino-nasal aspergillosis in dolichocephalic dogs

History
- Sneezing, nasal discharge and epistaxis all indicate nasal disease
- Known traumatic event
- Neurological signs: depression, obtundation, seizures, visual deficits

Clinical examination
Visual inspection
- Epistaxis
- Facial deformity
- Nasal discharge

Physical examination
- Deformity of nasal bones
- Lack of air movement through nostrils
- Neurological deficits

Laboratory findings
Haematology
- Typically unremarkable unless significant blood loss due to epistaxis causing regenerative anaemia

Serum biochemistry
- Usually unremarkable unless significant blood loss due to epistaxis causing hypoproteinaemia

Urinalysis
- Unremarkable

Imaging
- Skull radiographs to look for fractures, turbinate destruction or expansile lesions
- CT is preferred as cribriform plate integrity can be assessed

Special tests
- *Aspergillus* serology not very sensitive but specific
- Rhinoscopy with nasal biopsy

1.7 ANURIA/OLIGURIA

DEFINITION

Anuria is defined as a failure of the kidneys to produce urine; oliguria refers to cases with inadequate urine production. IRIS guidelines for acute kidney injury (AKI) define this in the context of fluid volume responsiveness over a 6-hour period; with anuria defined as no urine produced and oliguria < 1 ml/kg/hour after intravenous fluid therapy to correct dehydration and hypovolaemia. These definitions are useful as part of decision making on whether renal replacement therapy is required.

Failure to produce normal volumes of urine may also occur due to pre-renal causes (e.g. severe dehydration) and post-renal causes (e.g. bilateral ureteric obstruction, urethral obstruction, ruptured bladder). These are important exclusions before determining a renal cause for lack of urine production.

RELATED CLINICAL SIGNS

- Anuria is normally not the primary concern on presentation in patients; typically systemic causes of lack of glomerular filtration are the primary signs, including vomiting, anorexia, lethargy, or collapse related to potassium or central nervous system disturbances.
- Failure to produce urine due to post-renal causes is most commonly accompanied by stranguria and dysuria (*q.v.* section 1.19) except for ureteric causes, where abdominal pain and signs related to anuria may be the primary sign.

COMMON CAUSES

Infectious causes
- Leptospirosis
- Pyelonephritis

Toxins
- Ethylene glycol
- Grapes and raisins

Drugs
- NSAIDs

Vascular
- Severe hypotension or renal ischaemia, e.g. sepsis, multiple organ dysfunction, severe cardiac failure

Miscellaneous
- Cutaneous and renal glomerulovasculopathy (CRGV, 'Alabama rot')
- Hypercalcaemia

UNCOMMON CAUSES

Infectious
- *Babesia*
- *Leishmania*

Vascular
- Renal infarction

Miscellaneous
- Hyperviscosity, e.g. primary erythrocytosis, hyperglobulinaemia
- Myoglobinuria or haemoglobinuria

Drugs
- Radiographic contrast agents
- ACE inhibitors

Neoplasia
- Renal lymphoma likely bilateral if causing reduced glomerular filtration rate

DIAGNOSTIC APPROACH

1 Anuria or oliguria is usually detected in patients following identification of azotaemia on blood tests, or in systemically unwell patients where urine output is being monitored.
2 Exclude pre-renal causes by assessing hydration status, urinary specific gravity (if urine is available), and measuring urinary bladder size and body weight.
3 Response to intravenous fluid therapy (aim to correct hydration over a 12-hour period) can be monitored. Even with severe dehydration anuria is not anticipated.
4 Assess for post-renal causes by establishing history, passing a urinary catheter and renal imaging to assess bilateral ureteric obstruction (uncommon in dogs). Placement of a urinary catheter is also useful to enable ongoing urinary output monitoring.
5 Response to furosemide (furosemide stress test) following rehydration can be utilised to determine if functional renal tissue is intact. If the patient does not produce urine in spite of furosemide administration, prognosis for

renal recovery without renal replacement therapy is considered guarded.

Clinical clues
Predisposition
- Patients that are severely systemically unwell for any reason (e.g. sepsis, pancreatitis) may be vulnerable to anuric AKI
- Renal amyloidosis: Shar pei

History
- Assess drinking patterns prior to presentation (polyuria and polydipsia may be present in patients with hypercalcaemia-induced renal injury, or acute on chronic kidney disease)
- Exposure to toxins or drugs (especially NSAIDs) inducing renal injury
- Risk factors for AKI
  - CRGV: woodland environment, seasonality
  - Infectious disease: vaccination status, seasonality, wet environment, and lifestyle for risk of leptospirosis

Clinical examination
Visual inspection
- Assess for hydration status (eye position)
- Assess for evidence of concurrent systemic disease (e.g. jaundice in leptospirosis or pancreatitis)

Physical examination
- Abdominal pain or pyrexia: may increase suspicion of pyelonephritis
- Hydration (skin tent, mucous membrane moisture, body weight if recent measurements are available) and volume status (heart rate, mucous membrane colour)
- Skin wounds in patients with suspicion of CGRV

Laboratory findings
Haematology
- Leukocytosis with neutrophilia and monocytosis and left shift (band neutrophils and toxic change) may increase suspicion of infectious causes
- Moderate-marked poorly regenerative anaemia implies a more chronic process (acute on chronic disease) in the absence of comorbidities

Serum biochemistry
- Azotaemia is detected in most oligo/anuric patients, so the degree of azotaemia is not prognostic in AKI. However, failure to produce urine in response to fluid therapy is
- Potassium should be monitored closely in anuric patients (q2 hours); intervention may be indicated
- Urinalysis is important in discriminating between pre-renal and renal azotaemia; sediment analysis may detect calcium oxalate monohydrate (ethylene glycol), and may detect evidence of tubular injury (glucosuria esp. in leptospirosis, proteinuria) or increase the suspicion of pyelonephritis (active sediment examination)
- Urine cytology submitted in an EDTA tube may be useful in cases with a high suspicion of pyelonephritis
- Venous blood gas in ethylene glycol toxicity will display metabolic acidosis with a high anion gap and hypocalcaemia

Imaging
Plain radiographs
- Excluding radio-opaque uroliths as a cause of bilateral ureteric obstruction (uncommon in dogs cf. cats)

- In patients with hypercalcaemia to screen for neoplastic causes

Ultrasound
- Assess renal perfusion and architecture (small and irregular associated with more chronic disease, pyelonephritis may be detected by renal architectural change and renal pelvis dilation (although not 100% sensitive)), AKI cases may display hyperechoic renal cortices and perirenal retroperitoneal fluid
- In patients with hypercalcaemia to screen for neoplastic causes

Special tests
- Infectious disease testing, e.g. microscopic agglutination test (MAT) and blood or urine PCR for leptospirosis
- Pyelocentesis for cytology and culture in cases with a high suspicion of pyelonephritis
- Skin biopsy for histology may increase suspicion of CRGV
- Toxin screen including ethylene glycol on urine or blood

1.8 ATAXIA

DEFINITION

Ataxia is defined as uncoordinated voluntary movement. This occurs when there is a dysfunction of the elements of the nervous system that are responsible for coordination. Disorders that can present with ataxia include cerebellar dysfunction, vestibular system dysfunction, and loss of proprioception (sensory).

RELATED CLINICAL SIGNS

Cerebellar ataxia
- Can also present with vestibular dysfunction as this involves the cerebellum (flocculonodular lobe)
- Hypermetria

- Intention tremor
- Wide-based stance

Vestibular ataxia
- Bilateral vestibular ataxia presents without a head tilt and falling to both sides, wide excursions of the head, and an uncoordinated gait
- Falling/leaning to one side
- Head tilt
- Nystagmus

Proprioceptive (sensory) ataxia
- Abnormal placement of limbs, e.g. crossing over legs when walking, or pacing (forelimb and hindlimb strides at the same time), knuckling
- May stumble, e.g. stepping over objects

COMMON CAUSES

Cerebellar ataxia
- Infectious – protozoal (*Toxoplasma, Neospora*), *Angiostrongylus vasorum*
- Inflammatory – meningoencephalitis of unknown origin
- Neoplasia
- Vascular – haemorrhagic or thromboembolic stroke

Vestibular ataxia
Peripheral vestibular
- Cranial polyneuropathy (possible link with hypothyroidism)
- Idiopathic (old dog vestibular)
- Neoplasia
- Otitis media

Central vestibular (brainstem or cerebellar)
- Cerebellar disorders as above
- Inflammatory – meningoencephalitis of unknown origin
- Neoplasia
- Trauma

Proprioceptive (sensory) ataxia
- Degenerative disease, e.g. canine degenerative myelopathy (CDM)
- Drug-induced
- Fibrocartilaginous embolism (FCE)
- Intervertebral disc disease
- Neoplasia

UNCOMMON CAUSES

Cerebellar ataxia
- Cerebellar abiotrophy
- Storage disease
- Trauma

Vestibular ataxia
- Central vestibular (brainstem or cerebellar)
- Cerebellar disorders as above
- Drug-induced, e.g. metronidazole toxicity
- Hyperviscosity: erythrocytosis, hyperglobulinaemia including multiple myeloma
- Peripheral vestibular

- Storage disease
- Trauma

Proprioceptive (sensory) ataxia
- Inflammatory – meningomyelitis

DIAGNOSTIC APPROACH

Clinical clues
Predisposition
- Canine degenerative myelopathy is present in numerous breeds; German shepherd dogs (GSDs) are predisposed
- Cerebellar abiotrophy has been described in more than 40 breeds of dog; there are neonatal (e.g. beagles), juvenile (e.g. Airedale terrier) and adult onset (Bernese mountain dog) disorders
- Greyhounds are predisposed to thromboembolic cerebellar events (ischaemic stroke)

History
- Duration and progression of signs may aid in index of suspicion (acute onset improving increases suspicion of vascular or drug-induced, gradual onset progression may increase suspicion of degenerative or neoplastic disease, acute onset rapid progression may increase suspicion of inflammatory or infectious disease)

Clinical examination
Visual inspection
- Mentation (*q.v.* sections 1.3, 1.4) is expected to be impaired with central brainstem vestibular disorders

Physical examination
- Thorough examination to assess for multisystemic disease

Neurological examination
- Cerebellar: ipsilateral loss of proprioception and menace response, contralateral head tilt and direction of fast phase of nystagmus (paradoxical vestibular)
- Proprioceptive ataxia: abnormal conscious and unconscious proprioception
- Vestibular: head tilt and nystagmus

- In brainstem disorders consciousness may be reduced and other cranial nerves may be affected, e.g facial nerve (blink reflex) and glossopharyngeal and vagal nerves (gag reflex)
- Peripheral disorders may detect concurrent facial nerve abnormalities and Horner's syndrome

Ophthalmic examination
- May be useful to assess for infiltrative central nervous system disease, e.g. may detect papilloedema

Laboratory findings
Haematology
- Uncommon to detect changes except thrombocytopenia in haemorrhagic stroke

Serum biochemistry
- May detect causes of increased risk of thromboembolism: hepatic disease, hyperadrenocorticism, protein-losing enteropathy (PLE), protein-losing nephropathy (PLN)

Urinalysis
- Assess for PLN in dogs with thromboembolic stroke

Imaging
Plain radiographs
- Screen for disseminated neoplasia in cases with a high suspicion

Ultrasound
- Screen for disseminated neoplasia in cases with a high suspicion

Special tests
- Coagulation parameters (PT and aPTT) to assess for haemorrhagic stroke
- CSF tap to assess for cytology and biochemistry (inflammatory) and infectious disease (e.g. *Toxoplasma* and *Neospora* PCR)
- Infectious disease testing
  - *Toxoplasma* and *Neospora* serology
  - Baermann technique or AngioDetect® for *Angiostrongylus*
- Otoscopy and myringotomy in cases with suspicion of otitis media
- MRI scan to assess for central nervous system causes of ataxia

1.9 BLEEDING

DEFINITION

Bleeding may be observed due to excessive bruising or haemorrhage following no or minor trauma (e.g. blood sampling, minor surgery, teething or exercise) or due to disorders of the bleeding tissue. Bleeding diathesis means a tendency to bleed or bruise easily.

Haematoma is red or discoloured skin that does not blanch under pressure and occurs due to the presence of blood under the skin. These lesions can be defined by size; petechiae refers to haematomas < 3 mm and ecchymosis refers to haematomas > 1 cm. Purpura is a bleed 3 mm to 1 cm diameter but is not a term commonly used in veterinary medicine.

RELATED CLINICAL SIGNS

As with any cause of bleeding, causes can be divided into disorders of the organ affected or related to a disorder of haemostasis (systemic disease).

COMMON CAUSES

Disorders of affected organ
- Neoplasia, in particular haemangiosarcoma in any location or leiomyosarcoma in gastrointestinal haemorrhage
- Trauma
- Vasculitis, e.g. adder bite evenomation

Systemic disease

- *Angiostrongylus vasorum* infection causes a mixed haemostatic disorder: pulmonary or CNS bleeding may occur due to coagulopathy or migration of larvae
- Primary haemostatic disorders
  - Thrombocytopenia: immune-mediated thrombocytopenia (IMTP), consumptive (disseminated intravascular coagulation, DIC)
- Secondary haemostatic disorders
  - Vitamin K deficiency due to anticoagulant rodenticide toxicity
- Tertiary haemostatic disorders
  - Hyperfibrinolysis following surgery or major trauma in sighthounds

UNCOMMON CAUSES

Disorders of affected organ

- FB e.g. nasal FB for epistaxis
- Infection, e.g. *Angiostrongylus vasorum* for pulmonary haemorrhage

Systemic disease

- Primary haemostatic disorders
  - Thrombocytopathia (hyperviscosity due to hyperglobulinaemia (e.g. neoplasia, *Leishmania*), inherited disorders)
  - Thrombocytopenia (*Ehrlichia*, bone marrow disease)
  - von Willebrand factor deficiency
- Secondary haemostatic disorders
  - Liver dysfunction, e.g. chronic hepatitis
  - Vitamin K deficiency (cholestasis, congenital)
- Vasculitis, e.g. sepsis, anaphylaxis

DIAGNOSTIC APPROACH

Clinical clues

Predisposition

- Breed predispositions to IMTP and immune-mediated haemolytic anaemia (IMHA), e.g. cocker spaniels
- Sighthounds appear to have a disorder of hyperfibrinolysis, observed as excessive haemorrhage after trauma or major surgery

History

- Concurrent haemorrhage elsewhere to increase suspicion of systemic disorder
- Risk factors of trauma, adder bite envenomation or FB
- Travel history increases index of suspicion of vector-borne diseases including *Dirofilaria*, *Ehrlichia* and *Leishmania* infections

Clinical examination

Visual inspection

- Observe for demeanour, and evidence of haemorrhage elsewhere

Physical examination

- Thorough examination for evidence of haemorrhage elsewhere: skin, especially of the ventral abdomen, and gums, rectal examination for melaena

Laboratory findings

Haematology

- Assess platelet count
- Coagulation times (PT and aPTT) to assess for secondary haemostatic disorders
- Eosinophilia may be present in parasitic disease

Serum biochemistry

- Useful to screen for systemic disease

Imaging

Plain radiographs and ultrasound

- Evidence of organ changes, e.g. mass lesions such as splenic mass in haemoabdomen, and for multisystemic disease

Special tests

- CT with contrast to screen for infection, neoplasia when appropriate
- Haemostatic disorders
  - Baermann technique or Angiodetect® for *Angiostrongylus vasorum*
  - Buccal mucosal bleeding time to assess for thrombocytopathia
  - Testing for *Leishmania* and *Ehrlichia* infection as appropriate

- There is currently no available test to detect hyperfibrinolysis; as a result sighthound breeds are often treated empirically ahead of surgery or following haemorrhage (most commonly using the anti-fibrinolytic tranexamic acid)

- Thromboelastography and rotational thromboelastometry to assess clotting *in vitro*
- Toxicology to detect rodenticide
- von Willebrand factor antigen levels

1.10 BLINDNESS

DEFINITION

Blindness can occur due to disorders associated with pre-retinal, retinal, optic nerve, or central nervous system lesions. Pre-retinal disorders result in a failure of light to reach the retina (*q.v.* section 2.7), retinal disorders result in a failure to detect light, optic nerve lesions result in a failure to transmit information from the retina to the cortical brain, and central nervous system lesions result in a failure to process visual information and therefore a loss of conscious perception of sight.

RELATED CLINICAL SIGNS

- Duration of the onset of blindness may have a significant impact on the dog's ability to cope and therefore the clinical signs; dogs with a slow progression may have adapted in familiar environments and signs may be more subtle than in those that suffer acute onset blindness.
- With some disorders dogs may present with signs of ocular pain including blepharospasm (squinting), rubbing eyes, or ocular discharge.
- Dogs with central nervous system disorders or systemic diseases as a cause of the blindness may present with concurrent neurological or systemic signs respectively.
- With sudden acquired retinal degeneration syndrome (SARDS) dogs also present with clinical signs more typically associated with HAC including polyuria, polydipsia, polyphagia, excessive panting with muscle wastage and pot-bellied appearance.

COMMON CAUSES

Pre-retinal
- Cataracts: congenital, diabetic
- Corneal opacity, e.g. chronic dry eye, *q.v.* section 2.7
- Hyphaema
  - Coagulopathy
  - Hypertension
  - Uveitis
- Uveitis
  - Immune-mediated
  - Neoplasia
  - Systemic disease

Retinal
- Ivermectin toxicity can cause retinal oedema with folds (vision loss is temporary and resolves in 2–10 days)
- Retinal detachment (systemic hypertension, infectious, neoplastic, cataracts, lens luxation)
- SARDS

Optic nerve
- Optic neuritis: inflammatory, infectious, neoplastic

Central nervous system
- Inflammatory (meningoencephalitis of unknown origin)
- Neoplasia
- Post-ictal

UNCOMMON CAUSES

Pre-retinal
- Corneal opacity
  - Chronic superficial keratitis
  - Pigmentary keratitis
- Hyphaema
  - Intraocular neoplasia
  - Trauma
- Uveitis
  - Pigmentary uveitis
  - Uveodermatologic syndrome

Retinal
- Progressive retinal atrophy
- Retinal detachment (congenital, liquefied vitreous, optic nerve colobomas)

Optic nerve
- Optic nerve neoplasia: to cause blindness would involve the optic chiasm
  - Meningioma
  - Glioma
  - Lymphoma

Central nervous system
- Anaesthesia-related complication
- Hypertensive encephalopathy
- Hyperviscosity: multiple myeloma, erythrocytosis

DIAGNOSTIC APPROACH

Clinical clues
Predisposition
- Pigmentary keratitis: Pugs
- Chronic superficial keratitis (pannus): GSDs
- Uveodermatologic syndrome: Akitas and Arctic breeds
- Pigmentary uveitis: Golden retrievers
- Progressive retinal atrophy: Border collies, Irish setters, poodles

History
- Nature of onset of signs may be useful in prioritising differential diagnoses

- Progressive retinal atrophy affects rods first, so the dog may initially lose sight in dim light
- Signs of concurrent systemic disease may increase index of suspicion, e.g. DM, SARDS, and neoplasia or infectious disease
- Specific questions to assess for other signs of central nervous system disorders may be useful, in particular signs of forebrain disease (mentation change, incoordination, seizures)

Clinical examination
Visual inspection
- Mentation is expected to be impaired with central disorders

Physical examination
- Blood pressure: hypertension may be detected in increased intracranial pressure, hypertensive retinopathy, and hypertensive encephalopathy
- Pupillary light reflex is highly valuable in lesion localization: this will be impaired in pre-retinal, retinal and optic nerve disorders with fixed mydriatic pupils, whereas central lesions will result in a normal pupillary light reflex
- Thorough examination to assess for multisystemic disease

Neurological examination
- Focus on assessment of forebrain, i.e. response to nasal stimulation, mentation, proprioception

Ophthalmic examination
- Full ophthalmic examination to assess for pre-retinal lesions (corneal, lens, iris, vitreous changes), retinal lesions (retinal detachment), or optic nerve head changes (optic neuritis)

Laboratory findings
Haematology
- Useful to screen for systemic disease

Serum biochemistry
- Useful to screen for systemic disease
- Dogs with SARDS may have increased ALP enzyme activity but interpret results of ACTH stimulation and LDDS tests with caution in

these patients as there is a risk of false positives

Imaging

Plain radiographs
- Screen for disseminated neoplasia in cases with a high suspicion

Ultrasound
- Screen for disseminated neoplasia in cases with a high suspicion

Special tests
- Electroretinogram (ERG)
- Ocular paracentesis may be useful in cases with uveitis
- Ocular ultrasound may be useful to assess for evidence of intraocular neoplasia, FB or trauma
- MRI and CSF in cases with optic neuritis or central blindness

1.11 CONSTIPATION

DEFINITION

Infrequent and difficult or absent defaecation, with abnormal retention of faeces in the large intestine.

Obstipation is prolonged, intractable constipation in which faeces have become so firm that defaecation is no longer possible, and which ultimately leads to secondary degeneration of colonic musculature.

RELATED CLINICAL SIGNS

- Anorexia, lethargy and vomiting
- Dyschezia (pain or difficulty in defaecation), *q.v.* section 1.46
- Failure to pass faeces or small, hard, dry faeces
- Haematochezia if intraluminal cause
- Paradoxical diarrhoea (scant liquid faeces passed around the constipated mass)
- Tenesmus (straining to defaecate), *q.v.* section 1.46

COMMON CAUSES

Anorectal pain
- Anal furunculosis
- Anal sac impaction, abscess, cellulitis

Dietary
- Foreign material, e.g. bones, hair

- Excessive or insufficient fibre
- Inadequate water intake

Drug-induced
- Anticholinergics
- Barium
- Kaolin-pectin
- Opioids

Environmental
- Dehydration
- Hospitalization
- Inadequate exercise

Extraluminal obstruction
- Healed pelvic fracture
- Prostatic enlargement – hypertrophy, abscess

Intraluminal obstruction
- Perineal hernia and rectal diverticulum
- Rectal tumour

Neuromuscular disease
- Lumbosacral disease

Orthopaedic disease (pain and failure to posture)
- Injury to pelvis, hip or pelvic limbs
- Spinal (range of lumbo-sacral diseases)

Water-electrolyte abnormalities
- Dehydration
- Hypercalcaemia
- Hypokalaemia

UNCOMMON CAUSES

Anorectal disease
- Anal or rectal stricture
- Anal sac adenocarcinoma
- Atresia ani
- Atresia coli
- Pseudocoprostasis (faecal impaction due to matted hair)

Drug-induced
- Aluminium hydroxide
- Antihistamines
- Barium sulphate
- Diphenoxylate
- Diuretics
- Iron preparations
- Loperamide
- Phenothiazines
- Sucralfate
- Verapamil

Extraluminal obstruction
- Pelvic collapse due to nutritional bone disease
- Prostatic neoplasia
- Prostatic or paraprostatic cyst
- Sublumbar lymphadenopathy

Intraluminal obstruction
- Benign stricture
- FB other than bone or hair

Metabolic
- Hyperparathyroidism
- Hypothyroidism

Neuromuscular disease
- Bilateral pelvic nerve damage
- Dysautonomia
- Hirschsprung's disease (congenital megacolon)

DIAGNOSTIC APPROACH

1 Confirm constipation by abdominal and digital rectal palpation, and imaging.

2 Identify underlying cause through history, physical examination and proctoscopy.

Clinical clues
Predisposition
- Benign prostatic hypertrophy in uncastrated older dogs
- Prostatic carcinoma more common in castrated dogs
- Sedentary dogs on low-fibre diet

History
- Dysuria with prostatic disease
- Old pelvic trauma

Clinical examination
Visual inspection
- Anal furunculosis
- Dyschezia
- Hindleg weakness or pain with lumbosacral disease
- Haematochezia if intraluminal cause
- Pseudocoprostasis
- Tenesmus

Physical examination
- Abdominal palpation
  - Enlarged palpable intra-abdominal prostate
  - Faecal material in colon
  - Paraprostatic cyst
  - Pelvic deformity
- Digital rectal palpation
  - Anal sac disease
  - Dry, impacted faeces
  - Paraprostatic cyst
  - Pelvic canal narrowing
  - Perineal hernia and rectal diverticulum
  - Prostatic enlargement
  - Rectal stricture
  - Rectal mass

Laboratory findings
Usually unremarkable
- Hypercalcaemia with anal sac adenocarcinoma or lymphoma
- Hypokalaemia causing colonic muscle weakness

Imaging
Plain radiographs
- Old pelvic fractures
- Prostatomegaly

Contrast radiographs (barium enema)
- Rectal stricture
- Colonic/rectal tumour

Ultrasound
- Colonic tumour
- Prostatic disease
  - Abscess
  - Benign prostatic hypertrophy
  - Cyst or paraprostatic cyst
  - Neoplasia

Special tests
- Thyroid function tests
- Proctoscopy

1.12 CORNEAL OPACITY

DEFINITION

Focal or diffuse abnormality of the cornea preventing the transmission of light.
NB: Owners may mistake lenticular nuclear sclerosis and cataracts for corneal disease.

RELATED CLINICAL SIGNS

- Blindness, *q.v.* section 1.10
- Diffuse or focal abnormalities of corneal colour
- Blepharospasm and epiphora if ulceration

COMMON CAUSES

White
- Chemosis = corneal oedema
  - Interstitial/infectious keratitis
  - Ulcerative keratitis
- Hypopyon = infection in anterior chamber, often due to FB penetration
- Lipid

Brown/black pigment
- Chronic corneal irritation: ectopic cilia, aberrant hairs or eyelashes
- Pannus

Red
q.v. section 1.40

UNCOMMON CAUSES

White
- Crystalline: calcium
- Fibrosis
- Glaucoma

Brown/black pigment
- Congenital endothelial pigmentation
- Dermoid
- Iris prolapse
- Neoplasia: limbal melanoma
- Persistent pupillary membrane
- Ruptured iris cyst
- Sequestrum

Blue
- Chemosis
  - Canine adenovirus (CAV-1, and rarely CAV-2 live vaccine)
  - Glaucoma

Red
q.v. section 1.40

DIAGNOSTIC APPROACH

- Examine cornea
- Fluorescein staining
- Palpebral and corneal reflexes
- *q.v.* section 1.40

Clinical clues
Predisposition
- Hyperlipidaemia: Miniature schnauzers
- Pannus: Australian Shepherd, Belgian Tervuren, Border collie, Greyhound, GSD, Siberian Husky

History
- Other signs of hyperlipidaemia
- Other signs of hypothyroidism
- Previous corneal ulceration

Clinical examination
Visual inspection
- Blepharospasm and/or epiphora if ulcerated
- Chemosis = corneal oedema
- Corneal ulcer
- Ocular discharge

Physical examination
- Opacity covering part or all of the cornea

Laboratory findings
- Hyperlipidaemia: hypertriglyceridaemia and/or hypercholesterolaemia with lipid deposit

Imaging
- Full ophthalmological examination

Special tests
- Fluorescein staining
- Palpebral and corneal reflexes
- Schirmer tear test

1.13 COUGHING

DEFINITION

A sudden expiratory effort in an attempt to try and clear excess secretion or foreign material from the lungs, bronchi or trachea resulting in a sudden, noisy expulsion of air from the lungs.

RELATED CLINICAL SIGNS

Associated signs
- Dyspnoea/tachypnoea, *q.v.* section 1.18
- Exercise intolerance/collapse, *q.v.* sections 1.22, 1.51
- Halitosis, *q.v.* section 1.29
- Nasal/ocular discharge, *q.v.* section 1.32

COMMON CAUSES

Allergic/immune-mediated
- Reverse sneeze, sometimes mistaken for coughing

Cardiovascular
- Cardiomegaly with left atrial enlargement and bronchial compression
- Left-sided failure causing pulmonary oedema (dyspnoea rather than coughing)

Environmental irritants
- Dust
- Passive smoking

Infectious/inflammatory
- Acute or chronic inflammatory disease anywhere from pharynx to pulmonary tissue can stimulate coughing
- Acute secondary to infectious agents, e.g. infectious tracheobronchitis (kennel cough)
- Bronchopneumonia
- Canine infectious respiratory disease (CIRD) complex: 'kennel cough'
- Chronic bronchitis
- Inhalation pneumonia, secondary to oesophageal disease or GORD (aerodigestive syndrome)

Parasitic
- *Angiostrongylus vasorum* – regional variation in prevalence in UK

Pleural effusion
- Very rarely causes coughing; dyspnoea is more important sign, *q.v.* section 2.21

Physical/traumatic

- Collapsing trachea
- Inhalation pneumonia, secondary to oesophageal disease
- Inhaled/ingested FB
- Laryngeal paralysis: coughing when drinking
- Pulmonary haemorrhage

UNCOMMON CAUSES

Allergic

- Asthma (much more common in cats than dogs)
- Eosinophilic inflammatory respiratory diseases (pulmonary infiltrate with eosinophils) e.g. eosinophilic bronchitis/bronchopneumonopathy/pneumonia

Cardiovascular

- Non-cardiogenic pulmonary oedema
- Pulmonary thromboemboli
- Pulmonary oedema (cardiac origin)

Environmental irritants

- Chemical fumes
- Smoke inhalation from fire
- Potassium bromide
- Talcum powder

Infectious/inflammatory

- Abscess rarely
- Bronchiectasis
- Chronic pulmonary fibrosis, especially in WHWT
- Distemper
- Fungal (not in UK)
  - Blastomycosis
  - Coccidioidomycosis
  - Histoplasmosis
- Granulomatous disease
- Hilar lymph node enlargement
- *Pneumocystis* pneumonia

Neoplastic

- Mediastinal
- Metastatic (more commonly causes dyspnoea than cough)
- Primary

- Extrathoracic, e.g. rib/sternum/soft tissue
- Laryngeal
- Lymphosarcoma
- Tracheal

Parasitic

- *Angiostrongylus vasorum*; regional variation in prevalence in UK
- *Dirofilaria immitis* (not currently in UK)
- *Oslerus osleri* (lungworm)
- Others, e.g. *Crenosoma vulpis, Eucoleous, Filaroides hirthii, Paragonimus*
- Visceral larval migrans

Physical/traumatic

- Iatrogenic secondary to inhalation of liquids or solids, e.g. force feeding, barium administration

DIAGNOSTIC APPROACH

1 Determine whether this is an upper or lower airway problem from signs and physical examination.
2 Rule out cardiac disease.
3 Rule out oesophageal disease.
4 Investigate airway disease by radiography, laboratory analysis and endoscopy.

CLINICAL CLUES

Predisposition

- Brachycephalics have obstructive upper airway disease
- Idiopathic megaoesophagus: Great Dane, GSD, Irish setter
- Kennelled pets are at risk of CIRD
- Large/giant breed dogs
  - Dilated cardiomyopathy
  - Laryngeal paralysis
  - Megaoesophagus
  - Pneumonia
- Local outbreak of coughing consistent with CIRD
- *Oslerus* infection: young dogs
- *Pneumocystis* pneumonia: Cavalier King Charles spaniel (CKCS)

- Small dogs of mid- to old age likely to have:
  - Chronic mitral valve disease: CKCS
  - Chronic obstructive lung disease, e.g. chronic bronchitis
  - Collapsing trachea
  - Pulmonary interstitial fibrosis: WHWT

History
- Associated dyspnoea
  - Obstruction, and alveolar and pleural space disease
- Duration of cough
  - Acute (< 2 weeks duration) likely "kennel cough"
  - Chronic (> 2 weeks duration)
- Environment: flare factors for cough
  - Access to intermediate hosts of parasites
  - Cough associated with walking on collar and lead: collapsing trachea
  - Owners who are heavy smokers causing passive smoking
  - Potential exposure to other parasites if the dog has been outside of UK
  - Seasonality for allergic airway disease
- Nature of cough
  - Acute coughing can often be assumed to be infectious in origin, until proven otherwise
  - Haemoptysis with coagulopathy, FB, neoplasia or trauma
  - Non-productive moist or dry suggests upper airway
  - Productive/non-productive moist or dry suggests pulmonary
    - Animal may swallow excessively after coughing if productive
  - Regurgitation (and inhalation) in primary oesophageal disease
  - Terminal retch or vomiting can be confused with GI disease
  - "Wheezy" coughs suggest airway inflammation
- Response to therapy
- Timing of the cough
  - Any association with eating food/drinking fluids suggests larynx or oesophagus

Clinical examination
Visual inspection
- Audible respiratory sounds

- Dyspnoea, *q.v.* section 1.18
- Halitosis; often a feature with inhaled FBs, *q.v.* section 1.29
- Ocular/nasal discharge with allergic or infectious conditions, *q.v.* section 1.32
- Respiratory pattern, e.g. any abdominal effort
- Tachypnoea

Physical examination
- Palpation
  - Cough elicited by tracheal pinch if upper airway
  - Larynx, trachea and thorax for abnormalities
- Auscultation
  - Airway noise
    - Inspiratory: upper airway
    - Expiratory: lower airway
  - Localise origin
    - Trachea: abnormal respiratory sound
    - Thorax: adventitious respiratory sounds, e.g. crackles and wheezes
  - Presence of murmur

Laboratory findings
- Eosinophilia may be associated with parasitic diseases and eosinophilic immune-mediated disorders
- Faecal examination may reveal the presence of parasitic larvae
- Increased serum globulins may be seen in certain inflammatory conditions, e.g. granulomatous disease
- Leukocytosis in pulmonary inflammatory disease
- Often unremarkable if upper airway disease

Imaging
Thoracic radiographs
- Assess heart size for cardiomegaly, especially left atrium
- Assess tracheal diameter throughout its length: can do dynamic assessment under fluoroscopy for tracheal collapse
- Assess lung patterns as bronchial, interstitial, alveolar or mixed
- Assess for presence of mediastinal abnormalities

- Inflated radiographs under general anaesthesia may give more information
- Right lateral and dorso-ventral (DV) (lungs) or ventro-dorsal (VD) (heart) projections should be performed

Special tests
- Assessment of vocal fold movement under a light plane of anaesthesia
- Baermann technique for lungworms including *Angiostrongylus*

- Blood gas analysis (if available) – arterial to assess oxygenation
- Bronchoscopy
  - Bronchoalveolar lavage (BAL) for cytological examination and culture
- Cardiovascular examination: ECG, echocardiography
- Fine needle lung aspiration/biopsy
- Knott's test and/or serology for *Dirofilaria immitis*
- Nuclear scintigraphic studies of ventilation-perfusion
- Thoracocentesis
- Ultrasound of the larynx to assess for laryngeal paralysis

1.14 DEAFNESS

DEFINITION

Deafness, or the inability to perceive sound, can be divided into conductive or sensorineural deafness. Conductive deafness results from disorders affecting the transmission of sound from the environment to the tympanic membrane and ossicles of the inner ear. Sensorineural deafness results from disorders affecting the cochlear system, eighth cranial nerve, or central nervous system (brainstem and forebrain).

Presbycusis is the progressive and irreversible bilateral degeneration of the cochlea and associated structures and results in age-related irreversible sensorineural deafness.

RELATED CLINICAL SIGNS

- Dogs may be difficult to rouse from sleep or startled easily.
- Dogs with otitis externa or media may display discomfort: head shaking, scratching, pain on opening mouth.
- In congenital deafness puppies may not be as responsive to cries of littermates during play.

COMMON CAUSES

Conductive
- Otitis externa

- Otitis media

Sensorineural
- Congenital deafness; pigment and non-pigment associated
- Otitis interna
- Ototoxicity: gentamicin, furosemide, or topical chlorhexidine
- Presbycusis: degenerative, occurring with old age

UNCOMMON CAUSES

Conductive
- Hereditary ear canal atresia

Sensorineural
- Adult-onset hereditary deafness, e.g. Collie
- Anaesthesia associated
- Trauma

DIAGNOSTIC APPROACH

Clinical clues
Predisposition
- Congenital sensorineural deafness most commonly associated with white or merle coat colour: Boxer, Dachshund, Jack Russell terrier
- Otitis externa: Cocker spaniel
- Secretory otitis media: CKCS

History
- Dogs with significant brainstem or forebrain disease are likely to have more pertinent neurological findings and history
- History of exposure to ototoxic drugs: aminoglycosides, loop diuretics, erythromycin, cisplatin and carboplatin
- Older dogs with gradual-onset progressive deafness are most likely to have presbycusis

Clinical examination
Visual inspection
- Assessment of behaviour, mentation, and evidence of ear discomfort
- Assessment for response to sounds in the consulting room; can be challenging due to detection of vibrations
- Presbycusis results in loss of detection of high-pitched sounds first

Physical examination
- Dogs with otitis media or interna may have pain on opening jaw

Neurological examination
- Assessment for concurrent neurological deficits

Otoscopic examination
- Full otoscopy, including assessment of the tympanic membrane

Laboratory findings
Haematology
- Typically unremarkable, may be useful to screen for systemic disease

Serum biochemistry
- Typically unremarkable, may be useful to screen for systemic disease

Imaging
Plain radiographs
- Radiography of the head may detect mineralisation of the ear canal, and opacity within the bullae

Special tests
- Brainstem-auditory evoked response (BAER)
- CT scan
- MRI and CSF

1.15 DIARRHOEA

DEFINITION

An increase in the water content of faeces, with a consequent increase in their fluidity and/or volume and/or frequency.

Diarrhoea can be:
- Acute (sudden onset, often self-limiting) or chronic (arbitrarily > 3 weeks duration) which may be continuous or intermittent
- Caused by primary GI disease (disorders of the small or large intestine or both), or secondary to disease elsewhere
- Self-limiting or life-threatening
- Due to alterations in one or a combination of:
  - the osmotic content of the stool
  - intestinal secretion
  - intestinal mucosal permeability
  - motility

- The consistency of diarrhoea can vary from soft with some retention of form, through 'cow-pat', to completely watery
- Small intestinal (SI) diarrhoea is characteristically large volume, not increased in frequency and watery, and may contain melaena if there is bleeding, *q.v.* section 1.31
- Large intestinal (LI) diarrhoea is characteristically small volume, mucoid and may contain fresh blood (*q.v.* section 1.26). Dogs may show urgency, increased frequency of defaecation and straining (*q.v.* section 1.46); they may continue to strain after defaecation

RELATED CLINICAL SIGNS

- Abdominal discomfort (*q.v.* section 2.17.1), excessive borborygmi, flatus, and halitosis (*q.v.* section 1.29) are non-specific signs

- Anorexia (*q.v.* section 1.5) in the presence of diarrhoea is generally an indication of serious disease
- Severe, chronic diarrhoea may be a protein-losing enteropathy with consequent hypoalbuminaemia and ascites/oedema

- Signs of dehydration, particularly in acute diarrhoea
- Vomiting can be associated with both SI and LI diseases

1.15.1 ACUTE DIARRHOEA

DEFINITION

Acute diarrhoea generally occurs abruptly in a previously healthy dog and is typically profuse but self-limiting and of short duration. It will have been present continuously for less than two weeks, or intermittently for less than four weeks. In severe cases it may be haemorrhagic and can be life-threatening. It is frequently associated with vomiting, and often involves the whole GI tract.

RELATED CLINICAL SIGNS

- Associated vomiting
- Borborygmi
- Dehydration
- Weight loss is not a feature

COMMON CAUSES

Primary GI disease
Dietary
- Dietary indiscretion
  - Excess intake
  - Inappropriate food due to scavenging
  - Sudden change in diet
- Food intolerance
- Food poisoning – contamination of food by
  - live bacteria or bacterial toxins
  - mycotoxins

Drug/toxin
- Antimicrobials
- NSAIDs

Infection – Bacterial
- Acute haemorrhagic diarrhoea syndrome (AHDS), previously termed haemorrhagic gastroenteritis (HGE)

- *Campylobacter jejuni*; *C. upsaliensis* is more prevalent and may be non-pathogenic
- *Clostridium perfringens*: type A toxin (netF) may be the cause of AHDS
- *E. coli*

Infection – Parasitic
- *Ancylostoma* hookworms (not in UK)
- *Giardia*
- *Trichuris* whipworms (uncommon in UK)

Infection – Viral
- Coronavirus (usually mild, but has been associated in UK with acute, profuse vomiting)
- Parvovirus

Obstructive (surgical)
- Intussusception

Secondary, non-GI disease
- Acute pancreatitis
- Hypoadrenocorticism: not common but important

UNCOMMON CAUSES

Primary GI disease
Dietary
- Food hypersensitivity (true food allergy)

Drug/toxin
- ACE inhibitors
- Anthelmintics
- Anti-arrhythmics
- Anti-cancer agents, especially methotrexate
- Blue-green algae
- Digoxin
- Heavy metals

- Laxatives
- Organophosphates
- Phenylpropanolamine

Infection – Bacterial
- *Bacillus piliformis*
- *Campylobacter coli*
- *Leptospira*
- *Salmonella*: more likely if fed raw meat
- *Shigella*
- *Yersinia*

Infection – Parasitic
- Ascarids and cestodes: infection is common, but is rarely a cause of diarrhoea
- *Cryptosporidium*
- *Cystoisospora*: rarely primary pathogen, except in puppies
- *Strongyloides stercoralis*
- *Uncinaria stenocephala* hookworms

Infection – Rickettsial
- Salmon-poisoning disease, *Neorickettsia helminthica* and *elokominica* (geographically limited to Pacific Northwest, United States)

Infection – Viral (often mild)
- Astrovirus
- Bocavirus
- Circovirus: more severe disease reported occasionally
- Norovirus
- Rotavirus

Obstructive (surgical)
- FB: typically results in lack of faecal output but a partial obstruction may cause diarrhoea
- Incarcerated bowel loop: internal or external hernia
- Intestinal volvulus
- Linear FB
- Mesenteric torsion

Secondary, non-GI disease
- Acute hepatitis
  - Adenovirus (CAV-1, infectious canine hepatitis) can also cause diarrhoea
  - Leptospirosis
- AKI

- Canine distemper
- Diabetic ketoacidosis
- Pyometra

DIAGNOSTIC APPROACH

1 Differentiate between primary (GI) and secondary (non-GI) disease by history, physical examination and laboratory findings.
2 If secondary GI disease is present, investigate and treat underlying cause
3 If primary GI disease is present, differentiate by history, physical examination, laboratory findings and imaging those that require only symptomatic support (e.g. anti-diarrhoeals, fluid therapy) from life-threatening causes that require either:
- Intensive medical/supportive therapy
  - AHDS/HGE
  - Leptospirosis
  - Parvovirosis
  - Salmonellosis
  or
- Surgical correction
  - FB
  - Incarcerated bowel loop (internal or external hernia)
  - Intestinal volvulus
  - Intussusception
  - Linear FB
  - Mesenteric torsion

Clinical clues
Predisposition
- Raw feeding: risk of *Campylobacter*, *Salmonella*
- Unsanitary environment
- Unvaccinated
  - Dogs with distemper usually have concurrent respiratory signs, and dogs with leptospirosis usually have hepatic and renal problems as well
- Young, not fully immunocompetent

History
- Access to toxins
- Acute onset of diarrhoea, etc.
- Contact with infected dogs
- Drug administration

- Other signs, e.g. vomiting
- Presence of blood in diarrhoea
- Scavenging
- Vaccination status

Clinical examination
Visual inspection
- Dull and depressed versus bright and alert indicates greater need for definitive diagnosis and intensive treatment
- Faecal staining of perineum

Physical examination
- Systemic signs
  - Pyrexia with infectious/inflammatory disease
  - Signs of dehydration
    - Depression
    - Dry mucous membranes
    - Skin tenting
    - Slow capillary refill
    - Sunken eyes
    - Tachycardia
- Oral examination
  - Jaundice with hepatobiliary disease
  - Linear FB under tongue
  - Oral ulcers from acute uraemia
- Palpation
  - Abdominal pain: *q.v.* section 2.17.1
    - Cranial abdominal pain in pancreatitis
  - Bunching of intestines with linear FB
  - Fluid or gas-filled bowel loops
  - FB
  - Mesenteric lymphadenopathy
  - Sausage-shaped mass consistent with intussusception
- Rectal examination
  - Abnormal faecal material
  - Advanced ileo-colic intussusception
  - Evidence of diarrhoea
  - Evidence of melaena or haematochezia
  - Rectal prolapse

Laboratory findings
Haematology
- Eosinophilia may be seen with parasitism
- Haemoconcentration indicative of dehydration (NB: check total protein)

- Leukopenia in parvovirus infection (~60% of cases) or overwhelming sepsis
- Leukocytosis ± left shift with infectious/inflammatory disease
- Marked haemoconcentration with normal serum proteins suggests AHDS/HGE
- Pre-regenerative anaemia with peracute disease

Serum biochemistry
  Often unremarkable except for changes associated with dehydration, but helpful in ruling out non-GI diseases.
- Azotaemia may be pre-renal; check urine specific gravity (SG)
- Electrolyte abnormalities, especially hypokalaemia, inform choice of fluid therapy
- Hypoglycaemia sometimes seen in sepsis and in inadequate food uptake by puppies
- Non-GI diseases
  - Azotaemia in renal failure
  - Hyperkalaemia and hyponatraemia suggestive of hypoadrenocorticism
  - Increased liver enzyme activities secondary to intestinal inflammation, bacterial translocation, or because of primary hepatopathy
  - Lipase and canine pancreatic lipase (cPL) may be elevated in pancreatitis
- Serum proteins
  - Increased in dehydration
  - Decreased serum proteins may develop after rehydration in ulcerative/haemorrhagic diseases (AHDS/HGE, parvovirus)

Urinalysis
- Failure to concentrate urine fully is typical of hypoadrenocorticism
- Hypersthenuria in face of dehydration is appropriate
- Isosthenuria (SG 1.008–1.016) in face of dehydration is inappropriate, and indicates renal insufficiency

Faecal examination
- Bacterial culture may identify primary pathogen, and is indicated if there is haemorrhagic diarrhoea or pyrexia, but pathogenic bacteria can be found in the stool of healthy dogs
- Faecal cytology is of limited value. *Campylobacter*-like organisms and sporulating

Clostridia may be identified but are of uncertain significance
- Faecal SNAP® test or PCR for parvovirus
- Flotation tests to identify endoparasites
  - Baermann technique: *Strongyloides* larvae
  - Sodium nitrate, or formalin-ether: nematode and cestode ova
  - Sheather's sugar centrifugation: *Cryptosporidium*
  - Three zinc sulphate flotations 95% sensitive for the identification of *Giardia*
- SNAP® test for *Giardia*

Imaging
Radiographs
- Plain
  - FB
    - Free intra-peritoneal gas indicates perforated viscus
  - Intestinal distension with fluid or gas = ileus
    - Obstructive ileus with massively dilated stacked bowel loops
    - Physiological ileus is less severe and reflects inflammation or metabolic abnormalities
    - Mesenteric torsion causes distension of all intestinal loops
    - Strangulation causes dilation of one segment of intestine
    - Signs of obstruction

- Fluid- or gas-filled, dilated bowel loop(s)
  - 'Gravel' sign
    - Soft tissue density
    - Intussusception
- Contrast
  - Often no value over plain films in acute diarrhoea
  - Radiolucent FB

Ultrasound
- FB obstruction
- Hepatic and pancreatic pathology
- Intussusception: transverse double concentric ring with hyperechoic centre, or > 5 layers in longitudinal view of bowel loop
- Mesenteric lymphadenopathy

Special tests
- Basal cortisol or ACTH stimulation test
- Assay for *Clostridium (Cl.) perfringens* and *Cl. difficile* toxins
- Endoscopic biopsy (rarely indicated in acute disease)
- Exploratory laparotomy
- Scanning electron microscopy of faeces for virus particles
- Serology – haemagglutination inhibition after parvovirus infection
- SNAP® cPL: a negative result helps rule out pancreatitis; a positive result requires further investigation, i.e. Spec cPL, imaging

1.15.2 CHRONIC DIARRHOEA

DEFINITION

Diarrhoea is defined as chronic if:
- It has been present continuously for a minimum of 3 weeks, and has not responded to symptomatic treatment
  or
- If there is a pattern of recurrent episodes occurring over a period of > 4 weeks

RELATED CLINICAL SIGNS

- Ascites (*q.v.* section 2.5) occurs if a protein-losing enteropathy (PLE) causes significant (< 15 g/l) hypoalbuminaemia
- Polyphagia and weight loss in the presence of diarrhoea are suggestive of malabsorption
- Weight loss is characteristic of SI disease, but dogs with chronic LI disease may also lose weight if the owner repeatedly withholds food

COMMON CAUSES

Primary GI disease

- Antibiotic-responsive diarrhoea (ARD), formerly small intestinal bacterial overgrowth (SIBO)
- Bacterial infection, but some potential pathogens can be present in the faeces of healthy dogs
- Food intolerance
- Giardiasis
- CIE/IBD
  - Histological types
    - Lympho-plasmacytic enteritis (LPE) and/or colitis
    - Eosinophilic gastroenteritis (EGE)
  - Treatment-response types
    - Antibiotic-responsive enteropathy (ARE)
    - Food-responsive enteropathy (FRE)
    - Non-responsive enteropathy (NRE)
    - Steroid-responsive enteropathy (SRE)/immunosupressant-responsive enteropathy (IRE)
- Irritable bowel syndrome (functional diarrhoea)

Secondary non-GI disease

- Exocrine pancreatic insufficiency (EPI)
- Portal hypertension; typically with associated ascites
  - Chronic liver disease

UNCOMMON CAUSES

Primary GI disease

- Alimentary lymphoma
- Chronic intussusception
- Food allergy
- Granulomatous (histiocytic ulcerative) colitis (almost exclusively Boxer and French bulldog)
- Histiocytic disease (diffuse, infiltrative)
- Histoplasmosis (geographically limited to the Ohio Valley in the United States)
- CIE/IBD
  - Granulomatous enteritis
  - Immunoproliferative small intestinal disease (IPSID)

- Intestinal adenocarcinoma
- Lymphangiectasia
- Parasitic
  - Hookworm
    - *Ancylostoma caninum*; not in UK
    - *Uncinaria stenocephala*
  - *Strongyloides stercoralis*
  - Whipworm: *Trichuris vulpis*
- Prototothecosis
- Pythiosis (geographically limited to southern United States)
- Selective cobalamin malabsorption (Imerslund-Gräsbeck) *q.v.* section 5.7.1.2C
- Short-bowel syndrome

Secondary non-GI disease

- Chronic pancreatitis
- Gastrinoma (APUDoma)
- Hypoadrenocorticism
  - Classical, but acute presentation previously masked by symptomatic therapy
  - Atypical, i.e. normal electrolytes as only hypocortisolaemia
- Hyperthyroidism
  - Functional thyroid tumour
  - Raw feeding contaminated by exogenous thyroid tissue
- Portal hypertension
  - Cardiac tamponade
  - Portal vein thrombosis
  - Right-sided heart failure
- Renal disease

DIAGNOSTIC APPROACH

NB: Weigh and record weight for monitoring.
1. Rule out non-GI causes by history, physical examination and laboratory testing.
2. Rule out simple causes, such as diet-induced and parasitism from history and faecal examination, or empirical anti-parasiticide treatment.
3. Perform serum trypsin-like immunoreactivity (TLI) test to diagnose EPI *before* further investigations.
4. Anatomical localisation from history and faecal characteristics.

5 Suspect PLE from ascites due to hypoalbuminaemia.

6 Faecal culture is often unhelpful.

7 Cobalamin and folate to screen for malabsorption, *q.v.* sections 3.10, 3.15

8 Radiographs to screen for masses, partial obstruction, *q.v.* section 4.1.1

9 Ultrasound examination to examine bowel wall thickness and mucosal changes, and to identify masses

10 Endoscopic biopsy

11 Exploratory laparotomy and biopsy if endoscopy is unavailable or non-diagnostic, or if focal disease is found on imaging. Biopsy must always be performed, even if no gross abnormalities are found.

Clinical clues

Predisposition

- Clostridial enterotoxicosis in stressed (e.g. hospitalised) dogs
- EPI: GSD, Collie, Chow Chow, small terriers
- CIE/IBD
  - LPE: GSD, Shar pei, Soft-coated Wheaten terrier may also have concurrent PLN
  - EGE: GSD
  - Immunoproliferative small intestinal disease (IPSID): Basenji
- Granulomatous colitis: Boxer, French bulldog
- IPSID: Basenjis only
- Irritable bowel syndrome (IBS): toy breeds, working dogs
- Lymphangiectasia: Lundehund, Rottweiler, Yorkshire terrier
- Neoplasia in older dogs
- Selective cobalamin malabsorption (Imerslund-Gräsbeck syndrome): Australian shepherd, Beagle, Border collie, Giant schnauzer, Komondor

History

- Correlation of signs with specific food
- Drug administration
- Frequent mucoid diarrhoea ± haematochezia with tenesmus suggests colitis
- Full dietary history
- Melaena may indicate upper GI haemorrhage, and in association with diarrhoea suggests SI bleeding

- Mode of onset – abrupt versus gradual suggests infectious aetiology
- Other signs – vomiting, weight loss
- Previous surgery, especially intestinal resection
- Response to previous treatment

Clinical examination

Visual inspection

- Abdominal enlargement due to ascites or mass(es)
- Body condition score
- Demeanour
- Nature of faeces and style of defaecation help localise to SI or LI, but many are diffuse (mixed pattern diarrhoea)
- Pallor of mucous membranes due to blood loss anaemia
- Peripheral (ventral) oedema if severe hypoproteinaemia
- Poor-quality hair coat secondary to malabsorption
- Weight loss

Physical examination

- Palpation
  - Abdominal mass(es)
  - Abdominal pain
  - Ascites in PLE
  - Body condition score
  - Muscle condition score
  - Thickening of bowel loops suggests infiltration (IBD or lymphosarcoma)
- Rectal examination
  - Distal colonic mass or stricture
  - Evidence of melaena or haematochezia
  - Irregular mucosal texture due to inflammation or neoplasia

Laboratory findings

Haematology

- Eosinophilia sometimes seen in eosinophilic enteritis but many false positives and negatives. Consider parasitism or hypoadrenocorticism
- Haemoconcentration from intestinal fluid loss
- Leukocytosis (neutrophilia ± monocytosis) in severe inflammatory disease or perforation
- Lymphopenia with stress or lymphangiectasia

- Microcytic anaemia and thrombocytosis if chronic blood loss even if not visible
- Non-regenerative anaemia with chronic disease/malnutrition

Serum biochemistry
- Commonly unremarkable in primary, chronic GI disease
- Hyperkalaemia and hyponatraemia seen in hypoadrenocorticism and rarely in salmonellosis and whipworm colitis
- Hypocalcaemia in PLE
  - Total hypocalcaemia reflecting hypoalbuminaemia
  - Ionised hypocalcaemia reflecting malabsorption of calcium and vitamin D in PLE
- Hypocholesterolaemia is suggestive of malabsorption, especially lymphangiectasia
- Hypokalaemia of therapeutic importance
- Increased liver enzyme activities, secondary to intestinal inflammation
- Mild hypoproteinaemia if chronic GI bleeding
- Panhypoproteinaemia is typical in PLE, although severe inflammatory disease may cause raised globulins, e.g. IPSID in Basenji

Urinalysis
- Rule out proteinuria as the cause of hypoalbuminaemia

Faecal examination
- Faecal *Clostridium perfringens* and *Cl. difficile* toxins may give false positives
- Faecal culture may give false negatives and positives
- Faecal leukocytes on cytology indicate inflammation but are not specific
- Fungal culture and rectal cytology for histoplasmosis
- Occult blood test, but false positives are common
- Presence of undigested food is non-specific and unhelpful

Imaging
Radiographs
- Plain
  - To identify mass or FB or partial obstruction such as a chronic intussusception

- Contrast
  - 'Apple-core' sign with neoplasm causing partial obstruction
  - Barium follow-through studies generally unhelpful if just diarrhoea is present and plain radiographs are unremarkable
  - Barium enema is largely superseded by colonoscopy

Ultrasound
- Demonstrate free fluid or gas
- Identify masses, lymphadenopathy
- Measure bowel wall thickness

Special tests
- Basal cortisol + ACTH stimulation test if basal cortisol < 55 nmol/l
- Breath hydrogen for SIBO, but not readily available
- Canine CE-IBD test (Antech Diagnostics) – combination triple test for Anti-OmpC porins surface antigens, IgA antibodies, anti-canine calprotectin IgA antibodies and anti-gliadin IgA antibodies – not fully validated yet
- Exclusion diet trial
- Exploratory laparotomy and full-thickness biopsy
- Faecal alpha$_1$-protease inhibitor as a marker for a PLE (test only available in the United States)
- Faecal calprotectin as an inflammatory marker
- Faecal ELISA for *Giardia* antigen
- Folate and cobalamin to screen for SIBO, and infiltrative bowel disease
- Intestinal biopsy by endoscopy or laparotomy, *q.v.* section 5
  - Routine histology
  - Immunohistochemistry
  - PCR for antigen receptor rearrangements (PARR)
  - Histology-guided mass spectrometry (HGMS)
- Serum iron and total iron-binding capacity or serum ferritin to document iron deficiency
- Serum thyroxine, although hyperthyroidism in dogs is very rare
- Trypsin-like immunoreactivity (TLI)
- Vitamin D

1.16 DROOLING

DEFINITION

Dribbling of saliva from the mouth.

NB: Rabies should always be considered as a potential diagnosis in endemic areas before physical examination.

- Pseudoptyalism is drooling due to a failure to swallow normal amounts of saliva
- True ptyalism is increased production of saliva

RELATED CLINICAL SIGNS

- Drooling saliva from mouth
- Dysphagia
- Coughing, inappetence, etc. if non-pharyngeal disease
- Blood may be present with ulcerated oral lesions

COMMON CAUSES

Pseudoptyalism
- Anatomical abnormalities
  - Brachygnathism
  - Lip-fold deformities, especially in giant-breed dogs
- Oesophageal disease
  - Gastro-oesophageal reflux disease
  - Hiatal hernia
  - Obstruction: FB, stricture
  - Oesophagitis
- Oro-pharyngeal disease
  - Dental disease and malposition
  - Oral neoplasia
  - Oral ulcers
  - Oro-pharyngeal FB

Ptyalism
- Gingivitis
- Nausea, *q.v.* section 1.49
- Physiological
  - Anticipation of food (Pavlov reflex)
  - Increased ambient temperature
- Uraemia

UNCOMMON CAUSES

Pseudoptyalism
- Inability to close mouth
  - Botulism
  - Jaw fracture
  - Mandibular neuropraxia
    - trigeminal neuropraxia/neuritis
    - facial nerve paralysis
    - cranial nerve sheath tumours
  - Tetanus
- Masticatory myositis
- Myasthenia gravis
- Pharyngeal FB
- Tonsillar tumour: lymphoma, squamous cell carcinoma

Ptyalism
- Anaphylaxis
- Gastric tumour
- Infection
  - Candidiasis
  - Trench mouth
- Ingestion of toxic/irritant substances and plants
  - *Amanita*, Dumb Cane (*Dieffenbachia*), Philodendron, *Poinsettia*, toads, etc.
  - Caustics
  - Ivermectin
  - Metaldehyde
  - Metronidazole
  - Organophosphates
  - Trimethoprim-sulfa
- Neurological disease
  - Focal myasthenia gravis causing dysphagia and/or megaoesophagus
  - Seizure disorders
  - Vestibular dysfunction
- Rabies and pseudorabies (Aujeszky's disease)
- Salivary gland disease
  - Hypersialosis/sialoadenosis – phenobarbital responsive
  - Sialoadenitis
  - Salivary gland infarction
- Stomatitis
  - Eosinophilic stomatitis: CKCS

DIAGNOSTIC APPROACH

1 Distinguish oropharyngeal from oesophageal and gastric disease by the history
2 Examine oral cavity
3 Investigate for dysphagia, regurgitation and vomiting, *q.v.* sections 1.17, 1.41, 1.49

Clinical clues
- Concurrent dysphagia, regurgitation or vomiting
- Saliva staining of muzzle
- Blood-stained saliva if ulcerated

Clinical examination
Visual inspection
- Drooling saliva
- Lip-fold deformities

Physical examination
- Oral examination – may require sedation or GA
  - Dental diseases: tartar, gingivitis
  - FB
    - Solid FB between teeth, across hard palate or wedged in pharynx

- Linear FB around base of tongue
- Oral inflammation, masses or ulceration, *q.v.* section 5.1.1
- Uraemic breath
- General examination as for regurgitation and vomiting, *q.v.* sections 1.41 and 1.49

Laboratory findings
Haematology
- Typically unremarkable

Serum biochemistry
- Commonly unremarkable in primary oropharyngeal disease
- Azotaemia if uraemic

Urinalysis
- Typically unremarkable except isosthenuria in uraemia

Imaging
Radiographs
- To identify dental diseases and bony involvement with infection or neoplasia

Special tests
- Head CT

1.17 DYSPHAGIA

DEFINITION

Difficulty or inability to prehend, chew or swallow food due to:
- Pain
- Physical failure to open and close the jaws and swallow:
  - Anatomical/physical
  - Functional/neuromuscular

RELATED CLINICAL SIGNS

- Coughing and/or nasal discharge if secondary inhalation
- Drooling (hypersalivation or failure to swallow saliva)
- Extension or lowering of head and neck
- Failure to prehend food, dropping food from mouth
- Halitosis if retained food
- Pain on opening mouth

COMMON CAUSES

Structural or functional diseases of the mouth and/or temporo-mandibular joint and/or pharynx:
- Dental and/or periodontal disease
- FB usually wedged between dental arcades
- Mandibular fracture/luxation
- Oral neoplasia including tonsillar squamous-cell carcinoma, *q.v.* section 2.16
- Stomatitis and oral ulceration
- Pharyngitis/tonsillitis

- Retropharyngeal abscess or lymphadenopathy
- Temporal myositis

Oesophageal disorders
- More typically causes regurgitation, *q.v.* section 1.41

UNCOMMON CAUSES

- Cleft palate
- Craniomandibular osteopathy
- Cricopharyngeal achalasia
- Linear FB under the tongue
- Lingual frenulum disorder – 'tongue tie'
- Mandibular osteomyelitis
- Neuromuscular disorders
  - Botulism
  - Hypothyroid neuropathy
  - Mandibular neuropraxia
  - Muscular dystrophy
  - Myasthenia gravis
  - Peripheral neuropathy
  - Polyradiculoneuritis/tick paralysis
  - Tetanus
  - Trigeminal neuritis or sensory neuropathy
- Nutritional secondary hyperparathyroidism ('rubber jaw')
- Rabies and Aujeszky's disease (pseudorabies)
- Salivary gland disease
  - Hypersialosis/sialoadenosis – phenobarbital responsive
  - Sialoadenitis
  - Salivary gland infarction
- Temporo-mandibular joint disease: dysplasia/jaw locking, fracture/dislocation
- Uraemic stomatitis

DIAGNOSTIC APPROACH

1 Distinguish between regurgitation and vomiting.
2 Confirm difficulty in swallowing by observation.
3 Distinguish morphological causes from functional causes by oropharyngeal inspection and imaging.

CLINICAL CLUES

Predisposition
- Craniomandibular osteopathy: WHWT
- Muscular dystrophy: Bouvier, CKCS
- Trauma in younger dogs
- Uraemia, neoplasia in older dogs

History
- Concurrent signs of renal failure (anorexia, PU/PD), if uraemic ulcers
- Mandibular neuropraxia may follow excessive chewing of bones, etc. and leads to failure to close jaw
- Potential exposure to rabies is important outside UK
- Swollen painful muscles precede atrophy in temporal myositis
- Trauma (road traffic accident, or fall from height) can cause oral fractures/luxations

Clinical examination
Visual inspection
- Observe patient eating to confirm dysphagia and assess jaw motion

Physical examination
  NB: Rabies should always be considered as a potential diagnosis in endemic areas before physical examination.
- Auscultation
  - Chest for secondary inhalation pneumonia
  - Throat for upper airway obstruction
- Check extent of jaw tone, width of opening and presence of pain on opening mouth
- Check neurological function (jaw and tongue movements, gag reflex, trigeminal sensation) if no structural disease is obvious *before* sedation/GA
- Oral examination checking under tongue for linear FB complete examination may require sedation/GA
- Mandibular, retropharyngeal and cervical LNs if oral mass present
- Salivary glands for pain or swelling
- Temporal muscles for swelling or atrophy
- Tonsils may be hard if neoplastic

Laboratory findings
Haematology and serum biochemistry
- Creatine kinase activity increased in myositis
- Look for inflammatory and systemic diseases

Oral and pharyngeal sampling
- Swabs for culture rarely helpful
- Touch impressions, FNAs and biopsy for discrete lesions/masses and LNs

Imaging
Radiographs
- Plain
- Chest radiographs essential if oral mass present
- Head and neck radiographs only helpful for structural abnormalities
- Contrast
  - To assess swallowing function
  - Barium swallow, preferably with fluoroscopy, for functional dysphagia

Special tests
- Acetylcholine receptor antibody titre for myasthenia gravis
- CSF tap
- Electromyography (EMG) and muscle biopsy
- Thyroid function tests

1.18 DYSPNOEA/TACHYPNOEA

DEFINITION

Respiratory distress manifested as an inappropriate degree of breathing effort, reflected by changes in respiratory rate, rhythm and character.
- Exertional, paroxysmal or continuous
- Orthopnoea indicates breathing difficulty whilst in a recumbent position
- Tachypnoea refers to an increased rate of breathing but does not necessarily indicate dyspnoea; it may be seen with exercise, fear or pain

RELATED CLINICAL SIGNS

- Coughing may indicate airway or pulmonary disease, *q.v.* section 1.13
- Cyanosis, *q.v.* section 2.6
- Exercise intolerance, *q.v.* section 1.22
- Increased expiratory effort: lower airway obstruction
- Increased inspiratory effort: upper airway obstruction
- Lethargy
- Open-mouth breathing
- Pallor suggests anaemia or haemorrhage

COMMON CAUSES

Haematological disorders
- Anaemia

Lower airway disorders
- Bronchial disease
  - Chronic bronchitis
  - Eosinophilic bronchopneumopathy
- Left atrial enlargement causing bronchial compression
- Lungworm/heartworm
  - *Angiostrongylus*
  - *Dirofilaria*: not in UK
- Tracheal collapse

Mediastinal disorders
- Neoplasia

Peritoneal cavity disorders
- Ascites (severe)
- Gastric dilatation-volvulus (GDV)
- Organomegaly
- Pregnancy

Pleural/body wall disorders
- Diaphragmatic rupture
- Pleural effusion
- Thoracic wall trauma/pneumothorax

Pulmonary parenchymal disorders
- Allergic/immune-mediated disease, e.g. eosin-ophilic pneumonopathy
- Bronchiectasis
- Metastatic neoplasia
- Pneumonia
  - Aspiration
  - Infectious
  - Parasitic
- Pulmonary oedema
  - Heart failure
  - Neurogenic
    - Asphyxiation due to airway obstruction
    - CNS trauma
  - Shock
  - Toxic
- Pulmonary thromboembolism (PTE): increasingly common but probably still under-recognised
  - DIC
  - HAC
  - Heartworm
  - Neoplasia
  - PLE
- Trauma causing bleeding disorder

Upper airway disorders
Brachycephalic obstructive airway syndrome (BOAS)
- Everted laryngeal saccules
- Laryngeal collapse
- Over-long soft palate
- Stenotic nares
- Tracheal hypoplasia

Laryngeal disease
- Laryngeal oedema
- Laryngeal paralysis

Tracheal disease
- Collapse
- Tracheal FB

UNCOMMON CAUSES

Haematological disorders
- Methaemoglobinaemia

Lower airway disorders
Extraluminal intrathoracic tracheal and/or bronchial compression
- Heart base mass
- Lymphadenopathy

Tracheal diseases affecting thoracic trachea
- As for cervical trachea below

Mediastinal disorders
- Mediastinal mass
- Mediastinitis
- Pneumomediastinum

Nasal cavity obstruction
- Neoplasia
- Rhinitis, *q.v.* sections 1.32, 5.10.1

Peritoneal cavity disorders
- Organomegaly/morbid obesity

Pleural/body wall disorders
- Congenital body wall disorder
- Peritoneo-pericardial diaphragmatic hernia (PPDH)
- Thoracic wall trauma/neoplasia/paralysis

Pulmonary parenchymal disorders
- Broncho-oesophageal fistula
- Distemper
- Lung lobe torsion with pleural effusion
- Lungworm
  - *Crenosoma vulpis*
  - *Eucoleus aerophilus (Capillaria aerophila)*
- Non-cardiogenic pulmonary oedema
- Paraquat poisoning
- Primary pulmonary neoplasia
- Smoke inhalation

Upper airway disorders
Cervical tracheal disease
- Neoplasia very rarely
  - Chondrosarcoma
  - Lymphoma
  - Osteosarcoma
  - Squamous cell carcinoma
- Tracheal parasites:
  - *Filaroides hirthi*
  - *Oslerus osleri*
- Trauma or stricture

Laryngeal disease
- Laryngeal neoplasia

Miscellaneous
- Central nervous system disorder
- Fear/pain
- Hyperthyroidism causing tachypnoea
- Metabolic acidosis
- Obesity hypoventilation (Pickwickian) syndrome
- Peripheral nerve, neuromuscular, muscular disorder

DIAGNOSTIC APPROACH

1 The over-riding concern is not to make dyspnoea worse by investigations.
2 Determine whether there is inspiratory or expiratory dyspnoea or airway noise.
3 Check for upper airway obstruction and treat.
4 Characterise intra-thoracic disease by imaging and investigate appropriately.
5 Discrimination between cardiogenic and non-cardiogenic causes of dyspnoea
- History: suspicion of upper airway obstruction, electrocution, seizures for non-cardiogenic oedema
- Physical examination: heart murmur, jugular pulsation for cardiogenic oedema
- Evaluation for cardiac disease: cardiac size and pulmonary vasculature on radiographs, point of care ultrasound scan or echocardiography

Clinical clues
Predisposition
- BOAS: brachycephalics
- Congenital disorders usually less than 1 year old
- Idiopathic pulmonary fibrosis: WHWT
- Laryngeal paralysis: old, large-breed dogs, especially retrievers, setters
- Metastatic pulmonary neoplasia: usually older animals, e.g. haemangiosarcoma, mammary, prostatic
- Tracheal collapse: small-breed, middle-aged to old dogs
- Tracheal hypoplasia: BOAS breeds

History
- Environment/geographical location, e.g. access to potentially infectious/toxic agents
- History of trauma recent or old: undiagnosed diaphragmatic rupture
- Regurgitation or vomiting and consequent aspiration, *q.v.* sections 1.41 and 1.49

Clinical examination
Visual inspection
- Abnormal discharge, deformities or lesions
- Cyanosis
- Oculo-nasal discharge
- Orthopnoea suggests effusion or heart failure
- Pattern of dyspnoea, e.g. inspiratory vs expiratory
- Rate and rhythm of respiration
- Restrictive vs obstructive

Physical examination
- Palpation
  - Abdomen: feels 'empty' with ruptured diaphragm
  - Compressibility of the cranial mediastinum in small dogs; loss of 'spring' can suggest a mass lesion
  - Larynx/trachea
  - Ribs for evidence of trauma, fractures, masses
  - Thoracic wall percussion for alteration in resonance, e.g. increased with pneumothorax, decreased with thoracic fluid or consolidated tissue
- Auscultation
  - Airway noise suggests fluid or solid obstruction
  - Cardiac auscultation for arrhythmias, murmurs, tachycardia
  - Change in voice if disease of larynx or affecting recurrent laryngeal nerve
  - Crackles suggest small airway disease
  - 'Fluid line' with effusions: increased breath sounds dorsally and muffled ventrally
  - Heart sounds may be muffled with pleural or pericardial fluid
  - Normal or abnormal breath sounds localise airway obstruction
  - Wheezes suggest large airway disease
- Percussion
  - Dull

- Pleural or pericardial effusion
  - 'Fluid line' with effusions
  - Lung consolidation
- Hyper-resonant
  - Pneumothorax

- Nasal lesions, see nasal discharge/sneezing, *q.v.* sections 1.32, 1.43
- Ultrasonography to identify pulmonary/mediastinal mass lesions ± ultrasound-guided aspirate/biopsy

LABORATORY FINDINGS

- Bacterial bronchopneumonia: may be leukocytosis, left shift and degenerate neutrophils
- Coagulation panel helpful if bleeding disorder, disseminated intravascular coagulation
- Dark, brown blood with Heinz body anaemia suggests methaemoglobinaemia
- Eosinophilia may suggest parasitic disease or eosinophilic disorder
- Often within normal limits

IMAGING

- Airway disease, *q.v.* section 4.3
- Fluoroscopy to investigate dynamic airway collapse

SPECIAL TESTS

- Angiography
  - CT
  - Nuclear perfusion studies to investigate pulmonary vascular disease
- Blood gas analysis for pulmonary thromboembolism, plus tests of coagulation, metabolic disorders, and parenchymal diseases
- Bronchoscopy and BAL as for coughing if suspect airway ± pulmonary parenchymal disease
- Examination of laryngeal/pharyngeal region under anaesthesia
- Exploratory thoracotomy and lung biopsy
- Rhinoscopy, pharyngoscopy
- Specific tests for parasites
- Thoracocentesis and fluid analysis (cytology ± culture)

1.19 DYSURIA

DEFINITION

Dysuria (difficulty urinating) may be manifested as pollakiuria (frequently urinating small amounts) and/or stranguria (straining to urinate or pain on urination). Dysuria typically occurs with disorders of the lower urinary tract or its innervation.

RELATED CLINICAL SIGNS

Major signs
- Pollakiuria
  and/or
- Stranguria

Other potential signs
- Dyschezia
- Haematuria
- Nocturia

- Signs of systemic illness or neurological disease depending on the cause
- Urinary incontinence

COMMON CAUSES

Lower urinary tract disorders
- Bladder disorders
  - Bacterial cystitis
  - Neoplasia, e.g transitional (urothelial) cell carcinoma
  - Uroliths
- Urethral disorders
  - Neoplasia: transitional cell carcinoma of the bladder trigone
  - Uroliths
- Prostatic disorders
  - Prostatic carcinoma
  - Paraprostatic cysts, prostatitis, prostatic abscess in male entire dogs

Neurological causes

- Bladder atony
  - Secondary to lower motor neuron or upper motor neuron disorders
  - May occur due to urinary retention of any cause, and may impair recovery as it can be irreversible

UNCOMMON CAUSES

Lower urinary tract disorders

- Bladder disorders
  - Neoplasia: transitional cell carcinoma of the urethra
  - Polypoid cystitis
  - Sterile cystitis related to cyclophosphamide administration
- Urethral disorders
  - Proliferative urethritis
  - Urethral stricture
  - Transmissible venereal tumour
- Prostatic disorders
  - Benign prostatic hyperplasia: although common, it does not commonly cause dysuria
- Vaginal disorders
  - Neoplasia (leiomyoma, leiomyosarcoma)

Neurological causes
- Reflex dyssynergia
- Dysautonomia

Structural
- Perineal hernia with bladder retroflexion

DIAGNOSTIC APPROACH

Clinical clues
Predisposition
- Urinary incontinence, predisposing to bacterial cystitis is more likely with certain signalments
  - Urinary sphincter mechanism incompetence (USMI) can be detected in any dog, however most common in female neutered dogs
  - Young dogs, in particular Golden retrievers, increases the suspicion of ectopic ureter(s)

- Neuter status influences risk of prostatic disorders
  - Benign prostatic hyperplasia in male entire dogs
  - Prostatic carcinoma in male neutered dogs

History
- Pollakiuria should be discriminated from polyuria (increased volume of urination)
- In dogs with bacterial cystitis an emphasis should be placed on establishing risk factors that may have predisposed to the development of infection:
  - Anatomic causes
    - Juvenile vaginitis in puppies
    - Hooded vulva in female dogs
    - Urinary incontinence: ectopic ureter, USMI
  - Immunosuppression
  - Presence of systemic disease (HAC, DM)
- Concurrent dyschezia increases suspicion of an intrapelvic mass lesion: enlarged prostate or lymph nodes

Clinical examination
Visual inspection
- Measuring bladder size (using ultrasonography) following voiding may help establish whether the dog is able to void their bladder; if it remains large, obstructive and neurological causes are more likely
- Observing urination patterns can be informative: dogs with reflex dyssynergia typically initiate urination as normal; however, the urinary stream abruptly stops due to lack of synchrony between bladder contraction and urethral sphincter relaxation: the same pattern can also be observed with urethral obstruction

Physical examination
- Passing a urinary catheter to assess for ease of passing aids assessment for urethral obstructive disorders: can be done in conscious male dogs but likely requires sedation or anaesthesia for female dogs
- Rectal examination to assess the urethra, and prostate in male dogs
- Thorough examination for risk factors for development of bacterial cystitis should be performed in patients, in particular assessing

conformation: examine for hooded vulva, perivulval inflammation or urinary pooling in female dogs or prostatomegaly in male dogs

Neurological examination
- Ability to express bladder is useful in dogs with concurrent neurological deficits
- Assessment for concurrent neurological deficits

Laboratory findings
Haematology
- Useful to screen for systemic disease, uncommon to detect abnormalities

Serum biochemistry
- Useful to screen for systemic disease, may detect azotaemia in dogs with post-renal causes (urethral obstruction) or renal causes (extension of bacterial cystitis to pyelonephritis)

Urinalysis
- Urine culture (ideally from cystocentesis sample, otherwise interpret positive culture with caution)
- Urine cytology to assess for neoplastic cells
- Urine sediment for evidence of urinary tract infection or neoplastic cells
- Urine specific gravity to assess for polydipsia and polyuria

Imaging
Radiographs
May need to do an enema first to fully assess urinary system for uroliths. Ensure that the whole length of urethra is included; move hindlimbs cranially to assess perineal urethra in males.
- Assess for radiopaque uroliths, prostate
- Contrast studies: retrograde urethrogram (plain radiographs or fluoroscopy) and intravenous excretory urogram

Ultrasound
- Assess kidneys, ureters, urinary bladder and prostate

Special tests
- CT with contrast for urinary system assessment: intravenous urogram with iodinated contrast improves sensitivity for ectopic ureter compared to plain radiography
- Cystoscopy to assess urethra, bladder, and sites of implantation of ureters
- MRI and CSF for dogs with neurolocalisation
- Prostatic wash and fine needle aspiration for cytology and culture
- Urinary BRAF mutation analysis: presence of BRAF mutation detected in ~80% of dogs with transitional cell carcinoma
- Urodynamic pressure profilometry

1.20 DYSTOCIA

DEFINITION

Difficulty with vaginal delivery of fetuses; can result in morbidity and mortality for fetuses, neonates and bitch.

RELATED CLINICAL SIGNS

- Abnormal vulval discharge
- Failure for labour to start or progress
- Maternal distress
- Protracted straining, non-productive
- Stillborn or weak puppies

COMMON AND UNCOMMON CAUSES

- Fetal dystocia
  - Malpositioned/postured
  - Oversized
- Fetal/maternal dystocia
  - Mismatch of birth canal to fetal size, e.g. brachycephalic/hydrocephalic breeds
- Maternal dystocia
  - Abdominal wall defects (hernia)
  - Birth canal defects (stricture)
  - Metabolic disease
  - Poor lubrication in pelvic/birth canal

- Primary: no myometrial contractions
- Secondary: uterine inertia
- Severe vulvar oedema
- Uterine torsion

DIAGNOSTIC APPROACH

Clinical clues
Predisposition
- Abdominal wall defects, e.g. hernia
- Brachycephalic and hydrocephalic breeds
- Metabolic derangements in bitch, e.g.
  - DM
  - Hypocalcaemia
  - Hypoglycaemia
  - Hypovolaemia
  - Pre-eclampsia
  - Pregnancy toxaemia
  - Sepsis/systemic inflammatory response syndrome (SIRS)
- Obesity of bitch
- Pelvic canal narrowing, e.g. after fracture
- Poor condition of bitch
- Prolonged gestation can result in fetal overgrowth, e.g. small litters
- Some breed lines
- Uterine inertia, e.g. large litters
- Vaginal canal abnormalities (stricture, vaginal hyperplasia, oedema)

History
- Difficulty with previous labour
- Failure for labour to start on expected date
- Prolonged time between stages of labour
  - Stage 1, increased frequency and strength myometrial contractions and progesterone and temperature drops, normally 12–24 hours
  - Stage 2, co-ordination of abdominal and myometrial contractions and delivery of fetus, normally 8 hours
  - Stage 3, expulsion of placenta, normally 12–24 hours
- Prolonged time between delivery fetuses (normally < 1 hour)
- Stillborn or weak puppies

Clinical examination
Visual inspection
- Can be normal

- Abnormal vulval discharge e.g. green, malodorous, haemorrhagic
- Maternal distress: agitation, trembling, hyperpnoeic
- Nesting behaviour
- Persistent straining

Physical examination
- Can be normal, i.e. normothermia, and slight hypothermia can be normal
- Fatigue/weak
- Fetus stuck in birth canal
- Moderate to severe pain
- Muscle tremors/tetany
- Retention of placenta
- Vomiting

Laboratory findings
Haematology
- Mildly decreased HCT normal at due date

Serum biochemistry
- Hypocalcaemia can lead to uterine inertia
- Hypoglycaemia can lead to uterine inertia
- Mildly decreased total protein at due date

Urinalysis
- Glucose or ketones can indicate DM or pregnancy toxaemia

Imaging
Plain radiographs
- Evaluate litter size
- Assess relative fetal size
- Assess for obstruction/malposition

Ultrasound/Doppler
- Evaluate fetal viability
  - Normal fetal heart rate > 200 bpm
  - Fetal distress results in bradycardia

Special tests
- Review gestational length: error in expected due date could mean a lack of labour is normal
- Vaginal examination: digital or via scope to assess for obstruction and whether cervix is dilated
- Uterine pressure monitoring (tocodynamometry), if available

1.21 EPISTAXIS

DEFINITION

Haemorrhage from the nose or nasopharynx. Typically this drips out of the rostral nares but it can also be swallowed, especially with more caudal lesions.

RELATED CLINICAL SIGNS

- Bleeding from rostral nares
- Haematemesis or melaena due, respectively, to vomiting or passage of swallowed blood may occur
- Nasal disorders may have concurrent nasal discharge (serous, mucopurulent), sneezing, nasal depigmentation/deformities, or pawing at face may be observed
- Systemic causes may have concurrent evidence of haemorrhage (petechiae, ecchymoses, melaena, haematuria); although primary haemostatic disorders are most likely to be responsible for epistaxis, secondary haemostatic disorders may also occasionally present with epistaxis.

COMMON CAUSES

Nasal disease
- Chronic rhinitis
- FB
- Infection
  - Oronasal fistula
  - Periapical tooth root abscess
  - Sino-nasal aspergillosis
- Neoplasia: carcinoma, sarcoma, lymphoma

Systemic disease
- *Angiostrongylus vasorum* infection causing a mixed haemostatic disorder
- Hypertension
- Primary haemostatic disorders
  - Thrombocytopenia: IMTP, bone marrow disease
- Secondary haemostatic disorders
  - Vitamin K deficiency (rodenticide toxicity)

UNCOMMON CAUSES

Nasal disease
- Infection
  - *Leishmania*
  - Osteomyelitis
  - Parasitic (*Linguatula serrata*)
- Neoplasia (leiomyoma)
- Trauma

Systemic disease
- Primary haemostatic disorders
  - Hyperviscosity due to erythrocytosis, hyperglobulinaemia in leishmaniosis or myeloma
  - Thrombocytopenia: consumptive (DIC), *Ehrlichia*
  - Thrombocytopathia: inherited, e.g. Glanzmann's thrombasthenia, Scott syndrome
  - von Willebrand factor deficiency (congenital)
- Secondary haemostatic disorders
  - Liver dysfunction (chronic hepatitis, toxicity e.g. xylitol)
  - Vitamin K deficiency (cholestasis, congenital)

DIAGNOSTIC APPROACH

Clinical clues
- Bilateral is more likely chronic idiopathic rhinitis, aspergillosis or bleeding disorder
- Unilateral is more likely a FB neoplasia, oronasal fistula or dental disease

Predisposition
- Breed predispositions to IMTP, e.g. Cocker spaniels
- Dolichocephalic dogs are predisposed to sino-nasal aspergillosis
- Glanzmann's thrombasthenia: Great Pyrenees, Otterhound
- Older dogs are predisposed to nasal tumours and dental disease
- Scott syndrome (inherited thrombocytopathia): GSD

History
- Assessing for presence of unilateral or bilateral nasal discharge is useful in prioritising differential diagnoses
  - Unilateral is more likely a FB neoplasia, oronasal fistula or dental disease
  - Bilateral is more likely chronic idiopathic rhinitis, aspergillosis or bleeding disorder)
- History of other bleeding sites may be useful, e.g. haematuria
- Presence of nasal stertor increases suspicion of nasal FB or tumour
- Recent dental extractions may increase suspicion of oronasal fistula
- Risk of exposure to anticoagulant rodenticide
- Travel history: increases index of suspicion of vector-borne diseases including *Ehrlichia* and *Leishmania* infection

Clinical examination
Visual inspection
- Assess for presence of sneezing (increases suspicion of nasal disease)

Physical examination
- Blood pressure to assess for hypertension
- Evidence of haemorrhage elsewhere, especially skin of the ventral abdomen, and gums, and rectal examination for melaena
- Nasal planum depigmentation most common in fungal disease
- Examination of head conformation including ocular retropulsion for signs of deformity suspicious for neoplasia
- Oral examination to assess for dental disease and oronasal fistula

Ophthalmic examination
- Hypertensive retinopathy indicating target organ damage

Laboratory findings
Haematology
- Coagulation times (PT and aPTT)
- Platelet count

Serum biochemistry
- Useful to screen for systemic disease, in particular evidence of hyperglobulinaemia

Imaging
Plain radiographs
- Nasal turbinate destruction: tumour or aspergillosis
- Soft tissue opacity: tumour most likely but can also occur with fluid accumulation
- Sinus hyperostosis: aspergillosis

Special tests
- *Aspergillus* serology; specific but poorly sensitive test, i.e. positive result supports infection but negative result does not exclude infection
- Baermann technique or Angiodetect® for *Angiostrongylus vasorum*
- Buccal mucosal bleeding time to assess for thrombocytopathia
- CT scan with contrast to assess for nasal diseases
- DNA test
  - Glanzmann's thrombasthenia
  - Scott syndrome
- Testing for *Leishmania* and *Ehrlichia* infection as appropriate
- von Willebrand factor antigen

1.22 EXERCISE INTOLERANCE

DEFINITION

Exercise intolerance is the decreased ability to perform physical exercise at the normally expected level or duration for dogs of that age, size and muscle mass.

RELATED CLINICAL SIGNS

- Muscle weakness/wasting
- Musculoskeletal pain
- Panting/tachypnoea

- Prolonged recovery from exercise
- Pyrexia
- Reduced stamina at exercise
- Reluctance to exercise

COMMON CAUSES

Cardiovascular disease

q.v. sections 1.18, 1.51, 5.2

Endocrine disease

- HAC
- Hypoadrenocorticism
- Hypothyroidism

Generalised weakness

- Anaemia
- Chronic inflammation/infection/wasting
- Drugs, e.g. anticonvulsants, antihistamines, diuretics, vasodilators, anti-arrhythmics
- Neoplasia
- Obesity
- Pyrexia

Metabolic disease

- Hypercalcaemia
- Hypo-/hyper-kalaemia, *q.v.* section 3.23
- Hypo-/hyper-glycaemia, *q.v.* section 3.17
- Hyponatraemia, *q.v.* section 3.24

Muscular disease

- Inherited myopathies

Neurological/spinal disease

- Cervical spondylomyelopathy (wobbler)
- Intervertebral disc protrusion
- Vestibular disease

Neuromuscular disease

- Myasthenia gravis

Respiratory disease

- *q.v.* sections 1.18, 1.51

Skeletal disease

- Cruciate ligament disease/rupture
- Degenerative joint disease

UNCOMMON CAUSES

Endocrine disease

- Diabetic ketoacidosis
- Phaeochromocytoma

Metabolic disease

- Acidosis
- Hepatic encephalopathy
- Malignant hyperthermia

Miscellaneous

- Nutritional deficiency
- Parasitism

Muscular disease

- Exercise-induced hyperthermia, *q.v.* section 2.25
- Muscular dystrophy
- Polymyositis
- Scottie cramp

Neurological/spinal disease

- Botulism
- Cerebellar disease
- Cervical myelopathy
- Discospondylitis
- Dyskinesia
- Fibrocartilaginous embolism
- Narcolepsy/cataplexy
- Neoplasia
- Peripheral polyneuropathies
- Spinal trauma

Skeletal disease

- Hypertrophic osteopathy (Marie's disease)
- Immune-mediated polyarthritis (IMPA)
- Panosteitis

DIAGNOSTIC APPROACH

1. Thorough history to discern any other clinical signs apart from exercise intolerance which itself is non-specific.
2. Complete physical examination covering all body systems.
3. Exercise test once cardiorespiratory diseases and lameness have been ruled out.

Clinical clues

q.v. sections 1.44, 1.51

Predisposition
- Centronuclear myopathy: Labrador retriever
- Cervical spondylomyelopathy: Dobermann
- Exercise-induced hyperthermia: Border collie
- Mitochondrial myopathy: Clumber and Sussex spaniels
- Scottie cramp: Scottish terrier

Clinical examination

Visual inspection
- Normal at rest, but dyspnoea/tachypnoea after exercise
- Gradual slowing down or ataxic on exercise

Physical examination
- Musculoskeletal pain
- Hyperthermia

Laboratory findings

- Elevated creatine phosphokinase (CPK)/ aspartate aminotransferase (AST) in muscle disease e.g. polymyositis
  q.v. section 3.12

Imaging

q.v. sections 1.44, 1.51

Special tests

q.v. sections 1.44, 1.51
- DNA test for Labrador myopathy
- Malignant hyperthermia – exercise test will induce hyperlactacidaemia, hyperthermia, haemoconcentration mild respiratory alkalosis after a short period of exercise (*cf.* normal animals after long, strenuous exercise)
- Scottie cramp: administer serotonin antagonist to induce an episode in affected dogs, i.e. give 0.3 mg/kg orally of methysergide and exercise 2 hours later

1.23 FAECAL INCONTINENCE

DEFINITION

The involuntary passage of faecal material, due to an inability to retain faeces.
  The cause can be
- Anatomical, as the result of reduced capacity or compliance of the rectum
- Neurological sphincter mechanism incontinence

RELATED CLINICAL SIGNS

- Dyschezia
- Haematochezia
- Involuntary passage of faeces
- Perineal staining
- Tenesmus
- Other signs of neurological deficits

COMMON CAUSES

Anal disease
- Anal furunculosis
- Associated with constipation
  - perineal hernia
  - anal sac disease

Neurogenic sphincter mechanism incontinence
- Lumbosacral disease
  - Canine degenerative myelopathy (CDM)
  - IVDD

UNCOMMON CAUSES

Neurogenic sphincter incontinence
- Congenital malformation
- Previous local surgery
  - Attempted perineal hernia repair
  - Damage to anal sphincter during anal sacculectomy
  - Rectal pull-through procedure

- Fibrocartilaginous embolism (FCE)
- Polyneuropathy
- Sacrocaudal dysgenesis (brachycephalic breeds)
- Spina bifida
- Spinal arachnoid cysts
- Spinal trauma

Neoplasia

- Perineal, rectal or colonic

Myopathy

- Polymyopathy

DIAGNOSTIC APPROACH

1 Distinguish inappropriate defaecation (e.g. improper house training) from true incontinence by observing defaecation.
2 Rule out rectal/anal disease by the presence of straining and physical findings on digital rectal examination.
3 Evaluate local (anal tone) and general neurological function if there is no obvious anatomical cause.

Clinical clues

Predisposition
- Lumbosacral disease and canine degenerative myelopathy (CDM) classically in GSDs, but now recognised in numerous breeds
- Perineal hernia in intact male dogs

History
- Chronic progressive with most neurological disease except FCE and trauma

- Tenesmus, dyschezia and haematochezia with local rectal/anal disease

Clinical examination

Visual inspection
- Other neurological deficits – tail carriage, hindleg ataxia, etc.
- Perineal masses, bulges

Physical examination
- Postural reflex testing
- Rectal examination to determine anal tone and local disease

Laboratory findings
- Usually unremarkable

Imaging
Plain radiographs
- Plain
- Vertebral abnormality

Contrast radiographs
- Myelography is often inadequate to image lumbosacral disease
- Epidurography and MRI scan are preferred for lumbosacral disease

Special tests
- Biopsy of any mass(es)
- Electromyography
- Genetic test for superoxide dismutase mutation in some cases of degenerative myelopathy
- Lumbar CSF collection

1.24 FLATULENCE/BORBORYGMI

DEFINITION

Flatulence is the accumulation of gas within the GI tract. Borborygmi are rumbling/gurgling sounds caused by GI contractions mixing and moving fluid and gas.

Some gas production in the GI tract is a normal physiological process, but excess produc-

tion can be the result of GI disease or ingestion of non-absorbable fermentable substances.
- The gas may be:
  - Caused by bacterial fermentation
  - Gas diffusing from the blood
  - Swallowed air
  - The product of luminal chemical reactions (acid-alkali reactions)

- The presence of flatulence can be detected by finding abdominal distension or by auscultation
- Whilst eructation is the release of accumulated gas via the mouth, flatus is the release of gases via the anus. These are often odiferous because they contain volatile molecules such as ammonia, hydrogen sulfide, indoles, skatoles, volatile amines and short-chain fatty acids produced by bacterial metabolism.

RELATED CLINICAL SIGNS

- Abdominal discomfort
- Audible borborygmi
- Bloating
- Eructation (belching)
- Flatus

COMMON CAUSES

Aerophagia
- Dysphagia, *q.v.* section 1.17
- Dyspnoea, especially in BOAS, *q.v.* section 1.18
- Rapid/competitive eating

Diseases causing malabsorption and alterations in microbiome
- CIE/IBD
- Exocrine pancreatic insufficiency
- Intestinal dysbiosis/antibiotic-responsive diarrhoea/small intestinal bacterial overgrowth

Ingestion of non-absorbable substances
- Fermentable carbohydrates such as stachyose and raffinose found in soya and fermentable fibres

UNCOMMON CAUSES

- Administration of calcium carbonate to neutralise gastric acid or to treat hypocalcaemia, releasing carbon dioxide
- Diffusion of gas from the bloodstream

- Unimportant in dogs except in GDV
- Extreme exercise, causing aerophagia
- Ileus causing stasis of gut contents and secondary bacterial fermentation
- Ingestion of carbonated drinks
- Lactase deficiency: theoretical but never documented in dogs
- Lactulose

DIAGNOSTIC APPROACH

1 Obtain a full dietary history.
2 Auscultate and image chest if the dog is dyspnoeic.
3 Palpate and image the abdomen.
4 Investigate underlying causes of GI disease.

Clinical clues
The presence of audible borborygmi can be normal, especially in unfed dogs, with the sound mainly originating from gastric motility. As an isolated finding in an otherwise asymptomatic dog, increased borborygmi are not a concern. Excessive borborygmi in conjunction with flatus is abnormal, but the pattern of gut sounds is not pathognomonic for any specific disease.

Predisposition
- BOAS in brachycephalic dogs
- Chronic diarrhoea, *q.v.* section 1.15.2

History
- Audible gut sounds
- Concurrent diarrhoea
- Episodes of abdominal bloating and/or discomfort
- Repeated belching
- Odiferous flatus
- Soya-based food or unusual diet, e.g. beans, cabbage, lentils, Brussels sprouts

Clinical examination
Visual inspection
- Brachycephalic conformation
- Dyspnoea, tachypnoea
- Distended abdomen

Physical examination
- Abdominal distension or discomfort
- Borborygmi found on auscultation of abdomen
- Tympany on percussion in GD/GDV

Laboratory findings
- Usually unremarkable haematology and serum biochemistry except if significant primary GI disease
- Abnormal folate and/or cobalamin
- Low TLI in EPI

Imaging
Plain radiographs
- Alveolar pulmonary or pleural disease if dyspnoeic
- Gas-distended bowel loops

Ultrasound
- Excess intestinal gas

Special tests
- None

1.25 HAEMATEMESIS

DEFINITION

Vomiting of blood; *q.v.* section 1.49
  The blood can be:
- Due to a generalised bleeding problem
  or
- Swallowed from oral, nasal or respiratory bleeding
  or
- From gastric and/or upper GI ulceration

RELATED CLINICAL SIGNS

- Epistaxis, bleeding oral lesion or coughing if swallowing pulmonary blood
- Generalised bleeding if coagulation disorder
- Vomiting of fresh or changed blood
  - Large volumes and very fresh blood will appear bright red
  - After a few minutes in gastric acid, blood is changed and the dog will vomit brown granular material ('coffee grounds') which owners may not recognise as blood

COMMON CAUSES

Endocrine
- Hypoadrenocorticism (not common but important)

Gastric ulceration
- Acute and chronic gastritis ± CIE/IBD

- Abrasive gastric FB
- Gastric carcinoma
- NSAID-induced ulceration, especially if in combination with steroids
- Portal hypertension in end-stage liver disease
- Uraemic gastritis

Generalised bleeding problem
q.v. section 1.9
GI disease
- Acute pancreatitis
- Parvovirus infection

Swallowed blood
- Epistaxis, *q.v.* section 1.21
- Oral bleeding

UNCOMMON CAUSES

- AHDS/HGE

Duodenal ulceration
- Neoplasia

Gastric ulceration
- Gastric leiomyoma/sarcoma
- Gastric lymphoma
- Gastrinoma
- High-dose steroids: dexamethasone more commonly than prednisolone
- Mallory-Weiss tear: a gastric mucosal tear due to violent vomiting
- Mast cell tumour

- Post-GDV
- Pythiosis (not in UK)

Shock
- Hypovolaemia
- Septic shock
- Neurogenic shock

Swallowed blood
- Following haemoptysis – bleeding lung lesion, usually carcinoma
- Ingestion of blood
- Oesophageal disease
  - Neoplasia
  - Severe oesophagitis
  - Trauma
    - Ingested FB
    - Stick injury

DIAGNOSTIC APPROACH

1 Distinguish vomiting of gastric blood from a generalised bleeding problem or swallowed blood.
2 Treat symptomatically but investigate by imaging and endoscopy, etc. if severe or not improving.

Clinical clues
Predisposition
- Gastric carcinoma more common in 7- to 10-year-old Belgian shepherds (Tervuren), Bull terriers, Chow Chows and Collies

History
- Anorexia and weight loss if severe gastric ulceration and especially if gastric carcinoma
- Diarrhoea and weight loss with gastrinoma

- Known administration of NSAIDs or steroids, or exposure to infection or toxins

Clinical examination
Visual inspection
- Bleeding at other sites if generalised coagulopathy
- Epistaxis or oral bleeding
- 'Prayer position' if cranial abdominal pain due to ulceration or pancreatitis

Physical examination
- Skin mass(es) which may be a mast cell tumour
- Palpation
  - Cranial abdominal pain in acute pancreatitis, deep gastric ulceration
  - Cranial abdominal mass

Laboratory findings
- Anaemia and hypoproteinaemia if severe bleeding
- Microcytic anaemia with thrombocytosis if chronic bleeding and iron deficiency
- Leukocytosis if pancreatitis or peritonitis is associated with incipient or early ulcer perforation
- Amylase/lipase is unreliably increased in acute pancreatitis

Imaging
- *q.v.* section 1.49

Special tests
- Buccal mucosal bleeding time, clotting profile
- Spec cPL for pancreatitis
- As for vomiting, *q.v.* section 1.49

1.26 HAEMATOCHEZIA

DEFINITION

The presence of fresh blood in faeces.
- Usually an indicator of LI or perianal disease
- Rarely seen with SI haemorrhage, and only if this is massive and/or the rate of intestinal transit is increased

RELATED CLINICAL SIGNS

- Abnormal stool shape/size if rectal mass
- Concurrent diarrhoea, often with mucus if colitis
- Normal stool consistency with blood on surface if focal lesion, e.g. rectal polyp
- Passage of bright red, fresh blood

COMMON CAUSES

Anal disease
- Anal sac infection
- Anal sac adenocarcinoma
- Perianal adenoma

Generalised bleeding disorder
q.v. section 1.9

Generalised GI disease
- AHDS/HGE
- Bacterial enteritis

Large intestinal disease
- Colitis
  - Idiopathic CIE/IBD
  - Food-responsive enteropathy
- Foreign material, e.g., bones
- Ileo-colic intussusception
- Rectal prolapse
- Rectal polyps
- Colonic or rectal neoplasia

UNCOMMON CAUSES

Large intestinal disease
- Acute neurological trauma causing colonic ulceration/perforation
- Infection; whipworms and hookworms are more uncommon in the UK but more common in subtropical and tropical regions, and in countries where routine deworming is not practised
  - Amoebiasis: not in UK
  - *Ancylostoma* hookworms (rare in UK)
  - Histoplasmosis (restricted geographically, i.e., not in UK)
  - Prototheccosis
  - *Trichuris* whipworms
  - *Uncinaria* hookworms
- Blood vessel malformation (e.g. colonic angiodysplasia/vascular ectasia)
- Caecal inversion
- High-dose glucocorticoids
- Perianal carcinoma

DIAGNOSTIC APPROACH

1. Rule out generalised bleeding.
2. Localise problem to external anus or distal intestine.
3. Digital rectal examination.
4. Proctoscopy/colonoscopy.

Clinical clues
Predisposition
- Rectal prolapse is most common in young dogs with colitis

History
- Absence of diarrhoea helps rule out colitis
- Spotting of blood between bowel movements indicates anal disease or lesion close to anus

Clinical examination
Visual inspection
- Anal masses
- Bleeding at other sites if generalised
- Dyschezia if anal inflammation
- Protrusion of severe ileo-colic intussusception
- Rectal prolapse
- Tenesmus if inflammatory or neoplastic rectal disease

Physical examination
- Abdominal palpation
  - Colonic mass
- Digital rectal palpation
  - Anal sac disease
  - Rectal polyp or neoplasia

Laboratory findings
- Haematology and serum biochemistry usually unremarkable except for changes due to blood loss (anaemia, hypoproteinaemia)

Faecal examination
- Culture rarely helpful
- Parasitology for whipworms and hookworms

Imaging
- Sublumbar lymphadenopathy and/or periosteal reaction on lumbar vertebrae if metastasis from anal sac or rectal tumour
- Ultrasound examination limited by colonic gas

Special tests
- Barium enema (rarely performed)
- Proctoscopy/colonoscopy

1.27 HAEMATURIA AND DISCOLOURED URINE

DEFINITION

Haematuria may be observed as a gross change in urine colour or detected due to microscopic haematuria detected on dipstick or sediment analysis. Discolouration of urine can be caused by the presence of intact RBCs or free haemoglobin and other pigments including myoglobin.

RELATED CLINICAL SIGNS

- Haematuria or any change in urine colour may be the only clinical sign in some dogs.
- It may be in combination with signs of dysuria, *q.v.* section 1.19
- There may be concurrent evidence of systemic disease or bleeding diathesis. Some dogs with significant haemorrhage may even pass blood clots during their urine stream. As with any cause of bleeding, causes can be divided into disorders of the urinary tract or related to a disorder of haemostasis (systemic disease).
- Haematuria can be discriminated from haemoglobinuria (both will cause reddened urine) by sediment examination after allowing the urine to sediment, ideally, after centrifugation. Red blood cells will form a pellet whereas with haemoglobinuria the urine will remain tinged red with no pellet. A fresh sample should be examined as RBCs will lyse spontaneously in stored urine samples.

COMMON CAUSES – HAEMATURIA

Urinary tract disease
- Renal haemorrhage
  - Pyelonephritis
  - Trauma
- Bladder haemorrhage
  - Bacterial cystitis
  - Sampling method: cystocentesis sampling may result in mild bleeding into the sample
  - Trauma
  - Urolithiasis
- Urethral haemorrhage
  - Neoplasia (transitional cell carcinoma)
- Prostatic haemorrhage
  - Prostatic carcinoma (male neutered dogs)
  - Prostatitis (male entire dogs)
- Vaginal haemorrhage
  - Oestrus (female entire dogs)

Systemic disease
- Primary haemostatic disorders
  - Thrombocytopenia: IMTP
  - Thrombocytopathia: hyperviscosity due to hyperglobulinaemia, e.g. neoplasia, *Leishmania*
- *Angiostrongylus vasorum* infection causes a mixed haemostatic disorder

UNCOMMON CAUSES – HAEMATURIA

Urinary tract disease
- Renal haemorrhage
  - Idiopathic renal haemorrhage
  - Infarction

- Neoplasia
- Telangiectasia
- Urolithiasis
- Ureteral haemorrhage
  - Neoplasia
  - Urolithiasis
- Bladder haemorrhage
  - Neoplasia (transitional cell carcinoma)
  - Polypoid cystitis
  - Sterile cystitis (cyclophosphamide)
- Urethral haemorrhage
  - Proliferative/granulomatous urethritis
  - Urolithiasis
- Vaginal haemorrhage
  - Subinvolution of placental sites (SIPs), metritis (post whelping female entire dogs)
  - Pyometra (female entire dogs)
  - Neoplasia (leiomyoma, leiomyosarcoma)

Systemic disease

- Primary haemostatic disorders
  - Thrombocytopenia: IMTP, *Ehrlichia*, consumptive (DIC), bone marrow disease
  - Thrombocytopathia (congenital, hyperviscosity due to erythrocytosis)
  - von Willebrand factor deficiency (congenital)
- Secondary haemostatic disorders (rare cause of haematuria, body cavity bleeds more likely)
  - Vitamin K deficiency (rodenticide toxicity)
  - Liver dysfunction (chronic hepatitis, toxicity e.g. xylitol)
  - Vitamin K deficiency (cholestasis, congenital)

COMMON CAUSES – DISCOLOURED URINE

Red or brown urine – see haematuria

- Haemoglobinuria also
  - IMHA (intravascular haemolysis)
  - Heat stroke

Dark yellow urine

- Bilirubinuria, *q.v.* section 2.13
- Concentrated urine

UNCOMMON CAUSES – DISCOLOURED URINE

Red or brown urine – also see haematuria

- Haemoglobinuria
  - Blood transfusion reaction (acute haemolytic)
  - Paracetamol (acetaminophen) toxicity
  - Snake envenomation
  - Splenic torsion
- Myoglobinuria
  - Rhabdomyolysis
  - Severe muscle trauma

Dark yellow urine

- Food dyes
- Drugs

DIAGNOSTIC APPROACH

Clinical clues
Predisposition
- Breed predispositions to IMHA and IMTP, e.g. cocker spaniels

History
- Concurrent haemorrhage elsewhere: increases index of suspicion of systemic disorder
- Signs of dysuria: increases index of suspicion of urinary tract disorder
- Travel history: increases index of suspicion of vector-borne diseases including *Ehrlichia* and *Leishmania* infections

Clinical examination
Visual inspection
- Observe urination – occurrence of haematuria may prioritise differential diagnoses but this must be interpreted in combination with other investigations
  - Haematuria at the beginning of the urinary stream implies genital tract or urethral disorders
  - Haematuria throughout the duration of the urinary stream occurs with many disorders (renal, ureteral, bladder, or systemic disorders, occasionally urethral and prostatic

disorders can also result in reflux of blood into the bladder)

- Haematuria during the terminal phase suggests a ventral bladder wall lesion and can also occur with intermittent renal haemorrhage (as the blood is pooled in the ventral bladder and expelled at the end)
- Haemorrhage occurring independent of urination implies a disorder of the distal urethra or genital tract

Physical examination
- Abdominal palpation in particular to assess for renal pain or asymmetry where possible
- Evidence of haemorrhage elsewhere: skin especially of the ventral abdomen, and gums, rectal examination for melaena
- Rectal examination to assess urethra, as well as prostate in males
- Vaginal examination in female dogs

Laboratory findings
Haematology
- Coagulation times (PT and aPTT) in secondary haemostatic disorders
- Evidence of haemolysis (spherocytes, ghost cells), and regenerative anaemia in IMHA
- Low platelet count in IMTP

Serum biochemistry
- Screen for systemic disease
  - Azotaemia may be detected in pyelonephritis (renal) or ureteric or urethral disorders (post renal)

Urinalysis
- Haematuria on voided urine samples but not cystocentesis samples suggests a urethral or prostatic (male)/vaginal (female) disorder
- Sediment examination
  - Active sediment in the presence of urinary tract infection (diagnosis of bacterial cystitis should prompt assessment for risk factors rather than symptomatic treatment alone)
  - Presence of crystals: not diagnostic of urolithiasis but increases index of suspicion

- Neoplastic cells
- RBCs (ideally fresh sample as red blood cells may lyse, especially in dilute or alkaline urine, resulting in a false impression of haemoglobinuria)
- Urine cytology: as above, but submission of an EDTA-preserved urine sample may complement routine sediment examination

Imaging
Plain radiographs
- Assess for radiopaque uroliths, prostate, ensure length of urethra included; may need to do an enema first to fully assess urinary system for uroliths
- Contrast studies retrograde urethrogram (plain radiographs or fluoroscopy) and intravenous excretory urogram

Ultrasound
- Assess kidneys, ureters, urinary bladder and prostate

Special tests
- For haemolysis
  - Coombs' test to aid diagnosis of suspected IMHA
- For haemostatic disorders
  - Buccal mucosal bleeding time for thrombocytopathia
  - von Willebrand factor antigen
  - Baermann technique or Angiodetect® for *Angiostrongylus vasorum*
  - Testing for *Leishmania* and *Ehrlichia* infection as appropriate
- For urinary tract disorders
  - CT scan with contrast
  - Prostatic sampling (wash or fine needle aspirate)
  - Urocystoscopy – assessment of vagina, urethra, prostatic urethra, bladder and implantation of ureters. In idiopathic renal haemorrhage this identifies the kidney responsible for the haemorrhage (ideally carried out during haemorrhagic event).

1.28 HAEMOPTYSIS

DEFINITION

Haemoptysis refers to coughing up blood or bloody sputum.

RELATED CLINICAL SIGNS

- Haemoptysis may be observed in dogs with signs of significant respiratory disease (coughing, tachypnoea, dyspnoea) or may occur in combination with evidence of a bleeding diathesis.
- Melaena may occur concurrently due to swallowed blood or concurrent gastrointestinal haemorrhage.
- As with any cause of bleeding, causes can be divided into disorders of the respiratory system or related to a disorder of haemostasis (systemic disease).

COMMON CAUSES

Respiratory tract disease
- Lower airway haemorrhage
  - *Angiostrongylus vasorum* (lungworm)
  - FB
  - Parenchymal lung disease
  - Neoplasia
    - Carcinoma
    - Haemangiosarcoma
- Pharyngeal and/or laryngeal haemorrhage
  - FB (stick injury)
  - Trauma
- Tracheal haemorrhage
  - FB
  - Trauma

Systemic disease
- Primary haemostatic disorders
  - Thrombocytopenia: consumptive (DIC)
- Secondary haemostatic disorders
  - Vitamin K deficiency: rodenticide toxicity

UNCOMMON CAUSES

Respiratory tract disease
- Lower airway haemorrhage
  - Infectious pneumonia: fungal, bacterial, protozoal, viral
  - Inflammatory disease: chronic bronchitis, eosinophilic bronchopneumopathy
  - Neoplasia: histiocytic sarcoma
- Pharyngeal and/or laryngeal haemorrhage
  - Neoplasia
  - Post-nasal drip: nasal or nasopharyngeal haemorrhage, *q.v.* section 1.21
- Tracheal haemorrhage
  - Neoplasia; chondrocarcinoma arising from tracheal ring
- Parenchymal lung disease
  - *Dirofilaria* (heartworm, increased suspicion in travelled dogs)
  - Leptospirosis (described in mainland European cases more commonly than elsewhere)
  - Pulmonary oedema can result in pink sputum (cardiogenic and non-cardiogenic)
  - Pulmonary thromboembolism

Systemic disease
- Primary haemostatic disorders
  - Thrombocytopenia: IMTP, *Ehrlichia*, bone marrow disease
  - Thrombocytopathia: hyperviscosity due to hyperglobulinaemia, e.g. neoplasia, *Leishmania*
- Secondary haemostatic disorders
  - Liver dysfunction: chronic hepatitis, toxicity e.g. xylitol
  - Vitamin K deficiency: cholestasis, congenital

DIAGNOSTIC APPROACH

Clinical clues
Predisposition
- Breed predispositions to immune-mediated thrombocytopenia (e.g. cocker spaniels)

History
- Concurrent haemorrhage elsewhere to increase suspicion of systemic disorder
- Coughing to increase suspicion of respiratory tract disease
- Risk factors for FB, e.g. throwing sticks or stick chewing
- Travel history increases index of suspicion of vector-borne diseases, including *Dirofilaria*, *Ehrlichia* and *Leishmania* infections

Clinical examination
Visual inspection
- Observe nature of cough if present
- Observe respiratory pattern to increase suspicion of upper, lower respiratory tract or parenchymal disorder; also may increase suspicion for presence of pleural space disease

Physical examination
- Thorough oral examination, and thoracic auscultation
- Evidence of haemorrhage: petechiation, ecchymoses elsewhere
  - Mucous membranes: gums, prepuce, vulva
  - Rectal examination for melaena
  - Skin, especially of the ventral abdomen

Laboratory findings
Haematology
- Assess platelet count
- Coagulation times (PT and aPTT) to assess for secondary haemostatic disorders
- Eosinophilia may be present in parasitic disease

Serum biochemistry
- Useful to screen for systemic disease

Imaging
Plain radiographs
- Assess for evidence of pulmonary changes

Ultrasound
- Point of care ultrasound to assess for pleural effusion ± ascites; may be detected in secondary haemostatic disorders, in particular rodenticide toxicity and neoplasia

Special tests
- Arterial blood gas analysis
- Bronchoscopy and BAL
- CT with contrast, preferably before bronchoscopy
- Haemostatic disorders
  - Buccal mucosal bleeding time to assess for thrombocytopathia
  - von Willebrand factor antigen levels
  - Baermann technique or Angiodetect® for *Angiostrongylus vasorum*
  - Testing for *Leishmania* and *Ehrlichia* infection as appropriate
  - Toxicology to detect rodenticide
- Leptospirosis serology and PCR
- Pulmonary thromboembolism can be challenging to diagnose: D-dimers, thromboelastography, CT with contrast may increase suspicion
- Screening for *Dirofilaria* (antigen testing e.g. SNAP 4DX® test), antibody testing, blood smear from marginal ear vein, or modified Knott's test)

1.29 HALITOSIS

DEFINITION

Halitosis is offensive, foul-smelling breath emanating from the mouth or nose. Oral diseases predispose to bacterial proliferation in necrotic tissue or retained food particles.

RELATED CLINICAL SIGNS

- Coughing if inhalation pneumonia
- Offensive breath
- Oral pain may indicate periodontal disease, inflammation or neoplasia
- Retained food associated with masses, ulcers
- Vomiting and/or diarrhoea if GI disease

COMMON CAUSES

- Poor oral hygiene

Abnormal ingestive behavior or pica
- Coprophagy, the ingestion of faecal matter
- Fetid food/scavenging
- High protein meals

Oral diseases
- Dental tartar or periodontal disease
- Food retention in lip folds, etc.
- Oral FB
- Oral neoplasia – beware a non-healing gingival lesion after tooth loss
- Stomatitis/pharyngitis

UNCOMMON CAUSES

- Open-mouth breathing

Abnormal ingestive behaviour or pica
- Aromatic foods: garlic, onion
- Chemical burns secondary to the ingestion of caustic substances
- Electrical burns secondary to chewing on electric cords

Oral diseases
- Cleft palate
- Jaw malocclusion
- Wet hair in bearded breeds
- Xerostomia

Oral contact with contaminated site
- Balanoposthitis
- Impacted anal sacs

- Infected/necrotic skin lesions, etc.
- Vaginitis

Remote causes producing malodorous exhalation
- Diabetic ketoacidosis
- GI disease
  - Gastritis
  - Intestinal obstruction
  - Malabsorption
  - Obstipation
- Liver disease
- Nasal disease
  - Chronic rhinitis/sinusitis
  - FB
  - Fungal infection: sino-nasal aspergillosis
  - Neoplasia
- Oesophageal disease: megaoesophagus with food retention
- Pulmonary disease
  - Abscessation
  - Aspiration pneumonia
  - Bacterial bronchopneumonia
  - Bronchiectasis
  - Broncho-oesophageal fistula
  - Inhaled FB
  - Necrotic tumour
- Uraemia

DIAGNOSTIC APPROACH

- History will help localise source of smell
- Biochemistry for metabolic disease including DKA and uraemia
- Investigations as for dysphagia (*q.v.* section 1.17) if an oral cause suspected, starting with oral examination

---

1.30 HEAD TILT

DEFINITION

Head tilt involves tilting of the head to either side of the body, away from its orientation with the trunk and limbs. The dog may appear to be trying to prevent itself from falling, or struggling to retain a balanced posture as cerebellar or vestibular disorders are responsible.

RELATED CLINICAL SIGNS

Head tilt should be discriminated from head turn and is most easily assessed by examining the position of the eyes and ears relative to one another when looking at the dog face on.

Cerebellar disorder

- Falling/leaning to one side
- Hypermetria
- Intention tremor
- Nystagmus
- Wide-based stance

Vestibular disorder

- Falling/leaning to one side
- Nystagmus

COMMON CAUSES

Cerebellar disorder

- Infectious
  - *Angiostrongylus vasorum*
  - Protozoal: *Toxoplasma, Neospora*
- Inflammatory: meningoencephalitis of unknown origin
- Neoplasia
- Vascular: haemorrhagic or thromboembolic stroke

Vestibular disorder

- Central vestibular (brainstem or cerebellar)
  - Cerebellar disorders as above
  - Inflammatory: meningoencephalitis of unknown origin
  - Neoplasia
  - Trauma
- Peripheral vestibular
  - Cranial polyneuropathy (possible link with hypothyroidism)
  - Idiopathic (old dog vestibular)
  - Otitis media
  - Neoplasia

UNCOMMON CAUSES

Cerebellar disorder

- Cerebellar abiotrophy
- Storage diseases
- Trauma

Vestibular disorder

- Peripheral vestibular
- Trauma
- Central vestibular (brainstem or cerebellar)

- Cerebellar disorders as above
- Drug-induced, e.g. metronidazole toxicity
- Storage disease

DIAGNOSTIC APPROACH

Clinical clues

Predisposition
- Cerebellar abiotrophy has been described in more than 40 breeds of dog at different ages
  - Neonatal, e.g. beagles
  - Juvenile, e.g. Airedale terrier
  - Adult onset, e.g. Bernese mountain dog
- Greyhounds are predisposed to thromboembolic cerebellar events (ischaemic stroke)

History
- Duration and progression of signs may aid in index of suspicion
  - Acute onset but improving increases suspicion of vascular or drug-induced event
  - Acute onset with rapid progression may increase suspicion of inflammatory or infectious disease
  - Gradual, progressive onset may increase suspicion of degenerative or neoplastic disease

Clinical examination

Visual inspection
- Mentation is likely impaired with central brainstem vestibular disorders

Physical examination
- Thorough examination to assess for multisystemic disease

Neurological examination
- Cerebellar
  - Contralateral head tilt and direction of fast phase of nystagmus (paradoxical vestibular)
  - Ipsilateral loss of proprioception and menace response
- Vestibular
  - As above for cerebellar
  - With brainstem disorders consciousness may be reduced, and other cranial nerves may be affected (facial nerve – blink reflex, and glossopharyngeal and vagal nerves – gag reflex)

- With peripheral disorders may detect concurrent facial nerve abnormalities and Horner's syndrome

Ophthalmic examination
- May be useful to assess for infiltrative central nervous system disease, e.g. may detect papilloedema

Laboratory findings
Haematology
- Uncommon to detect changes, may identify thrombocytopenia in haemorrhagic stroke

Serum biochemistry
- Identify increased risks of thromboembolism: HAC, hepatic disease, PLE, PLN

Imaging
Plain radiographs
- Screen for disseminated neoplasia in cases with a high suspicion

Ultrasound
- Screen for disseminated neoplasia in cases with a high suspicion

Special tests
- Coagulation parameters (PT and aPTT) to assess for haemorrhagic stroke
- CSF tap to assess for cytology and proteins (inflammatory) or infectious (e.g. *Toxoplasma* and *Neospora* PCR)
- Infectious disease testing
  - Baermann technique or AngioDetect® for *Angiostrongylus*
  - *Toxoplasma* and *Neospora* serology
- Otoscopy and myringotomy in cases with suspicion of otitis media
- MRI to assess for CNS causes of head tilt

1.31 MELAENA

DEFINITION

Black, tarry faeces due to the presence of partially digested blood and or blood pigments, either from upper GI haemorrhage or swallowed blood.

RELATED CLINICAL SIGNS

- Dark, tarry faeces
  NB: Some medications (iron, metronidazole, tylosin, bismuth) can give faeces a dark colour, and the outside of an old faecal sample will become oxidized and become darker in appearance.
- Haematemesis
- Signs of hypovolaemia and/or anaemia if severe bleeding

COMMON CAUSES

Endocrine
- Hypoadrenocorticism (not common but important)

Generalised bleeding problem
q.v. section 1.9
Gastric neoplasia
- Gastric carcinoma
- Gastric leiomyoma/sarcoma

Gastric ulceration
- Abrasive gastric FB
- Acute and chronic gastritis
- NSAIDs
- Portal hypertension in end-stage liver disease
- Uraemic gastritis

Intestinal disease
- Inflammatory bowel disease

Intestinal neoplasia
- Adenocarcinoma
- Leiomyoma/sarcoma
- Lymphosarcoma

Swallowed blood
- Epistaxis
- Oral bleeding

UNCOMMON CAUSES

Gastric ulceration
- Gastrinoma (Zollinger Ellison syndrome)
- Mast cell tumour

Intestinal disease
- Chronic intussusception
- GI ischaemia
  - Infarction
  - Mesenteric avulsion
  - Shock
  - Vascular malformation
    - Angiodysplasia/vascular ectasia
    - AV fistula
  - Volvulus
- Polyps
- Severe hookworm infestation (not in UK)

Pancreatic disease
- Severe acute pancreatitis

Swallowed blood
- Haemoptysis

Severe oesophageal disease
- Neoplasia
- Oesophagitis

DIAGNOSTIC APPROACH

1 Any cause of haematemesis is likely to produce melaena and the diagnostic approach is similar, *q.v.* section 1.25
2 The presence of diarrhoea in association with melaena suggests intestinal disease.

Clinical clues
Predisposition
- *q.v.* section 1.25

History
- Diarrhoea and weight loss with intestinal disease, gastrinoma
- Epistaxis, bleeding oral lesion or coughing if swallowed blood
- Haematemesis if gastric lesion

Clinical examination
Visual inspection
- Passage of dark, tarry stool
- Staining of perineal region

Physical examination
- *q.v.* section 1.25

Palpation
- Abdominal discomfort/pain
- Abdominal mass

Digital rectal examination
- Confirms melaena

Laboratory findings
- Haematology and serum biochemistry consistent with blood loss, *q.v.* section 1.25

Imaging
- *q.v.* section 1.49

Special tests
- Occult blood test
  - Indicates presence of haemoglobin in faeces
  - This test is aimed at detecting microscopic bleeding and is unnecessary if there is overt melaena
  - Melaena is only identifiable visually when > 1 ml/kg blood enters the GI lumen
  - It cross-reacts with all dietary blood, and so the dog must be on a meat-free or hydrolysed diet for at least 72 hours before the test can be interpreted

1.32 NASAL DISCHARGE

DEFINITION

Nasal discharge is typically expelled from the external nares, and can be serous, mucopurulent or haemorrhagic, or combinations of these.

RELATED CLINICAL SIGNS

In some cases of nasal disease (in particular those within the caudal nasal chambers), the discharge may be swallowed or inhaled through post-nasal drip; in these cases dogs may also have a cough.
• Concurrent nasal depigmentation/deformities
• Coughing due to post-nasal drip and aspiration of nasal discharge
• If epistaxis present, may also have haematemesis or melaena due to swallowed blood
• Pawing at face
• Stertor or snoring due to reduced nasal airflow

COMMON CAUSES

• Chronic idiopathic rhinitis
• FB
• Infection
  • Sino-nasal aspergillosis
  • Tooth root abscess
  • Secondary to regurgitation with concurrent aspiration pneumonia
• Neoplasia (carcinoma, sarcoma, lymphoma)
  NB: If epistaxis, bleeding disorders should also be considered, *q.v.* section 1.21

UNCOMMON CAUSES

• Cleft palate
• Infection
  • Oronasal fistula
  • Osteomyelitis
  • Parasitic (*Linguatula serrata*)
• Neoplasia (leiomyoma)

• Trauma
• NB: Nasal disease can present secondary to reflux/regurgitation

DIAGNOSTIC APPROACH

The nature of the nasal discharge and its speed of onset suggest certain differential diagnoses but assessing for the presence of unilateral or bilateral nasal discharge is most useful in prioritising differential diagnoses.

Clinical clues
Predisposition
• Breed predisposition in sino-nasal aspergillosis suspected in Golden retrievers
• Dolichocephalic dogs are predisposed to sino-nasal aspergillosis
• Older dogs are predisposed to nasal tumours and dental disease

History
• Discharge
  • Bilateral: more likely chronic idiopathic rhinitis, aspergillosis or bleeding disorder
  • Unilateral: more likely FB neoplasia, oronasal fistula or dental disease
• Nasal stertor increases suspicion of nasal FB or tumour
• Recent dental extractions increase suspicion of oronasal fistula

Clinical examination
Visual inspection
• Presence of sneezing increases suspicion of nasal disease
• Stertor is suggestive of reduced nasal airflow

Physical examination
• Assess nasal airflow
  • Tissue or cotton wool to detect airflow at each nostril
  • Microscope slide and assess for condensation
  • Stethoscope and auscultate each side

- Examination of head conformation including ocular retropulsion for signs of deformity suspicious for neoplasia
- Examination of nasal planum for depigmentation (most common in fungal disease)
- Oral examination to assess for dental disease and oronasal fistulas

Laboratory findings
Haematology and serum biochemistry
- Useful to screen for systemic disease including coagulation profile, in particular for causes of epistaxis

Imaging
Plain radiographs
- Nasal turbinate destruction: tumour or aspergillosis

- Sinus hyperostosis (aspergillosis)
- Soft tissue opacity: tumour most likely but can also occur with fluid accumulation

Special tests
- *Aspergillus* serology: specific but poorly sensitive test, i.e. a positive result supports infection but a negative result does not exclude it
- CT scan with contrast to assess for nasal diseases
- Culture of nasal discharge is not useful; likely bacterial flora and positive *Aspergillus* culture is not diagnostic as it can be an environmental contaminant
- Nasal cytology (rarely useful) and tissue sample for histopathology
- Rhinoscopy to assess for nasal FB, tumours or aspergillosis

1.33 NYSTAGMUS

DEFINITION

Pathological nystagmus refers to inappropriate ocular movements; typically a slow phase in one direction; horizontal, vertical with a fast phase in the counter direction, or rotatory, and occurs due to a disorder of the vestibular system. This can be observed at rest (spontaneous nystagmus) or when the vestibular system is tested, e.g. putting the dog on its back (positional nystagmus).

Physiological nystagmus forms part of the oculocephalic reflex and is a normal response (e.g. when looking out of the window in a car). Blind dogs can have saccadic (quick, jerky) eye movements that do not reflect a vestibular disturbance.

RELATED CLINICAL SIGNS

Cerebellar disorders
- Falling/leaning to one side
- Head tilt
- Hypermetria
- Intention tremor
- Wide-based stance

Vestibular disorders
- Bilateral vestibular (more common in cats) presents without a head tilt but falling to both sides, wide excursions of the head, and an uncoordinated gait
- Falling/leaning to one side
- Head tilt

COMMON CAUSES

Cerebellar disorders
- Infectious:
  - *Angiostrongylus vasorum*
  - Protozoal (*Toxoplasma, Neospora*)
- Inflammatory: meningoencephalitis of unknown origin
- Vascular: haemorrhagic or thromboembolic stroke

Vestibular disorders
- Peripheral vestibular
  - Cranial polyneuropathy (possible link with hypothyroidism)
  - Idiopathic (old dog vestibular)
  - Otitis media
- Central vestibular (brainstem or cerebellar)
  - Cerebellar disorders as above

- Inflammatory: meningoencephalitis of unknown origin
- Neoplasia
- Trauma

UNCOMMON CAUSES

Cerebellar disorders
- Cerebellar abiotrophy
- Neoplasia
- Storage disease
- Trauma

Vestibular disorders
- Peripheral vestibular
  - Neoplasia
  - Trauma
- Central vestibular (brainstem or cerebellar)
  - Drug-induced, e.g. metronidazole toxicity
  - Cerebellar disorders as above
  - Storage disease
  - Congenital pendulous nystagmus (most common in Siamese cats but described in Belgian shepherds)

DIAGNOSTIC APPROACH

Clinical clues
Predisposition
- Cerebellar abiotrophy has been described in more than 40 breeds of dog at different ages
  - Neonatal, e.g. beagles
  - Juvenile, e.g. Airedale terrier
  - Adult onset, e.g. Bernese mountain dog
- Greyhounds are predisposed to thromboembolic cerebellar events (ischaemic stroke)

History
- Duration and progression of signs may increase index of suspicion
  - Acute onset but improving increases suspicion of vascular or drug-induced event
  - Acute onset with rapid progression may increase suspicion of inflammatory or infectious disease
  - Gradual progressive onset may increase suspicion of degenerative or neoplastic disease

Clinical examination
Visual inspection
- Mentation is likely impaired with central brainstem vestibular disorders

Physical examination
- Thorough examination to assess for multisystemic disease

Neurological examination
- Cerebellar
  - Ipsilateral loss of proprioception and menace response
  - Contralateral head tilt and direction of fast phase of nystagmus (paradoxical vestibular)
- Vestibular
  - As above for cerebellar, with brainstem disorders consciousness may be reduced, and other cranial nerves may be affected (facial nerve – blink reflex, and glossopharyngeal and vagal nerves – gag reflex)
  - With peripheral disorders may detect concurrent facial nerve abnormalities and Horner's syndrome

Ophthalmic examination
- May be useful to assess for infiltrative central nervous system disease, e.g. may detect papilloedema

Laboratory findings
Haematology
- Uncommon to detect changes
- Thrombocytopenia in haemorrhagic stroke

Serum biochemistry
- May detect causes of increased risk of thromboembolism (protein-losing nephropathy, protein-losing enteropathy, hepatic disease, hyperadrenocorticism)

Imaging
Plain radiographs
- Screen for disseminated neoplasia in cases with a high suspicion

Ultrasound
- Screen for disseminated neoplasia in cases with a high suspicion

Special tests
- Coagulation parameters (PT and aPTT) to assess for haemorrhagic stroke
- CSF tap to assess for cytology and proteins (inflammatory) or infectious (e.g. *Toxoplasma* and *Neospora* PCR)

- Infectious disease testing
  - Baermann technique or AngioDetect® for *Angiostrongylus*
  - *Toxoplasma* and *Neospora* serology
- Otoscopy and myringotomy in cases with suspicion of otitis media
- MRI to assess for CNS causes of head tilt

1.34 PARESIS/PARALYSIS

DEFINITION

Paresis is defined as weakness or partial loss of voluntary movement.

Paralysis (also known as -plegia) is the loss of voluntary movement and may be accompanied by a loss of sensory function.

Disorders may affect a single limb (monoparesis or monoparalysis), both pelvic limbs (paraparesis or paraplegia) or all four limbs (tetraparesis or tetraplegia).

RELATED CLINICAL SIGNS

- Weakness, incoordination or lack of voluntary movement in affected limbs
- There may also be a loss of sensation.
- Concurrent loss of urination, defaecation, and tail movement depending on localisation.

COMMON CAUSES

- Degenerative disease, e.g. canine degenerative myelopathy (CDM); previously termed canine degenerative radiculomyelopathy (CDRM)
- Fibrocartilaginous embolism (FCE)
- Intervertebral disc disease (IVDD)
- Neoplasia

UNCOMMON CAUSES

- Botulism
- Inflammatory: meningomyelitis
- Myasthenia gravis

- Nerve root tumour
- Polymyositis
- Polyradiculoneuritis (aka Coonhound paralysis)
- Protozoa: *Neospora*, *Toxoplasma*
- Tick paralysis (recognised in Australia, North America and South Africa but not in UK)

DIAGNOSTIC APPROACH

Clinical clues
- Duration and progression of signs will aid in index of suspicion
  - Acute onset but improving increases suspicion of vascular event
  - Acute onset and rapid progression may increase suspicion of inflammatory or infectious disease
  - Acute onset but stable may increase suspicion of FCE or IVDD
  - Gradual onset and progression may increase suspicion of degenerative or neoplastic disease
- Generalised weakness may be related to systemic disease, and must be excluded in these cases before assuming a neurological cause

Predisposition
- Dachshunds and many other breeds (e.g. Poodle, Cocker spaniel, Pekingese) are predisposed to IVDD
- CDM is present in numerous breeds: GSDs are predisposed and the condition has been linked to a mutation in the superoxide dismutase (SOD1) gene. Mutations in SOD1 have also been described in the Boxer, Chesapeake Bay Retriever, Pembroke Welsh Corgi, and Rhodesian Ridgeback.

History
- CDM is a slowly progressive condition affecting the hindlimbs and usually does not commence until at least 8 years of age
- Fibrocartilaginous embolism classically occurs acutely during vigorous exercise
- Monoparesis with marked muscle wastage and pain raises concerns of a nerve root tumour
- Neosporosis in young dogs affects the hindlimbs initially but can cause ascending paresis/paralysis

Clinical examination
Visual inspection
- Assess mentation and gait prior to examination

Physical examination
- Thorough examination to assess for multisystemic disease

Neurological examination
- FCE tends to causes lateralised signs and is normally not painful on examination
- IVDD can be localised as C1–C5, C6–T2, T3–L3, L4–S3 using spinal cord reflexes (limb and panniculus), proprioception, and assessment for spinal pain
- Polyradiculoneuritis typically causes an ascending (pelvic limbs affected first) paralysis, sensation is retained (dogs are unable to withdraw limbs but have a behavioural response to pedal withdrawal assessment), urination, defaecation and tail movement is usually preserved

Laboratory findings
Haematology and serum biochemistry
- Uncommon to detect changes
- CK and AST enzyme activities will be increased in polymyositis

Imaging
Plain radiographs
- Poorly sensitive and specific for CNS disease: contrast myelography in addition to radiography improves this
- May detect megaoesophagus in cases suspicious for myasthenia gravis; radiographs must be taken conscious as anaesthesia and sedation may cause false positives for megaoesophagus)

Ultrasound examination
- Screen for disseminated neoplasia in cases with a high suspicion

Special tests
- Acetylcholine receptor antibodies in cases suspicious for acquired myasthenia gravis
- CSF tap to assess for cytology and proteins (inflammatory) or infectious (e.g. *Toxoplasma* and *Neospora* PCR)
- Electrodiagnostics (EMG, nerve conduction velocities) in cases suspicious for peripheral nervous system, neuromuscular, or muscular disorders
- MRI scan (or CT ± contrast myelography) to assess for CNS causes of ataxia
- Muscle and nerve biopsies in cases suspicious for myositis or inflammatory/neoplastic neuropathy

1.35 PERINATAL DEATH

DEFINITION

Perinatal death is the sum of any stillborn puppies and puppies that die during the first week after birth, otherwise known as early neonatal mortality.

RELATED CLINICAL SIGNS

- Dead puppies < 1 week of age
- Stillborn puppies
- Vulval discharge
- Weak/fading puppies – failure to nurse, hypoglycaemic, weight loss, hypothermic

COMMON CAUSES

Infectious
- Canine herpes virus
- *Brucella canis/abortus*
- Mastitis
- Neonatal sepsis

Non-infectious
- Dystocia leading to fetal trauma
- Extended parturition, e.g. due to uterine inertia
- Fetal size/weight > 25% below average for breed reduces survival
- Large litters leading to pregnancy toxaemia
- Maternal neglect/illness

UNCOMMON CAUSES

Infectious
- Other bacterial infections: *Campylobacter*, *Salmonella*, enterotoxic *E. coli*, beta-haemolytic *Streptococci*, *Staphylococcus*, *Mycoplasma*, *Leptospira*
- Other viruses: parvovirus, rotavirus, coronavirus, distemper, canine adenovirus-1
- Parasitic/protozoal infections: *Cryptosporidium*, *Toxoplasma*, *Neospora*, *Leishmania*

Non-infectious
- Congenital anomalies/malformations, e.g. cleft palate
- Eclampsia
- Genetic causes
- Hypothyroidism in bitch
- Malnutrition/nutritional deficiency in bitch
- Maternal gestational DM

DIAGNOSTIC APPROACH

1 Review husbandry
2 Review previous breeding histry
3 Diagnostic testing – see special tests below

Clinical clues
Predisposition
- First litter
- Known genetic defects
- Large litters
- New dogs in kennels

History
- Problems with previous litters especially if in breeding kennels
  - Gastrointestinal signs
  - Respiratory signs
  - Other signs
- Vaccination status of bitch

Clinical examination
- Post mortem examination of dead puppies and placenta
- Vulval discharge

Laboratory findings
Haematology
- May indicate potential infection

Special tests
- Abortion PCR panel on placenta or fetal tissue
  - *Brucella canis*
  - *Campylobacter jejuni*
  - Canine distemper virus
  - Canine herpesvirus type 1 (CHV-1)
  - *Leptospira*
  - *Leishmania*
  - Minute virus (parvovirus type 1)
  - *Neospora*
  - *Salmonella*
  - *Toxoplasma*
- Culture (bacterial ± fungal) of placenta and fetal lung tissue
- Screening of bitch
  - Minimum data base
  - *Brucella* serology
  - Canine herpes virus serology
- Screening of stud dog
  - *Brucella* serology
  - Histopathology of placenta, liver, kidney, lung, heart and heart blood, brain, and any other lesional tissue(s)

PRESENTING COMPLAINTS

PRESENTING COMPLAINTS

1.36 POLYPHAGIA

DEFINITION

Eating in excess of normal caloric needs, either in response to a physiological or pathological increase in energy expenditure, or to a failure to absorb sufficient energy despite increased intake, or as an abnormal behaviour.

RELATED CLINICAL SIGNS

- Coprophagia (ingestion of faeces) and pica (bizarre intake) can be considered forms of polyphagia
- Increased appetite and even scavenging
- Weight gain or weight loss depending on underlying disease

COMMON CAUSES

Behavioural
- Boredom
- Competition
- Gluttony
- Highly palatable food
- Overfeeding

Drugs
- Anticonvulsants
- Glucocorticoids

Endocrine disease
- DM (non-ketotic)
- Hyperadrenocorticism (HAC)
- Hypothyroidism (eating in excess of requirement; not true increased intake)

GI disease
- EPI
- Intestinal malabsorption

Physiological
- Cold environment
- Increased exercise
- Lactation
- Poor-quality food
- Pregnancy

UNCOMMON CAUSES

Metabolic/endocrine disease
- Acromegaly
- Hyperthyroidism
  - Exogenous thyroid tissue contaminating raw food
  - Functional thyroid tumour (rare)
  - Iatrogenic
- Insulinoma (mild increase in appetite)
- SARDS

Drugs
- Amitraz
- Appetite stimulants
  - Capromorelin
  - Cyproheptadine
  - Diazepam (weak)
  - Mirtazapine
  - Progestagens

Neurological
- Psychogenic
- Destruction of satiety centre in hypothalamus (neoplasia, trauma)

Renal
- Protein-losing nephropathy without azotaemia may cause weight loss despite normal appetite; increased appetite is unusual

DIAGNOSTIC APPROACH

- Increases or decreases in weight in association with increased or decreased food intake can indicate the type of disease process
- If there is weight gain ± PU/PD, consider endocrinopathy
- If there is weight loss, first consider malabsorption, especially if diarrhoea is present

Clinical clues
Predisposition
- EPI and ARD/SIBO in GSDs
- Genetic mutation in Labradors: pro-opiomelanocortin (POMC) gene

History
- Weakness, lethargy and seizures
  - Insulinoma
- Weight gain
  - Drugs
  - HAC
  - Hypothyroidism
  - Insulinoma
  - Overeating
- Weight loss
  - Recent change in diet or physiological state
  - Ravenous appetite typical of EPI and benign causes of malabsorption
  - Coprophagia is seen most frequently in EPI and ARD/SIBO
  - Diarrhoea and weight loss
  - EPI and malabsorption
  - Physiological stress; exercise, lactation
  - Poor diet
- PU/PD
  - DM
  - HAC
  - Hyperthyroidism
    - Vomiting and diarrhoea, weight loss, tachycardia

Clinical examination
Visual inspection
- Emaciation if EPI or severe/prolonged malabsorption
- Pot belly and hair loss in HAC
- Overweight ± alopecia in endocrinopathy

Physical examination
- Normal if behavioural or physiological
- Weight gain or weight loss
- Abnormal body condition – loss of fat or lean muscle mass
- Hair loss in HAC
- Palpation
  - Ascites if severe hypoalbuminaemia (PLE, PLN)
  - Thin skin, pot-belly, secondary pyoderma and comedones in HAC
  - Thyroid mass if hyperthyroid

Laboratory findings
- Hypercholesterolaemia and high ALP activity in HAC
- Hyperglycaemia and glycosuria in diabetes mellitus
- Hypoalbuminaemia in PLE or PLN
- Hypoglycaemia in insulinoma
- Proteinuria in PLN

Imaging
- Adrenomegaly in HAC
- Altered hepatic echogenicity in endocrinopathy
- Hepatomegaly in endocrinopathy

Special tests
- Dynamic cortisol testing for HAC
- Folate /cobalamin for malabsorption
- Intestinal biopsies
- Serum insulin
- Serum T4
- cTLI test for EPI

1.37 POLYURIA/POLYDIPSIA (PU/PD)

DEFINITION

Polydipsia (PD) is a daily fluid intake of greater than 100 ml/kg/day.
Polyuria (PU) is a daily urine output of greater than 50 ml/kg/day.
Primary polyuria and secondary polydipsia is more common.

RELATED CLINICAL SIGNS

- Differentiate from urinary incontinence/increased frequency of urination (pollakiuria)
- Excessive fluid intake or urine output
- Nocturia is inappropriate urination at night that usually reflects increased volume due to PU/PD
- Other signs depend on the cause of PU/PD
- PU/PD may be the only clinical sign

COMMON CAUSES

Primary polydipsia
- Hepatic encephalopathy

Primary polyuria
Osmotic diuresis
- Diabetes mellitus
- Diuretic administration
- Fluid administration

Renal insensitivity to antidiuretic hormone (ADH) = Nephrogenic diabetes insipidus (NDI)
- Secondary NDI
  - Glucocorticoid administration
  - HAC
  - Hypercalcaemia
    - Malignancy: lymphoma, anal sac adeno-carcinoma, multiple myeloma
    - Primary hyperparathyroidism
  - Hypoadrenocorticism
  - Pyometra
  - Renal disease

UNCOMMON CAUSES

Primary polydipsia
- Acromegaly
- Diet: high sodium, low protein
- Exocrine pancreatic insufficiency/malabsorption (noted occasionally)
- Fever
- Neurological – lesion in the thirst centre of the hypothalamus
- Pain
- Psychogenic polydipsia

Primary polyuria
- Renal insensitivity to ADH
  - Primary NDI
  - Secondary NDI
    - Drugs
      - Diuretics
      - Phenobarbital
    - Hyperviscosity syndrome
    - Hypokalaemia
    - Jerky treats
    - Pyelonephritis
    - Renal medullary solute washout

- Osmotic diuresis
  - Dextrose infusion
  - Mannitol
  - Primary renal glucosuria
  - Fanconi's syndrome
  - Post-obstructive diuresis
- ADH deficiency = central diabetes insipidus (CDI)
  - Idiopathic
    - Congenital
    - Neoplastic
    - Trauma-induced

DIAGNOSTIC APPROACH

1 Confirm PU/PD by measuring water intake and urine SG, and distinguish from pollaki-uria or incontinence.
2 Rule out pyometra by history, physical examination, laboratory results and imaging.
3 Serum biochemistry to rule out renal disease, hypercalcaemia and diabetes mellitus.
4 Compare glycosuria with blood glucose: hyperglycaemia indicates diabetes mellitus; glycosuria with euglycaemia indicates Fanconi's disease or jerky treat ingestion.
5 Dynamic cortisol testing for HAC.
6 Water deprivation test to distinguish psychogenic polydipsia from diabetes insipidus (*q.v.* section 5.3.1) only when safe, i.e. after ruling out the above.

Clinical clues
Predisposition
- CDI is generally reported in middle-aged animals
- Fanconi syndrome in young Basenjis
- Feeding of jerky treats, causing glycosuria
- HAC is most common in middle-aged dogs
- Hypercalcaemia is commonly reported as part of a paraneoplastic syndrome e.g. lymphoma, anal sac adenocarcinoma, multiple myeloma
- Primary NDI is a congenital disease with animals presenting at a young age
- Primary renal glycosuria reported in Norwegian elkhound, Shetland sheepdog, Schnauzer

- Pyometra reported in bitches 1–3 months post-oestrus

History
- Differentiate polyuria from urinary incontinence or pollakiuria
- Entire females – oestrus activity – when was the last season?
- Is it appropriate polydipsia?
  - Environmental changes in temperature
  - Change in diet from moist to dry will increase water intake
- Owner should quantify the polydipsia – difficult in multi-animal households, this must be done in normal environment without external stresses
- Other clinical signs noticed by the owner suggesting any organ involvement
- Polyphagia in HAC and EPI

Clinical examination
Visual inspection
- Behavioural/neurological abnormalities, e.g. hepatic encephalopathy, pituitary neoplasms
- Body condition
- Dermatological changes, e.g. alopecia with HAC
- Panting – HAC

Physical examination
- Eyes
  - Cataracts: diabetes mellitus
  - Jaundice: hepatic disease
  - Corneal lipidosis: HAC
  - Papilloedema: pituitary mass
  - Retinal vessel tortuosity: hyperviscosity syndrome
- External genitalia for discharge, e.g. pyometra
- Oral cavity: ulceration/stomatitis secondary to uraemia
- Skin: hair coat for thin skin, comedones, hair loss in HAC

Palpation
- Lymph nodes for enlargement, e.g. lymphosarcoma
- Anal sac, mammary glands, thyroid gland area (parathyroid tumour) for masses causing paraneoplastic hypercalcaemia
- Hepatomegaly – diabetes mellitus (DM), hyperadrenocorticism, some liver diseases
- Kidneys – not usually easy to palpate in the dog – if enlarged consider neoplasia, pyelonephritis, portosystemic shunt (PSS)
- Uterine enlargement: pyometra

Auscultation
- Bradycardia with hyperkalaemia secondary to renal failure or hypoadrenocorticism
- Tachycardia with toxaemia, dehydration

Laboratory findings
Haematology
- Normal neutrophils, eosinophilia, lymphocytosis in hypoadrenocorticism
- Neutrophilia, eosinopenia, lymphopenia: stress leukogram in hyperadrenocorticism
- Neutrophilia with left shift: pyometra, sometimes in pyelonephritis
- Non-regenerative anaemia: CKD, hypoadrenocorticism, hepatic disease
- Erythrocytosis: hyperviscosity syndrome (distinguish from dehydration-elevating PCV)

Serum biochemistry
- Alanine aminotransferase
  - Increased with liver disease, toxaemia, e.g. pyometra
- Albumin
  - Decreased with liver disease, nephrotic syndrome
  - Increased with dehydration
- Alkaline phosphatase
  - Increased with HAC, liver disease
- Calcium
  - Decreased with CKD, hypoalbuminaemia
  - Increased with malignancy, hypoadrenocorticism, primary hyperparathyroidism, vitamin D toxicosis, CKD (esp. juvenile nephropathy)
- Cholesterol
  - Increased with HAC, DM, liver disease, nephrotic syndrome
- Creatinine and urea
  - Increased with CKD severe dehydration, hypoadrenocorticism, hypercalcaemia
- Globulin
  - Increased with hyperviscosity syndrome, liver disease

- Glucose
  - Increased with DM, acromegaly, HAC
  - Normal in renal glycosuria, jerky treat ingestion
- Phosphate
  - Decreased with primary hyperparathyroidism, malignancy-associated hypercalcaemia
  - Increased with CKD vitamin D toxicosis, severe dehydration, hypoadrenocorticism
- Potassium
  - Decreased: post-obstructional diuresis, diuretic administration, DM
  - Increased: CKD hypoadrenocorticism, severe diabetic ketoacidosis
- Sodium and chloride
  - Decreased: hypoadrenocorticism, ketoacidotic diabetic (psychogenic polydipsia)
  - Increased: primary nephrogenic diabetes insipidus, central diabetes insipidus, dehydration
- Total bilirubin
  - Increased: liver disease
- Urea
  - Decreased: liver disease

Urinalysis
- Sediment analysis for urinary tract infection (UTI)
- Urine specific gravity
  - Greater than 1.030 the dog is not likely to have a concentrating defect, polydipsia is to replace non-renal losses
  - 1.008–1.012 is isosthenuria, i.e. the same osmolality as plasma which, if the dog is dehydrated, suggests severe impairment of renal concentrating ability
  - Less than 1.007 (hyposthenuria) implies tubular function is present as urine is being actively diluted in response to polydipsia
- Urine chemistry analysis, e.g. glucose, ketones, excessive bilirubin, protein
- Urine culture
- Urine protein:creatinine (UPC) ratio to quantify proteinuria

Imaging
Abdominal radiographs
- Abnormal soft tissue masses, e.g. enlarged adrenal glands, spleen, mesenteric/sublumbar lymph nodes

- Liver size
  - Decreased with chronic liver diseases, PSS (± renomegaly)
  - Increased with DM, HAC or infiltrative disease
- Renal size
  - Decreased with chronic interstitial nephritis, juvenile nephropathy
  - Increased with pyelonephritis, congenital PSS, neoplasia, amyloidosis
- Uterine enlargement suggests pyometra

Thoracic radiographs
- Mediastinal lymph node involvement if hypercalcaemic
- Ultrasonography
- Assess renal, hepatic, adrenal tissues, etc.

Special tests
- Amino acid quantification in urine for identification of tubular disease, e.g. Fanconi's syndrome
- Fractional excretion of electrolytes
- Bone marrow aspirate in hypercalcaemic cases with no identifying cause to look for multiple myeloma
- Measurement of plasma ADH – not readily available
- Modified water deprivation test – never perform in azotaemic animals. It is advisable to completely rule out HAC before performing this test.
- Parathyroid hormone (PTH) and PTH-related peptide (PTHrp) assays if hypercalcaemic to distinguish primary hyperparathyroidism from lymphoma
- Rule out HAC: urine cortisol:creatinine ratio, ACTH stimulation test.
  If suggestive of hyperadrenocorticism, perform further tests: low-dose dexamethasone suppression test, high-dose dexamethasone suppression test, endogenous ACTH
- Tissue biopsy, e.g. liver, kidney, lymph node
- Urine and plasma osmolality: osmolality is not affected by particle size unlike the SG

1.38 PREPUTIAL DISCHARGE

DEFINITION

Visible material dripping from the prepuce or causing the dog to frequently lick the area. The material may be haemorrhagic or purulent. Dripping of urine is a sign of incontinence, *q.v.* section 1.48.

RELATED CLINICAL SIGNS

- Abnormal liquid dripping from prepuce: white, yellow or green exudate, or serosanguinous fluid
- Dog licking prepuce, with hair staining
- Dysuria, *q.v.* section 1.19
- Malodour
- Pyrexia, lethargy and pain with prostatitis or prostatic abscess

COMMON CAUSES

Haemorrhagic
- Penile or preputial tumour
  - Haemangiosarcoma
- Prostatitis
- Prostatic neoplasia
- Urinary tract bleeding
  - Balanoposthitis
  - Bleeding disorder
  - Paraphimosis and associated trauma: inability to retract penis into prepuce
  - Trauma, e.g. breeding attempt
    - Fracture of os penis
    - Haematoma
    - Laceration

Purulent
- Balanoposthitis
  - Bacterial infection
  - Herpes virus
- Preputial FB e.g. grass awn
- Phimosis: inability to extrude penis from prepuce

UNCOMMON CAUSES

Haemorrhagic
- Penile or preputial tumour
  - MCT
  - Melanoma
  - Papilloma
  - Squamous cell carcinoma
  - Transmissible venereal tumour (TVT)
- Urinary tract bleeding
  - Pyelonephritis
  - Urethral prolapse
  - Urethritis
  - Urolithiasis

Purulent
- Cystitis and/or urethritis
- Penile or preputial tumours: as above
- Prostatitis or prostatic abscess
- Phimosis or paraphimosis
- Seminal fluid

DIAGNOSTIC APPROACH

1 Determine whether discharge is associated with urination
2 Examine penis; full examination requires sedation or general anaesthesia (GA)
3 Digital rectal examination
4 Laboratory analysis of discharge and urine
5 Imaging
6 Biopsy of any penile/preputial lesions

Clinical clues
Predisposition
- None

History
- Signs of dysuria
- Licking of prepuce

Clinical examination
Visual inspection
- Preputial discharge: haemorrhagic or purulent

Physical examination
- Exteriorisation of penis
- Digital rectal examination

Laboratory findings
Haematology
- Often unremarkable

Serum biochemistry
- Often unremarkable

Urinalysis
- UTI

Imaging
Plain radiographs
- Pelvis, including lateral view with legs drawn forward to image urethra

Contrast radiographs
- Retrograde urethrogram

Ultrasound examination
- Prostate

Special tests
- Bacterial culture of discharge
  - *Acinetobacter*
  - *Bacillus*
  - *Corynebacterium*
  - *E. coli*
  - *Klebsiella*
  - *Mycoplasma*
  - *Proteus*
  - *Pseudomonas*
  - *Staphylococcus*
  - *Streptococcus*
- Biopsy
- Coagulation profile
- Cytology of discharge, mass or preputial smear
  - Neoplastic cells: mast cell tumour (MCT), TVT
  - Pus: bacteria and neutrophils

1.39 PRURITUS

DEFINITION

Itching: the sensation that provokes the desire to scratch.

RELATED CLINICAL SIGNS

- Brown discolouration of coat if repeated licking
- Scratching and licking
- Visible signs are the end result of persistent scratching
  - Alopecia
  - Erythema
  - Excoriation
  - Lichenification

COMMON CAUSES

- Acral lick granuloma
- Anal sac impaction causing perianal rubbing
- Atopy (inhaled allergens)
- Demodectic mange
- Dermatophytosis
- Fleas and flea-allergic dermatitis
- *Malassezia* infection
- Pyoderma
- Sarcoptic mange
- Superficial pyoderma

UNCOMMON CAUSES

- Calcinosis cutis
- *Cheyletiella*
- Contact dermatitis
- Drug eruptions
- Food allergy
- Harvest mites
- Lice
- Pemphigus erythematosus and foliaceous
- Psychogenic: self-mutilation
- Sporotrichosis
- Syringomyelia causes phantom scratching, so probably not pruritus

- Tapeworm segments causing perianal irritation
- *Uncinaria* larval migration causing pedal licking
- Urticaria

DIAGNOSTIC APPROACH

1 Identification of infectious agents by sellotape strips, skin scrapes, hair plucks, and bacterial and fungal cultures.
2 After failing to identify infectious causes, trial therapy for bacterial pyoderma, fleas and possibly also for *Sarcoptes*, is acceptable.
3 Intradermal skin testing or serology is performed to identify atopic reactions.
4 If negative for atopy, an exclusion food trial is indicated.

Clinical clues
Predisposition
- Atopy in French bulldog, WHWT
- Demodecosis in short-haired breeds, especially Shar pei, Bull terrier
- Infectious diseases in young dogs

History
- Contact with infected animals
- Effectiveness of flea control
- Owner with pruritus is suggestive of fleas, *Sarcoptes*, *Cheyletiella*, dermatophytosis
- Phantom scratching in CKCS with syringomyelia is not true pruritus

Clinical examination
Visual inspection
- Pruritic animals will scratch spontaneously, or the scratch reflex may be stimulated
- Presence of fleas or flea dirt
- Self-traumatic lesions

Physical examination
Inspection
- Excoriations, erythema, alopecia and lichenification
- Lesions secondary to self-trauma: erythema, excoriation, lichenification, hyperpigmentation
- Pinnae are often particularly sensitive in *Sarcoptes* infection
Palpation
- Thickened skin in areas of repeated self-trauma
Distribution of lesions
- Symmetric lesions involving:
  - Lumbosacral areas and thighs suggests fleas
  - Ear margins and elbows with sarcoptic mange
  - Face, feet and ventrum with atopy
  - Feet and ventrum with contact allergy
  - Face, ears and feet with food allergy
  - Face, ears, feet or multifocal with demodecosis
  - Face, feet, mucocutaneous junctions with autoimmune skin disease

Laboratory findings
- Blood tests usually unremarkable
  - Eosinophilia may be present in allergic skin disease

Special tests
- Skin examination
  - Bacterial ± fungal cultures
  - Hair plucks: *Demodex*, ringworm/dermatophytosis
  - Sellotape strips: *Cheyletiella* and *Malassezia*
  - Skin scrapes: *Sarcoptes*, *Demodex*
- Exclusion diet trial
- Intradermal skin tests
- *In vitro* allergy testing: only reliable for atopy, not food allergy
- Skin biopsy

1.40 RED EYE (AND PINK EYE)

DEFINITION

Erythema of the directly visible parts of the eye.

RELATED CLINICAL SIGNS

- Blepharospasm
- Chemosis (corneal oedema)
- Epiphora; mucoid/mucopurulent discharge
- Miosis if painful, except mydriasis in glaucoma
- Periorbital pain in glaucoma
- Photophobia
- Reddening of some or all of the structures of the anterior eye

COMMON CAUSES

- Conjunctivitis and/or blepharitis
  - Allergic/atopy
  - Bacterial
  - Keratoconjunctivitis sicca
  - Trauma
- Corneal ulceration
  - Ectopic cilia/distichiasis
  - Environmental irritants: dust, smoke
  - Exposure keratitis
  - Eyelid abnormalities: ectropion, entropion
  - FB
  - Trauma
- Ectopic cilia/distichiasis
- Ectropion
- Entropion
- Hyphaema and subconjunctival haemorrhage
  - Coagulopathy
  - Trauma
- Prolapse of nictitans gland ('cherry eye')
- Uveitis

UNCOMMON CAUSES

- Albinism: iris lacks normal pigment
- Conjunctivitis
  - Arthropod bites

- Chemical: acid, alkali, antiseptics, shampoos
- Distemper
- Plasma cell keratoconjunctivitis
- Dacryocystitis
- Episcleritis
  - Atopy
  - Nodular granulomatous episcleritis
- Glaucoma
- Hyphaema
  - Aberrant larva migrans (*Angiostrongylus*)
  - Envenomation
  - Lens luxation
  - Lymphoma
  - Neoplasia
  - Vasculitis
- Keratitis: bacterial, fungal
- Neoplasia
  - Haemangioma/haemangiosarcoma
  - Histiocytic disease
  - Mast cell tumour
  - Melanoma
  - Squamous cell carcinoma
- Neurological
  - Facial paralysis
  - Neurogenic keratoconjunctivitis sicca (KCS)
- Radiation
- *Thelazia* infection (only in imported dogs in the UK)
- Uveitis
  - Hyperviscosity syndrome
  - Hypertension
  - Immune-mediated
    - Idiopathic
    - Lens-induced, secondary to lens luxation
    - Pigmentary uveitis
    - Uveodermatological sydrome
    - Vaccine reaction: canine adenovirus
  - Metabolic
    - Hyperlipidaemia
    - Lens-induced in diabetes mellitus
    - Tyrosinaemia
  - Neoplasia: lymphoma, metastatic, primary
  - Scleritis
  - Systemic infection
    - Algal: *Prototheca*

- Bacterial: bacteraemia/septicaemia, *Bartonella, Borrelia, Brucella, Leptospira*
- Mycotic: aspergillosis, blastomycosis, coccidioidomycosis, cryptococcosis, histoplasmosis
- Parasitic: aberrant larval migration: *Angiostrongylus, Dirofilaria, Toxocara*
- Protozoan: *Hepatozoon, Leishmania, Toxoplasma*
- Rickettsial: *Ehrlichia*, Rocky Mountain spotted fever
- Viral: canine adenovirus 1
- Ulcerative keratitis

DIAGNOSTIC APPROACH

1. Physical examination to look for evidence of systemic disease.
2. Coagulation profile if hyphaema is present.
3. Laboratory investigation to rule in/out systemic disease: not necessary if local disease, particularly if only one eye is affected.
4. Full ophthalmological examination.

Clinical clues
Predisposition
- Cherry eye: Bulldogs
- Closed-angle glaucoma
- Exposure keratitis/ulceration: brachycephalics
- KCS in WHWT
- Pigmentary uveitis: Golden retriever
- Uveodermatological syndrome: Arctic breeds and Akita

History
- Known trauma
- Travel history for leishmaniasis

Clinical examination
Visual inspection
- Eyelid deformities
- Ocular discharge
- Erythema: diffuse or focal

Physical examination
- To look for evidence of systemic disease

Ophthalmic examination
- Erythema of conjunctival vessels primarily
  - Conjunctivitis
  - Corneal ulceration
  - Ectopic cilia
- Erythema of episcleral vessels primarily
  - Glaucoma – high intraocular pressure (IOP)
  - Uveitis – low IOP
- Focal erythema
  - Hyphaema
  - Masses

Laboratory findings
- Only indicated if systemic disease is suspected

Imaging
- Only indicated if systemic disease is suspected

Special tests
- Conjunctival cytology
  - Bacteria
  - Distemper inclusions
- Culture of conjunctival bacteria
- Direct and indirect ophthalmoscopy
- Fluorescein stain
- Slit lamp examination of anterior chamber
- Schirmer tear test
- Tonometry to measure intraocular pressure (IOP)

1.41 REGURGITATION

DEFINITION

Regurgitation is the expulsion of saliva and/or undigested food from the oesophagus out through the mouth.

It is exclusively a sign of oesophageal disease and is not part of the vomiting reflex. It is usually a passive process that predisposes to inhalation. However, it can be active, preceded by retching, if there is an acute obstruction (i.e. FB, recent stricture) causing oesophageal discomfort.

RELATED CLINICAL SIGNS

- Cachexia may develop in chronically mal-nourished cases
- Dog is usually keen to re-eat food unless there is pain on swallowing (e.g. oesophagitis)
- Pseudoptyalism occurs through inability to swallow saliva
- Secondary signs may develop from inhalation of regurgitated food
  - Coughing (inhalation)
  - Halitosis
  - Nasal discharge

COMMON CAUSES

Intra-luminal obstruction
- FB

Megaoesophagus
- Focal myasthenia gravis
- Idiopathic acquired
- Secondary megaoesophagus
  - Achalasia of lower oesophageal sphincter

Oesophagitis
- Gastric reflux
  - Acute and persistent vomiting
  - During anaesthesia
  - Hiatal hernia
  - Spontaneous reflux oesophagitis
- Ingestion
  - FB

UNCOMMON CAUSES

Extra-luminal obstruction
- Cranial mediastinal mass
- Peri-oesophageal abscess or mass
- Vascular ring anomaly, e.g., persistent right aortic arch

Intra-luminal obstruction
- Stricture
- Oesophagitis

Ingestive causes
- Caustics
- Hot liquids and food
- Irritants

Megaoesophagus
- Congenital idiopathic

Mural disease
- Diverticulum
- Gastro-oesophageal intussusception
- Primary neoplasia
  - Carcinoma
  - Leiomyoma/sarcoma
- Pythiosis
- *Spirocerca lupi* granuloma

Myopathies
- Dermatomyositis
- Dystrophin deficiency
- Polymyositis
- Systemic lupus erythematosus (SLE)
- Toxoplasmosis

Neuropathies/junctionopathies
- Bilateral vagal damage
- Botulism
- Brain stem disease
- Hydrocephalus
- Meningoencephalitis
- Dysautonomia: unlikely cause of oesophageal dysfunction, as striated muscle in dogs
- Generalised myasthenia
- Giant axonal neuropathy
- Peripheral neuropathy
  - Immune-mediated
  - Toxins: several outbreaks worldwide due to food contamination with unknown toxin
- Polyradiculoneuritis
- Tick paralysis

Toxins
- Anticholinesterase
- Acrylamide
- Botulism
- Food-related peripheral neuropathy
- Lead
- Thallium

Miscellaneous
- Distemper
- Glycogen storage disease Type II
- Hypoadrenocorticism
- Hypothyroidism; debatable whether a true cause or an association in older dogs
- Thymoma

DIAGNOSTIC APPROACH

1 Distinguish regurgitation from vomiting
2 Depending on clinical suspicion, investigate first by:
   - plain radiographs
   or
   - endoscopy
3. Fluoroscopic assessment of oesophageal motility, noting risk of inhaling barium
4. Special tests for causes of seondary megaoesophagus

Clinical clues
Predisposition
- Congenital megaoesophagus in Fox terrier, GSD, Irish setter
- Gastro-oesophageal intussusception in Shar pei breed
- Hiatal hernia seen in brachycephalics with BOAS, especially French bulldog and Pug, and in old dogs with laryngeal paralysis
- Idiopathic megaoesophagus is most common in GSD, Great Dane and Irish setter
- Persistent right aortic arch is most common in GSD and Irish setter and signs appear at weaning.
- Epidemic of megaoesophagus cases seen in countries where food has been contaminated by an unknown toxin causing a peripheral neuropathy

History
- It is essential to distinguish regurgitation from dysphagia and vomiting
  - Food prehension, chewing and swallowing are normal
  - Food is returned passively with no abdominal heave

- Food may be tubular in shape and should not be acidic or contain bile unless there is also gastro-oesophageal reflux
- Onset of signs at weaning with congenital megaoesophagus, diverticulum or vascular ring anomaly
- Recent history of ingestion of caustics or of a GA (with presumed reflux) may precede oesophagitis or stricture
- Regurgitation may occur immediately after eating or hours later, depending on whether the oesophagus is inflamed or dilated

Clinical examination
Visual inspection
- Depressed and dyspnoeic if inhalation pneumonia is present
- Dilated oesophagus may occasionally be seen ballooning in the left cervical area
- May regurgitate and re-eat food
- Nasal discharge and coughing if inhalation present

Physical examination
- Auscultation
  - May hear food/liquid slopping in dilated oesophagus
  - Moist lung sounds if inhalation pneumonia
  - Normal heart sounds with persistent right aortic arch (PRAA)
- Gag reflex may be absent if pharynx is also affected
- Halitosis if retention of food in megaoesophagus or inhalation pneumonia

Laboratory findings
Haematology
- Possible inflammatory leukogram with inhalation pneumonia

Biochemistry
- Usually unremarkable, unless patient is dehydrated

Imaging
Plain radiographs of conscious dog
- Dilated gas-filled oesophagus in megaoesophagus
   NB: Beware of over-interpretation of passive dilation under heavy sedation or GA

- Radio-dense FB
- Stricture not visible unless food accumulated proximally

Contrast radiographs: barium swallow after plain films
- Radiolucent FB
- Stricture
  NB: Risk of inhalation

Endoscopy
- To identify and potentially treat mural and intramural causes of regurgitation

NB: Risk of inhalation

Special tests
- Acetylcholine receptor antibody titre for focal myasthenia gravis
- Anti-nuclear antibody for SLE
- Basal cortisol or ACTH stimulation test for hypoadrenocorticism
- Creatine kinase for polymyositis
- Fluoroscopy
- Manometry
- Oesophagoscopy
- Thyroid function tests

1.42 SEIZURES

DEFINITION

An epileptic seizure is defined as manifestation of excessive synchronous, usually self-limiting electrical activity of neurons in the brain. This results in transient, typically short episodes with convulsions or focal motor, autonomic or behavioural features and is due to abnormal excessive and/or synchronous epileptic neuronal activity in the brain.

Seizures can be focal or generalised in nature.
- Focal seizures are less common and present with lateralised or regional signs, e.g. facial twitching, hypersalivation, or behavioural change
- Generalised seizures are characterised by bilateral involvement and typically result in tonic-clonic movements, loss of consciousness, and often have autonomic signs, i.e. urination, defaecation, salivation

RELATED CLINICAL SIGNS

Epileptic seizures can have up to three phases; prodrome, ictal, and post-ictal stages.
1 The prodrome is not commonly observed in dogs and is detected as disrupted behavior predictive of a seizure.
2 The ictal stage is the seizure itself.
3 The post-ictal period occurs after the seizure and may last hours to days; during this time

the dog may be disorientated and display abnormal behaviour such as aggression, compulsive walking, excessive drinking, eating, or vocalisation.

COMMON CAUSES

Extracranial causes
- Hypoglycaemia
  - Hepatic encephalopathy: PSS, chronic hepatitis
  - Hypoadrenocorticism
  - Insulinoma
  - Sepsis
  - Toxins, e.g. ivermectin, xylitol
  - Young toy-breed dogs

Intracranial causes
- Idiopathic
- Inflammatory: meningoencephalitis of unknown origin
- Neoplasia: meningioma, glioma
- Congenital: hydrocephalus

UNCOMMON CAUSES

Extracranial causes
- Electrolyte disturbances
  - Hypocalcaemia
  - Sodium derangements

- Hyperviscosity
  - Erythrocytosis
  - Hyperglobulinaemia
- Hypertensive encephalopathy
- Large/diffuse neoplasia
- Uraemia

Intracranial causes
- Degenerative, e.g. storage disease
- Infectious
  - *Angiostrongylus vasorum*
  - Bacterial empyema
  - Distemper
  - Fungal disease
  - *Toxoplasma* and *Neospora*
- Neoplasia
  - CNS lymphoma
  - Metastatic neoplasia
- Vascular: haemorrhagic or thromboembolic stroke

DIAGNOSTIC APPROACH

Clinical clues
Predisposition
- Idiopathic epilepsy is the most common intracranial cause of seizures in dogs aged 1–5 years
- Border collies and GSDs are predisposed to idiopathic epilepsy
- Middle-aged small- and toy-breed dogs are predisposed to meningoencephalitis of unknown origin

History
- Behaviour between seizures is important; dogs with idiopathic epilepsy would be expected to be normal after recovery from the post-ictal stage
- Duration and progression of neurological signs may aid in index of suspicion
  - Acute onset improving increases suspicion of vascular or toxin
  - Gradual onset progression may increase suspicion of degenerative or neoplastic disease
- Thorough history is important to discriminate between seizures, syncope, and movement disorders

- Movement disorders may cause abnormal movements in all four limbs, but consciousness tends to be preserved
- Syncope occurs more commonly during exercise or excitement and is normally characterised by brief, flaccid collapse with no post-ictal period

Clinical examination
Visual inspection
- Mentation may be impaired, additional signs of forebrain disease may be circling, head pressing, blindness and abnormal responsiveness

Physical examination
- Bradycardia and hypertension (Cushing's reflex) may be detected in dogs with increased intracranial pressure
- Thorough examination to assess for multisystemic disease

Neurological examination
- A full neurological examination should be performed
  - Normal between seizures if idiopathic epilepsy
  - Multifocal abnormalities are most suspicious for inflammatory, infectious or neoplastic disease
- The forebrain can be assessed with the menace response, proprioception, response to nasal stimulation, and observing mentation

Ophthalmic examination
- May be useful to assess for infiltrative central nervous system disease, e.g. may detect papilloedema

Laboratory findings
Haematology
- Uncommon to detect changes

Serum biochemistry
- Blood glucose to assess for hypoglycaemia as a cause (ideally close temporally to seizure)
- Electrolytes in particular calcium and sodium
- Evidence of hepatic dysfunction (low urea, albumin, cholesterol, glucose, increased bile acid stimulation test results and ammonia) or hepatic injury (increased enzyme activities)

Imaging

Plain radiographs
- Screen for disseminated neoplasia in cases with a high suspicion

Ultrasound
- Screen for disseminated neoplasia in cases with a high suspicion
- Assess for PSS; may be challenging to visualise

Special tests
- Fructosamine and serial fasted blood glucose measurement when suspicious of insulinoma

- CT angiogram to assess for portosystemic shunt and insulinoma
- MRI and CSF for cytology, proteins, and infectious disease PCR to assess for intracranial causes of seizures
- Toxicology in dogs with a high suspicion of toxin exposure
- Treatment trials with anti-epileptic drugs may be considered in cases where discrimination between a seizure and movement disorder is unclear and events are frequent

1.43 SNEEZING

DEFINITION

Classical sneezing is the forcible expulsion of air from the nose in an explosive spasmodic involuntary action resulting primarily from irritation of the nasal mucous membranes.

Reverse sneezing is forceful inspiration via the nose against a closed glottis, often occurring in paroxysms.

The differential diagnoses for sneezing and reverse sneezing are mostly shared, with the difference related to the location of the disorder, i.e. more caudal nasal disorders are more likely to present with reverse sneezing, but with a few exceptions noted below.

RELATED CLINICAL SIGNS

Sneezing is fairly simple for owners to recognise as it is very similar to sneezing in people. Reverse sneezing can be more distressing and harder to characterise, and can be mistaken for breathing difficulties by inexperienced owners.
- Concurrent nasal discharge: serous, mucopurulent, haemorrhagic or a mixture
- Coughing due to post-nasal drip and aspiration of nasal discharge
- Nasal depigmentation/deformities
- Pawing at face
- Stertor or snoring due to reduced nasal airflow

COMMON CAUSES

- Chronic idiopathic rhinitis
- Infection
  - Sino-nasal aspergillosis
  - Tooth root abscess
- Elongated soft palate causing reverse sneezing
- FB
- Neoplasia: carcinoma, sarcoma, lymphoma

UNCOMMON CAUSES

- Infection
  - Oronasal fistula
  - Osteomyelitis
  - Parasitic (*Linguatula serrata*, *Pneumonyssoides caninum*)
- Neoplasia (leiomyoma)
- Cleft palate
- Reverse sneezing may occur due to lower airway disease with irritation of the nasopharynx due to coughed-up secretions and with reflux

DIAGNOSTIC APPROACH

Clinical clues
Predisposition
- Breed predisposition in sino-nasal aspergillosis suspected in Golden retrievers

- Dolichocephalic dogs are predisposed to sino-nasal aspergillosis
- Older dogs are predisposed to nasal tumours and dental disease
- Reverse sneezing may occur in dogs with elongated soft palates, e.g. brachycephalic dogs, CKCS

Physical examination
- Assess nasal airflow
  - Tissue or cotton wool to detect airflow at each nostril
  - Microscope slide and assess for condensation
  - Stethoscope and auscultate each side
- Examination of head conformation including ocular retropulsion for signs of deformity suspicious for neoplasia
- Examination of nasal planum for depigmentation (most common in fungal disease)
- Oral examination to assess for dental disease and oronasal fistulas

Laboratory findings
Haematology and serum biochemistry
- Often unremarkable, but useful to screen for systemic disease

Imaging
Plain radiographs
- Nasal turbinate destruction: tumour or aspergillosis
- Soft tissue opacity: tumour is most likely but can also occur with fluid accumulation
- Sinus hyperostosis (*Aspergillus*)

Special tests
- *Aspergillus* serology: specific but poorly sensitive test, i.e. a positive result supports infection but a negative result does not exclude it
- CT scan with contrast to assess for nasal diseases
- Culture of nasal discharge is not useful; likely bacterial flora and positive *Aspergillus* culture is not diagnostic as it can be an environmental contaminant
- Nasal cytology (rarely useful) and tissue sample for histopathology
- Rhinoscopy to assess for nasal FB, tumours, or aspergillosis

---

1.44 STIFFNESS, JOINT SWELLING AND GENERALISED LAMENESS

DEFINITIONS

- Stiffness is a reduction in the range of joint movement and overall mobility.
- A joint swelling is enlargement of a synovial joint due to accumulation of fluid or soft tissue inflammation.
- Lameness is an abnormal gait resulting from partial loss of function or pain in a limb usually due to an orthopaedic problem.
- Generalised lameness affects two or more limbs and typically is related to systemic disease.
- Shifting lameness is when limbs are affected sequentially.

RELATED CLINICAL SIGNS

Stiffness, joint swelling, and generalised lameness may be identified together or in isolation.
- Abnormal or short-strided gait
- Change in mobility, e.g. reluctance to exercise, jump up/down onto furniture or climb/descend stairs
- Change in posture
- Joint swelling
- Tachycardia and tachypnoea may occur in the acute phase
- Weight shifting when standing
- Yelping or crying out, and sensitivity to touch due to pain

COMMON CAUSES

Spinal pain
- IVDD
- Steroid responsive meningitis arteritis (SRMA)

Musculoskeletal pain
- Cellulitis
- Degenerative joint disease (osteoarthritis)
- FB
- Fracture
- Immune-mediated polyarthritis (IMPA)
- Neoplasia: osteosarcoma
- Trauma

UNCOMMON CAUSES

Spinal pain
- Discospondylitis
- Nerve root tumour and other neoplasms of the spine

Musculoskeletal pain
- Aortic thromboembolism
- Metaphyseal osteopathy
- Myositis
- Osteomyelitis
- Panosteitis
- Septic joint

DIAGNOSTIC APPROACH

Clinical clues
Predisposition
- Breed predisposition
  - IVDD: Bassets, Dachshunds and, to a lesser extent, many other breeds, e.g. Cocker spaniel, Pekingese, Poodle
  - Metaphyseal osteopathy: Weimaraner
  - Osteosarcoma: large and giant breeds
  - SRMA: Beagle, Boxer, Whippet
- Juvenile dogs: SRMA, metaphyseal osteopathy and panosteitis
- Older dogs: neoplasia and degenerative joint disease

History
- Dogs with generalised lameness, in particular with inflammatory causes (IMPA), may present with signs of lethargy only; specific questions around normal behaviours may uncover more subtle signs of joint pain
- Lameness in multiple limbs is more difficult to detect than lameness in a single limb
- Spinal pain and abdominal pain can be difficult to discriminate; GI signs will aid this, i.e. in the absence of vomiting or diarrhoea, spinal pain would be considered more likely than abdominal pain
- Stiffness and significant lameness can be detected by owners, but joint swelling is not normally detected by owners

Clinical examination
Visual inspection
- Assess demeanour, ambulation, and navigating specific obstacles (e.g. stairs), and in some cases video recordings of the dog during episodes can be very useful
- Disorders involving multiple limbs can be more challenging than those affecting single limbs due to more subtle signs of lameness

Physical examination
During thorough examination pain may be localised; in some cases it may be important to pay attention for subtle signs of discomfort, e.g. lip licking
- Crepitus in degenerative joint disease
- Joint swelling and reduced range of movement
- Pyrexia is typically observed in steroid responsive meningitis arteritis, IMPA and metaphyseal osteopathy

Orthopaedic and neurological examinations
- To identify sites of pain and distinguish musculoskeletal causes of abnormal gait pain from neurological causes

Laboratory findings
Haematology and serum biochemistry
- Useful to screen for systemic inflammatory disease

Imaging

- Plain radiographs and abdominal ultrasound may be useful once pain is localised

Special tests

- Analgesia trial in the absence of suspicion of severe systemic disease
- Arthrocentesis cytology and culture for IMPA or septic joint

- C-reactive protein (CRP) may be increased in dogs with inflammatory disorders (SRMA, septic joint, IMPA)
- CSF cytology for SRMA
- Infectious disease screening in particular in travelled dogs: *Anaplasma*, *Ehrlichia*, *Leishmania*, and *Borrelia*
- Spec cPL can be increased in IVDD as well as pancreatitis, therefore may not aid in discriminating

1.45 STUNTING

DEFINITION

Stunting (retarded growth) is a reduced rate of growth resulting in a dog failing to attain the expected size, weight and/or height standards characteristic of a dog of the same age and breed.

RELATED CLINICAL SIGNS

- Proportionately small size or disproportionate stunting, i.e. normal body length but short limbs
- Signs of relevant organ dysfunction
  - Exercise intolerance
  - Neurological signs
  - Polyphagia
  - PU/PD
  - Vomiting and/or diarrhoea

COMMON CAUSES

- Congenital cardiac disease
- Chondrodystrophy
- Hepatic dysfunction
  - Congenital PSS
- Inadequate diet:
  - Underfeeding
  - Poor-quality food
- Malabsorption
  - Antibiotic-responsive diarrhoea (ARD or dysbiosis)
  - EPI

- Food-responsive enteropathy
- Parasitism: *Giardia*, hookworms
- Renal dysplasia

UNCOMMON CAUSES

- Achondroplasia and chondrodysplasia
- Congenital hypothyroidism
- Diabetes mellitus
- Endocarditis
- Food allergy
- Hepatic dysfunction
  - Glycogen storage disease
  - Lobular dissecting hepatitis
  - Portal vein hypoplasia: non-cirrhotic portal hypertension
- Hydrocephalus
- Hypoadrenocorticism
- Malabsorption
  - Chronic intussusception
  - CIE/IBD
- Oesophageal disease
  - Congenital megaoesophagus
  - Vascular ring anomaly
- Pituitary dwarfism
- Vitamin and mineral deficiencies
  - Vitamin A
  - Vitamin D
  - Vitamin B_{12}
    - Imerslund-Gräsbeck syndrome (selective cobalamin malabsorption)
    - Vegan diet
- Zinc deficiency

DIAGNOSTIC APPROACH

- Determine appetite
  - Anorexia suggestive of metabolic disease
  - Polyphagia suggestive of malabsorption or EPI
- Use other clinical signs to identify potential organ systems
- Serum biochemistry to identify metabolic causes
- Investigate specific organ systems

Clinical clues

Some breeds, such as Yorkshire terriers and poodles, have a range of normal sizes, but stunting can be recognised by comparison with unaffected littermates.

- Alopecia in pituitary dwarfism
- Chondrodystrophy is part of the normal breed standard in certain, short-legged breeds, and can cause type 1 IVDD
- Mental retardation can occur in untreated congenital hypothyroidism
- Disproportionate stunting is suggestive of chondrodysplasia or congenital hypothyroidism
- Dyspnoea/tachypnoea in inhalation pneumonia
- Intermittent forebrain signs due to hepatic encephalopathy or hydrocephalus
- Fibrous osteodystrophy (rubber jaw) in renal dysplasia

Predisposition
- ARD and EPI in GSDs
- Chondrodystrophy can be normal in several short-legged breeds: Dachshunds, Bassets
- Hydrocephalus in miniature and toy breeds: Chihuahua, Papillon, Yorkshire terrier
- Hydrocephalus in brachycephalics; Boston terrier, English bulldog, Pekingese
- Imerslund-Gräsbeck syndrome in Australian shepherd, Beagle, Border collie, Giant schnauzer, Komondor
- Inhalation pneumonia in brachycephalic breeds
- Pituitary dwarfism: GSD, Wolfdog (Czechoslovakian, Saarloos), Spitz, Miniature Pinscher, and Karelian Bear Dog
- Renal dysplasia in a wide range of breeds:

Alaskan Malamute, Bedlington terrier, Boxer, Bulldog, Chow Chow, Cocker Spaniel, Collie, Dobermann, Finnish Harrier, Golden and Labrador retriever, Great Dane, Irish Wolfhound, Keeshond, King Charles spaniel, Lhasa Apso, Miniature schnauzer, Norwegian Elkhound, Rhodesian Ridgeback, Rottweiler, Samoyed, Shih Tzu, Soft-coated Wheaten Terrier and Standard Poodle

History
- Failure to grow
- Signs associated with relevant organ system
  - GI signs and polyphagia in malabsorption
  - PU/PD in DM, PSS, renal dysplasia

Clinical examination
Visual inspection
- Abnormal behaviour and obtundation in hepatic encephalopathy or hydrocephalus
- Shortened legs in chondrodystrophy
- Small size: proportionate or disproportionate?

Physical examination
- Domed skull and/or open fontanelle in hydrocephalus
- Small size
- Underweight

Laboratory findings
- Abnormalities associated with relevant organ system, e.g. azotaemia with renal dysplasia
- Hyperglycaemia and glycosuria if diabetes mellitus

Imaging
Abnormalities associated with relevant organ system

Radiographs
- Poor bone mineralization
- Pneumonia
- Shortened limb bones
- Small kidneys

Ultrasound
- Abnormal kidneys with renal dysplasia
- PSS ± renomegaly

Special tests
- Cobalamin for B_{12} deficiency
- DNA test for Imerslund-Gräsbeck syndrome
- DNA test for pituitary dwarfism
- Dynamic bile acids for PSS
- IGF for pituitary dwarfism (growth hormone assay not commercially available)
- TLI for EPI

1.46 TENESMUS AND DYSCHEZIA

DEFINITION

- Tenesmus is straining to defaecate or urinate.
- Dyschezia denotes pain or difficulty in defaecation and is often associated with tenesmus in distal LI and/or perianal disease.
- Faecal tenesmus is straining to pass faecal material.
- Urinary tenesmus is straining to pass urine, *q.v.* section 1.19

RELATED CLINICAL SIGNS

Primary signs
- Signs of pain
  - Circling repeatedly before attempting defaecation
  - Stopping straining abruptly and/or crying out during attempted defaecation
- Tenesmus: straining to pass faecal material or after defaecation
  - Straining after defaecation if there is colono-rectal inflammation or mass
  - Straining before passing stool and may ultimately pass small volume feces or liquid if constipated

Associated signs
- Anorexia and vomiting if severely constipated
- Blood and mucus mixed in faeces if colitis
- Blood on surface of faeces if focal bleeding lesion, e.g. polyp
- Distorted faecal shape if rectal mass/stricture present

COMMON CAUSES

- All causes of constipation, *q.v.* section 1.11
- Anal sac
  - Abscess/perineal cellulitis
  - Anal sacculitis
  - Impaction
- Colorectal disease
  - With diarrhoea
    - Acute colitis
    - Chronic colitis
  - Without passing stool
    - Colitis
    - Constipation
- Pelvic fracture
- Perineal disease
  - Anal furunculosis
  - Perineal hernia and rectal diverticulum
- Benign prostatic hypertrophy
- Spinal cord injury

UNCOMMON CAUSES

- Anorectal stricture
  - Inflammatory
  - Non-accidental injury
  - Post-surgical
- Anal sac adenocarcinoma
- Colorectal disease
  - With fresh blood and/or faecal deformation (indented or ribbon-shape)
    - Rectal polyp
    - Rectal tumour
- Idiopathic megacolon
- Paraprostatic cyst

- Pseudocoprostasis
- Prostatic carcinoma
- Rectal FB
- Vulval mass

DIAGNOSTIC APPROACH

1 Distinguish between urinary and faecal tenesmus by history and observation.
2 Examine perineum and perform rectal examination if faecal.
3 Look for underlying cause of constipation.

Clinical clues
Predisposition
- Anal sac adenocarcinoma: middle-aged female dogs
- Perineal hernia: male entire dogs

History
- Confirm whether dyschezia or dysuria is cause of tenesmus by observation and physical examination

Clinical examination
Visual inspection
- Observe defaecation and urination to distinguish which is associated with straining
- May strain and cry out, stop, walk around and try again
- Pseudocoprostasis visible

Physical examination
- Abdominal palpation
  - Distended abdomen
  - Enlarged, firm colon if constipated
  - Full bladder if obstructed

- Small bladder if cystitis/urethritis
- Anal furunculosis
- Perineal swelling

Rectal examination
- Anal sac disease
- Constipation
- Pain
- Perineal hernia
- Prostatomegaly
- Rectal mass
- Stricture: benign strictures are rare, neoplasia more likely
- Vulval mass

Laboratory findings
- Haematology and serum biochemistry usually unremarkable

Imaging
Plain radiographs
- Extent of colonic impaction
- Identifies:
  - Abnormal faecal material (e.g. bones) if constipated
  - Pelvic bone and some spinal lesions
  - Pelvic mass
  - Prostatic enlargement
  - Sublumbar lymphadenopathy

Ultrasound
- Colonic masses
- Prostatic enlargement

Special tests
- Barium enema
- Colonoscopy
- Advanced imaging: myelogram, CT, MRI

1.47 TREMORS

DEFINITION

Tremors are involuntary, repetitive, rhythmic, muscular oscillations. They can be generalised or affect single body parts.

RELATED CLINICAL SIGNS

- Circumstance of occurrence is useful; intention tremors are those that occur during voluntary movement, only when standing (orthostatic tremor), and idiopathic head tremors can be terminated by distracting the dog.

- In addition to tremors depending on aetiology
  - Ataxia
  - Generalised seizures
  - Vestibular dysfunction
- Marked sustained tremors may cause hyperthermia due to sustained muscle contractions.

COMMON CAUSES

Cerebellar disease
- Corticosteroid responsive tremor syndrome (formerly known as white hairy shaker syndrome)
- Meningoencephalitis of unknown origin

Idiopathic
- Idiopathic head tremor
- Senile-related tremor

Metabolic disease
- Hepatic encephalopathy
- Non-specific
  - Anxiety
  - Pain
- Toxins
  - Tremorgenic mycotoxin
  - Chocolate toxicity

UNCOMMON CAUSES

Cerebellar disease
- Abiotrophy
- Congenital (hypoplastic)
- Infectious, e.g. *Toxoplasma* or *Neospora* infection
- Neoplasia
- Storage disease
- Vascular: thromboembolic or haemorrhagic

Miscellaneous
- Distemper
- HAC-induced myoclonus
- Hypoaldosteronism
- Hypocalcaemia
  - Eclampsia
  - Hypoadrenocorticism
- Primary orthostatic tremor

- Toxin induced
  - Metaldehyde

DIAGNOSTIC APPROACH

Clinical clues
Predisposition
- Corticosteroid responsive tremor syndrome: small toy-breed types
- Idiopathic head tremor: Boxers, English bulldogs and Dobermanns
- Nursing bitches at risk of hypocalcaemia
- Orthostatic tremor: large-breed dogs
- Older dogs, especially small breed dogs, predisposed to senile tremor

History
- Circumstance of tremor
  - If localised consider cerebellar disorders
  - Voluntary movement more likely intention tremor
- Risk of exposure to toxins, including mouldy food contaminated by tremorgenic mycotoxin
- Systemic disease or pain if behavioural causes of tremor are suspected

Clinical examination
Visual inspection
- Assess demeanour, ambulation, and navigating specific obstacles, e.g. stairs, etc.
- In some cases video recordings of the dog during episodes can be very useful

Physical examination
- Thorough examination for signs of systemic disease or pain
- Full neurological examination

Laboratory findings
Haematology and serum biochemistry
Useful to screen for systemic inflammatory disease
- Evidence of hepatic dysfunction and/or injury: albumin, cholesterol, glucose, bilirubin, liver enzyme activities, and a bile acid stimulation test
- Hypoglycaemia: insulinoma
- Hypocalcaemia: eclampsia

Imaging
- Unremarkable in most cases

Special tests
- ACTH stimulation test for hypoadrenocorticism

- Analgesia trial in the absence of suspicion of severe systemic disease
- LDDS test for HAC where clinical signs are present
- MRI and CSF tap cytology for cerebellar disorders

1.48 URINARY INCONTINENCE

DEFINITION

Urinary incontinence is the loss of voluntary control of urination with consequential unconscious urinary leaking. This must be discriminated from nocturia (urinating overnight) or inappropriate urination (e.g. behavioural or during excitement or apprehension).

Urinary incontinence may occur due to a failure to store urine (storage disorders), or due to an inability to completely void the bladder during conscious urination and resultant urinary leaking (overflow incontinence).

Urinary incontinence may present as constant leaking, or occurrence may be related to specific circumstances (lying down, or during activity).

RELATED CLINICAL SIGNS

- Neurological disease depending on the cause
- Systemic illness
- Urinary tract infection: haematuria, pollaki-uria, pungent urine

COMMON CAUSES

Storage disorders
- Detrusor hyperreflexia/instability (urge incontinence)
  - Calculi
  - Infection: urethritis
  - Neoplasia
  - Polyps
- Ectopic ureter
- Urethral sphincter mechanism incompetence (USMI)
- Urinary tract infection

Overflow incontinence
- Partial obstruction
  - Neoplasia
  - Prostatic disease (abscess, paraprostatic cyst, benign prostatic hyperplasia, neoplasia)
  - Urethritis
  - Urolithiasis
- Neurogenic (brainstem or spinal cord disorders)

UNCOMMON CAUSES

Storage disorders
- Persistent urachus
- Ureterocoele
- Urethrovaginal or urethrorectal fistula

Overflow incontinence
- Detrusor atony
- Detrusor urethral dyssynergy
- Dysautonomia

DIAGNOSTIC APPROACH

Clinical clues
Predisposition
- Neuter status influences risk of prostatic disorders
  - Neutered dogs are most likely to have carcinoma
  - Entire dogs are most likely to have benign prostatic hyperplasia, abscess, or paraprostatic cysts
- USMI can be detected in any dog, however most common in female neutered dogs
- Young dogs, in particular Golden retrievers, increase suspicion of ectopic ureter

History
- Assess for polyuria and polydipsia
- Concurrent dyschezia increases suspicion of intrapelvic mass lesion (enlarged prostate or lymph nodes)
- In dogs with bacterial cystitis an emphasis should be placed on establishing risk factors that may have predisposed to the development of infection:
  - Anatomical causes (juvenile vaginitis in puppies, hooded vulva in female dogs, urinary incontinence (e.g. ectopic ureter, USMI)
  - Presence of systemic disease (hyperadrenocorticism, diabetes mellitus)
  - Immunosuppression
- Urination in inappropriate places whilst the dog is conscious and aware is likely behavioural unless there is a UTI or severe PU/PD

Clinical examination
Visual inspection
- Measuring bladder size (using ultrasonography) following voiding may help establish whether the dog is able to void their bladder (if this remains large, obstructive and neurological causes are more likely)
- Urination pattern
  - Dogs with reflex dyssynergia or urethral obstruction typically try to initiate urination as normal; however, any urinary stream stops abruptly due to lack of synchrony between bladder contraction and urethral sphincter relaxation or obstruction

Physical examination
- Conformation risk factors for development of bacterial cystitis
  - Hooded vulva, perivulval inflammation or urinary pooling in female dogs
  - Prostatomegaly in male dogs
- Rectal examination to assess the urethra, and prostate in male dogs
- Passing a urinary catheter (can be done in conscious male dogs but likely requires sedation or anaesthesia for female dogs), to assess for ease of passing aids assessment for urethral obstructive disorders

Neurological examination
- Assessment for concurrent neurological deficits
- Ability to express bladder useful in dogs with concurrent neurological deficits

Laboratory findings
Haematology
- Typically unremarkable; it may be useful to screen for systemic disease

Serum biochemistry
- Useful to screen for systemic disease, may detect azotaemia in dogs with post-renal causes (urethral obstruction) or renal causes (extension of bacterial cystitis to pyelonephritis)

Urinalysis
- Cytology to assess for neoplastic cells
- Culture: ideally from cystocentesis sample, otherwise interpret positive culture with caution
- Sediment for evidence of urinary tract infection (pyuria) or neoplastic cells
- Urine specific gravity to assess for polydipsia and polyuria

Imaging
Plain radiographs
- Assess for radiopaque uroliths, prostate, ensure length of urethra included, may need to do an enema first to fully assess urinary system for uroliths
- Contrast studies retrograde urethrogram (plain radiographs or fluoroscopy) and intravenous excretory urogram
- Bladder may be intrapelvic in urinary sphincter mechanism incompetence

Ultrasound
- Assess kidneys, ureters, urinary bladder and prostate

Special tests
- CT with contrast for urinary system assessment (improves sensitivity for ectopic ureter compared to plain radiography)

- Cystoscopy to assess urethra, bladder, and implantation of ureters
- MRI and CSF for dogs with neurolocalisation
- Prostatic wash and fine needle aspiration for cytology and culture

- Urinary BRAF: assess urine for presence of BRAF mutation detected in a high proportion of dogs with transitional cell carcinoma
- Urodynamic pressure profilometry

1.49 VOMITING

DEFINITION

Vomiting (emesis) is a reflex act characterised by forceful expulsion of gastric ± small intestinal contents from the stomach, and co-ordinated by the vomiting centre in the medulla.

The multiple afferents to the vomiting centre mean vomiting can be caused by primary GI disease or disease elsewhere in the dog. Vomiting can be acute (sudden onset, often self-limiting) or chronic (arbitrarily > 3 weeks' duration)

RELATED CLINICAL SIGNS

- Changes in appetite and weight loss
- Expulsion of gastric contents:
  - Digested or undigested food
  - Bile and mucus
  - Blood, *q.v.* section 1.25
- Preceded by nausea
  - Frequent swallowing/gulping/retching
  - Hypersalivation, *q.v.* section 1.16
  - Lip-licking
  - Restlessness/anxiety
- Repeated contractions of abdominal wall
- Signs of dehydration
- Tremors if ingested tremorgenic mycotoxin, *q.v.* section 1.47

COMMON CAUSES

Acute vomiting
Primary GI disease
- Acute haemorrhagic diarrhoea syndrome (AHDS)/haemorrhagic gastroenteritis (HGE), *q.v.* section 1.15.1
- Dietary indiscretion
  - Adverse reaction to a natural component in food, e.g. histamine

- Change in diet
- Scavenging: garbage intoxication, mycotoxins
- Over-indulgence
- Gastric foreign body
- Intestinal obstruction: FB, intussusception
- Parvovirus infection
- Gastric dilatation-volvulus – ineffective attempts to vomit

Secondary, non-GI disease
- Acute pancreatitis
- AKI and post-renal obstruction
- Diabetic ketoacidosis
- Drugs: chemotherapy agents, digoxin, morphine, NSAIDs
- Hypoadrenocorticism: not common, but too important to be overlooked
- Pyometra
- Toxins, e.g. ethylene glycol, mycotoxins, plant alkaloids
- Vestibular disease, motion sickness

Chronic vomiting
Primary GI disease
- Chronic gastritis
  - Enterogastric reflux (bilious vomiting syndrome)
  - *Helicobacter*
  - Idiopathic
- Gastric ulceration
  - NSAIDs
- Inflammatory bowel disease/chronic inflammatory enteropathy

Secondary, non-GI disease
- Chronic pancreatitis
- Hypercalcaemia
- Uraemia

UNCOMMON CAUSES

Acute vomiting

Primary GI disease
- Distemper
- Intestinal volvulus
- Peritonitis
- Psychogenic

Secondary, non-GI disease
- Acute hepatitis
- Anaphylaxis
- Diaphragmatic rupture
- Heat stroke
- Leptospirosis
- Prostatitis
- Septicaemia/endotoxaemia
- Sialoadenitis/salivary gland infarction

Chronic vomiting

Primary GI disease
- Chronic hypertrophic pylorogastropathy (CHPG)/gastric antral mucosal hypertrophy
- Gastric ulceration
  - Gastric carcinoma
  - Gastrinoma
  - Gastric mast cell tumour: gastric
- Gastroparesis
  - Visceral myopathy: leiomyositis
  - Visceral neuropathy
  - Mesenteric ganglionitis
- Hiatal hernia: can cause regurgitation and/or vomiting
- Obstipation
- *Physaloptera* (not in UK)
- Pyloric stenosis
- Pythiosis (not in UK)

Secondary, non-GI disease
- Acute and chronic hepatitis
- Cholecystitis
- Dysautonomia
- Gall bladder mucocoele
- Hepatoencephalopathy
- Histamine release from remote MCT
- Hyperthyroidism
- Hypertriglyceridaemia
- Hypocalcaemia
- Intracranial disease
  - Encephalitis

- Head trauma
- Meningitis
- Raised intracranial pressure
  - Hydrocephalus
  - Space-occupying lesion: cyst, neoplasia
- Salmon-poisoning (not in UK)
- Sialoadenosis: phenobarbitone-responsive
- Swallowed blood from oral bleeding or epistaxis

DIAGNOSTIC APPROACH

1 Distinguish vomiting from regurgitation by clinical clues below.
2 Rule out secondary causes of vomiting by history, physical exam and minimum laboratory database.
3 Treat acute vomiting symptomatically unless surgical disease is suspected.
4 Investigate chronic vomiting by laboratory tests, imaging and endoscopy.

CLINICAL CLUES

Predisposition
- Gastric carcinoma: 7- to 10-year-old Collies, Belgian shepherds and Bull terriers
- Intussusception is more common in immature dogs
- Parvovirus infection is more likely in young, unvaccinated dogs
- Pyloric stenosis is seen most often in brachycephalic dogs and soon after weaning
- Pyometra and diabetes mellitus are more common in middle-aged to older unspayed females
- Salivary gland infarction in Jack Russell terriers
- Scavenging is more common in Labradors
- Tremors associated with mycotoxin ingestion

History
- Access to garbage, or history of roaming
- Lethargy and weight loss in hypoadrenocorticism
- Metoestrus phase for pyometra
- Systemic illness if secondary vomiting, e.g. PU/PD in diabetes mellitus

- Timing of vomition: more frequent and sooner after feeding the more acute and nearer to the stomach the cause

Clinical examination
Visual inspection
- Distinguish vomiting from regurgitation by presence of prodromal nausea and abdominal contractions/heaves
- Inspect content of vomit: bile, partially digested food, worms, blood
- 'Prayer position' with cranial abdominal pain, *q.v.* section 2.17.1

Physical examination
- Assess degree of dehydration
- Borborygmi: absence of gut sounds indicates ileus and possible peritonitis
- Bradycardia if hypoadrenocorticism
- Enlarged salivary glands in sialoadenosis/sialoadenitis/infarction
- Jaundice if hepatopathy
- Pale mucous membranes and tachycardia if bleeding gastric ulceration
- Palpation
  - Abdominal masses
  - FB
  - Pain if pancreatitis, peritonitis or gastric ulceration

Laboratory findings

Haematology
- Inflammatory leukogram if pyometra, pancreatitis, peritonitis or deep gastric ulceration
- Neutropenia if parvovirus infection or acute peritonitis (bowel perforation)
- PCV dramatically increased in AHDS/HGE
- PCV increased in dehydration

Serum biochemistry
- Amylase and lipase unreliably increased in pancreatitis
- Azotaemia and isosthenuria in uraemia
- Electrolyte disturbances if prolonged vomiting
- Hyperglycaemia and glycosuria if diabetes mellitus
- Hyponatraemia/hyperkalaemia in hypoadrenocorticism

Imaging
Radiographs
Plain
- Abdominal fluid (peritonitis)
- Abdominal mass
- Abnormalities of other organs
- Free abdominal gas (GI perforation)
- Obstructive GI gas pattern
- Pyometra
- Radiopaque FB

Contrast
- Low yield
- Only indicated if plain films are unremarkable and supportive lab studies are non-diagnostic

Ultrasound
- Abnormalities of other organs
- Abdominal masses
- FB
- Gastric tumour
- Intussusception

Special tests
- ACTH stimulation test
- Gastroscopy is only indicated in chronic vomiting after ruling out systemic disease, and for FB removal
- Exploratory laparotomy
- GI biopsy
- Spec cPL

1.50 VULVAL DISCHARGE

DEFINITION

Increased volume of mucoid discharge or change in nature of discharge, e.g. purulent or haemorrhagic.

RELATED CLINICAL SIGNS

- Attractive to other males
- Excessive licking of vulva
- Hair staining in perineum

- Increased volume mucoid discharge or purulent or haemorrhagic discharge
- Pollakiuria/discomfort on urination
- Staining of bed/carpet/hair in perineum
- Scooting
- ± PU/PD
- ± Incontinence
- ± Pruritus
- ± Systemic illness

COMMON CAUSES

- Abortion/miscarriage
- Endometritis/pyometritis
- Ovarian remnant syndrome
- Pseudopregnancy
- Reproductive cycle, e.g. proestrus/oestrus
- Vulvovaginitis

UNCOMMON CAUSES

- Congenital/structural anomalies
  - Vestibulo/vaginal stenosis
  - Septal bands
  - (Pseudo)hermaphroditism
- Stump pyometritis
- Sub-involution of placental sites (SIPS) post-partum
- Vaginal FB
- Vaginal/uterine neoplasia
- Secondary to systemic disease e.g. DM, HAC
- Secondary to infection e.g. *Brucella canis*, herpes virus, transmissible venereal tumour

DIAGNOSTIC APPROACH

The reproductive status of the bitch (intact, nulliparous, post-partum, multiparous or neutered) will rule in/out many of the potential diagnoses.

Clinical clues
Predisposition
- Atrophic or juvenile vulva with excessive skin folds and perivulvar dermatitis
- Exposure to hormone products can increase discharge

- Haemorrhagic discharge more suggestive of neoplasia, systemic bleeding disorder, proestrus or SIPS
- Overweight dogs with urinary incontinence and excessive skin folds and urine scalding
- Vulval discharge seen in intact and especially breeding bitches, more than neutered females

History
- Accompanying signs, e.g. attractive to males, pain, pollakiuria
- Details of recent oestrus in entire females
- In neutered females review if any signs of oestrus present, in case of ovarian remnant
- Malodorous purulent/sanguinous discharge typically associated with bacterial infection
- May be systemically well; lethargy/inappetence/pyrexia with systemic disease
- Other clinical signs suggestive of systemic disease or venereal disease
- PU/PD in DM and HAC
- Sterile inflammation is normally mucoid and non-malodourous
- Vaginitis is more common in spayed females

Clinical examination
Visual inspection
- Excessive licking/grooming
- Nature of vulval discharge: colour, smell, volume
- Staining of perivulval hair
- Swelling of vulva

Physical examination
- Assess vulval conformation, e.g. hooded vulva
- Inflamed vulval membranes
- Inflamed, moist, erythematous perivulvar skin
- Vulval discharge

Laboratory findings
Haematology
- Anaemia post-partum or with SIPS
- Leukocytosis ± left shift ± toxic neutrophils with infections such as pyometra
- Leukopenia in some cases of pyometra

Serum biochemistry
- Unremarkable unless systemic illness

Urinalysis
- Identify concurrent urinary tract infection

Imaging
Plain radiographs
- Evidence of enlarged uterus with pyometra

Ultrasound
- Evidence of changes to the uterus
- Evaluate for ovarian disease: cysts/neoplasia/remnant
- Evaluate for concurrent urinary tract disease

Special tests
- *Brucella canis* serology
- Coagulation profile if bleeding for evidence of systemic bleeding disorder

- Ovarian remnant investigations
  - Anti-mullerian hormone
  - Laparoscopy/laparotomy
  - Progesterone
  - Vaginal cytology
- Progesterone testing for stage of oestrus
- Retrograde vagino-urethrogram
- Vaginal investigations for nodules, masses, FB, strictures
  - Biopsy
  - Culture for aerobic and *Mycoplasma* culture: normally mixed flora present
  - Cytology: assess stage of cycle or evidence of ovarian remnant
  - Digital rectal palpation
  - Vaginoscopy and cystoscopy

1.51 WEAKNESS, COLLAPSE AND SYNCOPE

DEFINITIONS

Weakness is a state of lacking strength, firmness, or vigour.
- Can be due to:
  - lassitude/fatigue, which is a lack of energy or
  - generalised muscle weakness; asthenia is a true reduction in muscle tone
- Collapse is a transient or persistent loss of postural tone in one of more limbs
- Syncope is a collapse due to cardiac disease and is caused by deprivation of energy substrates, either oxygen or glucose, which briefly impairs cerebral metabolism
  - Episodes are usually transient with either flaccid muscles or opisthotonus, but other causes of collapse can be more sustained
  - Most commonly results from impaired cerebral blood flow

RELATED CLINICAL SIGNS

Weakness
- Cachexia
- Generalised muscle weakness

Collapse
- Muscle flaccidity
- Transient loss of consciousness

Signs related to underlying disease
- Altered appetite
- Altered defaecation
- Congestive heart failure
- Cough
- Cyanosis
- Dysphagia
- Dyspnoea/tachypnoea
- Lameness
- PU/PD
- Stertor
- Vomiting
- Weight loss or gain

COMMON CAUSES

Weakness is a non-specific sign and the causes are too numerous to list. Causes of collapse are listed.

Cardiovascular disease
Acquired disease
- Dilated cardiomyopathy

- Arrhythmogenic right ventricular cardiomyopathy

Arrhythmia
- Bradyarrhythmia
  - Mobitz type 2 second degree or third-degree atrioventricular (AV) block
  - Sick-sinus syndrome
- Tachyarrhythmia
  - Supraventricular tachycardia
  - Ventricular tachycardia

Congenital disease
- Aortic stenosis
- Pulmonic stenosis

Pericardial disease
- Pericardial effusion
  - Idiopathic haemorrhage
  - Right auricular haemangiosarcoma

Vascular
- Vasovagal syncope
  (aka reflex-mediated syncope, neurocardiogenic syncope, situational syncope)
  - Combination of bradycardia and vasodilation
  - Triggered by excitement, cough, emesis, urinating, defaecating, etc.

Endocrine/metabolic
- Hypoadrenocorticism
- Hypoglycaemia

Haematological
- Acute blood loss anaemia (e.g. ruptured splenic mass)
- Immune mediated haemolytic anaemia
- Erythrocytosis increasing blood viscosity

Neurological
- Vestibular disease

Orthopaedic disease
- Fracture
- Osteoarthritis

Respiratory tract disease
- Hypoxia secondary to:
  - *Angiostrongylus vasorum*

- BOAS
- Pleural effusions
- Pulmonary fibrosis
- Tracheal collapse

UNCOMMON CAUSES

Cardiovascular disease
Acquired disease
- Myxomatous mitral valve disease after major chordae tendinae rupture

Congenital disease
- Right to left shunting disorders (patent ductus arteriosus [PDA], ventricular septal defect [VSD])

Pericardial disease
- Effusive constrictive pericarditis
- Heart base tumour/chemodectoma
- Mesothelioma

Vascular
- Carotid sinus hypersensitivity e.g. brachycephalic dogs, carotid sinus inflammation/neoplasia
- Iliac thrombosis

Endocrine/metabolic
- Hyperkalaemia
- Hypokalaemia
- Hypocalcaemia
- Hyponatraemia/hypernatraemia: only if rapid changes in sodium
- Hypothyroidism
- Phaeochromocytoma

Iatrogenic
- Drug administration, e.g. phenothiazines, drugs with effects on systemic BP

Neurological
- Exercise-induced collapse
- Increased intra-cranial pressure (e.g. space occupying lesion)
- Movement disorders
- Narcolepsy/cataplexy

Other
- Myasthenia gravis causes weakness
- Pain
- Pyrexia

Respiratory tract disease
- Non-cardiogenic pulmonary oedema
- Pulmonary thromboembolism
- Tracheal/bronchial FB

DIAGNOSTIC APPROACH

1 History – collapse episodes should be documented and recorded where possible
2 Confirm the presence or absence of respiratory signs.
3 Rule out orthopaedic disease with physical examination.
4 Rule out haematological and metabolic disease by laboratory testing.
5 Investigate suspected cardiac disease.

Clinical clues
- Distinguish syncope from seizures
  - Does the dog go flaccid or develop opisthotonus (syncope) or have tonic movements (seizure)?
  - Is there a rapid recovery (syncope) or a prolonged post-ictal period (seizure)?
  - Is the dog normal between episodes?
  - Is the dog otherwise unwell?

Predisposition
- Auricular haemangiosarcoma and pericardial haemorrhage: GSD
- Aortic stenosis: Boxer, Golden retriever, Newfoundland
- Arrhythmogenic right ventricular cardiomyopathy: Boxer
- Dilated cardiomyopathy (DCM): large- and giant-breed dogs
- Heart-based tumours: Boxer
- Hypoxia and vasovagal syncope: brachycephalic dogs with BOAS
- Idiopathic pericardial haemorrhage: giant-breed dogs, Golden retriever
- Pulmonary fibrosis: WHWT
- Sick sinus syndrome: Schnauzer and WHWT
- Tracheal collapse: Yorkshire terriers

History
- Characterisation of type of collapse
  - Association with
    - Exercise or excitement: cardiovascular, respiratory
    - Feeding or starvation: endocrine, metabolic
    - Rest or waking: neurological
- Duration of event
- Altered behaviour before or after episode – neurological
- Mucous membrane colour during episode
  - Cyanosis: cardiovascular, respiratory
  - Pallor: cardiovascular, respiratory, haematological
- Frequency of episodes
  - Continuous weakness: endocrine/metabolic
  - Episodic collapse: cardiovascular, respiratory
- Behaviour during collapse
  - Flaccid or opisthotonus ± urination: cardiovascular syncope
  - Tonic-clonic movements, hypersalivation, urination, defaecation: neurological
- Differentiate from seizures; this is important and sometimes difficult
- Drug/chemical/parasite exposure
- Familial history of congenital heart disease, seizures
- Other clinical signs reflect underlying disease, e.g. polydipsia, altered appetite, dysphagia, vomiting, polyuria, incontinence, altered defaecation, respiratory signs, weight loss or gain suggestive of concurrent disease

Clinical examination
Visual inspection
- Brachycephalic conformation
- Gait abnormalities
- Respiratory pattern
- Weight loss

Physical examination
- Mucous membrane colour and capillary refill time
- Neurological system including reflexes, etc.
- Skin for any evidence of endocrinopathies

Auscultation
- Assess for any pulse deficit/arrhythmia

- Abnormal percussion suggesting fluid/consolidation in thoracic cavity
- Abnormal respiratory noise/effort
- Cardiac evaluation for murmurs, etc.

Palpation
- Abdominal palpation for evidence of ascites, masses
- Femoral arteries for pulse
- Lymph nodes
- Musculoskeletal system
- Peripheral pulse volume and rhythm

Laboratory findings
Haematology
- To assess for anaemia or erythrocytosis
NB: In acute blood loss the PCV may remain normal for 12–24 hours
- Check total proteins in conjunction

Serum biochemistry
- To assess in particular:
  - Glucose
  - Electrolytes/ions (sodium, potassium, calcium, magnesium)
  - Muscle enzyme activities (CPK, AST) increased by muscle disease and prolonged seizure
  - Blood urea
  - Liver enzyme activities (ALT, ALP)
  - Proteins

Urinalysis
- Proteinuria predisposing to hypercoagulable state leading to thromboembolism

Imaging
Plain radiographs
- Inspiratory films to assess cardiac size and lung fields
- Expiratory films or fluoroscopy to assess dynamic airway collapse
- Skeletal radiographs may be indicated by the results of physical examination

Ultrasound
- Abdomen
  - Adrenal glands
  - Free fluid
  - Masses
  - Urinary obstruction
- Thorax
  - B lines
  - Free fluid or air
- Echocardiography

Special tests
- Acetylcholine receptor antibody titres or edrophonium response test if myasthenia gravis suspected
- ACTH stimulation to investigate hypoadrenocorticism
- Baermann technique or Angiodetect® for *Angiostrongylus vasorum*
- Blood gas analysis: resting, pre- and post-exercise
- Blood glucose
  - High normal/increased insulin in face of hypoglycaemia is diagnostic for insulinoma
  - Hypoglycaemia with xylitol toxicity
- CT for more detailed assessment of lungs and abdominal structures; contrast can help identify abnormalities
- ECG: in clinic and Holter monitor or event recorder
- Echocardiography with bubble study in suspected cardiac disease
- Electromyography (EMG), nerve conduction velocities, and muscle and nerve biopsies in investigation of neuromuscular disease
- Exercise testing
- Liver function tests, e.g. bile acids
- MRI and CSF analysis for suspected neurological causes of syncope or true seizures
- Respiratory tract investigation e.g. bronchoscopy and BAL
- Serum lactate: resting, pre- and post-exercise
- Thyroid function tests to investigate hypothyroidism

1.52 WEIGHT GAIN/OBESITY

DEFINITION

Weight gain occurs through the accumulation of fat, muscle mass or fluid, or by the growth of large masses.

Obesity is an abnormal accumulation of body fat and develops when caloric intake is increased and/or energy use is decreased.

- Any increase > 15% over ideal body weight is considered overweight
- Obesity is usually defined as an increase in body fat such that body weight is 20% greater than ideal
- Obesity predisposes to significant health risks
  - Cardiovascular disease
  - Diabetes mellitus
  - Orthopaedic disease: cruciate ligament disease, degenerative joint disease and osteoarthritis, IVDD

RELATED CLINICAL SIGNS

- Increased appetite
- Increased body mass
  - Ascites
  - Increased fat deposition
  - Large mass
- Lethargy/exercise intolerance

COMMON CAUSES

- Decreased exercise
  - Inactive lifestyle
  - Limited by orthopaedic (especially osteoarthritis) or cardiorespiratory disease (especially BOAS)
- Dietary
  - High-calorie diets
  - Overeating/overfeeding
- Drugs
  - Corticosteroids
  - Phenobarbital
  - Progestagens
- Genetic predisposition: pro-opiomelanocortin (POMC) mutation

- Hepatosplenomegaly
- HAC
- Hypogonadism, especially in bitches after ovariohysterectomy
- Hypothyroidism
- Pregnancy

UNCOMMON CAUSES

- Acromegaly
- Increased abdominal organ size
- Insulinoma
- Large mass (e.g. lipoma, haemangiopericytoma, granulosa cell tumour)
- Peripheral oedema/ascites
- Pyometra

DIAGNOSTIC APPROACH

1 Record weight and body condition score.
2 If an increase in body weight is noted which cannot be reduced by decreasing dietary intake or if there are concurrent clinical signs, a pathological cause should be sought.
3 If overfeeding can be ruled out, and there is no obvious fluid accumulation or mass, an endocrinopathy is most likely.

Clinical clues
Predisposition
- Acromegaly in dogs in metoestrus or treated with progesterone
- Genetic predisposition in Labradors and Flat-coat retrievers with POMC mutation
- HAC in middle-aged to older dogs
- Hypogonadism after neutering
- Hypothyroidism
- Insulinoma in middle-aged to older bitches
- Osteoarthritis in older dogs

History
- Administration of progesterone or recent oestrus in acromegaly
- Increased appetite in HAC, diabetes mellitus, insulinoma

- Lethargy in hypothyroidism
- PU/PD in HAC
- Recent mating in pregnancy
- Recent oestrus before pyometra

Clinical examination

Visual inspection
- Alopecia in hypothyroidism and HAC
- Obesity

Physical examination
- Abdominal mass if neoplasia
- Ascites
- Enlarged uterus or foetuses in pregnancy
- Increased subcutaneous fat and thickened skin in hypothyroidism
- Increased appetite in HAC, insulinoma
- Intra-abdominal fat accumulation and a pot belly characteristic of HAC
- Subcutaneous oedema
- Thin skin in HAC
- Tubular structure if pyometra
- Weakness and/or seizures in hypoglycaemia caused by insulinoma

Laboratory findings

Haematology
- Inflammatory leukogram sometimes in pyometra
- Stress leukogram in HAC

Serum biochemistry
- Hyperglycaemia and glycosuria in diabetes mellitus
- Hypoalbuminaemia if ascites/oedema
- Increased ALP activity in HAC

Imaging
- Adrenal mass(es)
- Hepatosplenomegaly
- Occult thoracic and abdominal masses
- Pregnancy and pyometra

Special tests
- DNA test for POMC mutation not yet available commercially
- Dynamic cortisol testing
- Raised serum insulin in face of hypoglycaemia
- Increased IGF-1 in acromegaly
- Thyroid function tests

1.53 WEIGHT LOSS

DEFINITION

A dog will lose weight when its energy use or loss exceeds its energy intake and can, therefore, occur with increased use or loss, or with decreased intake or absorption, or with both. A loss of more than 10% of body weight is considered significant.

RELATED CLINICAL SIGNS

- Reduced body condition
  - Cachexia denotes extreme weight loss resulting from metabolic derangements with associated weakness and depression, and often cannot be corrected by increasing dietary energy intake alone
  - Emaciation is severe weight loss and equates to approximately > 20% loss of body weight when bony prominences become noticeable
- Loss of muscle mass will occur in cachexia, but loss in the absence of loss of fat suggests inflammatory myopathies or muscular dystrophy
- Other signs may be associated with the primary cause,
  e.g. diarrhoea in malabsorption, dyspnoea in cardiac failure, pyrexia, etc.

COMMON CAUSES

Normal to increased appetite,
q.v. section 1.36
Physiological
- Exercise
- Lactation

- Planned weight loss programme
- Pregnancy (weight gain later)

Pathological
- Malabsorption
  - ARD/SIBO
  - EPI
  - Mild IBD/CIE
- Non-ketotic DM
- Regurgitation, *q.v.* section 1.41
- Vomiting, *q.v.* section 1.49

Decreased appetite
Any condition causing anorexia,
q.v. section 1.5
- Chronic kidney disease
- Fever
- Dysphagia and regurgitation: tries to eat but cannot swallow, *q.v.* section 1.41
- Heart failure (cardiac cachexia)
- Hypoadrenocorticism
- Ketoacidotic diabetes mellitus
- Malabsorption
  - Severe CIE/IBD
- Liver disease
- Neoplasia (cancer cachexia)
- Pain

UNCOMMON CAUSES

Normal to increased appetite
- Chronic blood loss
- Cold environment
- Hyperthyroidism
  - Dietary: raw food containing thyroid tissue
  - Iatrogenic
  - Rare functional tumour
- Fanconi syndrome
- Malabsorption
  - Bile salt malabsorption
  - Lymphangiectasia
  - Short bowel syndrome
- Poor quality food
- Protein-losing nephropathy
- Systemic fungal infections, especially histoplasmosis
- Temporal myositis
- TMJ disease

- Underfeeding
  - Accidental lack of food
  - Errors when calculating energy requirements
  - Malicious withholding of food
- Widespread skin burns

Decreased appetite
- Malabsorption
  - Alimentary lymphoma
- Oral disease
  - Oral neoplasia
  - Severe dental disease
  - TMJ dysplasia
  - Temporal muscle myositis
- Severe intestinal parasitism
- Severe pyoderma

DIAGNOSTIC APPROACH

1 Record weight, body condition score and muscle score.
2 The differential diagnoses can be subdivided by whether the dog wants to eat or has a reduced or absent appetite.
3 Weight loss simply due to lack of food intake causes an expected weight loss of ~2% body weight per week.
4 Weight loss in excess of 2% body weight per week indicates increased energy loss or usage.
5 Other signs may help localise the organ system involved and direct investigations.

Clinical clues
Predisposition
- Congestive heart failure (CHF) in small breeds (especially CKCS) with valvular endocardiosis, and large breeds with DCM
- EPI in Collies, GSDs
- Internal malignancies most commonly in Boxer, Flat coat retriever, Bernese mountain dog
- Malabsorption through lymphangiectasia in Lundehund, Rottweiler, Yorkshire terrier
- PLE ± PLN in Soft-coated wheaten terrier

History
- Abnormal faeces in malabsorption and EPI

- Cough/dyspnoea/ascites in CHF
- Inadequate intake identified in history
- Increased appetite in malabsorption and EPI

Clinical examination
Visual inspection
- Bony prominences and ribs obvious when emaciated
- Jaundice if liver disease

Physical examination
- Neurological examination
- Palpable goitre with functional thyroid mass
- Palpable mass if intra-abdominal neoplasia

Laboratory findings
Haematology
- Anaemia suggests chronic blood loss
- Eosinophilia suggests parasitism
- Leukocytosis suggests inflammation or infection

Serum biochemistry
- Azotaemia if renal disease
- Glycosuria and hyperglycaemia if diabetes mellitus
- Hypoproteinaemia suggests PLE, PLN or liver disease
- Increased liver enzyme activities ± hyperbilirubinaemia if liver disease
- Proteinuria if PLN

Faecal examination for parasites

Imaging
- CHF
- Occult thoracic and abdominal masses
- To identify effusions

Special tests
- Bronchoscopy

- Cardiac evaluation
  - Cardiac biomarkers
  - Electrocardiography
  - Echocardiography
  - Holter monitoring
- Calcium status
  - Ionised calcium
  - Parathyroid hormone
  - Parathyroid hormone-related protein
  - Vitamin D
- Endocrine testing
  - Fructosamine
  - Basal cortisol ± ACTH stimulation testing
  - Total thyroxine ± free thyroxine (free T4)
- Intestinal evaluation
  - Folate and cobalamin
  - Endoscopic or surgical intestinal biopsy for malabsorption
  - Serum TLI for EPI
- Neuromuscular evaluation
  - Acetylcholine receptor antibodies
  - Cerebrospinal fluid analysis
  - Muscle and nerve biopsy
  - *Toxoplasma* and *Neospora* serology
  - 2M antibody for masticatory myositis
- Nutritional evaluation of the diet
- Pancreatic testing
  - DGGR lipase – not pancreas-specific
  - Spec cPL
  - TLI
- Renal evaluation
  - Glomerular filtration rate
    - Exogenous creatinine clearance
    - Iohexol clearance
  - Symmetric dimethylarginine (SDMA)
  - Urine protein:creatinine ratio
- Therapeutic trials
  - Antiparasitic medication
  - Exclusion diet

SECTION 2
PHYSICAL ABNORMALITIES

In this section, significant findings from the physical examination are listed alphabetically.

- Each problem is defined.
- Common and uncommon causes are suggested for each problem.
- Related clinical signs are listed.
- For each problem a logical diagnostic approach is suggested.
  - Key findings to look for in the history and physical examination are noted; not all will be present in every case.
  - Laboratory findings that aid the diagnosis are noted.
  - Key results of imaging are noted.
  - Special tests that may confirm the diagnosis are listed.

2.1 ABDOMINAL ENLARGEMENT

DEFINITION

Distension of the abdomen by fat, fluid, gas, or organ enlargement, and/or by weakness of the abdominal musculature.
- The causes can be remembered by the mnemonic of the 6 Fs:
  - Faeces/food
  - Fat
  - Fetus
  - Flatus
  - 'Flotsam' (i.e. masses), *q.v.* section 2.2
  - Fluid
- Ascites is the accumulation of free fluid within the peritoneum that may be a low-protein transudate, high-protein modified transudate or an exudate, or which may contain blood, bile, chyle, pus or urine, *q.v.* section 2.5
- Any fluid or gas accumulation may be intraluminal or free, intraperitoneal

RELATED CLINICAL SIGNS

- Acute enlargement with gas accumulation, e.g. in gastric dilatation-volvulus (GDV) and ruptured organ/viscus
- Chronic, progressive enlargement in most cases
- Dyspnoea or tachypnoea when large fluid accumulation prevents normal respiratory excursions
- Signs related to dysfunction of relevant organ or specific cause of the distension, e.g. obstruction

COMMON CAUSES

Abdominal wall musculature weakness
Hyperadrenocorticism (HAC): pot-belly appearance compounded by fat redistribution and hepatomegaly

Faeces
Constipation/obstipation

Fat
- Diabetes mellitus (DM)
- HAC
- Obesity

Fluid
Ascites, *q.v.* section 2.5
- Exudate
- High-protein, modified transudate
- Low-protein transudate

Haemoperitoneum
- Coagulopathy
- Haemangiosarcoma of liver/spleen
- Traumatic rupture of liver/spleen

Intraluminal
Pyometra

Uroperitoneum
Traumatic rupture of bladder

Gas
Gastric dilatation/volvulus

Mass(es)
q.v. section 2.2
Pregnancy

UNCOMMON CAUSES

Abdominal wall musculature weakness
- Large umbilical hernia
- Malnutrition
- Primary myopathy
- Rupture of prepubic tendon

Fat
Intra-abdominal lipoma

Fluid
Bile peritonitis
Rupture of gall bladder or bile duct(s)

Notes on Canine Internal Medicine, Fourth Edition. Victoria L. Black, Kathryn F. Murphy, Jessie Rose Payne, and Edward J. Hall.
© 2022 John Wiley & Sons Ltd. Published 2022 by John Wiley & Sons Ltd.

Chylous effusion
• Congestion: right heart failure
• Lymphangiectasia ± concurrent chylothorax
• Neoplasia, in particular phaeochromocytoma
• Trauma

Haemoperitoneum
• Peliosis
• Rupture of splenic haematoma

Septic peritonitis
Nocardia/Actinomyces

Uroperitoneum
Traumatic rupture of kidney or ureter

Gas
Pneumoperitoneum
• Penetrating wound
• Post-operative
• Ruptured viscus

Intestinal enlargement
• Dysautonomia
• Food bloat from overeating
• Visceral myopathy (leiomyositis) or neuropathy (mesenteric ganglionitis)

Mass(es)
q.v. section 2.2

DIAGNOSTIC APPROACH

1 Identify free fluid and organomegaly/mass by abdominal palpation and ballottement.
2 Confirm by radiographs, ultrasound and abdominocentesis.
3 Investigate causes of fluid accumulation or organ enlargement, *q.v.* sections 2.2, 2.5

Clinical clues
Predisposition
• Enlarged bladder in breeds predisposed to intervertebral disc disease (IVDD)
• GDV in large/giant, deep-chested dogs
• Haemangiosarcoma in middle-aged German shepherd dogs (GSDs)
• Pancreatic carcinoma in geriatric dogs

History
• Anorexia, collapse and vomiting if uroperitoneum
• Collapse/shock (recurrent/intermittent) if ruptured haemangiosarcoma
• Exercise intolerance with right or congestive heart failure, or cardiac tamponade
• Ingestion of large amount of food, usually stolen, causing food bloat
• Lack of urination if uroperitoneum or urethral obstruction
• Overflow urinary incontinence with atonic bladder
• Possibility of mating if pregnant
• Polyuria/polydipsia (PU/PD) if pyometra
• Pyometra in older unspayed bitches a few weeks after oestrus
• Unproductive retching in GDV

Clinical examination
Visual inspection
• Distended abdomen
• Movement of free fluid
• Tachypnoea/dyspnoea if right heart failure

Physical examination
• Ballottement of free fluid or masses
• Icterus if pancreatic mass obstructing common bile duct or bile peritonitis
• Jugular pulses if right heart failure or cardiac tamponade
• Muffled heart sounds if cardiac tamponade
• Presence of enlarged organ or mass
• Pyrexia if peritonitis or large mass with necrotic centre
• Rectal palpation may reveal paraprostatic cyst
• Tympany if gas
NB: Beware fat redistribution with abdominal muscle weakness in HAC, which can feel like free fluid.

Laboratory findings
Haematology
• Inflammatory leukogram if septic peritonitis or large necrotic mass
• Regenerative (or pre-regenerative) anaemia if bleeding mass

Serum biochemistry
- Azotaemia and hyperkalaemia if uroperitoneum or urinary obstruction
- Raised liver enzyme activities with primary hepatopathy or secondary to inflammatory disease elsewhere in abdomen

Imaging
Plain radiographs
- Abdominal mass
- Chest radiographs should be taken if ascites is present to look for metastatic and cardiac disease; abdominal radiographs will be non-diagnostic due to the presence of fluid
- Dilation and compartmentalization in GDV
- Excessive gastric food accumulation in food bloat
- Fetal skeletons after day 45 of pregnancy

- Loss of detail if free intraperitoneal fluid, and therefore not very helpful in ascites
- Uterine enlargement in pyometra and pregnancy

Ultrasound
- Abdominal mass(es)
- Free fluid
- Organ enlargement/infiltration
- Pyometra or pregnancy
- Torsion of splenic pedicle

Special tests
- Abdominocentesis
- Coagulation profile
- Exploratory laparotomy
- Fine needle aspirate (FNA) or Tru-Cut biopsy of abdominal mass

2.2 ABDOMINAL MASSES

DEFINITION

A solid structure (enlarged organ or discrete mass) within the abdomen identified by palpation, imaging or exploratory surgery.
- Abdominal enlargement (q.v. section 2.1) is not always present as it depends on the size of the mass
- Associated fluid accumulation may be noted
- Prostatomegaly (q.v. section 2.23) will only present as an abdominal mass if it is large enough to move from the pelvic canal

RELATED CLINICAL SIGNS

Signs related to dysfunction of relevant organ

COMMON CAUSES

Gastrointestinal (GI)
- Constipation / obstipation
- Intussusception
- Large foreign body (FB): corn cob, peach stone, pebble
- Reactive mesenteric lymphadenomegaly

Liver
q.v. section 2.8

Spleen
q.v. section 2.28

Uterus
- Pregnancy
- Pyometra

UNCOMMON CAUSES

GI
- Gastric neoplasia: must be large to be palpable
  - Adenocarcinoma
  - Leiomyoma/sarcoma
- Intestinal neoplasia
  - Adenocarcinoma
  - GI stromal tumour (GIST)
  - Histiocytic sarcoma
  - Leiomyoma/sarcoma
  - Lymphoma
- Mesenteric lymphadenomegaly
  - Lymphoma

Gonads
- Ovarian carcinoma
- Tumour of retained testicle
  - Leydig cell
  - Seminoma
  - Sertoli cell

Liver
q.v. section 2.8

Kidney
- Congenital porto-systemic shunt (PSS)
- Neoplasia
  - Carcinoma
  - Haemangiosarcoma
  - Lymphoma
  - Metastatic disease
  - Nephroblastoma
  - Sarcoma

Pancreas
- Adenocarcinoma
- Chronic fibrosing pancreatitis

Spleen
q.v. section 2.28

Uterus
- Leiomyoma/sarcoma
- Mummification

DIAGNOSTIC APPROACH

1 Identify organomegaly/mass by abdominal palpation and ballottement.
2 Confirm by radiographs and ultrasound.
3 FNA, incisional biopsy or excise suspected neoplastic masses

Clinical clues
Predisposition
- Haemangiosarcoma in middle-aged GSDs
- Nephroblastoma in young dogs
- Pancreatic carcinoma in geriatric dogs

History
- Collapse/shock (recurrent/intermittent) if ruptured haemangiosarcoma

- Haemolysis with splenic torsion
- Possibility of mating if pregnant
- PU/PD if pyometra
- Pyometra in older unspayed bitches a few weeks after oestrus

Clinical examination
Visual inspection
- Distended abdomen, especially if associated fluid accumulation
- Feminisation if Sertoli cell tumour in retained testicle
- Very large masses may distort the body wall

Physical examination
- Ballottement of free fluid or masses
- Icterus if pancreatic mass obstructing common bile duct or bile peritonitis
- Presence of enlarged organ or mass
- Pyrexia if large mass with necrotic centre
- Rectal palpation to rule in/out prostate as abdominal mass
  NB: Beware fat redistribution with abdominal muscle weakness in HAC, which can feel like free fluid.

Laboratory findings
Haematology
- Inflammatory leukogram if large necrotic mass
- Regenerative (or pre-regenerative) anaemia if bleeding from mass

Serum biochemistry
Increased liver enzyme activities with primary hepatopathy or secondary to inflammatory disease elsewhere in abdomen or hormonal disease

Imaging
Plain radiographs
- Abdominal mass
- Chest radiographs to look for metastatic disease
- Fetal skeletons after day 45 of pregnancy
- Loss of detail if free intraperitoneal fluid, and therefore not very helpful in ascites
- Uterine enlargement in pyometra and pregnancy

Ultrasound
- Abdominal masses
- Free fluid
- Organ enlargement/infiltration
- Pyometra or pregnancy
- Torsion of splenic pedicle

Special tests
- Abdominocentesis
- Coagulation profile
- Exploratory laparotomy
- FNA or Tru-Cut biopsy of abdominal mass

2.3 ABNORMAL LUNG SOUNDS

DEFINITION

Areas of dullness
Areas where normal bronchovesicular sounds cannot be heard
- Areas of dullness can be focal or across all rib spaces dorsal or ventral to a line
- Can be due to pleural fluid, pneumothorax or soft tissue structures without normal air entry

Crackles
High-pitched, brief, discontinuous lung sounds that can resemble popping sounds or a crisp packet being scrunched up
- Can be inspiratory, expiratory or both; inspiratory is more common
- Can be coarse or fine
  - Coarse crackles often occur when there are excessive intraluminal secretions in the large upper airways
  - Fine crackles often occur when an obstruction prevents the smaller airways from opening immediately, the crackle occurs as the airway opens up; the obstruction may be due to cellular infiltrate or fluid accumulation within the pulmonary interstitial spaces, or severe interstitial fibrosis

Wheezes
'Musical' sounds that, compared to crackles, are much longer in duration
- Result from vibrations of airway walls due to increased resistance to airflow – resistance can be due to reactive or thickened airways or airway compression from pulmonary disease

RELATED CLINICAL SIGNS

- Cough
- Cyanosis
- Exercise intolerance/lethargy
- Haemoptysis
- Syncope
- Varying degrees of dyspnoea and tachypnoea

COMMON CAUSES

Areas of dullness
Focal
- Neoplasia
- Pneumonia

Dorsal to a line
Pneumothorax, *q.v.* section 2.22

Ventral to a line: pleural effusion
- Chylothorax (can be modified transudate or exudate)
  - Idiopathic
  - Traumatic thoracic duct rupture
- Exudate
  - Neoplasia
    - Mediastinal: lymphoma
    - Pulmonary masses
  - Pyothorax
    - Migrating FB
    - *Nocardia*, *Actinomyces*
- Haemothorax
  - Coagulopathy
  - Neoplasia
  - Trauma

PHYSICAL ABNORMALITIES

- Modified transudate
  - Neoplasia
  - Pericardial effusion and tamponade
  - Transudate (hydrothorax)
- Hypoalbuminaemia
  - Hepatic failure
  - Protein-losing enteropathy (PLE)
  - Protein-losing nephropathy (PLN)

Crackles

- Bronchitis (chronic bronchitis or eosinophilic bronchopneumopathy)
- Pulmonary oedema
  - Cardiogenic
  - Non-cardiogenic
    - Electrocution (e.g. secondary to chewing electrical cords)
    - Near choking
    - Near drowning
    - Smoke inhalation
- Pneumonia and bronchopneumonia
  - Aspiration
  - Bacterial
  - Viral
- Pulmonary fibrosis

Wheezes

- Bronchitis (chronic bronchitis or eosinophilic bronchopneumopathy)

UNCOMMON CAUSES

Areas of dullness
Focal
- Atelectasis
- Lung lobe torsion
- Ruptured diaphragm with organ entrapment

Dorsal to a line
- Pneumothorax, *q.v.* section 2.22

Ventral to a line: pleural effusion,
q.v. section 2.21
- Chylothorax
  - Congenital
  - Dirofilariasis
  - Jugular vein thrombosis (after cannulation)
  - Neoplasia
  - Right-sided congestive heart failure (less commonly primary cardiac *cf.* cat)

- Exudate
  - Neoplasia
    - Heart base
    - Mediastinal: thymoma
    - Mesothelioma
    - Rib chondrosarcoma, osteosarcoma
  - Pyothorax
    - Penetrating wound (chest wall or oesophagus)
    - Parapneumonic effusion, i.e. extension of pulmonary infection
  - Sterile inflammation
    - Dirofilariasis
    - Lung lobe torsion; can occur secondary to other primary cause of effusion
    - Eosinophilic pulmonary granulomatosis
    - Ruptured diaphragm with organ entrapment
    - Pancreatitis (small volume)
    - Walled-off abscess
- Haemothorax
  - Lung lobe torsion, when lung lobe becomes necrotic
  - Necrotic neoplasm
    - Mesothelioma
    - Thymus
- Modified transudate
  - Right-sided congestive heart failure (rare)
  - Vasculitis
  - Post-partum (small volume)
  - Pulmonary thromboembolism (PTE) (small volume)
  - Pyometra (small volume)
  - Ruptured diaphragm
  - Secondary to abdominal surgery (small volume)
- Transudate (hydrothorax)
  - Right-sided congestive heart failure (rare)

Crackles
- Non-cardiogenic pulmonary oedema
  - Acute respiratory distress syndrome (ARDS)
  - Sepsis
  - Snake bites
  - Upper airway obstruction
- Fungal pneumonia and bronchopneumonia
- Pulmonary hypertension

Wheezes
- Neoplasia causing obstruction to small airways
- Pulmonary hypertension

DIAGNOSTIC APPROACH

1 Percussion
   - Hyper-resonant: pneumothorax
   - Dull: pleural effusion, consolidated lung, mass
2 Thoracic ultrasound to look for pleural effusion or B lines and basic cardiac assessment.
3 If effusion is present, obtain a sample of effusion for analysis after ruling out generalised coagulopathy.
4 Thoracic imaging (after thoracocentesis if required); radiographs initially, but computer tomography (CT) may be more sensitive.
5 Bronchoscopy ± bronchoalveolar lavage.
6 Identify the underlying cause from fluid analysis and imaging results.

Clinical clues
Predisposition
- Cardiogenic pulmonary oedema secondary to dilated cardiomyopathy in middle-aged, large-breed dogs
- Cardiogenic pulmonary oedema secondary to myxomatous mitral valve disease in older, small-breed dogs
- Idiopathic chylothorax in Afghan hound, Borzoi
- Migrating FB e.g. grass awn in working spaniels
- Pulmonary fibrosis in West Highland White terrier (WHWT)

History
- Access to anticoagulant rodenticide
- Chewing of electrical cables/near drowning/strangulation/smoke inhalation
- Coughing
- Jugular catheterisation
- Previous trauma causing penetrating wound, pneumothorax or ruptured diaphragm
- Signs of underlying causes of hypoalbuminaemia

Clinical examination
Visual inspection
- Dyspnoea, tachypnoea
- Evidence of generalised bleeding

- Jugular pulsation with right-sided congestive heart failure
- Respiratory effort, including phase of respiration where effort is increased
  - Upper respiratory tract disease: increased inspiratory effort ± noise
  - Lower respiratory tract disease: increased expiratory effort ± noise

Physical examination
- Palpation
  - Chest wall mass
  - Displacement of apex beat by intrathoracic mass
  - Displacement of trachea from midline of thoracic inlet by intrathoracic mass
  - Jugular thrombosis
- Auscultation
  - Arrhythmias with dilated cardiomyopathy (DCM) (not all cases)
  - Crackles
  - Dull lung sounds – either focally, ventrally or dorsally
  - Murmurs with myxomatous mitral valve disease and some cases of DCM
  - Wheezes
- Percussion
  - Pleural effusion: dull ventrally
  - Pneumothorax: hyper-resonant dorsally

Laboratory findings
Haematology
- Inflammatory leukogram if pyothorax or necrotic tumour

Serum biochemistry
- Changes characteristic of underlying systemic disease

Urinalysis
- Proteinuria if PLN

Imaging
Plain radiographs
Performed after ultrasound to rule out pleural effusion; drain effusions first to get best-quality radiographs. Need to assess patient stability when restraining for radiographs.
- Dorso-ventral (DV), left lateral and right lateral ideally to assess:

- bronchial, interstitial or alveolar patterns
- cardiac silhouette
- displacement of normal intra-thoracic structures
- pulmonary venous distension
- soft tissue opacities within lung fields
- Cardiogenic pulmonary oedema diagnosis requires presence of all three:
  1 Cardiomegaly
  2 Interstitial or alveolar pattern; initially peri-hilar in dogs but will spread with increased severity
  3 Pulmonary venous distension
- Lung lobe torsion causes displacement of mainstem bronchi
- Mediastinal mass seen as soft tissue density cranial to heart and displacing trachea dorsally
- Pleural fluid
  NB: Intrathoracic fat or skin fold may mimic effusion.
  - Obscured cardiac and diaphragmatic outline
  - Pleural fissure lines
  - Retraction of lung lobes from thoracic wall
  - Ultrasound is a safer modality to detect effusions, and can detect smaller volumes than radiographs
- Pneumothorax
  - Lung lobe atelectasis/collapse (appearing more radiopaque than normal) – there may be a space between collapsed lungs and pleura
  - Lifting of the cardiac silhouette from the sternum

Ultrasound
- Absence of glide sign is suggestive of pneumothorax

- Echocardiography to assess for structural cardiac causes
- Identification of mass
- Identify pleural fluid and B lines implying fluid within alveolar spaces
- Used to guide thoracocentesis, FNA and needle biopsy

Special tests
- Analysis of pleural fluid
  - Cell numbers and morphology
    - Lymphocytes (chylothorax, lymphoma, thymoma)
    - Neoplastic cells
    - Neutrophils
      - Degenerate: pyothorax
      - Non-degenerate: inflammation, neoplasia
  - Culture
  - Fluid cholesterol < serum, and fluid triglyceride > serum if chylothorax
  - Gram stain for pyothorax
  - Packed cell volume (PCV)
  - Protein
  - Specific gravity (SG)
- Bronchoscopy
- Bronchoalveolar lavage
  - Cytology
  - Culture/ PCR
  - Lungworm testing
- Coagulation profile
- CT may be required in cases where thoracic radiographs are unremarkable
- Exploratory thoracotomy
- FNA and needle biopsy
- Thoracocentesis
  - May be negative if loculated or thick exudate

2.4 ARRHYTHMIAS

DEFINITION

An abnormal, irregular heart rhythm.
- Arrhythmias can take the form of single abnormal beats, paroxysms (short bursts) or sustained rhythm disturbances

- Arrhythmias can have a primary cardiac cause or can be secondary to systemic diseases
- Arrhythmias are broadly grouped into
  - Bradyarrhythmias

- Heart rate is too slow, generally less than 60 bpm
  - Atrioventricular block (first, second and third)
  - Sick sinus syndrome
  - Persistent atrial standstill
- Tachyarrhythmias:
  - Heart rate is too fast, generally greater than 180 bpm
    - Atrial fibrillation
    - Supraventricular premature complexes
    - Supraventricular tachycardia
    - Ventricular premature complexes
    - Ventricular tachycardia
    - (Accelerated idioventricular rhythm)

RELATED CLINICAL SIGNS

No clinical signs may be evident.
- Lethargy
- Intermittent collapse episodes
- Signs of congestive heart failure
  - Tachypnoea
  - Dyspnoea
  - Abdominal distension
- Signs related to underlying disease, e.g. vomiting with hypoadrenocorticism

COMMON CAUSES

Bradyarrhythmias
- Primary cardiac
  - Myocardial fibrosis
- Elevated vagal tone
  - Gastrointestinal disease
  - Increased intracranial pressure
  - Mediastinal disease
  - Upper respiratory tract obstruction/brachycephalic conformation
- Drugs
  - Digoxin
  - Beta blockers
  - Alpha 2 agonists
- Metabolic disturbances
  - Hyperkalaemia (hypoadrenocorticism, urinary obstruction)
  - Hypothyroidism

Tachyarrhythmias
- Primary cardiac
  - Arrhythmogenic right ventricular cardiomyopathy (ARVC)
  - DCM
  - Myxomatous mitral valve disease
- Metabolic disturbances
  - Acidosis
  - Hypercalcaemia
  - Hypokalaemia
  - Hypoxia
- Others
  - Hypotension
  - Infection
  - Pain
  - Pyrexia
  - Renal failure
  - Splenic disease

UNCOMMON CAUSES

Bradyarrhythmias
- Primary cardiac
  - Myocarditis
  - Neoplastic infiltration of the conduction system
- Elevated vagal tone
  - Increased intra-cranial pressure
  - Mediastinal mass
  - Vagal nerve damage
- Drugs
  - Calcium channel blockers
  - Narcotics
  - Procainamide
- Metabolic disturbances
  - Hyperkalaemia: urinary rupture and uroperitoneum
  - Hypocalcaemia
  - Hypothermia

Tachyarrhythmias
- Primary cardiac
  - Myocarditis
  - Neoplastic infiltration of the conduction system
  - Inherited ventricular arrhythmias of the GSD

- Bypass tract-mediated supraventricular tachycardia (orthodromic atrioventricular (AV) reciprocating tachycardia)
- Drugs
  - Atropine
  - Glycopyrrolate
  - Theobromine (chocolate poisoning)
  - Thyroxine
- Metabolic disturbances
  - Alkalosis
  - Hyperthyroidism
  - Hypocalcaemia
  - Hypomagnesaemia
- Other
  - Phaeochromocytoma

DIAGNOSTIC APPROACH

- ECG is required to further characterise the arrhythmia
- Full cardiac evaluation (echocardiography, blood pressure measurement, 24-hour ECG Holter monitoring) if underlying disease is not found
- Full drug history is important
- Laboratory testing to rule out metabolic disturbances
- Some arrhythmias are transient and related to obvious disease states, and can be ignored
- Treat the arrhythmia if it is causing, or likely to cause, clinical signs

Clinical clues
Predisposition
- ARVC: Boxers
- Bypass tract-mediated supraventricular tachycardia: Labradors, Boxers
- DCM: large-breed dogs
- Myxomatous mitral valve disease: older, small-breed dogs
- Pronounced sinus arrhythmia with first-degree AV block and sinus pauses can be commonly found in brachycephalic patients
- Sick sinus syndrome in Miniature schnauzer and WHWT
- Third-degree atrioventricular block is more common in older dogs

History
- Episodes of syncope/lethargy
- Drug exposure
- Signs of underlying disease
- GI disease: vomiting and diarrhoea
- Hypoadrenocorticism: collapse, vomiting, diarrhoea, weight loss
- Hypothyroidism: lethargy, coat changes, weight gain
- Intracranial disease: neurological deficits
- Urinary obstruction: collapse, vomiting, dysuria

Clinical examination
Visual inspection
Episodes of weakness/collapse/syncope

Physical examination
- Auscultation
  - Arrhythmias may be intermittent or persistent
  - May hear a murmur secondary to underlying cardiac disease
- Hypothermia
- Palpation
  - Altered pulse rate and quality
- Pyrexia if endocarditis

Laboratory findings
Haematology
- Often unremarkable
- Inflammatory leukogram may be seen with endocarditis
- Normocytic, normochromic anaemia in hypothyroidism

Serum biochemistry
- Increases in ALT activity, urea and creatinine may be seen if there is sustained reduction in cardiac output
- Hypocalcaemia
- Hyperkalaemia and azotaemia if urinary obstruction
- Hyperkalaemia and hyponatraemia if hypoadrenocorticism

Urinalysis
- Generally unremarkable

Imaging
Plain radiographs
- Size and shape of heart
- State of pulmonary vasculature
- Presence of pulmonary oedema
- Presence of any intrathoracic mass

Ultrasound examination
- Thoracic ultrasound
  - Presence of pleural effusion
- Echocardiography
  - Blood flow and turbulence
  - Size of heart chambers
  - State of cardiac muscle
- Abdominal ultrasound
  - Presence of ascites

- Assess spleen, liver, adrenals, bladder for arrhythmia triggers

Special tests
- ACTH stimulation test
- Atropine response test
- Blood cultures
- Blood pressure (BP) measurement
- Electrophysiology studies
- Exercise test
- Lyme serology
- Neurological examination
- Serum digoxin concentration
- Thyroid function tests
- Troponin I
- 24-hour Holter ECG
- 24-hour urinary catecholamines

2.5   ASCITES

DEFINITION

Ascites is the accumulation of free fluid within the peritoneal cavity.

It can be due to the accumulation of:
- low-protein transudate – due to hypoalbuminaemia (< 15 g/l)
- high-protein modified transudate – due to portal hypertension
- exudates – due to septic and non-septic inflammation

or may contain:
- bile
- blood
- chyle
- urine

RELATED CLINICAL SIGNS

- Abdominal distension is most likely with transudate or non-septic exudate; other signs usually occur with other causes of ascites before large volumes can accumulate
- Concurrent pleural effusion and/or subcutaneous oedema may be present if hypoalbuminaemic
- Respiratory embarrassment if massive ascites

- Signs related to primary cause of fluid accumulation, e.g. jaundice in liver failure

COMMON CAUSES

Blood
- Generalised clotting factor disorder
- Ruptured haemangiosarcoma
- Traumatic splenic or hepatic rupture

Low-protein transudate (hypoalbuminaemia)
Hepatic disease
- Chronic hepatitis/cirrhosis, but often with concurrent portal hypertension

Protein-losing enteropathy
- Chronic inflammatory enteropathy (CIE), inflammatory bowel disease (IBD)

Protein-losing nephropathy
- Glomerulonephritis

High-protein, modified transudate (portal hypertension)
Cardiac tamponade (pericardial effusion)
- Idiopathic pericardial haemorrhage
- Right atrial haemangiosarcoma

Hepatic disease
- Chronic hepatopathy/cirrhosis

Right-sided heart failure
- DCM
- Valvular heart disease

Exudate – inflammatory
Non-septic
- Carcinomatosis
- Pancreatitis

Septic
- GI perforation
- Ruptured pyometra

Urine
- Ruptured bladder

UNCOMMON CAUSES

Blood
- Amyloidosis
- Iatrogenic following FNA or biopsy
- Peliosis

Low-protein transudate
Hepatic disease
- Congenital PSS (NB: no portal hypertension present)
- Portal vein thrombosis

Protein-losing enteropathy (PLE)
- Alimentary lymphoma
- Lymphangiectasia
- Systemic aspergillosis in immunosuppressed dogs
- Histoplasmosis (not in UK)
- Pythiosis and other phycomycoses (not in UK)

Protein-losing nephropathy (PLN)
- Renal amyloidosis

High-protein, modified transudate (portal hypertension)
Cardiac tamponade
- Heart-base tumour
- Restrictive pericarditis

Caudal vena cava (CVC) compression/obstruction
- Caval syndrome (dirofilariasis)
- Cor triatrium dexter
- 'Kinked' CVC
- CVC thrombosis

Liver disease
- Lobular dissecting hepatitis
- Non-cirrhotic portal hypertension (idiopathic juvenile hepatic fibrosis) due to portal vein hypoplasia

Non-septic
- Mesothelioma

Post-hepatic obstruction
- *Angiostrongylus*
- Budd-Chiari syndrome
- Diaphragmatic rupture and liver entrapment
- *Dirofilaria*
- Intra-cardiac neoplasia
- Veno-occlusive disease

Exudate – inflammatory
Bile
- Gallstones and/or cholecystitis causing spontaneous perforation of biliary tract
- Perforated proximal duodenal ulcer
- Rupture of biliary mucocoele
- Traumatic rupture of gall bladder or extra-hepatic biliary tree

Chyle (lymphatic obstruction or leakage)
- Intestinal obstruction
- Lymphangiectasia
  - Idiopathic
  - Obstruction
    - Right heart failure
    - Phaeochromocytoma

Non-septic
- Pansteatitis

Septic
- *Nocardia/Actinomyces*
- Penetrating wound
- Ruptured abscess
- Volvulus/infarction of GI tract

Urine
• Ruptured kidney and/or ureters

DIAGNOSTIC APPROACH

1 Distinguish free fluid from other causes of abdominal enlargement (*q.v.* section 2.1) by ballottement ± ultrasound examination
2 Abdominocentesis for fluid collection, and classification based on laboratory analysis, cytological examination and culture

	Transu-date	Modified transu-date	Exu-date
Specific gravity	< 1.017	1.017–1.025	> 1.025
Protein (g/l)	< 25	25–60	> 25
Nucleated cells/mm³	< 1,000	< 7,000	> 7,000
Cytology			Neutro-phils

3 Investigation of relevant organ system depending on specific type of fluid and other clinical signs
• For bile peritonitis, compare fluid:serum bilirubin
• For modified transudate, check for right heart failure, cardiac tamponade, liver disease and neoplasia
• For septic exudate, perform bacterial culture, measure fluid glucose and lactate and look for intracellular bacteria
• For transudate, check causes of hypoalbuminaemia, especially PLE and PLN
• For uroabdomen, compare fluid:serum creatinine

Clinical clues
Predisposition
• Cardiac tamponade in large-/giant-breed dogs
• Chronic liver disease in certain pure-bred dogs, e.g. Dobermann, Cocker spaniel, GSD
• DCM in giant-breed dogs

• CIE/IBD in GSD, Shar pei
• Lymphangiectasia in toy breeds and Rottweiler

History
• GI signs and hypoalbuminaemia consistent with PLE
• Intermittent weakness/collapse consistent with recurrent haemorrhage from bleeding haemangiosarcoma or idiopathic pericardial haemorrhage
• Previous trauma
• Signs consistent with liver disease – anorexia, encephalopathy, jaundice, etc.

Clinical examination
Visual inspection
• Abdominal enlargement
• Dyspnoea if massive ascites
• Extended jugular pulse suggestive of right heart failure
• Jaundice if bile peritonitis

Physical examination
• Fluid wave on ballottement
• Hepatojugular reflux in right heart failure
• Muffled heart sounds if cardiac tamponade
• Murmur if primary valvular disease or advanced DCM
• Weak peripheral pulse if DCM or cardiac tamponade

Laboratory findings
Haematology
• Regenerative anaemia if recurrent bleeding from haemangiosarcoma
• Inappropriate numbers of nucleated RBCs suggest splenic pathology
• Leukocytosis, and perhaps a degenerative left shift, if septic peritonitis

Serum biochemistry
• Azotaemia and hyperkalaemia if uroabdomen
• Hyperbilirubinaemia if liver disease or ruptured biliary tree
• Hypocalcaemia secondary to hypoproteinaemia
• Hypoproteinaemia

PHYSICAL ABNORMALITIES

	Albumin	Globulin
Protein-losing enteropathy	Low	Low (increased if severe inflammatory disease)
Protein-losing nephropathy	Low	Normal
Liver disease	Low	Normal/increased

Serum bile acids to assess hepatic function

Imaging
Radiographs
Plain
- Abdominal films are generally unhelpful due to loss of detail by free abdominal fluid
- Chest radiographs to evaluate pleural effusion, heart silhouette and lung patterns
  Contrast
- Barium meal can outline position of stomach and hence indicate liver size

Ultrasound
- Abdominal masses

- Free fluid
- Heart function
- Hepatic and splenic abnormalities
- Pericardial effusion

Special tests
- Abdominal fluid analysis
  - Cell count
  - Cholesterol < serum, and triglyceride > serum if chyloabdomen
  - Cytology – sepsis, neoplasia
  - Creatinine > serum indicates uroperitoneum
  - Glucose < plasma indicates sepsis
  - Gram stain for bacteria: septic peritonitis
  - PCV/RBC count for haemoperitoneum
  - Protein
  - Specific gravity
- Coagulation times
- Knott's and occult heartworm test
- Endoscopic intestinal biopsy
- Exploratory laparotomy and hepatic or intestinal biopsy
- FNA of intrabdominal mass
- Pericardiocentesis

2.6 CYANOSIS

DEFINITION

A bluish colour, most visible in the mucous membranes, nail beds and hairless skin, caused by excessive desaturation of haemoglobin in the blood. Adequate levels of haemoglobin are present, but inadequate levels of oxygenation. Oxygen saturations are usually less than 75% for cyanosis to be obvious.

The origin of cyanosis can be:
- Central, from arterial hypoxaemia
  - Problems with oxygenation (respiratory disease) or a right-to-left shunt of blood within the circulation so deoxygenated blood mixes with oxygenated blood
  - Respiratory disease is a more common cause of cyanosis than cardiac shunts

- Peripheral due to low tissue oxygenation despite normal arterial oxygen saturation
  - Methaemoglobinaemia
  - Local circulatory problems (vasoconstriction, arterial or venous obstruction)

RELATED CLINICAL SIGNS

- Visual detection of cyanosis is notoriously unreliable; severe hypoxaemia can exist without cyanosis
  - In general at least 50 g/l or 5% of haemoglobin must be desaturated for cyanosis to be visible
  - When Hb concentration is normal, the PaO_2 must be below 50 mmHg

- When Hb concentration is low (anaemia), the PaO_2 must be even lower to produce 50 g/L of reduced-Hb
- When Hb concentration is high (erythrocytosis), cyanosis will occur at a PaO_2 above 50 mmHg, but erythrocytosis may also be a consequence of hypoxaemia
- Dyspnoea and tachypnoea
- Exercise intolerance, weakness, syncope
- Extremities are cold and cyanotic
- Cyanosis can be generalised or localised to one area of the body

COMMON CAUSES

Central
Pulmonary disease
- Brachycephalic obstructive airway disease
- Laryngeal paralysis
- Metastatic pulmonary neoplasia
- Pleural effusion
- Pneumothorax
- Pulmonary oedema – cardiac and non-cardiac
- Pulmonary thromboembolism (PTE)

Neurological – depressed respiration
Anaesthesia

Peripheral
Physiological
- Cold exposure
- Shock (intense peripheral vasoconstriction rather than true cyanosis)

UNCOMMON CAUSES

Central
Pulmonary disease
- Asthma (rare in dog cf. cat)
- Atelectasis
  - Compression following ruptured diaphragm
  - Lung lobe torsion
- Collapsing trachea (severe)
- Laryngeal oedema

- Laryngeal neoplasia
- Lung lobe consolidation
- Pneumonia (severe)
- Primary pulmonary neoplasia (extensive)
- Pulmonary fibrosis
  - Idiopathic progressive interstitial fibrosis
  - Paraquat poisoning

Cardiovascular disease
- Reverse PDA: differential cyanosis, i.e. only caudal mucous membranes are cyanotic
- Reverse VSD
- Tetralogy of Fallot

Neurological – depressed respiration
- Central nervous system (CNS) disease affecting medulla or upper cervical spinal cord
- Increased intracranial pressure

Peripheral
Arterial obstruction
- Thromboembolism
  - HAC
  - Hypoalbuminaemia: PLE or PLN
  - Immune-mediated haemolytic anaemia (IMHA)
- Tourniquet application

Methaemoglobinaemia
- Congenital haemoglobin abnormality
- Paracetamol (rare cf. cat)

Venous obstruction
- Thrombophlebitis
- Tourniquet

DIAGNOSTIC APPROACH

1. History and physical examination to identify drug exposure and cardiorespiratory disease.
2. If localised cyanosis, examine regional pulse.
3. Arterial blood gas to determine oxygen saturation levels.
4. Echocardiography.

PHYSICAL ABNORMALITIES

Clinical clues

Predisposition

- Congenital cardiovascular disease in puppies
  - Patent ductus arteriosus: Poodle, Cocker spaniel, GSD
  - Tetralogy of Fallot: English Bulldog and Keeshond
- Idiopathic interstitial pulmonary fibrosis: WHWT

History

- Neurological signs with CNS disease
- Hindlimb collapse at exercise with reverse patent ductus arteriosus (PDA)

Clinical examination

Visual inspection

- Cyanotic mucous membranes
- Dyspnoea and tachypnoea

Physical examination

- Differential cyanosis, i.e. pink oral mucous membranes, but cyanotic caudally (prepuce, vulva), in a young animal with a reverse PDA
- Neurological deficits
- Stridor
- Palpation
  - Absent pulses in thromboembolism
  - Weak pulses in congestive heart failure
- Auscultation
  - Muffled heart sounds with pneumothorax
  - Murmurs
  - Pulmonary adventitious sounds
  - Stridor

Laboratory findings

Haematology

- Brown discolouration of blood that does not turn red on shaking with air suggests methaemoglobinaemia
- Erythrocytosis secondary to hypoxaemia

Serum biochemistry

- Hypoalbuminaemia in PLE, PLN

Urinalysis

- Proteinuria in PLN

Imaging

Plain radiographs

- Cardiac silhouette to assess generalised or localised cardiomegaly
- Pneumothorax
- Pulmonary parenchymal disease

Ultrasonography

- To assess for pleural effusion
- Echocardiography to assess for acquired and congenital cardiac defects (may require bubble study) and pulmonary hypertension

Special tests

- Blood gas analysis
  - Calculate alveolar-arterial oxygen difference
  - Measure PaO_2
- CT for PTE
- Coombs' test
- Faecal analysis for *Angiostrongylus*

2.7 EYE LESIONS

DEFINITION

Abnormalities of the eye visible either to the naked eye or with ophthalmoscopic examination.

Changes may be a sign of systemic illness or local disease affecting one or more parts of the eye:

1 Cornea: opacity due to focal or diffuse abnormality preventing the transmission of light, *q.v.* section 1.12

2 Anterior chamber: accumulation of blood, fibrin, lipids or WBCs

3 Iris: atrophy, inflammation, abnormal pigmentation or neoplasia

4 Lens: diffuse or focal loss of transparency

5 Vitreous: diffuse or focal loss of transparency

6 Retina: changes in attachment, pigmentation, tapetal reflection or vascularity usually only visible with ophthalmoscopy, and potentially resulting in blindness, *q.v.* section 1.10

RELATED CLINICAL SIGNS

- Aqueous flare caused by fibrinous deposits in anterior uveitis
- Blepharospasm and epiphora if ocular pain
- Diffuse or focal changes in colour, opacity or size of the eyeball, cornea, anterior chamber, pupil (iris), lens, vitreous or retina
- Reduced visual acuity, especially in low ambient light (night blindness), or total blindness *q.v.* section 1.10
- Strabismus and nystagmus (*q.v.* section 1.33) indicate vestibular and/or intracranial disease

COMMON CAUSES

Cornea
q.v. section 1.12

Anterior chamber (aqueous humor)
- Anterior uveitis
  - Idiopathic
  - Secondary to systemic inflammatory disease
- Hypopyon (infection in anterior chamber)
  - FB penetration
- Hyphaema
  - Coagulopathy (thrombocytopenia)
  - Trauma

Iris
- Abnormal colouration
  - Merle – normal but can be associated with other congenital defects, e.g. coloboma
- Anisocoria
  - Asymmetric iris atrophy – gives false appearance of dilated pupil
  - Unilateral Horner's syndrome – miosis of affected eye, *q.v.* section 2.9
- Miosis
  - Anterior uveitis
  - Bright ambient light
  - Horner's syndrome, *q.v.* section 2.9
  - Ocular pain
  - Opioids
- Mydriasis
  - Atropine
  - Bilateral iris atrophy, giving false appearance of dilated pupils

- Closed-angle glaucoma
- Dark environment
- Fear/stress (sympathetic tone)
- Optic neuritis
- Retinal blindness: pupillary light responses (PLRs) will be intact with cortical blindness, but menace response will be absent
  - Retinal degeneration
  - Retinal detachment

Lens opacities
- Cataracts
  - DM
  - Genetic
  - Lens luxation: inherited, traumatic
- Lenticular nuclear sclerosis

Vitreous
- Asteroid hyalosis
- Floaters due to posterior vitreal detachment

Retina
- Detachment
  - Chorioretinitis – often occurs with anterior uveitis
  - Systemic hypertension
- Retinal atrophy/degeneration/dysplasia/dystrophy
  - Glaucoma
  - Inherited
  - Trauma
- Vascular tortuosity and/or haemorrhage
  - Chorioretinitis

UNCOMMON CAUSES

Cornea
- *q.v.* section 1.12

Anterior chamber (aqueous humor)
- Anterior uveitis: fibrinous deposits causing aqueous flare
  - Infection
    - Brucellosis
    - Distemper
    - Ehrlichiosis
    - Intraocular larva migrans
    - Systemic mycoses
    - Prototshecosis

- Septicaemia
- Toxoplasmosis
- Lens luxation
- Trauma
- Uveo-dermatologic syndrome
- Hyphaema
  - Intra-ocular neoplasia
- Hypopyon
  - Lymphoma
  - Infection
- Lipaemia

Iris
- Abnormal colouration
  - Albinism
  - Ocular melanosis
- Anisocoria
  - Any uncommon cause of unilateral mydriasis or miosis listed below
  - CNS diseases
- Miosis
  - Iridocyclitis
  - Organophosphate poisoning
  - Posterior synechiae (can also cause mydriasis)
- Mydriasis
  - Bromide toxicosis
  - Coloboma
  - Diffuse iris mass – lymphoma, diffuse melanoma
  - Dysautonomia
  - Exposure to toxic plants containing muscarinic alkaloids
  - Intracranial disease
  - Iris hypoplasia
  - Posterior synechiae (can also cause miosis)
  - Proptosed eyeball
  - Retrobulbar haemorrhage
  - Retrobulbar neoplasia

Lens opacities
- Electric shock
- Hypocalcaemia
- Nutritional

Vitreous
- Haemorrhage due to retinal detachment
- Hyalitis
  - Numerous infectious agents
  - Penetrating injury

Retina
- Detachment
  - Dysplasia
  - Hereditary/congenital
  - Neoplasia
- Haemorrhage
  - Thrombocytopenia
- Infectious chorioretinitis
  - Agents as for anterior uveitis
- Optic disc swollen and protuberant with fuzzy edge
  - Increased intracranial pressure; inconsistent sign
  - Optic neuritis
- Sudden acquired retinal degeneration syndrome (SARDS)
- Vascular tortuosity and/or haemorrhage
  - Hyperviscosity
    - Primary erythrocytosis (polycythaemia vera)
    - Multiple myeloma, particularly Waldenström's macroglobulinaemia (IgM myeloma)
- Vitamin E deficiency

DIAGNOSTIC APPROACH

- Examine cornea
- Fluorescein staining
- Full ophthalmoscopic examination
- Palpebral and corneal reflexes
- Schirmer tear test

Clinical clues
- Bilateral changes are more likely with metabolic and inflammatory conditions; unilateral changes are more likely with neoplasia or trauma
- Cataracts block the tapetal reflection whereas lenticular nuclear sclerosis does not
- Diabetic cataracts often develop rapidly
- Unilateral Horner's syndrome is characterised by anisocoria (miosis of affected eye), ptosis, enophthalmos and prominent nictitans *q.v.* section 2.9

Predisposition
- Cataracts in DM
- Coloboma: Australian shepherds and collies

- Idiopathic Horner's syndrome common in Golden retrievers
- Inherited retinal atrophy/degeneration/dysplasia/dystrophy in a large number of pure-bred dogs
- Iris hypoplasia: Dalmatians
- Lenticular nuclear sclerosis in older dogs
- Merle colouration: sheepdogs
- Ocular melanosis: Cairn terriers
- Uveodermatologic syndrome: Akitas and Arctic breeds

History
- Gradual or sudden-onset blindness
- Previous corneal ulceration or trauma
- Signs of diabetes mellitus: PU/PD, etc.
- Signs of hypothyroidism: lethargy, etc.

Clinical examination
Visual inspection
- Abnormal corneal or iris colour
- Blepharospasm and/or epiphora if ulcerated
- Buphthalmos in open-angle glaucoma
- Changes in pupil size or pigmentation
- Chemosis
- Cloudy appearance to pupil in lenticular nuclear sclerosis
- Corneal ulcer
- Increased tapetal reflectivity with retinal atrophy
- Ocular discharge
- White lipid deposits in cornea

Physical examination
- Abnormal colouring or opacity of part of the ocular light path
  NB: Cataracts, but not lenticular sclerosis, impair visualization of tapetal reflection
- Abnormal pupillary light reflexes

- Chorioretinitis manifests as retinal oedema, retinal vascular changes (e.g. tortuosity or vasculitis, intraretinal, preretinal or vitreal hemorrhages), and retinal detachment; vision may be impaired
- Exophthalmos in brachycephalics and with retrobulbar lesion
- Melanocytic tumours are diagnosed based on typical appearance and clinical signs: changes in iris color and/or a visible mass raised from the surface of the iris are typical. Additional signs may include:
  - Dyscoria
  - Glaucoma secondary to uveitis
    - Retinal detachment and blindness may also be noted in advanced stages
    - Raised intraocular pressure in glaucoma
  - Hyphaema
  - Uveitis in advanced stages
- Raised intraocular pressure in glaucoma

Laboratory findings
- Hyperglobulinaemia or erythrocytosis with hyperviscosity syndrome
- Hyperglycaemia and glucosuria with diabetic cataracts
- Hyperlipidaemia: hypertriglyceridaemia and/or hypercholesterolaemia with lipid deposit

Imaging
- Full ophthalmic examination
- Ultrasound examination of posterior chamber and retrobulbar space

Special tests
- Pharmacological testing (topical pilocarpine, phenylephrine)
- Thyroid function tests
- Tonometry

2.8 HEPATOMEGALY

DEFINITION

Hepatomegaly is enlargement of the liver.
- The normally sized liver lies within the costal arch and is generally not palpable

- An enlarged liver is palpable and/or visible on radiographs (*q.v.* section 4.1.1)
NB: Young animals have relative hepatomegaly normally.

RELATED CLINICAL SIGNS

- Enlarged liver may cause abdominal enlargement with a pot-belly appearance
- May be asymptomatic
- Rapid, shallow breathing through chest compression if massive
- Signs related to underlying cardiac, endocrine or liver disease

COMMON CAUSES

Generalised
Congestion
- Pericardial tamponade
- Right heart failure: DCM, tricuspid regurgitation

Infiltrative disease
- Extramedullary haematopoiesis
- Primary neoplasia
  - Haemangiosarcoma
  - Hepatocellular carcinoma
- Metastatic neoplasia
- Nodular hyperplasia
- Reticuloendothelial hyperplasia (chronic infectious/inflammatory diseases)
  - IMHA
  - Immune-mediated thrombocytopenia (IMTP)

Drugs
- Barbiturates
- Iatrogenic steroid administration

Endocrinopathy
- Hepatic lipidosis
  - DM
  - Obesity
- Steroid hepatopathy
  - HAC
  - Iatrogenic

UNCOMMON CAUSES

- Neoplasia

Generalised
Congestion
- Budd-Chiari-like syndrome (occlusion of hepatic veins): very rare and most reported cases are actually CVC thrombosis
- Caudal vena caval obstruction
  - Caval syndrome (dirofilariasis)
  - Cor triatrium dexter
  - 'Kinked' CVC (post-traumatic adhesions)
  - CVC thrombosis
- Diaphragmatic rupture entrapment
- Extrahepatic bile duct obstruction

Infiltrative disease
- Amyloidosis
- Lipid storage disease
- Lysosomal storage diseases
- Neoplasia
  - Biliary carcinoma/cholangiocarcinoma
  - Hepatoma
  - Histiocytic sarcoma and malignant histiocytosis
  - Lymphoma
  - Mast cell tumour (MCT)
  - Metastatic disease

Inflammation
- Acute hepatitis
- Infectious canine hepatitis
  - *Leptospira*
  - Cholangiohepatitis
- Chronic hepatitis (microhepatica more common)
- Fungal granuloma
- Idiosyncratic drug reaction
- Reticuloendothelial hyperplasia (chronic infectious/inflammatory diseases)
  - Systemic bacterial, fungal and rickettsial diseases

Focal
- Abscess(es)
- Cyst(s) and biliary pseudocyst(s)
- Haematoma
- Hepatic AV fistula
- Liver lobe torsion
- Neoplasia
  - Biliary cystadenoma/cholangiocarcinoma

DIAGNOSTIC APPROACH

1 Determine from history and clinical signs whether cardiac disease, drug administration or endocrinopathy is likely, and investigate accordingly.
2 If significantly anaemic or thrombocytopenic investigate causes other than liver disease first.
3 Investigate primary liver disease by laboratory testing, ultrasound examination, FNA and biopsy.

Clinical clues
Predisposition
• Acute hepatitis: unvaccinated dogs
• Barbiturate or glucocorticoid usage
• DCM and pericardial disease: large/giant breeds
• DM: older, unspayed bitches
• HAC: older dogs
• Hepatocellular carcinoma: Scottish terriers
• IMHA: Cocker spaniel, English Springer spaniel, poodles, Old English sheepdog (OESD), Collies
• IMTP: Cocker spaniel, Miniature and Toy poodles, OESD
• Lipid storage disease: Fox terriers (not reported in UK)
• Nodular hyperplasia: dogs ≥ 8 years

History
• Anorexia or polyphagia
• Drug administration: treated epilepsy
• PU/PD in DM and HAC
• Weakness/collapse in cardiac or pericardial disease

Clinical examination
Visual inspection
• Pot belly

Physical examination
• Enlarged liver, palpable beyond costal arch
• Findings related to underlying disease, e.g. alopecia in HAC

Laboratory findings
Haematology
• Changes related to underlying disease

Serum biochemistry
• Changes related to underlying disease, e.g., hyperglycaemia in DM
• Increases in liver enzyme activities are non-specific
  • Primary liver disease: inflammatory, neoplastic or toxicosis
  • Reactive hepatopathy

Urinalysis
• Glycosuria ± ketonuria in DM
• Hyposthenuria in HAC

Imaging
Plain radiographs
• Cardiac silhouette
• Enlarged liver
• Primary or metastatic neoplastic disease

Ultrasound examination
• Adrenal glands
• Echocardiography
• Liver architecture

Special tests
• Knott's and occult heartworm test
• Dynamic cortisol testing
• Coombs' test
• Bone marrow examination
• Liver FNA and/or biopsy for inflammatory and neoplastic liver disease

2.9 HORNER'S SYNDROME

DEFINITION

Horner's syndrome refers to the combination of clinical signs observed as a result of oculosympathetic nerve dysfunction. They include miosis (small pupil), ptosis (drooping upper eyelid), enophthalmos (sunken eye), third eyelid protrusion and, less commonly, conjunctival hyperaemia, and reduced nasal secretion.

PHYSICAL ABNORMALITIES

Horner's syndrome occurs as a result of a disruption of sympathetic innervation to the eye and surrounding adnexa. Dysfunction of the central, preganglionic, and postganglionic nerves results in first-, second- and third-order Horner's syndrome, respectively.

Relevant nerve fibres originate in the hypothalamus and travel via midbrain and spinal cord, where they then synapse with preganglionic neurons at the cranial thoracic segments (C8–T4) before exiting the spinal cord, becoming the sympathetic trunk. This travels through the mediastinum to the level of thoracic inlet where it joins the vagus nerve becoming the vagosympathetic trunk. The vagosympathetic trunk courses through the cervical region then, at the head, the vagus and sympathetic trunk separate, and the sympathetic trunk terminates at the cranial cervical ganglion ventromedial to the tympanic bulla. Here the preganglionic neurons synapse with postganglionic neuron, which then proceeds to innervate the eye.

RELATED CLINICAL SIGNS

- Any concurrent clinical signs depend on the location of nerve dysfunction.
  - First-order disorders (hypothalamus, brainstem, spinal cord) may present with signs of concurrent brainstem (obtundation, cranial nerve disorders) or spinal cord (paraparesis, paraplegia) dysfunction.
  - Second-order disorders may have concurrent brachial plexus signs (e.g. monoparesis), mediastinal or thoracic disorders (e.g. tachypnoea, regurgitation, dysphagia, coughing), or cervical signs (e.g. laryngeal paralysis).
  - Third-order disorders may result in concurrent VII and VIII cranial neuropathies, causing facial nerve paralysis or vestibular disease, respectively.

COMMON CAUSES

First-order (central)
- Fibrocartilaginous embolism (spinal cord)

Second-order (preganglionic)
- Idiopathic
- Mediastinal, pulmonary or cervical neoplasia
- Brachial plexus trauma (avulsion)

Third-order (postganglionic)
- Idiopathic (may be observed with concurrent facial nerve paralysis or vestibular disease)
- Otitis media or interna

UNCOMMON CAUSES

First-order (central)
- Infectious (neospora)
- Trauma
- Meningoencephalitis of unknown origin

Second-order (preganglionic)
- Trauma

Third-order (postganglionic)
- Iatrogenic, e.g. post total ear canal ablation (TECA)
- Neoplasia

DIAGNOSTIC APPROACH

Clinical clues
Predisposition
- Golden retrievers are predisposed to idiopathic Horner's syndrome
- Idiopathic Horner's syndrome is most common in dogs aged 5–8 years but can occur at any age

History
- Duration of onset of signs may be useful in prioritising differential diagnoses
- Assess for other signs of CNS disorders, in particular signs of brainstem disease: mentation change, incoordination
- Assess for other signs of intrathoracic disease or megaoesophagus, e.g. cough or regurgitation, respectively
- Assess for history of ear disease that may increase suspicion of otitis media, e.g. history of topical ear medications

Clinical examination

Visual inspection

- Mentation is likely impaired with central nervous disorders, *q.v.* section 1.4

Physical examination

- Assess for multisystemic disease
- Otoscopy to assess for evidence of otitis externa with extension to otitis media
- Thorough auscultation to assess for respiratory disease

Neurological examination

- Focus on assessment of brainstem (signs of facial nerve paralysis or vestibular dysfunction in particular)

Laboratory findings

Haematology and serum biochemistry

- Useful to screen for systemic disease

Imaging

Plain radiographs

- Thoracic radiographs to screen for pulmonary and mediastinal disorders
- Head radiographs to screen for bulla lesions

Special tests

- Phenylephrine response test: apply 1% phenylephrine topically and monitor for pupil dilation; if this occurs within 20 minutes the lesion is likely to be third-order (postganglionic)
- CT scan to assess cervical and thoracic structures when high suspicion of neoplasia
- MRI and cerebrospinal fluid (CSF) in cases with suspicion of central disorder

2.10 HYPERTENSION

DEFINITION

Hypertension, or increased blood pressure (BP), is detected either by intra-arterial catheterisation (gold standard), or, more practically, indirectly using Doppler or oscillometric techniques.

Measurement of BP should be carried out using a standardised approach, with attempts to minimise patient anxiety (e.g. 5–10 minutes acclimatisation). The dog should be in lateral or ventral recumbency to minimise the difference in vertical height between the cuff and the heart base.

Interpretation of an increased BP must take into account the patient demeanour and circumstance.

- Normotensive; no target organ damage (TOD) risk: systolic BP < 140 mmHg
- Prehypertensive; minimal risk of TOD: systolic BP 140–159 mmHg
- Hypertensive; moderate risk of TOD: systolic BP 160–179 mmHg
- Severely hypertensive; high risk of TOD: systolic BP > 180 mmHg

RELATED CLINICAL SIGNS

Hypertension has negative consequences for multiple organs; in particular TOD can affect

- Kidneys: progression of chronic kidney disease (CKD), persistent proteinuria
- Eyes: retinopathy, most commonly exudative retinal detachment
- Brain: encephalopathy
- Heart: left ventricular hypertrophy
- Blood vessels: haemorrhage, e.g. epistaxis, stroke

COMMON CAUSES

- Acute kidney injury (AKI)
- CKD
- Hyperadrenocorticism
- Situational hypertension

UNCOMMON CAUSES

- Cushing's reflex (increased intracranial pressure resulting in hypertension and bradycardia)

- Diabetes mellitus
- Iatrogenic
  - Desoxycorticosterone pivolate (DOCP)
  - Toceranib phosphate (Palladia)
  - Erythropoiesis-stimulating agents
- Idiopathic (primary) hypertension
- Phaeochromocytoma
- Primary hyperaldosteronism

DIAGNOSTIC APPROACH

Clinical clues
Predisposition
- Sighthounds are recognised to have higher BP relative to other breeds (10–20 mmHg higher during hospitalisation), likely to be situational hypertension
- Higher prevalence of hypertension in Shetland sheepdogs than reported in other breeds

History
- Signs suspicious for AKI or CKD
- Signs suspicious for HAC

Clinical examination
Visual inspection
- Assess demeanour to allow for interpretation of BP measurement results, i.e. consideration of situational hypertension
- Evidence of haircoat and conformation changes suspicious for HAC
- If obtunded, complete neurological examination to assess for suspicion of increased intracranial pressure

Physical examination
- Thorough examination to assess for multisystemic disease
- Femoral pulses when considering aortic thromboembolism

Ophthalmic examination
- Retinal changes supportive of target organ damage

Laboratory findings
Haematology, serum biochemistry
- To screen for renal disease and evidence supportive of hyperadrenocorticism

Urinalysis
- To assess for urine concentration (useful for renal disease and HAC) and presence of proteinuria

Imaging
Plain radiographs and ultrasound
- Adrenal gland imaging to assess for suspicion of HAC or phaeochromocytoma
- Renal imaging to assess for evidence of AKI or CKD

Special tests
- Testing for hyperadrenocorticism (urine cortisol creatinine ratio [UCCr], low-dose dexamethasone suppression [LDDS] test, ACTH stimulation test)
- Testing for phaeochromocytoma (urine and plasma normetanephrines)
- Testing for hyperaldosteronism (renin aldosterone ratio)
- MRI ± CSF where suspicion of increased intracranial pressure, consider administration of mannitol

2.11 HYPOTENSION

DEFINITION

Hypotension, or low blood pressure, is defined as a systolic blood pressure of less than 90 mmHg, although a systolic blood pressure of 90–100 mmHg is likely to be subnormal based on studies assessing blood pressure in healthy dogs.

RELATED CLINICAL SIGNS

Systolic blood pressure < 80 mmHg may impair vital organ blood supply, with resultant signs of organ dysfunction, e.g. AKI.

Hypotension is most commonly associated with shock. Accompanying signs are likely to include concurrent signs of shock depending on the cause:
- Hypovolaemia: tachycardia and pallor
- Distributive shock: congested mucous membranes with delayed capillary refill time initially)

COMMON CAUSES

- Cardiogenic shock
  - Heart failure (dilated cardiomyopathy, degenerative mitral valve disease)
- Distributive shock
  - Sepsis
- Hypovolaemic shock
  - Anaesthesia-induced
  - Haemorrhage
  - Fluid losses (vomiting and diarrhea)

UNCOMMON CAUSES

- Distributive shock
  - Vasodilation due to mast cell degranulation or anaphylaxis
- Cardiogenic shock
  - Bradyarrhythmias
  - Atrial fibrillation
  - Ventricular tachycardia
- Obstructive shock
  - Gastric dilatation-volvulus (GDV)
  - Pericardial effusion
- Vagal stimulation
  - Intra-abdominal disease (in particular gastrointestinal)

DIAGNOSTIC APPROACH

Clinical clues
Predisposition
- Golden retrievers are predisposed to idiopathic pericardial effusion
- Giant-breed deep-chested dogs are predisposed to GDV

History
- Assess for suspicion of hypovolaemic, distributive, or cardiogenic shock

Clinical examination
Visual inspection
- Assess respiratory pattern and effort (useful for causes of shock)

Physical examination
- Thorough examination to assess for evidence of systemic disease
- Assess for jugular pulsation as a sign of volume overload suspicious for cardiogenic shock or pericardial effusion

Laboratory findings
Haematology, serum biochemistry and urinalysis
- Useful to screen for systemic disease

Imaging
Plain radiographs and ultrasound
- Useful to screen for systemic disease and cardiac disorders

Special tests
- Intravenous fluid response: crystalloid fluid bolus in dogs with a low suspicion of cardiogenic shock
- Echocardiography
- Electrocardiogram (ECG)

2.12 HYPOTHERMIA

DEFINITION

Subnormal body temperature (T < 37.9°C), or hypothermia, may occur due to environmental factors or to a failure of the patient to generate adequate body heat due to illness, injury, or drugs.

RELATED CLINICAL SIGNS

Animals that are hypothermic due to environmental factors:
- Initially shiver and seek heat to warm themselves; this reaction to cold stops as the body temperature drops below 34.4°C
- Below 34.4°C thermoregulation is impaired and vasodilation occurs
- Below 31.1°C the hypothalamus no longer generates a thermoregulatory response to the body temperature. This occurs in conjunction with severe central nervous system depression along with severe systemic consequences (cardiovascular, respiratory, immunological).

COMMON CAUSES

- Drug-induced, especially general anaesthesia
- Severe shock: cardiogenic, distributive, hypovolaemic
- Hypothyroidism

UNCOMMON CAUSES

- Aortic thromboembolism; hypothermia if based on rectal temperature
- Environmentally induced hypothermia (exposure): rare in UK
- Hypothalamic dysfunction (trauma, inflammatory)
- Uraemic hypothermia

DIAGNOSTIC APPROACH

Clinical clues
Predisposition
- Hypothyroidism: Boxers, Dobermanns and Golden retrievers

- Small patients or those with low body condition are particularly vulnerable to hypothermia

History
- Assess for clinical suspicion of shock
- Assess for clinical suspicion of hypothyroidism

Clinical examination
Visual inspection
- Mentation is likely impaired with CNS disorders affecting the hypothalamus
- Evidence of haircoat changes suspicious for hypothyroidism

Physical examination
- Thorough examination to assess for multisystemic disease
- Examine for femoral pulses when considering aortic thromboembolism

Laboratory findings
Haematology and serum biochemistry
- Useful to screen for systemic disease, renal disease, and evidence supportive of hypothyroidism (mild non-regenerative anaemia, hypercholesterolaemia)

Imaging
Plain radiographs and ultrasound
- Screen for causes of shock when appropriate
- Ultrasound scan aorta to assess for thrombus

Special tests
- Thyroid panel (T4, TSH, free T4)

2.13 ICTERUS/JAUNDICE

DEFINITION

Jaundice (syn. icterus) is the yellow discolouration of tissues caused by excess bilirubin. 'Blue jaundice' is a colloquial term for cyanosis, *q.v.* section 2.6.
- Jaundice can be caused by:
  - Massive haemolysis (pre-hepatic jaundice)

- Liver dysfunction (hepatic jaundice)
- Failure of biliary flow into the intestine (post-hepatic jaundice) because of either biliary obstruction or biliary rupture and leakage leading to bile peritonitis

NB: Jaundice is not seen in congenital PSS.

RELATED CLINICAL SIGNS

- Elastic tissues are most discoloured when hyperbilirubinaemia is present, but ante mortem jaundice is most easily recognised in the sclera, then the mucous membranes, and then the skin.
- Jaundice in the plasma can be detected when serum bilirubin concentrations exceed 25 µmol/l, but tissue jaundice cannot be detected until serum concentrations exceed 40–50 µmol/l.

COMMON CAUSES

Prehepatic jaundice
- IMHA; primary or secondary to drugs, bacterial infection or neoplasia
- Babesiosis: currently rare in UK except in travelled dogs, but common in endemic subtropical areas, especially South Africa and southern United States related to the distribution of the tick vector, *Dermacentor*

Hepatic jaundice
- Bacterial cholangitis/cholangiohepatitis
- Chronic hepatitis, including copper hepatotoxicosis
- Cirrhosis
- Leptospirosis

Post-hepatic jaundice
- Acute pancreatitis
- Gall bladder mucocoele with sludge in bile ducts

UNCOMMON CAUSES

Prehepatic jaundice
- *Clostridium perfringens* releasing phospholipase during bacteraemia

- Caval syndrome in dirofilariasis
- Congenital porphyria
- *Mycoplasma haemocanis*, usually only after splenectomy
- Incompatible blood transfusion
- Onion poisoning
- Phosphofructokinase (PFK) deficiency
- Resorption of large haematoma or haemoperitoneum (probably doesn't cause jaundice)
- Zinc toxicosis

Hepatic jaundice
- Acute infectious canine hepatitis (ICH)/canine adenovirus 1 (CAV-1)
- Drugs – idosyncratic reaction
- Hepatic neoplasia (diffuse): primary, infiltrative (lymphoma) or metastatic
- Hepatocutaneous syndrome (Swiss cheese liver): rarely causes jaundice
- Juvenile hepatic fibrosis/non-cirrhotic portal hypertension/portal vein hypoplasia
- Lobular dissecting hepatitis
- Sepsis causing intrahepatic cholestasis

Post-hepatic jaundice
- Bile duct carcinoma
- Chronic fibrosing pancreatitis
- Cholelithiasis (gall stones)
- Duodenal FB obstructing major duodenal papilla
- Pancreatic carcinoma
- Ruptured gall bladder or extrahepatic bile ducts
  - Cholelithiasis
  - Iatrogenic – GB aspiration when obstructed
  - Necrotising cholecystitis
  - Trauma
- Stricture of major duodenal papilla

DIAGNOSTIC APPROACH

The three forms of jaundice are distinguished by history, clinical signs, laboratory analysis and ultrasound examination, and investigated and treated accordingly.

1 If jaundice is pre-hepatic, the dog must be anaemic; normal or only mildly decreased haematocrit rules out haemolytic disease.

2 Differentiate hepatic and post-hepatic causes by ultrasound examination.
3 Liver biopsy if primary hepatic cause.

Clinical clues
Predisposition
- Chronic hepatitis: Cocker spaniel, Retriever, Standard poodle
- Copper-associated chronic hepatitis: Bedlington terrier, WHWT, Dobermann, Skye terrier
- Gall bladder mucocoele: Border terrier, Shetland sheepdog
- Hepatocellular carcinoma: Scottish terrier
- IMHA: Cocker spaniel, English Springer spaniel, Poodle, OESD, Collie
- PFK deficiency: Springer spaniel

History
- Prehepatic
  - Dark urine from hyperbilirubinaemia ± haemoglobinuria if intravascular haemolysis
  - Jaundice after exertion in PFK deficiency
- Hepatic
  - Dark urine from hyperbilirubinaemia
  - Lameness or reluctance to walk with hepatocutaneous syndrome
  - Often have other signs of liver disease (PU/PD, ascites, hcpatoencephalopathy)
- Post-hepatic
  - May have signs of the primary disease, e.g. vomiting and pain in acute pancreatitis, or remarkably few signs if there is a chronic progressive obstruction (e.g. chronic pancreatitis, pancreatic carcinoma)
  - Dark urine from hyperbilirubinaemia
  - Pale, acholic faeces if complete biliary obstruction
  - Previous episodes of pancreatitis if chronic fibrosing pancreatitis
  - Trauma if ruptured biliary tree (may have occurred more than 1 week previously)

Clinical examination
Visual inspection
- Distended abdomen if ascites, hepatomegaly or bile peritonitis
- Jaundiced sclera
- Weakness

Physical examination
- Hyperkeratotic, cracked footpads in hepatocutaneous syndrome
- Jaundiced mucous membranes, and pale if underlying anaemia
- Jaundiced skin in areas of thin hair or when hair is parted

Auscultation
- Haemic murmur if anaemic
- Tachycardia, tachypnoea if anaemic

Palpation
- Abdominal pain with acute hepatitis, GB mucocoele and pancreatitis
- Ascites
- Hepatomegaly, q.v. section 2.8
- Pancreatic mass

Laboratory findings
Haematology
- Inflammatory leukogram in acute hepatitis, pancreatitis
- Mild normocytic, normochromic anaemia if liver disease or post-hepatic
- Regenerative anaemia (anisocytosis, polychromasia, reticulocytosis) in pre-hepatic causes
- Spherocytosis, microagglutination and sometimes leukocytosis in IMHA
- Severe anaemia if haemolysis ± spherocytosis, autoagglutination

Serum biochemistry
- Hypoglycaemia, hypoalbuminaemia, hypocholesterolaemia, increased ALT and ALP activities in liver disease
- Lipase and canine pancreatic lipase (cPL) sometimes increased in pancreatitis; DGGR [1,2-o-dilauryl-rac-glycero-glutaric acid-(6'-methylresorufin)] lipase not highly specific
- Increase in ALP >> ALT activity plus hypercholesterolaemia in extra-hepatic biliary obstruction
- Increased serum bilirubin
  NB: Distinguishing the type of jaundice by determining the relative amounts of conjugated and unconjugated bilirubin (Van den Bergh test) is unreliable and should not be attempted.

Urinalysis

- Absence of urobilinogen in biliary obstruction
- Bilirubinuria > 2+
- Dilute or isosthenuric urine in severe hepatic disease
- Haemoglobinuria in IMHA
- Urate crystals in chronic liver disease

Imaging
Radiography

- Hepatomegaly, *q.v.* section 2.8
- Hepatosplenomegaly if IMHA, lymphosarcoma
- Loss of detail if ascites or bile peritonitis
- Microhepatica if chronic hepatitis/cirrhosis

Ultrasound

- Ascites
- Diffuse change in echogenic density (cf. spleen and kidney) if infiltrated (e.g. lymphosarcoma)
- Dilated extrahepatic biliary tree if post-hepatic obstruction
- Disorganised or nodular echogenicity if primary or metastatic neoplasia
- Irregular outline and echogenicity in chronic hepatitis/cirrhosis
- Obstructive mass in pancreas

Special tests

- Abdominocentesis if ascitic
- Coombs' test and slide agglutination for IMHA
- Dark field urine examination for *Leptospira*
- Exploratory laparotomy ± pancreatic biopsy
- Liver biopsy ± culture
- Spec cPL for pancreatitis

2.14 LYMPHADENOPATHY

DEFINITION

Lymphadenopathy is any change in lymph node size or consistency, detected on palpation or imaging. This may affect one lymph node, a chain, or a more generalised disorder.

RELATED CLINICAL SIGNS

- The underlying cause of lymphadenopathy likely results in clinical signs rather than lymph node change alone, e.g. lethargy and inappetence in autoimmune and neoplastic causes
- Severe lymphadenomegaly may result in:
  - Dyspnoea, especially if enlarged retropharyngeal lymph nodes
  - Venous obstruction, e.g. caval syndrome with facial swelling in dogs with large mediastinal lymph nodes

COMMON CAUSES

- Neoplasia
  - Round cell: lymphoma
  - Metastatic: carcinoma, sarcoma, mast cell tumour
- Infectious disease
  - Vector-borne diseases: *Ehrlichia*, *Leishmania* (common worldwide, but not in UK)
- Reactive hyperplasia
  - Dental disease
  - Immune-mediated polyarthritis (IMPA)
  - Skin disease
  - Wound

UNCOMMON CAUSES

- Immune-mediated disease
  - Pyogranulomatous lymphadenitis
- Infectious disease
  - Mycobacterium (*M. bovis*, *M. tuberculosis*)
  - *Toxoplasma*
  - Vector-borne diseases: *Anaplasma*, *Bartonella*, *Brucella*, *Cryptococcus*, systemic aspergillosis
- Juvenile cellulitis (puppy strangles)
- Neoplasia
  - Round cell: histiocytic sarcoma, leukaemia

DIAGNOSTIC APPROACH

Clinical clues
Predisposition
- Middle-aged to older dogs predisposed to neoplasia
- Springer spaniels are predisposed to pyogranulomatous lymphadenitis

History
- Duration of onset of signs may be useful in prioritising differential diagnoses
- Multiple enlarged lymph nodes are highly suggestive of multicentric lymphoma
- Travel history and exposure to ticks may influence suspicion of vector-borne disease

Clinical examination
Visual inspection
- Assess for cutaneous changes: may increase suspicion of *Leishmania* or reactive hyperplasia, depending on pattern of distribution
- Juvenile cellulitis presents with classic facial changes: initially facial swelling, then development of papules and pustules with lymphadenomegaly

Physical examination
- Examine region distal to single lymph node or chain of nodes for primary lesion
- Thorough examination to assess for multisystemic disease

Laboratory findings
Haematology and serum biochemistry
- Useful to screen for systemic disease

- Hypercalcaemia may be detected in neoplasia (anal sac adenocarcinoma, lymphoma) and pyogranulomatous lymphadenitis

Imaging
Plain radiographs and abdominal ultrasound
- Radiographs and abdominal ultrasound to screen for sites of inflammation or neoplasia

Special tests
- Bone marrow aspirate or core biopsy for neoplastic disease (if cytopenias are present) or infectious disease
- FNA or incisional/excisional biopsy of lymph nodes for cytology, histopathology and additional tests on tissue biopsies as appropriate
  - Culture
  - Flow cytometry and PCR for antigen receptor rearrangements (PARR) to characterise lymphoma
  - PCR for infectious disease, e.g. mycobacteria, *Leishmania*, *Ehrlichia*
  - Special stains, e.g. periodic acid schiff (PAS) for fungal disease, Ziehl-Neelsen stain for acid-fast bacteria in particular mycobacteria
- Infectious disease screening as appropriate
  - SNAP® 4Dx for *Anaplasma*, *Borrelia*, *Dirofilaria*, *Ehrlichia*
  - Serology and PCR for *Bartonella*, *Leishmania*, *Leptospira*
  - PCR for *Babesia*, *Bartonella*, *Leishmania*, *Leptospira* and *Toxoplasma*

2.15 MURMUR

DEFINITION

Murmurs, which may be innocent or pathological, are sounds produced by vibrations due to turbulence of blood.

q.v. section 5.2, Cardiovascular system, for more details.

2.16 ORAL MASSES

DEFINITION

Abnormal proliferative tissue in the oral cavity, which may be inflammatory, benign or malignant. Be aware that non-healing lesions and/or spontaneous tooth loss may have an underlying neoplastic condition.

RELATED CLINICAL SIGNS

May be asymptomatic, or show signs of:
- Drooling, *q.v.* section 1.16
- Dysphagia, *q.v.* section 1.17
- Facial swelling or deformity
- Halitosis, *q.v.* section 1.29
- Oral bleeding: blood staining of saliva
- Tooth loss

COMMON CAUSES

Benign hyperplasia
- Focal fibrous gingival hyperplasia

Benign tumours
- Odontogenic fibroma (epulides)
- Acanthomatous ameloblastoma

Malignant neoplasia
- Fibrosarcoma
- Malignant melanoma
- Squamous cell carcinoma

UNCOMMON CAUSES

- Calcinosis circumscripta
- Craniomandibular osteopathy ('Lion jaw', 'Westie jaw')
- Cysts
  - Developmental
  - Inflammatory
- Eosinophilic granuloma (rare cf. cat)
- Peripheral giant cell granuloma
- Pyogenic granuloma
- Sublingual salivary mucocoele (sialocoele) in mouth (ranula)

Benign tumours
Non-odontogenic
- Melanocytoma
- Ossifying fibroma
- Osteoma
- Papilloma
- Plasmacytoma

Odontogenic
- Ameloblastoma
- Ameloblastic fibroma/dentinoma/odontoma
- Amyloid-producing odontogenic tumour
- Complex and compound odontomas
- Odontoma/hamartoma
- Peripheral odontogenic fibroma
- Odontogenic myxoma/myxofibroma
- Ossifying fibroma

Malignant neoplasia
- Epitheliotropic lymphoma affecting mucous membranes
  - MCT
- Multilobular tumour of bone/osteochondrosarcoma
- Peripheral nerve sheath tumour
- Osteosarcoma

DIAGNOSTIC APPROACH

1 Head and chest radiographs to assess bony invasion and metastasis.
2 Biopsy of mass lesion.
3 FNA of mandibular lymph nodes.
4 Attempt complete surgical excision if not performed when biopsied initially.

Clinical clues
Predisposition
- Calcinosis circumscripta can be in tongue (more typically over joints): GSD
- Craniomandibular osteopathy: Cairn and Scottish terriers and especially WHWT
- Eosinophilic granuloma: Cavalier King Charles spaniel (CKCS)
- Gingival hyperplasia and epulides: brachycephalic breeds, especially Boxer

- Gingival hyperplasia associated with periodontal disease
- Papillomatosis in young dogs

History
- Difficulty eating and drooling
- Facial deformity
- Oral bleeding

Clinical examination
Visual inspection
- Blood-stained saliva
- Drooling
- Facial swelling/deformity

Physical examination
- Displacement and/or loss of teeth
- Mandibular lymphadenopathy
- Oral mass itself, which may be ulcerated

Laboratory findings
- Usually unremarkable

Imaging
Plain radiographs
- Head
  - Local bone destruction
  - Soft tissue mass
- Chest
  - Metastatic disease

Special tests
- CT of skull
- FNA and/or biopsy
- FNA regional lymph nodes (LNs) (mandibular, retropharyngeal, cervical)
- Imaging of lungs to look for metastatic disease

2.17   PAIN

DEFINITION

Pain is the unpleasant emotional experience associated with potential or actual tissue damage. It can be challenging to recognise in dogs, with difficulties in appreciating the presence of pain, discriminating from other causes of abnormal behaviour and, in some cases, localising the source.

2.17.1   ABDOMINAL PAIN

DEFINITION

The sensation of pain caused by stimulation of nerve fibres within the abdomen, manifested either through changes in a patient's behaviour or identified by abdominal palpation. Mild pain is often termed 'discomfort'.
- Abdominal pain is caused by distension, chemical or infectious inflammation, smooth muscle spasm, or ischaemia of the abdominal viscera and/or peritoneal space
- An 'acute abdomen' is the sudden onset of severe abdominal pain, often resulting in shock, that can indicate a life-threatening emergency and often requires surgical intervention

- Somatic pain (e.g. pancreatitis, peritonitis) tends to be sharper and more painful than visceral pain and may be localised on palpation; visceral pain tends to be dull and diffuse, and can't be localised
- Painful lesions of the abdominal wall (e.g. bruising, cellulitis, muscle rupture), and thoracolumbar spinal pain may falsely give the appearance of intraperitoneal pain

RELATED CLINICAL SIGNS

- Abdominal distension or tucked-up abdomen
- Diarrhoea
- Grunting/groaning

- Occasional adoption of 'prayer position' if cranial abdominal pain
- Resentment of abdominal palpation
- Restlessness, pacing, trembling
- Vomiting

COMMON CAUSES

Any abdominal organ and/or the peritoneum may be involved.

Endocrine
- Hypoadrenocorticism (uncommon but important)

Gastrointestinal
- Acute gastroenteritis
  - Acute haemorrhagic diarrhoea syndrome (AHDS)/haemorrhagic gastroenteritis (HGE)
  - Parvovirus infection
- CIE/IBD
- Colitis
- Constipation
- FB obstruction
- GDV
- Gastric ulceration: more likely the deeper the ulcer
- Intestinal spasm, usually associated with acute gastroenteritis
- Intussusception
- Neoplasia

Pancreatic
- Acute pancreatitis and associated peritonitis

Splenic
- Ruptured splenic haematoma, haemangioma, haemangiosarcoma with bleeding
- Traumatic rupture

Urogenital
- Acute prostatitis
- Lower urinary tract infection
- Urethral obstruction

UNCOMMON CAUSES

Gastrointestinal
- Colonic torsion
- Flatulence (severe)
- Gastric food engorgement (food bloat)
- Intestinal incarceration in internal, inguinal or umbilical hernia
- Intestinal volvulus
- Ischaemia or infarction
- Obstipation

Hepatobiliary
- Abscessation
- Acute hepatitis
- Cholecystitis
- Cholelithiasis with or without obstruction
- Gallbladder mucocoele
- Leptospirosis
- Liver lobe torsion
- Portal vein thrombosis

Pancreatic
- Abscess
- Ischaemia

Peritoneal
- Carcinomatosis, although often non-painful
- Pansteatitis
- Peritonitis
  - *Actinomyces* or *Nocardia* infection
  - Adhesions
  - Dehiscence of surgical intestinal wound
  - Iatrogenic perforation
    - Gastric ulcer from non-steroidal anti-inflammatory drug (NSAID) administration
  - Ruptured biliary tract
  - Spontaneous perforation of GI tract
    - Intestinal neoplasia
    - Perforated gastric ulcer from remote mast cell tumour
    - Colonic ulcers in acute CNS disease
  - Traumatic perforation/rupture of GI tract
    - Avulsion of mesenteric vessels leading to ischaemic perforation
    - Migrating FB, e.g. cocktail stick, grass awn
    - Surgical dehiscence

Splenic
- Splenitis
- Torsion of splenic pedicle

Toxins and drugs
- Lead and other heavy metals
- NSAIDs and other ulcerogenic drugs

Urogenital
- AKI
- Acute prostatitis
- Dystocia
- Lower urinary tract infection
- Metritis
- Ovarian cyst
- Pyelonephritis
- Renolithiasis
- Ruptured kidney
- Ruptured pyometra
- Ruptured ureter/bladder
- Testicular torsion: more common in cryptorchids
- Ureterolithiasis/ureteral obstruction
- Uterine torsion

DIAGNOSTIC APPROACH

1 Manage any shock if an acute abdomen.
2 Appropriate analgesia.
3 Abdominal imaging.
4 Distinguish benign causes that can be managed medically from conditions needing urgent surgery through minimum database and imaging.
5 Exploratory surgery.

Clinical clues
- Anorexia and vomiting are common concurrent problems
- Foreign content in any vomitus may indicate cause
- Lack of defecation and empty rectum on digital examination suggestive of obstruction
- 'Prayer' position suggests cranial abdominal pain, i.e. gastric ulceration, pancreatitis
- Shock if acute haemorrhage, hypovolaemia, endotoxaemia or intestinal obstruction

- Spinal pain may appear abdominal in origin, either because pain is referred or simply because abdominal palpation causes painful spinal movement

Predispositions
- GDV in large/giant, deep-chested dog breed: Great Dane, Wolfhound, Irish setter
- Intestinal volvulus: Bloodhounds, GSDs with EPI
- Older dogs are more likely to have neoplastic disease
- Pancreatitis in middle-aged, female overweight dogs, especially toy breeds, including Miniature schnauzer
- Splenic torsion: GSDs and Great Danes
- Testicular torsion in cryptorchids
- Young dogs are more likely to have an infectious cause or hypoadrenocorticism

History
- Dietary indiscretion precipitating pancreatitis
- Ingestion of foreign plant material or toxins
- Intermittent GI signs in hypoadrenocorticism
- Large meal and exercise before GDV
- NSAID administration
- Previous episodes of FB ingestion
- Pyometra in older unspayed bitches after oestrus
- Trauma: signs may be delayed by hours or days following known trauma

Clinical examination
Visual inspection
- Lethargic or collapsed
- Stilted gait, arched back or reluctance to move
- Tucked-up or distended abdomen
- Unproductive attempts to vomit in GDV
- Vocalisation

Physical examination
- Abdominal palpation:
  Slow gentle palpation is required to overcome abdominal splinting due to anxiety at being handled. A systematic approach is needed to palpate every organ and identify masses or

organomegaly and/or ascites. Localisation of pain may indicate somatic rather than visceral pain.

- Absence of bladder if ruptured
- Caudal mass/pain in cryptorchid with testicular torsion
- Hepatomegaly if liver is palpable beyond the costal arch and hepatic masses may be pedunculated
- Hollow, tympanitic viscus on percussion in GDV
- Pain: cranial abdominal if gastric/pancreatic
  - May vomit on palpation if severe peritonitis
  - Some dogs (e.g. Labradors) are quite stoical and may only manifest a small expiratory grunt on palpation; others may vocalise
  - Splinting of abdominal wall
- Splenomegaly or mass, which may be moveable caudally
- Digital rectal examination to palpate prostate for pain response and asymmetry
- Inguinal or umbilical hernias swollen and painful if intestinal loops are incarcerated
- Jaundice if bile peritonitis or biliary obstruction
- Mucous membranes
  - Pale and prolonged capillary refill if distributive or haemorrhagic shock
  - Brick red if septic shock
- Pyrexia
- Tachycardia

Laboratory findings
Haematology
- Anaemia if severe/recurrent bleeding
- Degenerative left shift if overwhelming sepsis (e.g. ruptured GI tract)
- Inappropriate number of nucleated red blood cells (nRBCs) in lead poisoning
- Leukopenia (neutropenia) with no left shift in parvovirus
- Neutrophilia and left shift in inflammatory disease

Serum biochemistry
- Azotaemia if ruptured urinary tract, AKI

- Increased amylase and lipase may be seen in pancreatitis but unreliable

Urinalysis
- Haematuria if urinary tract trauma
- Pyuria in pyelonephritis, prostatitis

Imaging
Plain radiographs
- Abdominal effusion
- Free intraperitoneal gas if GI perforation
- GDV
- Obstructed bowel loops
- Intestinal volvulus
- FB
- Splenic mass

Ultrasound
- Abdominal effusion
- Biliary obstruction and/or cholelithiasis
- Gall bladder mucocoele
- Intra-abdominal neoplasia
- Pancreatitis
- Splenic mass or congestion if torsion present

Special tests
- Abdominocentesis, *q.v.* section 2.5
  - Bacterial culture
  - Bilirubin concentration
  - Creatinine gradient (fluid:serum concentration ratio) in cases of urinary tract rupture. NB: Urea concentration is not so helpful as it equilibrates across the peritoneum.
  - Cytology, especially looking for intracellular bacteria
  - Glucose (decreased) and lactate (increased) are suggestive of septic peritonitis
  - Protein content
- Contrast GI study: use iodinated contrast if perforation is suspected
- Gastroscopy if gastric ulceration is suspected
- Excretory urogram and retrograde (vagino-) urethrogram
- Exploratory laparoscopy/laparotomy
- Pancreatic lipase
- Retrograde (vagino)-urethrogram

2.17.2 GENERALISED PAIN

DEFINITION

Pain that is difficult or impossible to localise or occurs in multiple sites.

RELATED CLINICAL SIGNS

- Altered behaviour may be observed:
  - Aggression
  - Avoiding specific activities, e.g. going up/down stairs, jumping on/off furniture, walking on slippery surfaces
  - Inappetence
  - Reluctance to exercise or reduced activity levels
  - Yelping or crying out
- There may be localised signs, e.g. lameness or hunched posture. In the acute phase there may be tachycardia and tachypnoea.

COMMON CAUSES

- Abdominal pain, *q.v.* section 2.17.1
- Spinal pain
  - IVDD
  - Steroid-responsive meningitis-arteritis (SRMA)
- Musculoskeletal pain
  - Cellulitis
  - Degenerative joint disease
  - FB
  - IMPA
  - Neoplasia: osteosarcoma
  - Trauma

UNCOMMON CAUSES

- Abdominal pain, *q.v.* section 2.17.1
- Musculoskeletal pain
  - Aortic thromboembolism
  - Metaphyseal osteopathy
  - Myositis
  - Nerve root tumour
  - Osteomyelitis

- Panosteitis
- Septic joint
- Spinal pain
  - Discospondylitis
  - Neoplasia

DIAGNOSTIC APPROACH

1 Manage any shock.
2 Appropriate analgesia.
3 Identify systemic disease through clinical signs and laboratory testing.
4 Perform relevant imaging.

Clinical clues
Predisposition
- Elbow and hip dysplasia in large breeds
- Juvenile dogs predisposed to SRMA and metaphyseal osteopathy
- Older dogs are predisposed to tumours and degenerative joint disease
- Osteosarcoma in large/giant breeds
- Panosteitis: GSDs

History
- Spinal pain and abdominal pain can be difficult to discriminate; GI signs will aid this. In the absence of vomiting or diarrhoea spinal pain would be considered more likely than abdominal pain.

Clinical examination
Visual inspection
- Assess demeanour, ambulation, and navigating specific obstacles (e.g. stairs); in some cases video recordings of the dog during episodes can be very useful

Physical examination
- A full orthopaedic and neurological examination may be valuable
- During thorough examination pain may be localised, but in some cases it may be important to pay attention for subtle signs of discomfort

- Pyrexia is typically observed in SRMA, IMPA and metaphyseal osteopathy

Laboratory findings
Haematology and serum biochemistry
- Useful to screen for systemic inflammatory disease

Imaging
Plain radiographs and abdominal ultrasound
- May be useful once pain is localised

Special tests
- Analgesia trial in the absence of suspicion of SRMA severe systemic disease
- Arthrocentesis cytology for IMPA or septic joint
- CSF cytology for SRMA
- cPL can be elevated in IVDD and with SI obstruction as well as pancreatitis and therefore may not aid in discrimination

2.18 PALLOR

DEFINITION

Pallor is paleness of the skin or mucous membranes such as conjunctiva or oral mucous membranes. It can be transient due to circulatory disturbance or persistent due to anaemia.

RELATED CLINICAL SIGNS

- Collapse
- Generalised or regional pallor
- Lethargy
- Tachypnoea/dyspnoea
- Weakness

COMMON CAUSES

- Anaemia, *q.v.* section 3.30.1
- Decreased peripheral perfusion
  - Pain
  - Shock
  - Syncope
  - Vasoconstriction

UNCOMMON CAUSES

- Drugs/toxins, e.g. adder bite, NSAIDs
- Regional, e.g. thromboembolic disease

DIAGNOSTIC APPROACH

Clinical clues
Predisposition
- None

History
- Non-specific secondary signs are typically noticed by owners, e.g. weakness, lethargy, reduced exercise tolerance or collapse

Clinical examination
Visual inspection
- Collapsed
- Lethargic
- Weak

Physical examination
- Absent pulses with regional pallor due to thromboembolism
- Altered pulse strength, e.g. weak with hypovolaemic shock
- Cool extremities with vasoconstriction/shock
- Evidence of blood loss
- Paralysis of limb with thromboembolism
- Prolonged capillary refill time with shock, normal with anaemia
- Regional or generalised pallor of membranes
- Tachycardia
- Tachypnoea

Laboratory findings

Haematology

- Extremely useful to differentiate between anaemia and hypoperfusion
  - Anaemic dogs will have decreased PCV/HCT, haemoglobin (Hb) and RBC count

Serum biochemistry

- In anaemic animals secondary to blood loss, proteins may be decreased depending on time elapsed since blood loss occurred
- In hypoperfused dogs, changes secondary to organ dysfunction and hypoperfusion/hypo-volaemia may be present, e.g. elevated urea, creatinine, SDMA

Urinalysis

- Useful alongside haematology and biochemistry to interpret organ function, evidence of dehydration

Imaging

- *q.v.* sections 5.2 and 5.4

Special tests

- BP is usually normal with anaemia and low with hypoperfusion

2.19 PERINEAL LESIONS

DEFINITION

Abnormal swelling or tissue in the perineal region.

RELATED CLINICAL SIGNS

- Constipation
- Dyschezia
- Dysuria with retroflexed bladder
- PU/PD
- 'Scooting' on rear
- Spotting blood
- Swelling
- Tenesmus

COMMON CAUSES

- Anal furunculosis
- Anal sac conditions; may develop sequentially
  - Impaction
  - Sacculitis
  - Abscess
- Perianal adenomas (circumanal, hepatoid tumours)

UNCOMMON CAUSES

- Anal sac adenocarcinoma (ASAC)
- *Dipylidium caninum* proglottids
- Hypospadia
- Ileo-colic intussusception, severe enough to pass through anus
- Malignant melanoma
- Mast cell tumour
- Myiasis
- Perianal adenocarcinoma
- Perineal hernia ± rectal diverticulum
- Pseudocoprostasis
- Protruding recto-anal polyp
- Pythiosis
- Rectal prolapse
- Rectocutaneous fistula
- Retroflexed bladder within perineal hernia
- Squamous cell carcinoma

DIAGNOSTIC APPROACH

1 Observation of perineal region.
2 Digital rectal examination; may require anaesthesia if painful lesion.
3 Serum ionised calcium if anal sac mass.
4 Imaging followed by FNA and/or (excisional) biopsy if suspected neoplasia.

Clinical clues

Predisposition
- Anal furunculosis: GSDs
- Anal sac impaction: CKCS and other toy breeds
- ASAC: Cocker spaniels
- Perianal adenocarcinomas: Alaskan Malamutes, Bulldogs, and Siberian Huskies; should always be suspected in castrated males as they are not hormone-dependent.
- Perianal adenomas occur in entire male dogs: Cocker spaniels, Pekingese, Samoyeds and Siberian Huskies
- Perineal hernia in entire male dogs, but can occur in females

History
- Dietary history of wet food with little fibre resulting in anal sacs not emptying during defaecation
- Straining to defecate

Clinical examination

Visual inspection
- Swelling
- Mass with or without ulceration

Physical examination
- Abnormal tissue

- Digital rectal exam to identify anal sac disease and perineal hernia, and to determine extent of any mass
- Perianal adenomas are non-painful, slow-growing masses, and can be single or multiple. They can ulcerate and become infected.
- Perianal adenocarcinomas grow rapidly, are larger and firmer, ulcerate and adhere to underlying tissues

Laboratory findings
Often unremarkable
- Inflammatory leukogram with anal sac abscess
- Paraneoplastic hypercalcaemia with ASAC

Imaging

Radiographs
- Sublumbar periosteal reaction and enlarged sublumbar LNs with anal sac adenocarcinoma
- Thoracic radiographs for metastasis check

Ultrasound
Sublumbar lymphadenopathy

Special tests
None, but surgical correction of intussusception and perineal hernia confirm the diagnosis

---

2.20 PERIPHERAL OEDEMA

DEFINITION

Peripheral oedema is an excess of interstitial fluid in body tissues and may be localised or generalised. Oedema causes swelling that 'pits' under light pressure, i.e. depression caused by pressure dissipates only slowly.

RELATED CLINICAL SIGNS

- Ascites, hydrothorax, hydropericardium, and pulmonary oedema represent oedema occurring in a specific location (q.v. section 2.5) and often occur before generalised peripheral oedema develops

- Generalised peripheral oedema should appear symmetrical but can occur anywhere although initially it occurs most often ventrally and in distal limbs
- Localised oedema affects only one part of the body, e.g head, single limb

COMMON CAUSES

Generalised oedema
Decreased capillary oncotic pressure (hypoalbuminaemia)
- PLE
- PLN
- End-stage chronic liver disease

Increased capillary hydrostatic pressure
• Cardiac tamponade
  • Idiopathic pericardial haemorrhage
  • Right atrial haemangiosarcoma
• Over-zealous fluid administration
• Right heart failure

Increased vascular permeability
• Urticarial angio-oedema

Localised
Increased capillary hydrostatic pressure
• Tourniquet, e.g. bandage, collar
• Venous obstruction
  • Thrombophlebitis

Increased vascular permeability
• Insect bite
• Local infection/cellulitis
• Thrombophlebitis

UNCOMMON CAUSES

Generalised
• Inappropriate ADH secretion
• Myxoedema (hypothyroidism)

Decreased capillary oncotic pressure
(hypoalbuminaemia)
• Severe burns

Increased capillary hydrostatic pressure
• Dirofilariasis
• Restrictive pericarditis

Increased vascular permeability
• Sepsis
• Vasculitis

Localised
Increased capillary hydrostatic pressure
• Abscess/granuloma
• Arteriovenous fistula
• Neoplasia
• Venous thrombosis

Increased vascular permeability
• Mast cell tumour

• Severe burns
• Snake bite
• Vasculitis

Lymphatic obstruction (variable localization)
• Congenital (inherited) lymphoedema
  • Aplasia or hypoplasia
  • Hyperplasia with absent LNs
• Lymphangiectasia
• Lymphangioma/sarcoma
• Lymphangitis/lymphadenitis
• Lymphocysts
• Occlusion of cranial vena cava, causing oedema of head and neck
  • Dirofilariasis (caval syndrome)
  • Mediastinal neoplasia
    • Lymphoma
    • Thymoma
  • Neck neoplasia
    • Lymphoma
    • Thyroid carcinoma
  • Thrombosis
• Pelvic region neoplasia causing oedema of hindlimbs
• Post-surgical

DIAGNOSTIC APPROACH

1 Determine whether oedema is localised or generalised by physical examination.
2 If localised, investigate local lymphatic system and evidence for insect bite, tumours, etc.
3 With generalised peripheral oedema, check serum albumin, and investigate any cause of hypoalbuminaemia.
4 If normal serum proteins, rule out right heart and pericardial disease before investigating lymphatic and vascular systems.

Clinical clues
Predisposition
• Dirofilariasis in travelled dogs in UK, and in dogs native to endemic areas
• Idiopathic pericardial haemorrhage in large-/giant-breed dogs
• Right atrial haemangiosarcoma in GSDs

History
- Acute onset cranial oedema with anorexia, respiratory distress, and weakness in caval syndrome
- Gradual/fluctuating oedema with neoplasia and congenital lymphoedema
- Sudden onset of oedema with right heart failure, pericardial disease

Clinical examination
Visual inspection
- Swelling of limb(s) and/or trunk and/or head

Physical examination
- Pitting oedema
- Right-sided cardiac murmur with caval syndrome

Laboratory findings
Haematology
- Anaemia in caval syndrome
- Inflammatory leukogram suggests inflammation ± infection

Biochemistry
- Hepatic and renal dysfunction in caval syndrome
- Hypoalbuminaemia
- Increased liver enzyme activities and bile acids suggests liver disease

Urinalysis
- Haemoglobinuria in caval syndrome
- Proteinuria suggests PLN

Imaging
- Radiography to demonstrate mass, increase in organ size, or body fluid accumulation
- Ultrasonography to demonstrate fluid in various body cavities

Special tests
- Abdominocentesis, thoracocentesis, pericardiocentesis
- Angiography
- Biopsy
- Knott's test or occult heartworm antigen test
- Lymphangiography

2.21 PLEURAL EFFUSION

DEFINITION

An accumulation of fluid in the pleural space. The accumulated fluid can be:
- Transudate (hydrothorax) due to hypoalbuminaemia
- Modified transudate
- Exudate due to septic (pyothorax) or non-septic inflammation
  or may contain:
- Blood (haemothorax)
- Chyle (chylothorax)

RELATED CLINICAL SIGNS

- Abnormal lung sounds, *q.v.* section 2.3
- Cyanosis, *q.v.* section 2.6
- Exercise intolerance/lethargy, *q.v.* section 1.22
- Varying degrees of dyspnoea and tachypnoea, *q.v.* section 1.18

COMMON CAUSES

Chylothorax
NB: rare compared to other causes of pleural effusion but most common cause of chylothorax
- Idiopathic
- Traumatic thoracic duct rupture

Exudate
Neoplasia
- Mediastinal lymphoma

Pulmonary masses
- Adenocarcinoma

Pyothorax
- Migrating FB

Haemothorax
- Bleeding disorder

- Neoplasia, especially haemangiosarcoma
- Trauma

Modified transudate
- Congestive heart failure including pericardial effusion secondary to cardiac tamponade
- Neoplasia

• Transudate (hydrothorax)
- Hypoalbuminaemia
  - Hepatic failure
  - PLE
  - PLN

UNCOMMON CAUSES

Chylothorax
- Congenital
- Constrictive pleuritis
- Dirofilariasis
- Jugular vein thrombosis (after cannulation)
- Neoplasia
- Post-pacemaker implantation
- Right heart failure (rare cause of effusion cf. cat)

Exudate
Neoplasia
- Cranial mediastinal thymoma
- Heart base tumour
- Mesothelioma
- Rib chondrosarcoma, osteosarcoma

Pyothorax
- *Actinomyces, Nocardia*
- Oesophageal perforation
- Penetrating wound (chest wall or oesophagus)
- Parapneumonic effusion, i.e. extension of pneumonia
- Ruptured pulmonary abscess
- Tuberculosis

Sterile inflammation
- Bile pleuritis: ruptured biliary tree through diaphragmatic rupture
- Dirofilariasis
- Lung lobe torsion; can occur secondary to other primary cause of effusion

- Eosinophilic pulmonary granulomatosis
- Ruptured diaphragm with organ entrapment
- Pancreatitis (small volume)
- Systemic lupus erythematosus (SLE)
- Walled-off abscess

Haemothorax
- *Angiostrongylus*
- Lung lobe torsion when lung lobe becomes necrotic
- Necrotic neoplasm
  - Mesothelioma
  - Thymus

Modified transudate
- Lung lobe torsion
- Right heart failure (uncommon *cf.* cat)
- Ruptured diaphragm with organ entrapment
- Vasculitis

Small volume
- Pancreatitis
- Post-partum
- PTE
- Pyometra
- Secondary to abdominal surgery
- SLE

DIAGNOSTIC APPROACH

1 Confirm clinical suspicion of pleural effusion by imaging.
2 Obtain sample of effusion for analysis after ruling out coagulopathy.
3 Repeat imaging after drainage, having used chest drain if large volume.
4 Identify underlying cause from fluid analysis and imaging results.
5 Further investigations depend on type of effusion, e.g investigate causes of hypoalbuminaemia.

Clinical clues
Predisposition
- Idiopathic chylothorax in Afghan hound, Borzoi
- Migrating FB (e.g. grass awn) in working spaniels

History
- Access to anticoagulant rodenticide
- Coughing
- Jugular catheterisation
- Previous trauma causing penetrating wound or ruptured diaphragm
- Signs of underlying GI or liver disease

Clinical examination
Visual inspection
- Dyspnoea, tachypnoea
- Evidence of generalised bleeding

Physical examination
Auscultation
- Muffled lung sounds ventrally; fluid line may be discernible

Palpation
- Chest wall mass
- Displacement of apex beat by intrathoracic mass
- Displacement of trachea from midline of thoracic inlet by intrathoracic mass
- Jugular thrombosis

Percussion
- Dull ventrally; fluid line discernible

Laboratory findings
Haematology
- Inflammatory leukogram if pyothorax or necrotic tumour

Serum biochemistry
- Changes characteristic of underlying systemic disease

Urinalysis
- Proteinuria if PLN

Imaging
Plain radiographs,
q.v. section 4.3
- DV (and standing lateral) preferred if lateral recumbency causes dyspnoea
- Lateral recumbent radiograph taken after thoracocentesis

- Lung lobe torsion causes displacement of mainstem bronchi
- Mediastinal mass
  - Associated effusion may obscure mass
  - Soft tissue density cranial to heart and displacing trachea dorsally
- Pleural fluid
  - 50–100 ml is the minimum amount of fluid that can be detected
  - Pleural fissure lines
  - Retraction of lung lobes from thoracic wall
  - Obscured cardiac and diaphragmatic outline

  NB: Intrathoracic fat or skin fold may mimic effusion.

Ultrasound examination
- Better contrast between fluid and soft tissue if performed before thoracocentesis
- Echocardiography
- Identification of mass
- Used to guide thoracocentesis, FNA and needle biopsy

Special tests
- Aerobic and anaerobic culture
- Analysis of pleural fluid
  - Cell numbers and morphology
    - Lymphocytes (chylothorax)
    - Neoplastic cells
    - Neutrophils
      - Degenerate: pyothorax
      - Non-degenerate: neoplasia
  - Cholesterol concentration > serum, and triglyceride concentration < serum if chylothorax
  - Gram's stain for pyothorax
  - PCV
  - Protein
  - Specific gravity
- Coagulation profile
- Exploratory thoracotomy
- FNA and/or needle biopsy of masses
- Lymphangiography
- Spec cPL
- Thoracocentesis
  - May be negative if loculated or thick exudate

2.22 PNEUMOTHORAX

DEFINITION

An accumulation of air in the pleural space. This may occur due to direct communication with the external environment or via an air leak due to intrathoracic pathology.

RELATED CLINICAL SIGNS

- Abnormal lung sounds, *q.v.* section 2.3
- Collapse
- Cyanosis
- Dyspnoea
- Exercise intolerance/lethargy
- Hyper-resonant percussion
- Tachycardia
- Tachypnoea

COMMON CAUSES

- Trauma
  - Blunt trauma to thorax causing lung damage through acute pressure changes
  - Penetrating thoracic wall trauma
  - Traumatic rib fractures lacerating lung lobe(s)
NB: Beware of radiographic artefact misinterpreted as pneumothorax.
  - Over-development
  - Over-exposure

- Over-inflation
- Skin folds
- Hypovolaemia

UNCOMMON CAUSES

- Spontaneous
  - Airway obstruction
  - Migrating FB
  - Neoplasia
  - Oesophageal perforation
  - Pneumonia: bacterial, fungal
  - Pulmonary abscess
  - Ruptured bulla(e)
  - Tracheal trauma, e.g. bite wound; pneumomediastinum more likely
- Iatrogenic
  - Cardiopulmonary resuscitation
  - Chest drain leak
  - FNA or transcutaneous biopsy
  - Over-inflation during bronchoscopy
  - Over-inflation of endotracheal tube; pneumomediastinum more likely
  - Mechanical ventilation
  - Thoracocentesis
  - Thoracotomy

DIAGNOSTIC APPROACH

q.v. section 5.10.5B

2.23 PROSTATOMEGALY

DEFINITION

Enlargement of the prostate gland.
   As the normal prostate size is related to the dog's size, enlargement is defined by:
- Movement to an intra-abdominal position
- Relationship to height of pelvic canal on rectal examination; normal is one-third
- Ultrasonographic measurement
   An enlarged prostate on palpation may demonstrate:

- Abnormal shape: asymmetric, loss of median raphé
- Abnormal texture: fluctuant, hard, irregular
- Adherence to pelvic floor
- Pain

COMMON CAUSES

- Acute prostatitis
- Benign prostatic hypertrophy/hyperplasia (BPH)

- Chronic prostatitis
- Prostatic abscess
- Prostatic carcinoma or transitional cell carcinoma/urothelial carcinoma (TCC/UC)

UNCOMMON CAUSES

- *Brucella canis*: not endemic in UK but consider in imported dogs
- *Leishmania*
- Paraprostatic cyst
- Prostatic neoplasia
  - Lymphoma
  - Metastatic disease
- Prostatic cyst
- Squamous metaplasia

RELATED CLINICAL SIGNS

- Caudal abdominal pain
- Constipation
- Deformed stool (ribbon-shape)
- Dripping blood from penis
- Dysuria
- Fever
- Haematuria
- Hind limb lameness
- Hind limb oedema
- Intermittent haemorrhage from penis, not associated with urination
- Urinary and/or faecal tenesmus

DIAGNOSTIC APPROACH

1 Assess prostate size and structure by abdominal and rectal palpation.
2 Image prostate by ultrasound and/or positive contrast retrograde urethrogram/contrast CT.
3 Urine culture.
4 Biopsy: FNA, prostatic wash, catheter suction biopsy, needle biopsy.

Clinical clues
Predisposition
- *Brucella canis* in imported stud dog
- BPH in older intact dog

- Prostatic carcinoma is more common in castrated dogs

History
- Signs of urinary tract infection, dysuria and tenesmus

Clinical examination
Visual inspection
- Blood may drip from penis between urinations
- Dysuria
- Haematuria
- Tenesmus

Physical examination
- Pyrexia if prostatitis or prostatic abscess, or brucellosis
- Signs of feminism and testicular tumour if squamous metaplasia

Rectal palpation
- Enlarged prostate ± abnormal texture/ structure
- Pain: prostatitis or prostatic abscess
- Orchitis, epididymitis or lymphadenopathy in brucellosis

Laboratory findings
Haematology
- Inflammatory leukogram if prostatitis or prostatic abscess
- Usually unremarkable

Serum biochemistry
- Usually unremarkable
- Azotaemia if urinary obstruction

Urinalysis
- Abnormal cells in prostatic carcinoma (cytology better than sediment analysis)
- Haematuria sometimes in BPH, prostatic cyst, carcinoma
- Pyuria in prostatitis

Imaging
Plain radiographs
- Caudal abdominal mass – prostate, paraprostatic cyst or distended bladder

- Sublumbar lymph node enlargement with periosteal reaction on lumbar vertebral bodies with prostatic neoplasia
- Thoracic radiographs for metastatic disease
  Contrast radiographs
- Assymetric position of urethra if neoplasia or cyst
- Extravasation of contrast on retrograde urethrogram if prostate is diseased

Ultrasound examination
  Prostate size and changes in echoarchitecture
  - Abscess

- Cyst(s)
- Neoplasia
- Paraprostatic cyst(s)

Special tests
- BRAF gene mutation test for TCC/UC
- *Brucella* serology (RSAT and 2ME-RSAT)
- Canine prostate specific arginine esterase: non-specific marker of prostatic disease
- *Leishmania* serology
- Prostatic wash or ejaculate for culture and cytology
- (Ultrasound-guided) FNA and Tru-cut biopsy

2.24 PULSE ABNORMALITIES

DEFINITION

The peripheral pulse reflects the difference between the systolic and diastolic pressure.
  Hyperdynamic peripheral pulse:
- A large difference between the systolic and diastolic pressure
- Due to a high output state (increase in cardiac output with decreased vascular resistance) or conditions that cause a decrease in diastolic pressure
  Weak/absent peripheral pulse
- A small difference between the systolic and diastolic pressure
- Due to poor cardiac output or obstruction in peripheral vessel
- May have intermittent weak pulses (known as pulse deficits)

RELATED CLINICAL SIGNS

May have no clinical signs or:
- Acute onset hindlimb paresis
- Congestive heart failure
- Murmur
- Syncope/weakness/lethargy

COMMON CAUSES

Hyperdynamic
- Anaemia

- Bradyarrhythmias
- Exercise/excitement
- Patent ductus arteriosus
- Pyrexia

Weak/absent
- Atrial fibrillation
- Cardiac arrest
  - Asystole
  - Electromechanical dissociation
- Cardiac tamponade: may feel *pulsus paradoxus*, i.e. a decrease in pulse quality during inspiration and increase in pulse quality in expiration
- DCM
- Hypovolaemia
- Tachyarrhythmias: may get deficits with single premature beats, whereas sustained arrhythmias are likely to cause weak pulses

UNCOMMON CAUSES

Hyperdynamic
- Aortic endocarditis causing severe aortic insufficiency

Weak/absent
- (Femoral) arterial thromboembolism

DIAGNOSTIC APPROACH

Hyperdynamic pulses
- Assess mucous membranes for evidence of anaemia
- Auscultate heart for murmurs and arrhythmias
- Echocardiography may be required
- Measure rectal temperature for evidence of pyrexia

Weak/absent pulses
- Abdominal imaging to assess for thromboembolism
- Assess for evidence of hypovolaemia (tachycardia, pale mucous membranes, delayed capillary refill time, skin tent)
- Auscultate heart for murmurs, arrhythmias and dull heart sounds
- Echocardiography likely required as cannot rule out dilated cardiomyopathy based on the absence of a heart murmur
- Investigations into diseases that cause a hypercoagulable state (protein-losing conditions, hyperadrenocorticism, pancreatitis, immune-mediated anaemia/thrombocytopenia, systemic inflammation, neoplasia) via hematology, biochemistry and urinalysis ± thoracic/abdominal imaging if evidence of thromboembolism

Clinical clues
Predisposition
- DCM more common in older large-breed dogs
- Patent ductus arteriosus: females, Cocker spaniel, Poodle and GSD
- Pericardial effusion more common in older patients
- Subaortic stenosis increases the chances of developing aortic endocarditis
- Thromboembolism in HAC

History
- Arterial thromboembolism causes an acute onset painful loss of use of one or more limbs
- Episodes of syncope may be reported with tachyarrhythmias or bradyarrhythmias
- Signs of HAC, *q.v.* section 5.3.4A

Clinical examination
Visual inspection
- May be tachypnoeic/dyspnoeic with any disease that has led to congestive heart failure
- Pale mucous membranes, prolonged capillary refill time, skin tent with hypovolaemia
- Pale mucous membranes with anaemia

Physical examination
Auscultation
- Aortic endocarditis murmur will be diastolic (insufficiency) and/or systolic (obstruction)
- Dilated cardiomyopathy patients may not have a murmur
- May hear flow murmur at the left base with anaemia
- PDA murmur is continuous
  Palpation
- Hepatomegaly and abdominal effusion with bradyarrhythmias, pericardial effusion or tachyarrhythmias due to venous congestion

Laboratory findings
Haematology
- Assess for IMHA and thrombocytopenia in cases with arterial thromboembolism
- May see inflammatory leukogram with endocarditis
- Rule in/out anaemia as a cause of hyperdynamic pulses

Serum biochemistry
- Increase in ALP and ALT activities with HAC
- Signs of reduced cardiac output (pre-renal azotaemia, increased ALT activity) with tachyarrhythmias, bradyarrhythmias and cardiac tamponade
- May see hypoalbuminemia with protein-losing conditions predisposing to thrombus formation

Urinalysis
- Assess for proteinuria/infection as a cause for hypercoagulable state

Imaging
Plain radiographs
- Globoid cardiac silhouette with pericardial effusion

- Cardiomegaly may be seen with anaemia, dilated cardiomyopathy, patent ductus arteriosus, aortic endocarditis, tachyarrhythmias and bradyarrhythmias – depending on severity of changes, may also see pulmonary venous congestion and interstitial/alveolar patterns if in congestive heart failure
- Assess for pulmonary neoplasia as a trigger for arterial thromboembolism
- Look for cause of anaemia/pyrexia

Ultrasound

- Abdominal ultrasound to assess for ascites, arterial thromboembolism, adrenal size, pancreatic appearance, cause of anaemia/pyrexia, presence of splenic/hepatic disease triggering tachyarrhythmias

- Echocardiography to assess for pericardial effusion, chamber size, systolic function, evidence of endocarditis and presence/absence of a patent ductus arteriosus
- Thoracic ultrasound to assess for B-lines implying fluid within the alveolar space or pleural effusion

Special tests

- ACTH stimulation test, LDDS test, UCCR
- Bone marrow assessment
- cPL
- Coombs' test
- Cytology of any effusions
- ECG – in clinic and 24-hour ECG Holter monitor
- Pericardiocentesis with fluid analysis
- Troponin I

2.25 PYREXIA AND HYPERTHERMIA

DEFINITIONS

Hyperthermia

Hyperthermia (> 39.2°C) is an increased body temperature due to a failure of the individual to dissipate generated heat; this may occur due to a failure of thermoregulation, or increased environmental temperature, or a combination of both. Dogs are vulnerable to heatstroke when core body temperature is > 41°C and can suffer from negative effects of an increased temperature above this. At a temperature > 41.5°C direct cytotoxicity occurs as enzymes are no longer able to function.

Pyrexia

Pyrexia or fever, in contrast to hyperthermia, is defined as an increased body temperature (> 39.2°C) that occurs due to alteration of the thermoregulatory set point in the anterior hypothalamus in response to endogenous or exogenous pyrogens. Pyrexia is a highly conserved physiological adaptive response that, in the short term, confers an evolutionary advantage, particularly when combating infectious disease.

RELATED CLINICAL SIGNS

Hyperthermia

Animals that are hyperthermic will be seeking to dissipate heat. Dogs will often display panting, seeking cool surfaces and may display signs of anxiety (pacing, restlessness). Dogs with heatstroke may display the negative effects of this elevated temperature, i.e. vomiting, diarrhoea, collapse, abnormal consciousness and/or seizures, and bleeding diatheses.

Pyrexia

In contrast, pyrexic animals do not seek to dissipate heat, and are more likely to be lethargic and inappetant. Attempts to cool the patient by external environmental cooling are futile.

Pyrexia in conjunction with dyspnoea (e.g. pneumonia) can be more challenging to discriminate from hyperthermia, especially in brachycephalic dogs where there may be both hyperthermia and pyrexia.

COMMON CAUSES

Hyperthermia
Risk factors for development of hyperthermia:
- Excessive physical activity or stress
- Hot especially humid environments
- Obesity
- Pain
- Prolonged seizures or muscle tremors
- Upper airway obstruction: brachycephalic obstructive airway syndrome (BOAS), laryngeal paralysis

Pyrexia
- Immune-mediated disease
  - IMPA
  - SRMA
- Infectious disease
  - Cholangiohepatitis
  - Migrating FB
  - Pneumonia (aspiration, bronchopneumonia, FB)
  - Prostatitis
  - Pyelonephritis
  - Pyometra
  - Pyothorax
  - Specific infectious diseases: *Bordetella bronchiseptica*, *Leptospira*, *Neospora*, parvovirus, *Toxoplasma*
  - Traumatic wound
- Neoplasia
  - Any large tumour burden (especially lymphoma, large masses)
- Miscellaneous inflammatory
  - Metaphyseal osteopathy
  - Pancreatitis

UNCOMMON CAUSES

Hyperthermia
- Malignant hyperthermia
  - Drug-induced, especially general anaesthesia with halothane
  - Exercise-induced due to genetic mutation

Pyrexia
- Immune-mediated disease
  - IMHA, but pyrexia uncommon

- Inflammatory brain disease, but pyrexia uncommon
- Panniculitis and pansteatitis
- Pyogranulomatous lymphadenitis
- Infectious disease
  - Discospondylitis, e.g. *Brucella*, migrating FB
  - Endocarditis, e.g. *Bartonella*, haematogenous infection
  - Septic arthritis:
    - haematogenous infection
    - implant-related infection
    - vector-borne disease
  - Opportunistic infections to immune disorders, e.g. metaphyseal osteomyelitis in Border collies with trapped neutrophil syndrome, cyclic haematopoiesis or selective cobalamin deficiency
  - Vector-borne infections (*Anaplasma*, *Babesia*, *Borrelia*)
- Miscellaneous inflammatory
  - Panosteitis
  - Splenic torsion

DIAGNOSTIC APPROACH

- Distinguish hyperthermia from pyrexia.
- In patients where there is suspicion of stress-induced hyperthermia, admit and monitor temperature, or discharge the dog and provide the owner with a thermometer to allow home monitoring.
- In heatstroke, monitor vital parameters (coagulation times, renal function, etc.) whilst actively cooling.
- In pyrexia, investigate underlying cause whilst potentially reducing body temperature with paracetamol or appropriate NSAIDs.

Clinical clues
Predisposition
- Border collies and Springer spaniels are thought to have a genetic basis for exercise-induced malignant hyperthermia
- Juvenile dogs are most likely to have immune-mediated disorders (e.g. SRMA, metaphyseal osteopathy)

History

- Dogs with pyrexia are more likely to be sedentary and lethargic. Detailed history may help to gain clues regarding the cause of pyrexia, e.g. dogs with IMPA may have subtle signs of joint pain, *q.v.* section 2.17.2
- Excitable, active dogs or brachycephalic dogs with a history of vigorous exercise especially in hot, humid environments will increase suspicion of hyperthermia
- Travel history, exposure to ticks and vaccination and lifestyle history may influence suspicion of infectious disease

Clinical examination

Visual inspection

- Observation of the dog in the consulting room may help in discriminating between pyrexia and hyperthermia: dogs with hyperthermia more likely to have a higher energy state and display attempts to dissipate heat
- Careful observation of the dog's interaction with the environment may help with clues for causes of pyrexia, including thorough assessment for lameness or neck movement

Physical examination

- Thorough examination to assess for multisystemic disease or source or pain
  - Assess for a novel heart murmur (may increase suspicion of endocarditis)
  - Assess for joint effusions (may increase suspicion of polyarthritis or septic joint)
  - Assess in puppies for bone pain, especially periarticular (may increase suspicion of metaphyseal osteopathy)
  - Neurological examination in patients with suspicion of discospondylitis, and inflammatory brain disease
- Orthopaedic examination in patients with suspicion of polyarthritis and septic joint

Laboratory findings

Haematology and serum biochemistry

- Haematology may be useful to assess for inflammatory disease but not in hyperthermia
- Biochemistry is useful to screen for systemic disease and organ involvement as underlying cause of pyrexia or damage caused by hyperthermia

Imaging

Plain radiographs and ultrasound

- Screen for infectious, inflammatory or neoplastic disorders
- Spine for evidence of discospondylitis

Special tests

- Arthrocentesis for cytology ± culture to assess for IMPA and septic joints
- cPL to assess for pancreatitis, may be elevated in other causes of inflammatory disease
- C-reactive protein to assess for inflammatory disease; also useful to monitor individual patients
- CSF sampling for cytology and proteins for SRMA
- Echocardiography and troponins to assess for endocarditis
- Infectious disease screening as appropriate
  - SNAP® 4Dx for *Anaplasma, Borrelia, Dirofilaria, Ehrlichia*
  - PCR for *Babesia*
  - PCR for *Leptospira*
  - Serology or PCR for *Bartonella*
- Prostatic wash for cytology and culture in male entire dogs with suspicion of prostatitis

2.26   SKIN LESIONS

DEFINITION

A range of lesions can be caused by primary skin diseases or occur secondarily as signs of systemic illness often in conjunction with alopecia (*q.v.* section 1.2) and skin pigment changes (*q.v.* section 2.27). Pruritic skin conditions (*q.v.* section 1.39) can produce lesions through self-trauma. Primary infective, inflammatory, immune-mediated and neoplastic skin conditions can produce visible lesions.

Primary lesions
Macules and patches
- A macule is small patch of skin (< 1 cm) that is altered in colour (pigmented, depigmented or purpuric), but is not elevated
- A patch is a larger area of colour change, with a smooth surface

Nodules
A palpable/raised, solid lesion greater than 1 cm in diameter, usually originating in the dermal or subcutaneous tissue

Papules and plaques
- A papule is a small (< 1 cm), raised, solid, erythematous eruption in the epidermis caused by inflammation, oedema and hypertrophy
- A plaque is a circumscribed, elevated, solid lesion that is greater than 1 cm in diameter and is usually broader than it is thick

Pustules
Small circumscribed or larger asymmetric eruptions on the skin, initially filled with an inflammatory/suppurative exudate, but often ruptured leaving an epidermal collarette

Scaling
The loss of the outer layer of the epidermis in large, scale-like flakes

Vesicles and bullae
A vesicle is a small, superficial, circumscribed blister less than 1 cm in diameter and filled with clear, serous, haemorrhagic, or purulent fluid; a bulla is a large, raised, circumscribed blister that is > 1 cm in diameter and contains clear, serous, haemorrhagic, or purulent fluid, but are seen rarely as they rupture easily

Wheals
An urticarial reaction causing circumscribed, erythematous raised papules or plaques, often transient and usually with a flat surface associated with allergy-related inflammation

Secondary lesions
Crusting
Dried exudate (serum, blood or pus) on the skin surface, often trapping scale

Erosions and excoriations
- Erosions are circumscribed losses of epidermal layers above the basement membrane typically caused by scratching, rubbing or biting
- Excoriations are superficial erosions

Furunculosis
- A skin infection forming lumps and pus
  - A furuncle (abscess) forms when a hair follicle and surrounding tissue become infected.
  - A carbuncle (deep pyoderma) is made up of multiple furuncles and goes much deeper into the skin.

Hyperkeratosis
- Increased thickness of the stratum corneum

Lichenification
- Thickening of the skin with exaggerated skin markings caused by chronic inflammation or friction, and usually accompanied by hyperpigmentation, q.v. section 2.27

Ulcer
- A circumscribed loss of the epidermis and extending into at least the upper dermis and may be associated with draining tracts from furunculosis

RELATED CLINICAL SIGNS

- Alopecia
- Erythema
- Malodour
- Pigment changes, q.v. section 2.27
- Primary lesions: scaling, papules, pustules, nodules, vesicles
- Pruritus, q.v. section 1.39
- Secondary lesions: crusting, erosions/excoriations, hyperkeratosis, lichenification and ulcers

COMMON CAUSES

Macules (and patches)
- Blood extravasation: ecchymoses, petechiation
- Freckles

PHYSICAL ABNORMALITIES

- HAC
- Hypothyroidism
- Healed superficial erosions

Nodules
Inflammation
- Bacterial infection:
  - Subcutaneous abscess
- Fungal infection
  - Dermatophytosis (ringworm)
- Granuloma:
  - Acral lick granuloma
  - Callus and hygroma
  - Insect bite
- Leishmaniasis; common in Mediterranean climate zones, and imported dogs in the UK

Epithelial neoplasia
- Apocrine adenoma/carcinoma
- Basal cell tumour
- Perianal gland adenoma/adenocarcinoma, *q.v.* section 2.19
- Pilomatrixoma
- Sebaceous adenoma/carcinoma
- Sweat gland tumours
- Trichoepithelioma
- Viral papillomatosis

Round cell neoplasia
- Histiocytoma
  - MCT
- Plasmacytoma

Mesenchymal neoplasia
- Lipoma

Non-inflammatory, non-neoplastic
- Benign nodular sebaceous hyperplasia
- Cysts
  - Dermoid
  - Epidermoid
  - Follicular
- Polyp
- Seroma
- Tail gland hyperplasia

Papules and plaques
Immune-mediated
- Atopy
- Flea allergic dermatitis

Infection
- Dermatophytosis
- Impetigo
- *Leishmania*
- Sarcoptic mange
- Superficial pyoderma

Pustules
- Acne
- Demodecosis
- Dermatophytosis
- Pyoderma
  - Impctigo
  - Superficial pyoderma

Scaling
Primary and inherited disorders of keratinisation
- Acne
- Nasal hyperkeratosis

Secondary scaling
- Allergic/immune-mediated
  - Atopy
  - Flea allergic dermatitis
- Environmental
  - Physical or chemical damage
- Infectious/parasitic
  - Bacterial pyoderma
  - Cheyletiellosis
  - Demodecosis
  - Dermatophytosis
  - Fleas
  - Leishmaniasis (not common in UK yet)
  - *Malassezia*
  - Pyoderma
  - Sarcoptic mange
- Metabolic/hormonal
  - HAC
  - Hypothyroidism

Vesicles and bullae
- None: all uncommon

Wheals (urticaria)
- Environmental allergens
- Insect bites and stings
  - MCT

PHYSICAL ABNORMALITIES

UNCOMMON CAUSES

Macules (and patches)
- Sertoli cell tumour
- Vitiligo (depigmented patches)

Nodules
Inflammation
- Angiogenic oedema
- Infection
  - Bacterial
    - Actinomycosis
    - Botryomycosis (cutaneous bacterial pseudomycetoma)
    - Leproid granuloma syndrome
    - Nocardiososis
    - Opportunistic mycobacteriosis
    - Tuberculosis
  - Fungal
    - Blastomycosis
    - Coccidioidomycosis
    - Cryptococcosis
    - Eukaryotic mycetoma
    - Histoplasmosis
    - Phaeohyphomycosis
    - Prototheccosis
    - Pythiosis
    - Lagenidiosis
    - Sporotrichosis
    - Zygomycosis
  - Parasitic
    - *Cuterebra*
    - *Dirofilaria repens*
    - Dracunculiasis
    - Neosporosis
- Histiocytosis
- Nodular cutaneous amyloidosis
- Nodular dermatofibrosis
- SLE
- Sterile nodular panniculitis
- Urticaria
- Vesicular lupus erythematosus (LE)
- Xanthoma

Epithelial neoplasia
- Keratoacanthoma
- Polyp
- Squamous cell carcinoma

Melanocyte neoplasia
- Malignant melanoma

Round cell neoplasia
- Lymphoma
  - Epitheliotropic
  - Lymphomatoid granulomatosis
  - Non-epitheliotrophic
- Histiocytic sarcoma
- Plasmacytoma

Mesenchymal neoplasia
- Fibropruritic nodule
- Fibrous histiocytoma
- Dermatofibroma
- Fibrolipoma
- Fibroma/fibropapilloma/fibrosarcoma
- Hamartoma/haemangioma/haemangiosarcoma
- Haemangiopericytoma
- Leiomyoma/sarcoma
- Liposarcoma
- Lymphangioma/sarcoma
- Myxosarcoma
- Schwannoma

Metastatic
- A variety of carcinomas

Non-inflammatory, non-neoplastic
- Benign nodular sebaceous hyperplasia
- Calcinosis circumscripta
- Fibroadnexal dysplasia
- Follicular cysts
- Haematoma
- Naevi
- Urticaria pigmentosa

Papules and plaques
Immune-mediated
- Contact dermatitis
- Dermatomyositis
- Drug reaction
- Eosinophilic plaques
- Food hypersensitivity
- Pemphigus foliaceous
- Squamous cell carcinoma
- Subcorneal pustular dermatosis
- Sterile eosinophilic pustulosis

Infection
- Calcinosis cutis
- Cheyletiellosis
- Chin pyoderma
- Pediculosis
- Trombiculiasis

Metabolic
- Xanthoma

Neoplasia
- Epitheliotropic lymphoma
- Papilloma

Pustules
- Linear immunoglobulin A (IgA) dermatosis
- Panepidermal pustular pemphigus
- Pemphigus foliaceous
- Subcorneal pustular dermatosis
- Sterile eosinophilic pustulosis

Scaling
Exfoliative dermatoses
- Parapsoriasis
- Toxic epidermal necrolysis

Primary and inherited disorders of keratinisation
- Ear margin dermatosis
- Idiopathic seborrhoea
- Epidermal dysplasia
- Follicular dysplasia
- Follicular hyperkeratosis and parakeratosis
- Footpad hyperkeratosis
  - Distemper
  - Superficial necrolytic dermatitis (SND), also known as metabolic epidermal necrosis, or necrolytic migratory erythema
    - Glucagonoma
    - Hepatocutaneous syndrome
- Icthyosis
- Lethal acrodermatitis
- Lichenoid psoriasiform dermatosis
- Nasodigital hyperkeratosis
- Schnauzer comedo syndrome
- Sebaceous adenitis
- Vitamin A-responsive dermatosis
- Zinc-responsive dermatosis
  - Type 1 in Alaskan breed

- Type 2 in fast-growing large-breed dog
- Type 3 due to dietary deficiency

Secondary scaling
- Allergic/immune-mediated
  - Contact hypersensitivity
  - Drug eruption
  - Food hypersensitivity
  - Pemphigus foliaceous
  - SLE
  - Thymoma
- Environmental
  - Low humidity
- Infectious/parasitic
  - Pediculosis
- Metabolic/hormonal
  - Diabetic dermatopathy
  - Growth hormone-responsive dermatosis
  - Hyperandrogenism
  - Hypopituitarism
  - Male feminizing syndrome
  - Intestinal malabsorption
  - Necrolytic migratory erythema
  - Oestrogen-responsive dermatosis
  - Pancreatic carcinoma
  - Sertoli cell tumour
  - Superficial necrolytic dermatitis/necrolytic migratory erythema
    - Glucagonoma
    - Hepatocutaneous syndrome
  - Testosterone-responsive dermatosis
- Tail gland hyperplasia

Vesicles and bullae
Rarely seen because of early rupture due to self-trauma, leaving erosions or ulcers.
- Bullous pemphigoid
- Cutaneous burns
- Cutaneous drug eruptions
- Epidermolysis bullosa
- Erythema multiforme
- Topical chemicals
- Pemphigus complex
  - Pemphigus erythematosus
  - Pemphigus foliaceous
  - Pemphigus vulgaris
- SLE

Wheals (urticaria)
- Contact dermatitis

- Drug reaction
- Food allergic reactions
- Physical factors
  - Pressure
  - Cold
  - Exercise
- Snake venoms
- Vaccines

DIAGNOSTIC APPROACH

1 Identification of infectious agents by sello-tape strips, skin scrapes, hair plucks, and bacterial and fungal cultures.
2 After failing to identify infectious causes, trial therapy for bacterial pyoderma, fleas and possibly also for *Sarcoptes*, is acceptable.
3 Intradermal skin testing or serology is performed to identify atopic reactions.
4 If negative for atopy, an exclusion food trial is indicated.
5 Skin biopsy.

Clinical clues
Predisposition
- Atopy: French bulldog, WHWT
- Comedones: Miniature schnauzer
- Demodecosis: short-haired breeds
- Lethal acrodermatitis: Bull terrier, Miniature Bull terrier
- Lichenoid psoriasiform dermatosis: Springer spaniels
- Linear IgA dermatosis: Dachshunds
- Zinc-responsive dermatosis: Alaskan breeds, e.g. Siberian Husky and Alaskan Malamute, but also reported in Dobermann and Great Dane

History
- Hair loss/alopecia
- Increased shedding
- Pruritus
- Skin flakes (dandruff)

Distribution of lesions
q.v. section 1.39 for clues from distribution of pruritic lesions

Claw
- Bacterial infection
- Dermatophytosis

- *Leishmania*
- Melanoma
- Squamous cell carcinoma
- Symmetrical lupoid onychodystrophy
- Trauma
- Vasculitis

Ear margins
- Bullous pemphigoid
- Canine leproid granuloma syndrome
- Drug reactions
- Insect bite dermatitis
- Lupus erythematosus: discoid, systemic (SLE), vesicular cutaneous
- Pemphigus: erythematosus, foliaceous and vulgaris
- Sarcoptic mange/scabies
- Solar dermatitis
- Squamous cell carcinoma
- Vasculitis

Facial
- Discoid lupus erythematosus
- Early familial dermatomyositis
- Eosinophilic furunculosis
- Juvenile cellulitis
- Pemphigus: erythematosus, foliaceous
- Pyoderma: chin, mucocutaneous, nasal
- Uveodermatologic syndrome

Interdigital pododermatitis
- Atopy
- Bacterial infections
- Contact dermatitis
- Demodecosis
- Dermatophytosis
- Food hypersensitivity
- Interdigital pyogranuloma
- *Malassezia*
- Trombiculiasis
- Uncinaria hookworm

Nasal depigmentation
- Bullous pemphigoid
- Contact dermatitis
- Cutaneous, epitheliotropic lymphoma
- Lupus erythematosus: discoid, systemic (SLE), vesicular cutaneous
- Nasal aspergillosis
- Pemphigus: erythematosus, foliaceous and vulgaris

- Uveodermatologic syndrome
- Vitiligo

Nasodigital hyperkeratosis
- Cutaneous horn
- Corns
- Distemper
- Familial footpad hyperkeratosis
- Hepatocutaneous syndrome
- Hereditary nasal parakeratosis of Labradors
- Idiopathic nasodigital hyperkeratosis
- Leishmaniasis
- Pemphigus foliaceous
- SLE
- Zinc-responsive dermatosis

Oral lesions
- Bullous pemphigoid
- Candidiasis
- Contact dermatitis
- Cutaneous drug reaction
- Eosinophilic granuloma
- Epitheliotropic lymphoma
- Erythema multiforme
- Lupus erythematosus: systemic (SLE), vesicular cutaneous
- Melanoma
- Pemphigus vulgaris
- Squamous cell carcinoma
- Vasculitis

Scrotal lesions
- Bullous diseases
- Contact dermatitis
- Cutaneous histiocytosis
- Cuterebriasis
- Erythema multiforme
- Fixed pigmented erythema
- Frostbite
- Intertrigo
- Lupus erythematosus: systemic (SLE), vesicular cutaneous
- *Malassezia*
- Neoplasia
  - MCT
  - Melanoma
  - Squamous cell carcinoma
- Solar damage
- Superficial necrolytic dermatitis

- Trauma
- Vascular hamartoma

Clinical examination
Visual inspection
- Alopecia
- Pruritus
- Skin pigmentation

Physical examination
Internal organs
- Hepatomegaly in endocrine diseases
- Muscle atrophy in HAC
  Skin
- Alopecia
- Crusting
- Erosions
- Erythema
- Macules and patches
- Nodules
- Papules and plaques
- Pigment changes
- Pustules
- Scaling
- Thick skin: acral lick dermatitis, callus, hypothyroidism (myxoedema)
- Thin skin: HAC
- Ulcer
- Vesicles and bullae
- Wheals

Laboratory findings
Haematology
- Usually unremarkable in primary skin disease

Serum biochemistry
- Unremarkable unless underlying endocrine/metabolic disease

Imaging
- Generally not indicated as likely to be unremarkable unless there is an underlying medical condition
- 'Swiss cheese liver' associated with hepatocutaneous syndrome

Special tests
- DNA test for lethal acrodermatitis
- Immunohistochemistry of skin biopsies

2.27 SKIN PIGMENTATION CHANGES

DEFINITION

Abnormal skin and/or hair coat colour, which may be congenital or acquired, and may be localised or generalised.

RELATED CLINICAL SIGNS

- Alopecia, *q.v.* section 1.2
- Change in skin and/or coat colour
- Changes in iris colour and coloboma, *q.v.* section 2.7
- Changes in skin thickness and lichenification
- Deafness, *q.v.* section 1.14
- Pruritus, *q.v.* section 1.39

COMMON CAUSES

Blue
- Cyanosis, *q.v.* section 2.6

Black
Hyperpigmentation/melanosis
NB: Skin hyperpigmentation may be associated with skin thickening and hair loss but can also be clinically insignificant.
- Chronic inflammation/pruritus
  - Atopy (chronic)
  - Chronic trauma
  - Demodecosis
  - Flea allergic dermatitis
  - *Malassezia* infection
  - Superficial pyoderma
- Comedones: blocked follicles with surface melanin (blackheads)
- Endocrine
  - HAC
  - Hypothyroidism
  - Sertoli cell tumour
- External causes
  - Chronic friction, e.g., collars
- Lentigo: pigmented macules (freckles)
- Melanoma
- Naevus (mole)
- Normal areas of skin pigmentation
- Recurrent/seasonal flank alopecia

Brown
Areas of chronically wet hair due to tear or saliva overflow, or repeated licking of feet, due to the presence of porphyrins in saliva and bacterial activity
Hypopigmentation (pale, pink or merle)
- Anaemia, *q.v.* section 3.30.1
- Depigmentation
  - Discoid lupus erythematosus (DLE)
  - Breed-related leukoderma/vitiligo
  - Follicular infections causing leukotrichia
- Merle
  - Normal for some breeds

Red/purple (blood, haemoglobin)
- Papules and macules, *q.v.* section 2.26
- Petechiation, ecchymoses, haematoma, *q.v.* section 1.9

Yellow
Jaundice, *q.v.* section 2.13

UNCOMMON CAUSES

Black
Hyperpigmentation/melanosis
NB: Melanoplakia is focal melanosis of the mucous membranes and tongue.
- Acanthosis nigricans
- Chronic inflammation/pruritus
  - Contact dermatitis
  - Dermatomycosis/ringworm
  - Food-allergic dermatitis
  - Sarcoptic mange
- Endocrine
  - Alopecia X
  - Hyperoestrogenism
  - Male feminising syndrome
- External causes
  - Drugs
    - Minocycline
    - Mitotane
  - Radiation therapy
  - UV light exposure; tanning of exposed areas
- Lentigo profusa
- Neoplasia

- Basal cell tumour
- Malignant melanoma
- Urticaria pigmentosa-like disease
- Post-chemotherapy hair regrowth

Hypopigmentation (pale, pink or merle)
- Albinism
- Cold environment causing vasoconstriction
- Depigmentation
  - Acquired idiopathic hypopigmentation of the nose
  - Age-related greying
  - Aspergillosis (nasal planum)
  - Dermatomyositis
  - Immune-mediated
    - Bullous pemphigoid
    - SLE
    - Canine uveodermatological (Vogt-Koyanagi-Harada-like) syndrome
  - Leukoderma/vitiligo
    - Copper deficiency
    - Freezing, frost-bite
    - Nasal contact with p-benzyl hydroquinone in rubber food bowls
    - Radiation therapy
    - Severe necrosis and scarring
    - Solar dermatitis (nasal planum)
    - Zinc deficiency
  - Leukotrichia, same as leukoderma plus
    - Clipping of black hair (temporary)
    - Periocular leukotrichia (Aguirre syndrome)
- Neoplasia
  - Epitheliotropic lymphoma
  - Squamous cell carcinoma including multicentric SCC in situ (Bowen's disease)
- Merle
  - Cyclic haematopoiesis
  - Waardenburg-Klein syndrome
- Piebaldism
- Tyrosinase deficiency

Red/purple (blood, haemoglobin)
- Carbon monoxide poisoning
- Cutaneous phlebectasia (telangiectasis)
- Erythema multiforme
- Erythrocytosis

Yellow
- Acquired aurotrichia; black hair turns golden

- Excessive carotene ingestion
- Quinacrine

DIAGNOSTIC APPROACH

1 Perform physical examination to map colour changes.
2 Differentiate broken hairs (self-trauma) from hair loss if alopecic.
3 Rule in/out pruritic skin diseases by history and trichogram, q.v. section 1.39.
4 Pattern recognition from skin appearance, colour and lesion distribution.
5 Recognition of related heritable changes (e.g., deafness, merle iris).
6 Dermatological investigations: cytology (sellotape strips), scrapes, culture.

Clinical clues
Predisposition
- Acquired aurotrichia: Miniature schnauzers
- Acquired idiopathic hypopigmentation of the nose: Arctic breeds, GSDs, Poodle, retrievers
- Cyclic haematopoiesis: grey and pale merle collies
- DLE: Collies and GSDs
- Dermatomyositis: Beauceron shepherd, Collies, Shetland sheepdog
- Lentigo profuse: Pugs, mainly on the ventral skin
- Merle colouration: Collies, Great Dane
  - Concurrent deafness or ocular changes associated with merle and piebald colours
- Nasal aspergillosis: dolichocephalic dogs
- Post-chemotherapy hair regrowth: Old English sheepdogs regrow darker puppy coat
- Saliva staining due to drooling, q.v. section 1.16
- Seasonal flank alopecia: most common in Airedale terriers, Boxers, English bulldogs, French bulldogs, and Schnauzers
- True acanthosis nigricans: Dachshunds
- Vitiligo: Belgian tervuren, Dobermann and Rottweiler
- Uveo-dermatological (Vogt-Koyanagi-Harada-like) syndrome: Akitas, Samoyeds and Siberian huskies
- Waardenburg-Klein syndrome: Boxer, Dachshund and Shetland sheepdog

History

- Drooling
- Known traumatic event
- Repetitive licking
- Neurological signs: depression, obtundation, seizures, visual deficits
- Vitiligo develops in young adult dogs

Clinical examination

Visual inspection

- Alopecia, *q.v.* section 1.2
- Changes in pigmentation (hyper- and hypo-) of exposed skin or hair colour

Physical examination

- Changes in pigmentation (hyper- and hypo-) of skin or hair
- Changes in skin thickening
- Skin lesions, *q.v.* section 2.26

Laboratory findings

Haematology

- Usually unremarkable unless severely anaemic or underlying endocrine disease

Serum biochemistry

- Usually unremarkable unless underlying endocrine disease or jaundiced

Urinalysis

- Unremarkable except in jaundice

Imaging

- Unremarkable unless underlying systemic disease

Special tests

- Skin biopsy
- Immunohistochemistry for immune-mediated skin diseases

PHYSICAL ABNORMALITIES

2.28 SPLENOMEGALY

DEFINITION

Enlargement of the spleen; the enlargement may be focal or generalised.
The spleen can often be identified on palpation by its mobility and shape.

- The normal size of the spleen is quite variable, and a large spleen is normal for a GSD
- An enlarged spleen is generally palpable and/or visible on imaging (*q.v.* section 4.1)

RELATED CLINICAL SIGNS

- There may be no clinical signs
- Abdominal distension
- Abdominal enlargement
- Acute abdomen: rupture and intraperitoneal bleeding, splenic torsion
- Intermittent weakness/collapse from splenic haemorrhage or torsion
- Non-specific signs: anorexia, lethargy
- Signs related to underlying cause

COMMON CAUSES

Diffuse enlargement

- Barbiturate anaesthesia
- Lymphoma
- Reactive, including extra-medullary haematopoiesis in IMHA

Focal mass(es)

- Haematoma
- Neoplasia
  - Haemangioma
  - Haemangiosarcoma
  - Lymphoma
- Nodular hyperplasia

UNCOMMON CAUSES

Diffuse enlargement

- Amyloidosis
- Congestion
  - GDV
  - Portal hypertension

PHYSICAL ABNORMALITIES

- Splenic thrombosis
- Splenic torsion
- Phenothiazines
- Splenic torsion
- Infection/inflammation
  - Babesia
  - Brucellosis
  - Ehrlichiosis
  - Blastomycosis
  - Sporotrichosis
  - Leishmaniosis
  - Splenitis: secondary to systemic bacterial infection, e.g. endocarditis, bacteraemia/septicaemia
- Hypereosinophilic syndrome
- Necrotising
  - Salmonellosis
  - Splenic infarction
  - Splenic torsion
  - Splenic tumour
  Neoplasia
  - Leukaemia
  - Malignant histiocytosis
  - Myeloproliferative disease
  - Systemic mastocytosis

Focal mass(es)
- Fibrohistiocytic nodules
- Focal infection
  - Migrating FB
  - Penetrating wound
- Splenic neoplasia
  - Non-angiomatous sarcomas: fibrosarcoma, leiomyosarcoma, osteosarcoma
  - Haematoma
  - Histiocytic sarcoma

DIAGNOSTIC APPROACH

1 Confirm palpable cranial abdominal orga-nomegaly as splenic in origin by imaging.
2 Identify underlying infectious/inflammatory diseases causing reactive splenomegaly by laboratory testing.
3 Rule out bleeding disorders.
4 FNA.
5 Exploratory laparotomy and biopsy or removal.

CLINICAL CLUES

Predisposition
- Haemangiosarcoma in middle-aged GSDs
- Nodular hyperplasia in old dogs
- Malignant histiocytosis in Bernese Mountain dog
- Splenic torsion in large/giant dogs

History
- Barbiturate administration
- Intermittent weakness/collapse from splenic haemorrhage or torsion
- Signs related to underlying disease

Clinical examination
Visual inspection
- Abdominal enlargement
- Haemoglobinuria sometimes seen in splenic torsion

Physical examination
- Ascites if portal hypertension or ruptured spleen
- Splenomegaly
  - Focal
  - Generalised

Laboratory findings
Haematology
- Anaemia
  - Inappropriate number of normoblasts
  - Microangiopathic haemolytic anaemia (presence of schistocytes) in primary splenic pathology
  - Regenerative due to haemorrhage
- Leukocytosis if inflammatory/infectious disease

Serum biochemistry
- Changes reflecting underlying disease
- No specific changes for primary splenic disease

Urinalysis
- Haemoglobinuria sometimes seen in splenic torsion

Imaging
Plain radiographs
- Splenomegaly
- Metastatic disease

Ultrasound examination
- Splenic parenchymal changes
  - Altered echogenicity and homogeneity
  - Mass(es)
  - Vasculature

- Hepatic metastasis
- Lymphadenopathy
- Peritoneal fluid

Special tests
- Exploratory laparotomy
- FNA

2.29 STOMATITIS

DEFINITION

Stomatitis is inflammation of the oral mucosa. It may be generalised or localised to one area of the mouth or to one structure within the mouth, e.g. chelitis and glossitis are inflammation of the lips and tongue, respectively. Severe inflammation can cause oral ulceration

RELATED CLINICAL SIGNS

- Blood-stained saliva
- Drooling, *q.v.* section 1.16
- Dysphagia, *q.v.* section 1.17
- Halitosis, *q.v.* section 1.29
- Pain on eating

COMMON CAUSES

Local disease
- Benign and malignant oral tumours, *q.v.* section 2.16
- Cheilitis due to lip conformation allowing drooling
- Chronic ulcerative paradental stomatitis (chronic ulcerative paradental stomatitis [CUPS], 'Kissing ulcer')
- FB trauma (e.g. stick injury)
- Stomatitis/gingivitis associated with periodontal disease

Systemic disease
- Uraemia

UNCOMMON CAUSES

Local disease
- Candidiasis
- Eosinophilic stomatitis
- Lymphoplasmacytic stomatitis (rare cf. cat)

Contact stomatitis
- Chemical/caustic ingestion
- Electrical burns
- Oak Processionary moth caterpillar
- Necrotic stomatitis ('trench mouth') due to spirochaetal infection
- Thermal burns

Systemic disease
- Autoimmune diseases
  - Bullous pemphigoid
  - Lupus (SLE)
  - Pemphigus foliaceous, vulgaris
- Canine distemper
- Ciclosporin causing gingival hyperplasia
- Cyclic haematopoiesis
- Diabetes mellitus
- Drug reaction
- Heavy metal toxicity
- Radiation mucositis, following radiotherapy of oral or nasal tumours
- Toxic epidermal necrolysis
- Trigeminal sensory neuropathy allowing dog to inadvertently bite its tongue
- Vasculitis
- Xerostomia (dry mouth), including Sjögren-like syndrome

DIAGNOSTIC APPROACH

1 Laboratory testing for underlying systemic disease – crucial if uraemia is suspected.
2 Complete oral examination – may require GA.
3 Remove any obvious cause (e.g. FB) or biopsy any suspect lesions.
4 Radiograph teeth and tooth roots to diagnose dental disease.
5 Radiograph skull if there is suspected bone involvement.
6 Appropriate dental care if no other cause is detected.
   NB: Be aware that non-healing lesions and/or spontaneous tooth loss may have an underlying neoplastic condition, *q.v.* section 2.16.

Clinical clues
Predisposition
- Candidiasis in xerostomia or immunosuppression or prolonged antibiosis
- Chemical burns in dogs given caustic emetics (washing soda crystals, hydrogen peroxide)
- Cyclic haematopoiesis in grey and pale merle collies
- Distemper in unvaccinated dogs
- Electrical burns in puppies chewing electric cords
- Eosinophilic stomatitis in CKCS
- Thermal burns in greedy dogs stealing hot food

History
- Drug administration
- Known electrocution
- Vaccination status

Clinical examination
Visual inspection
- Dysphagia when observed eating

- Evidence of saliva staining
- Facial swelling/deformity
- Halitosis evident, although not visible

Physical examination
- CUPS of buccal mucous membranes where they touch ('kiss') dental plaque and calculus
- Erythema of lingual or buccal mucous membranes
- FB
- Lesions at other mucocutaneous junctions in pemphigus
- Small white plaques characteristic of candidiasis
- Plaque and calculus
- Ulceration of mucous membranes or mucocutaneous junction

Laboratory findings
Haematology
- Usually unremarkable

Serum biochemistry
- Azotaemia in uraemia
- Hyperglycaemia in diabetes mellitus

Imaging
Plain radiographs
- Local bone destruction suggesting osteomyelitis or infiltrative neoplasia
- Usually unremarkable unless significant dental disease

Special tests
- Antinuclear antibody (ANA)
- FNA regional LNs
- Touch impressions and/or biopsy ± immunohistochemistry

2.30   STRIDOR AND STERTOR

DEFINITIONS

Stridor
Stridor is increased upper respiratory tract noise which has a high-pitched reverberating quality and is related to laryngeal and, less

commonly, oropharyngeal and tracheal disorders.

Stertor
Stertor is increased upper respiratory tract noise which has a low-pitched snoring quality

and is related to nasal, nasopharynx, and soft palate disorders, *q.v.* sections 1.43 and 5.10.

RELATED CLINICAL SIGNS

Stridor
- Epistaxis
- Nasal discharge
- Reverse sneezing
- Sneezing

Stertor
- Voice change (high-pitched bark)
- Variable dyspnoea and orthopnoea

COMMON CAUSES

Stridor
- Laryngeal paralysis
  - Degenerative neuropathy
  - Pulmonary neoplasia
  - Laryngeal collapse

Stertor
- Brachycephalic obstructive airway syndrome (BOAS); one or more of:
  - Elongated soft palate
  - Everted laryngeal saccules
  - Laryngeal collapse
  - Stenotic nares
  - Tracheal hypoplasia
- Nasal FB
- Nasal tumour
- Sinonasal aspergillosis

UNCOMMON CAUSES

Stridor
- Laryngeal paralysis
  - Congenital
  - Hypothyroidism
  - Lead poisoning
  - Myasthenia gravis
  - Traumatic
- Laryngeal infiltrative disease
  - Inflammatory

- Neoplasia: lymphoma, MCT, tonsillar carcinoma

Stertor
- Oronasal fistula
- Dental abscess

DIAGNOSTIC APPROACH

1 Distinguish the type of sound and its likely origin.
2 Visual examination of throat.
3 Imaging of pharynx and cranial neck.
4 If safe, examination of region upper airway examination under light plane of anaesthesia:
- to assess laryngeal function
- to assess soft palate length and laryngeal saccule eversion
- to identify and sample any masses

Clinical clues
Predisposition
- Congenital laryngeal paralysis: Bouvier des Flandres, Bull terriers, and Dalmatian
- Degenerative polyneuropathy which often first affects the larynx: Labrador retrievers

History
- Functional upper respiratory tract disorders (e.g. laryngeal paralysis) are likely to be exacerbated by exercise, heat and stress
- Sneezing, reverse sneezing and nasal discharge or epistaxis increase suspicion of nasal FB, infectious disease (abscess, aspergillus, oronasal fistula) or neoplasia

Clinical examination
Visual inspection
- Assess for nasal discharge (unilateral or bilateral)
- Assess for response to gentle exercise

Physical examination
- Thorough examination to assess for multisystemic disease
- Neurological examination to assess for polyneuropathy

PHYSICAL ABNORMALITIES

Laboratory findings
Haematology and serum biochemistry
- Useful to screen for systemic disease

Imaging
Plain radiographs and abdominal ultrasound
- Thoracic radiographs in laryngeal paralysis to screen for neoplastic causes
- Nasal radiographs as appropriate in workup for nasal disorders

Special tests
Stertor
- *Aspergillus* serology: specific but poorly sensitive test, i.e. positive result supports infection but negative result does not exclude it
- CT scan with contrast to assess for nasal diseases
- Culture of nasal discharge is not useful; likely bacterial flora, and positive *Aspergillus* culture is not diagnostic
- FNA or biopsy any mass
- Nasal cytology (rarely useful) and tissue sample for histopathology
- Rhinoscopy to assess for nasal FB, tumours, or *Aspergillus*

Stridor
- Acetylcholine receptor antibodies for acquired myasthenia gravis
- Electrodiagnostics (EMG and nerve conduction studies) to assess for peripheral neuropathy
- Total thyroxine and cTSH for hypothyroidism

SECTION 3

LABORATORY ABNORMALITIES

In this section laboratory abnormalities of haematology, serum biochemistry and urinalysis are listed alphabetically.

• The abnormality is defined.
• Causes are listed, and the likely degree of severity is suggested.
• The diagnostic interpretation for the abnormality is given.
• Adjunctive tests that may help confirm the diagnosis are given.

3A BIOCHEMICAL TESTS

3.1 ACID–BASE

Measurement of acid–base status is increasingly available using patient-side blood gas analysis, providing useful information in terms of any metabolic and respiratory disorders that may be present. Normal pH range in a dog is approximately 7.35—7.46.

- Acidaemia is defined as a lower than normal blood pH.
- Acidosis is a process of accumulation of acid or loss of base, resulting in gain of H$^+$ ions.
- Alkalaemia is higher than normal blood pH.
- Akalosis is a process of accumulation of base or loss of acid, resulting in loss of H$^+$ ions.
- An acidosis or alkalosis may be:
  - Primary, i.e. responsible for derangement in acid-base balance
  or
  - Secondary, i.e. a compensatory response to the primary derangement in an attempt to normalise the pH
- An acidosis may be:
  - Respiratory: detected by an increase in pCO$_2$
  or
  - Metabolic: a more negative base excess or decrease in bicarbonate
- An alkalosis may also be:
  - Respiratory: detected by a decrease in pCO$_2$
  or
  - Metabolic: an increase in base excess or increase in bicarbonate
- The anion gap may be useful when further interrogating acid–base disturbances
  - Anion gap = (Na$^+$ + K$^+$) – (Cl$^-$ + HCO$_3^-$)

COMMON CAUSES

Acidosis
- Metabolic acidosis
  - Hyperchloraemic (normal anion gap) metabolic acidosis
    - Vomiting and diarrhoea

- High anion gap metabolic acidosis
  - Acute kidney injury (AKI) or chronic kidney disease (CKD)
  - Diabetic ketoacidosis
- Respiratory acidosis
  - Hypoventilation
    - Airway obstruction, e.g. laryngeal paralysis
    - General anaesthesia
    - Neurological disease
    - Pleural space disease, i.e. pneumothorax, pleural effusion

Alkalosis
- Metabolic alkalosis
  - Compensation for respiratory acidosis
  - Hypochloraemia: excessive gastrointestinal losses of chloride-rich fluid, in particular high gastrointestinal obstruction (functional due to ileus or mechanical) resulting in vomiting and loss of hydrogen chloride-rich fluid
- Respiratory alkalosis
  - Hyperventilation
    - Anxiety
    - Hypoxaemia (respiratory disease, anaemia)
    - Pain
  - Compensation for metabolic acidosis

UNCOMMON CAUSES

Acidosis
- Metabolic acidosis
  - Hyperchloraemic (normal anion gap) metabolic acidosis
    - Compensation for respiratory alkalosis
    - Dilutional acidosis (large volume of fluid administration)
    - Renal tubular acidosis
  - High anion gap metabolic acidosis
    - Ethylene glycol toxicity
    - Lactic acidosis

Notes on Canine Internal Medicine, Fourth Edition. Victoria L. Black, Kathryn F. Murphy, Jessie Rose Payne, and Edward J. Hall.
© 2022 John Wiley & Sons Ltd. Published 2022 by John Wiley & Sons Ltd.

- Respiratory acidosis
  - Hypoventilation
    - Late pulmonary parenchymal disease
    - Neurological disease (reduced respiratory drive)
  - Poor tissue perfusion
  - Compensation for metabolic alkalosis

Alkalosis
- Metabolic alkalosis
  - Gain of base or bicarbonate (iatrogenic)
  - Renal loss of hydrogen – primary hyperaldosteronism
- Respiratory alkalosis
  - Hyperventilation
    - Hypoaxaemia (carbon monoxide poisoning)

DIAGNOSTIC SIGNIFICANCE

Acidaemia results in reduced cardiac output, arrhythmias, depression and, in more chronic cases, bone demineralisation.

Alkalaemia results in tetany, seizures, weakness, and, in more chronic cases, polyuria and polydipsia.

Adjunctive tests
- Electrolytes
- Serum biochemistry
  - Beta hydroxybutyrate if high anion gap metabolic acidosis or confirmed diabetic
- Phosphate

3.2 AMMONIA

Ammonia is produced by deamination of amino acids (and urea) by:
- Endogenous metabolism, especially in muscle
- Enterocyte and metabolism of glutamine
- Intestinal bacterial fermentation of dietary protein and urea

Increases are a component of the metabolic derangement causing hepatic encephalopathy. Ammonia of intestinal origin is cleared from the portal blood by conversion in the liver to urea. Increase in ammonia production is likely post-prandially or if there is gastrointestinal (GI) bleeding or constipation but increases in the systemic circulation will only occur if there is a congenital porto-systemic shunt (PSS) or acquired shunts or the liver is significantly diseased.

COMMON CAUSES

Decreased
Anorexia

Increased
- Congenital PSS
- Secondary, acquired PSS
  - Chronic hepatitis/cirrhosis

UNCOMMON CAUSES

Decreased
- Antibacterial therapy
- Lactulose administration
- Restricted protein diet
- Starvation

Increased
- Ammonium chloride ingestion (ammonia tolerance test)
- Inherited selected cobalamin deficiency (Imerslund-Gräsbeck syndrome), *q.v.* sections 3.10, 5.7.1.2C
- Physiological
  - High protein meal/post-prandial
    - Early increase is likely enterocyte metabolism of glutamine
    - Late increase is likely colonic fermentation
- Secondary, acquired PSS
  - Lobular dissecting hepatitis
  - Strenuous exercise
- Urea enzyme cycle deficiency

ARTEFACT

Increased
- Delay in sample analysis
- Delayed plasma separation

- Fluoride/oxalate anticoagulants
- Haemolysis

DIAGNOSTIC SIGNIFICANCE

- Decreased ammonia is of no clinical significance
- Indicator of hepatic dysfunction and/or congenital and acquired porto-systemic shunting
- Prone to artefact if analysis delayed, or with point-of-care analysis
  - Measurement of blood ammonia is problematic as it is very unstable and is not routinely undertaken. Arterial blood samples are preferable to venous blood samples and heparinised or EDTA-anticoagulated plasma samples are preferable to serum. Because of its chemical instability and leakage from RBCs, whole blood samples should be kept on ice, then separated within 15 minutes of collection. Separated samples to be assayed for ammonia as soon as possible

after sample collection and maintained at 4°C (or on ice) until assayed within 3 hours.
- Test sensitivity can be increased by an ammonia tolerance test, where NH_4Cl is given by gavage. However, it can cause vomiting and precipitate hepatoencephalopathy and is rarely done. A 6-hour post-prandial ammonia measurement is safer but less sensitive.
- Weak correlation with degree of hepatoencephalopathy

ADJUNCTIVE TESTS

- DNA tests for Imerslund-Gräsbeck syndrome if cobalamin is decreased
- Dynamic bile acids: more easily applicable in practice
- Hepatic imaging
  - CT angiography
  - Ultrasound
- Liver biopsy
- Serum cobalamin

3.3 AMYLASE AND LIPASE

Increased serum activities of the enzymes amylase and lipase have been considered markers of pancreatitis. However, they are often unreliable markers.

COMMON CAUSES

Marked increase
- Pancreatitis

Mild increase
- Decreased glomerular filtration
- Hyperadrenocorticism (HAC) or exogenous glucocorticoids (lipase)
- Non-specific GI disease
- Pancreatitis

UNCOMMON CAUSES

Marked increase
- Pancreatic neoplasia
- Pancreatic necrosis

Mild increase
- Liver disease
- Pancreatic duct obstruction
- Pancreatic neoplasia
- Pancreatic necrosis

DIAGNOSTIC SIGNIFICANCE

- Amylase is not specific to the pancreas; starch digestion (amylase-like activity) is also catalysed by the SI brush border enzyme sucrase-isomaltase
- Increases in lipase activity more than 4 times the reference interval are considered significant but merely support the diagnosis of pancreatitis in dogs with typical signs
- Neither amylase nor lipase activity is pancreas-specific
  - Lipase activity is found in gastric secretions and in the liver
  - Lipase activity assayed using DGGR [1,2-o-dilauryl-rac-glycero glutaric acid-

(6'-methylresorufin)] ester as the substrate is considered to be more specific than other enzymatic assays, but is not completely organ-specific
- Other factors affect serum amylase and lipase activity
  - Decreased GFR (with azotaemia) is likely in any dog with acute vomiting, and then raised activities must be interpreted with caution
  - Lipase activity is increased by exogenous steroids

ADJUNCTIVE TESTS

- Canine pancreatic lipase (cPL) is an immuno-assay for pancreas-specific lipase and a more sensitive and specific test for pancreatitis than conventional enzyme assays, *q.v.* section 3.21
- Exploratory laparotomy and pancreatic biopsy
- Ultrasound examination of pancreas
- Use of glucocorticoids and HAC should be assessed if signs are not typical of pancreatitis

3.4 AZOTAEMIA

Azotaemia refers to increased accumulation in the blood of nitrogen-rich end products of protein metabolism. The most commonly measured markers of this are urea and creatinine. Azotaemia usually develops due to failure of renal clearance of these compounds as a result of a reduced glomerular filtration rate (GFR) and can occur due to pre-renal, renal, or post-renal causes. Increased urea can also occur due to non-renal causes, *q.v.* section 3.29.

Uraemia refers to the pathological and clinical signs that develop as a consequence of azotaemia.

COMMON CAUSES

Pre-renal
- Renal hypoperfusion
  - Dehydration
  - Cardiogenic shock, e.g. congestive heart failure
  - Hypovolaemic shock, e.g. haemorrhage, vomiting and diarrhoea, hypoadrenocorticism,
- Increase in urea alone
  - Gastrointestinal haemorrhage
  - Recent meal, especially high protein meal

Renal
- AKI
  - Hypoperfusion
  - Iatrogenic, e.g. NSAIDs, diuretics
  - Toxin
- CKD degenerative

Post-renal
- Urethral obstruction
- Urinary tract rupture: bladder

UNCOMMON CAUSES

Pre-renal
- Renal hypoperfusion
  - Distributive shock, e.g. sepsis
  - Diuretic therapy
  - Obstructive shock, e.g. gastric dilatation-volvulus (GDV), pericardial effusion
- Increase in urea alone
  - Increased catabolism, e.g. fever

Renal
- AKI
  - Hypercalcaemia
  - Pyelonephritis
- CKD
  - Glomerulonephritis
  - Renal dysplasia

Post-renal
- Ureteric obstruction
- Urinary tract rupture: ureter or urethra

DIAGNOSTIC SIGNIFICANCE

- Dogs with azotaemia and USG > 1.030 should be investigated for pre-renal causes of azotaemia

- In dehydration, urea may overestimate renal functional impairment. Urea-to-creatinine ratio is used for this reason in man, but does not perform well in dogs in discriminating between pre-renal and renal causes of azotaemia
- Renal dysfunction will not be detected by increases in urea and creatinine until 75% of glomeruli are compromised
- Response to intravenous fluid therapy or management of congestive heart failure may be necessary to discriminate between pre-renal and renal causes of azotaemia as pre-renal disorders may result in urine specific gravity (USG) < 1.030 due to concurrent disorders
- Signs of uraemia are not expected in mild azotaemia

ADJUNCTIVE TESTS

- Albumin (in glomerular disease), *q.v.* section 3.27
- Blood gas analysis (acid base), *q.v.* section 3.1
- Calcium (total and ionised), *q.v.* section 3.7
- Haematology (haematocrit), *q.v.* section 3.30
- Potassium and sodium, *q.v.* sections 3.23 and 3.24
- Symmetric dimethylarginine (SDMA), *q.v.* section 3.25
- Serum phosphate, *q.v.* section 3.22
- Urinary tract imaging, *q.v.* section 5.12
- Urine protein:creatinine (UPC) ratio, *q.v.* section 3.36
- USG, *q.v.* section 3.37

NB: Renal biopsy is rarely justified if a dog is already azotaemic

3.5 BILE ACIDS

Bile acids are synthesised in the liver, secreted in bile and then undergo enterohepatic recycling, being absorbed in the ileum, then removed from the portal circulation by the liver to be re-secreted. Therefore, finding increased bile acids in the peripheral circulation is indicative of hepatic dysfunction or porto-systemic shunting or both.

The sensitivity of the test is improved by taking a sample two hours after a meal, where gall bladder contractions will have increased the bile acid pool being recycled.

CAUSES

Decreased
- Cholestyramine (bile salt binder)
- Delayed gastric emptying
- Malabsorption and rapid intestinal transit
- Ileal resection

NB: End-stage liver disease does not cause decreased bile acids

Marked increases
- Cholestatic disease
- Porto-systemic shunting

- Congenital PSS
- Microvascular dysplasia (portal vein hypoplasia)
- Secondary PSS: acquired shunts due to primary hepatopathy
- Severe hepatocellular dysfunction

NB: Administration of ursodeoxycholic acid (UDCA) will only increase serum bile acids if there is significant liver dysfunction or porto-systemic shunting

Mild increases
Mild hepatocellular dysfunction

Secondary hepatic disease
- Steroid hepatopathy
  - HAC
  - Iatrogenic
- Vacuolar hepatopathy
  - Inflammatory or neoplastic disease elsewhere

ARTEFACT

- Haemolysis: falsely decreases
- Icterus: doesn't interfere but pointless test if the patient is jaundiced
- Lipaemia: falsely increases

DIAGNOSTIC SIGNIFICANCE

- Bile acid testing is superfluous if the patient is icteric
- Bile acids > 30 µmol/l are always associated with hepatic pathology, but this can be primary hepatic disease or a secondary (vacuolar) hepatopathy.
- Decreased bile acids are not clinically significant
- Marked increases in bile acids (>~80 µmol/l) are associated with significant (usually primary) hepatic dysfunction, but the concentrations correlate poorly with the degree of dysfunction and do not allow progression or resolution of disease to be evaluated
  - Hepatocellular and cholestatic disease more typically produces increased resting concentrations, with less increase post-prandially
- Portosystemic shunting typically causes a low/normal resting bile acid concentration and markedly increased post-prandial values
- Pre- and post-prandial bile acid concentrations < 25 µmol/l are not clinically significant

ADJUNCTIVE TESTS

- Blood ammonia
- Hepatic ultrasound
- Liver biopsy
- Serum proteins and liver enzyme activities
- Urinary bile acids; more sensitive in hepatopathies than PSS

3.6 BILIRUBIN

Increased bilirubin causes jaundice and can be caused by:
- Massive haemolysis (pre-hepatic)
- Liver dysfunction (hepatic)
- Failure of biliary flow into the intestine (post-hepatic) because of either biliary obstruction or biliary rupture and leakage leading to bile peritonitis

q.v. section 2.13

3.7 CALCIUM

Total serum calcium exists in three states:

1 Inorganic (~5%)
2 Ionised: physiologically active (~50%)
3 Protein-bound (~45%), but depends on serum albumin concentration

Ideally, ionised calcium should be measured when assessing calcium status. However, the test may not be readily available in practice due to assay requirements.

3.7.1 HYPERCALCAEMIA

An increase in ionised calcium is clinically significant and can sometimes be seen with a normal total calcium. Therefore, consider measurement of ionised calcium where signs can fit.

Total serum calcium concentration may also appear increased if serum albumin concentration is also increased, as the amount of bound calcium is increased.

COMMON CAUSES

Marked
- Malignancy, associated with production of parathyroid hormone (PTH)-related protein, PTHrP
  - Anal sac adenocarcinoma (ASAC)
  - Lymphoma

Mild
- CKD
- Dehydration/haemoconcentration/hyperproteinaemia

- Hypoadrenocorticism
- Physiological in young growing dogs

UNCOMMON CAUSES

Marked

- Granulomatous disease, e.g. blastomycosis (not in UK), angiostrongylosis, panniculitis, sterile nodular skin disease (pyogranulomatous), mycobacteria infection
- Malignancy (PTHrP production)
  - Mammary tumours
  - Sarcomas
  - Carcinomas
- Primary hyperparathyroidism (including breed-related in Keeshond)
- Vitamin D toxicosis
  - Calcipotriene ointment (psoriasis medication)
  - Cholecalciferol rodenticide
  - Dimethyl sulphoxide (DMSO) treatment of calcinosis cutis
  - Over-supplementation
  - Plants with leaves containing cholecalciferol, e.g. day-blooming jessamine, *Solanum*

Mild/moderate

- Dietary excess
- Idiopathic (rare in dog)
- Osteolytic disease
  - Multiple myeloma
  - Primary and metastatic bone tumours
  - Septic osteomyelitis

ARTEFACT

- Hyperlipaemia
- Laboratory error
- Non-fasted sample

DIAGNOSTIC SIGNIFICANCE

- Concurrent hypophosphataemia suggests primary hyperparathyroidism or malignancy-associated hypercalcaemia
- Concurrent hyperphosphataemia suggests CKD, vitamin D toxicosis or hypoadrenocorticism
- Concurrent azotaemia suggests dehydration, kidney disease or hypoadrenocorticism

- Dogs with primary hyperparathyroidism may be asymptomatic initially
- Hyperkalaemia suggests AKI or hypoadrenocorticism
- If ionised calcium cannot be measured, adjustments should be made for the albumin concentration
- If there is no history of vitamin D overdose, and the anal sacs are normal on palpation, the most likely diagnosis is lymphoma, but if lymphoma cannot be identified and/or a parathyroid mass can be demonstrated by ultrasound, measurement of PTH to assess for primary hyperparathyroidism is indicated
- Lytic bone disease is usually obvious clinically or at least radiographically
- Marked hypercalcaemia in the presence of azotaemia is more likely cause than effect

ADJUNCTIVE TESTS

- Basal cortisol or ACTH stimulation test to screen for hypoadrenocorticism
- Fine needle aspirate (FNA) and/or biopsy of lymph nodes
- Ionised calcium to assess physiological calcium concentration
- Radiographs/ultrasonography/CT for lymphadenopathy, internal organomegaly (liver/spleen/kidney) and bone lesions, neck lesions (parathyroid nodules)
- Rectal examination for ASAC
- Serum albumin concentration to estimate true total calcium
- Serum phosphate, urea, creatinine, SDMA and USG
- Serum PTH
- Serum PTHrP
- Urinalysis
- 25-hydroxy vitamin D
- 1,25-dihydroxy vitamin D (Calcitriol)

If all other tests negative
- Bone marrow aspirate

3.7.2 HYPOCALCAEMIA

A decrease in ionised calcium is clinically significant. Total serum calcium concentration may appear to be decreased if serum albumin concentration is also decreased, as the proportion of bound (physiologically inactive) calcium is decreased.

COMMON CAUSES

- Acute or chronic kidney injury/disease
- Critical illness/sepsis
- Eclampsia: pregnancy/parturition/lactational
- Hypoproteinaemia (hypoalbuminaemia)
- Primary hypoparathyroidism

UNCOMMON CAUSES

- Alkalosis
- Calcitonin treatment
- Ethylene glycol toxicity
- Excess dietary phosphate
- Fanconi's syndrome and renal tubular acidosis
- Hyperadrenocorticism
- Hypovitaminosis D
- Intravenous phosphate administration/phosphate enemas
- Malabsorption
- Massive transfusion
- Muscle necrosis
- Necrotising pancreatitis
- Nutritional secondary hyperparathyroidism (low-calcium diet)
- Parathyroidectomy
- Renal secondary hyperparathyroidism
- Thyroid C cell tumour (calcitonin-secreting)

ARTEFACT

- EDTA contamination
- Citrate contamination

DIAGNOSTIC SIGNIFICANCE

Unless ionised calcium can be measured, adjustments should be made for the albumin concentration.
- Clinical signs of hypocalcaemia include tremors, twitching and tetanic muscle contraction
- Eclampsia typically occurs during peak lactation, a few weeks after parturition
- Hypocalcaemia in the presence of azotaemia is likely secondary to primary renal disease

ADJUNCTIVE TESTS

- Ionised calcium to assess physiological calcium concentration
- Renal parameters: creatinine and urea, SDMA, USG
- Serum albumin to indicate true calcium
- Serum phosphate increased in renal failure and vitamin D toxicosis
- PTH concentrations
- Tests for pancreatitis, e.g. pancreatic lipase, abdominal ultrasound
- Vitamin D metabolites

3.8 CARDIAC BIOMARKERS

Cardiac biomarkers (NT-proBNP, troponins) can be used to increase or decrease the index of suspicion for cardiac disease in the absence of systemic disease, but cannot be used to make a definitive diagnosis due to wide breed and individual variations present.

3.8.1 N-TERMINAL PRO B-TYPE NATRIURETIC PEPTIDE (NT-PROBNP)

- Pro B-type natriuretic peptide (proBNP) is released in response to myocardial stretch, volume overload or pressure overload

- proBNP is cleaved to the biologically active B-type natriuretic peptide (BNP) and the inactive N-terminal (NT)-proBNP
  - BNP causes vasodilation, increases GFR and inhibits renin
  - NT-proBNP has a longer half-life than BNP and so is easier to measure

COMMON CAUSES

Marked increase
- Structural cardiac disease: acquired and congenital

Mild increase

- Azotaemia
- May be normal due to individual or breed variation, e.g. Labradors often have NT-proBNP above upper reference interval
- Structural cardiac disease: acquired and congenital
- Systemic hypertension

UNCOMMON CAUSES

Marked increase

- Pulmonary hypertension
- Sustained arrhythmias

Mild increase

- Pulmonary hypertension
- Sustained arrhythmias

DIAGNOSTIC SIGNIFICANCE

- A combination of increased NT-proBNP and increased troponin I (*q.v.* section 3.8.2) can be used to identify patients that would benefit from further screening for dilated cardiomyopathy (DCM)
- NT-proBNP increases with increasing disease severity in myxomatous mitral valve disease and dilated cardiomyopathy, the biggest increase being in the 6 months before the development of congestive heart failure
- NT-proBNP can distinguish cardiac vs noncardiac causes of respiratory distress, but the time taken to get results may mean that this is not an appropriate test to run in all cases
- Significant breed and individual variation is reported

ADJUNCTIVE TESTS

q.v. section 3.8.2
- Blood pressure
- Echocardiography
- Renal parameters
- 24-hour ECG Holter monitoring

3.8.2 TROPONIN I

Troponin I, troponin C, troponin T and tropomyosin form a complex that attaches to the actin filaments within myocardial cells. Binding of calcium to the troponin-tropomyosin complex causes a conformational change in the complex. This allows the myosin filaments to interact with the actin filaments and so causes myocardial contraction.

COMMON CAUSES

Marked increase

- Myocarditis
- Critically ill patients

Mild increase

- GDV
- Heatstroke
- IMHA
- Leptospirosis
- Meningoencephalitis
- Myocarditis
- Pancreatitis
- Systemic inflammatory response syndrome (SIRS)
- Snake envenomation
- Structural cardiac disease (acquired and congenital)
- Systemic inflammation

UNCOMMON CAUSES

Marked increase

- Myocardial trauma
- Sustained arrhythmias

Mild increase

- Babesiosis
- Ehrlichiosis
- Hypoadrenocorticism
- Hyperadrenocorticism
- Leishmaniasis
- Neoplasia
- Parvoviral enteritis
- Pyometra

LABORATORY ABNORMALITIES

DIAGNOSTIC SIGNIFICANCE

- An increase in serum troponin I implies myocardial cell damage
- The combination of increased and increased troponin I and NT-proBNP (*q.v.* section 3.8.1)

can be used to identify patients that would benefit from further screening for DCM

ADJUNCTIVE TESTS

q.v. section 3.8.1

3.9 CHLORIDE

Chloride is an important contributor to plasma osmolality and acid–base balance. Calculating corrected chloride allows interrogation of the underlying cause of chloride derangement; a normal corrected chloride implies changes in free water (chloride change in conjunction with sodium), whereas an abnormal corrected chloride implies an acid–base disorder.

Corrected chloride = (normal sodium ÷
    measured sodium) × measured chloride

3.9.1 HYPERCHLORAEMIA

COMMON CAUSES

Increased plasma osmolality (normal corrected chloride)
q.v. section 3.24.1

Acid–base disturbance (increased corrected chloride)
- Hyperchloraemic metabolic acidosis (due to loss of bicarbonate)
  - AKI
  - CKD
  - Proximal and distal tubular acidosis (renal)
- Iatrogenic – administration of high chloride-containing medications (hypertonic saline)

UNCOMMON CAUSES

Increased plasma osmolality (normal corrected chloride)
q.v. section 3.24.1

Acid–base disturbance (increased corrected chloride)
- Compensatory metabolic acidosis (retention of chloride due to renal excretion of bicarbonate related to respiratory alkalosis)
  - Respiratory alkalosis due to hypocapnia or hyperventilation

ARTEFACT

- Potassium bromide therapy

DIAGNOSTIC SIGNIFICANCE

- There are no clinical signs associated directly with hyperchloraemia

ADJUNCTIVE TESTS

- Blood gas analysis (acid–base), *q.v.* section 3.1
- Potassium, *q.v.* section 3.23
- Sodium, *q.v.* section 3.24

3.9.2 HYPOCHLORAEMIA

COMMON CAUSES

Decreased plasma osmolality (normal corrected chloride)
q.v. section 3.24.2

Acid–base disturbance (decreased corrected chloride)
- Iatrogenic – administration of drugs, including furosemide
- Hypochloraemic metabolic alkalosis

- Excessive gastrointestinal losses of chloride-rich fluid, in particular high gastrointestinal obstruction (functional due to ileus or mechanical) resulting in vomiting and loss of hydrogen chloride-rich fluid

bicarbonate related to respiratory acidosis)
- Respiratory alkalosis due to hypercapnia or hypoventilation

UNCOMMON CAUSES

Decreased plasma osmolality (normal corrected chloride)
q.v. section 3.24.2

Acid–base disturbance (decreased corrected chloride)
- Compensatory metabolic alkalosis (excretion of chloride due to renal retention of

DIAGNOSTIC SIGNIFICANCE

- There are no clinical signs associated directly with hypochloraemia

ADJUNCTIVE TESTS

- Blood gas analysis (acid–base), *q.v.* section 3.1
- Potassium, *q.v.* section 3.23
- Sodium, *q.v.* section 3.24

3.10 COBALAMIN

Cobalamin (vitamin B_{12}) is a dietary vitamin found in meat, fish, milk, cheese and eggs. It is absorbed in the ileum by a complex receptor-mediated process involving binding to intrinsic factor secreted by the gastric mucosa and pancreatic ducts. Large daily oral supplements can also be absorbed by a non-receptor-mediated process.

Cobalamin is usually measured concurrently with folate as markers of intestinal malabsorption.

COMMON CAUSES

Decreased
- Exocrine pancreatic insufficiency
- Distal small intestinal disease
  - Any chronic enteropathy
    - Alimentary lymphoma
    - Chronic inflammatory enteropathy (CIE)/inflammatory bowel disease (IBD)
    - Intestinal dysbiosis
    - Idiopathic (formerly termed antibiotic-responsive diarrhoea, ARD, or small intestinal bacterial overgrowth, SIBO)
    - Secondary to CIE

Increased
Iatrogenic
- By injection
- By large daily oral dosing

UNCOMMON CAUSES

Decreased
- Anorexia
- Atrophic gastritis (theoretical)
- Cobalamin deficiency
  - Cobalamin deficiency of the Shar pei
  - Inherited selected cobalamin deficiency (Imerslund-Gräsbeck syndrome): Australian shepherd, Beagle, Border collie, Giant schnauzer, Komondor, *q.v.* section 5.7.1.2C
- Dietary deficiency (vegan diet)

ARTEFACT

Decreased
- Antibiotics if bioassay used (decreased)
- Prolonged exposure to light (decreased)
- Prolonged storage

LABORATORY ABNORMALITIES

DIAGNOSTIC SIGNIFICANCE

Decreased
- Marker for severe/chronic infiltrative small intestine (SI) disease, and an indicator for the need to supplement
- Can occur in exocrine pancreatic insufficiency (EPI), which should always be tested for, *q.v.* section 3.28

Increased
- No known diagnostic significance nor deleterious effects reported in dogs

ADJUNCTIVE TESTS

- DNA test for inherited selected cobalamin deficiency (Imerslund-Gräsbeck syndrome)
- Plasma homocysteine: increased in hypocobalaminaemia
- Methylmalonic acid (blood or urine): increased when intracellular cobalamin is depleted
- Canine trypsin-like immunoreactivity (cTLI) for EPI, *q.v.* section 3.28
- Intestinal imaging, *q.v.* section 4.1
- Intestinal biopsy
- Serum folate, *q.v.* section 3.15

3.11 CORTISOL (BASAL)

Cortisol deficiency (hypoadrenocorticism) and excess (hyperadrenocorticism, HAC) is associated with Addison's and Cushing's disease, respectively. However, basal serum concentrations fluctuate and cannot be used to definitively diagnose either condition. Dynamic cortisol tests must be used, *q.v.* section 5.3.4
NB: Changes in the antibody used in the assay in 2021 will lead to revised reference intervals.

COMMON CAUSES

Decreased
- Hypoadrenocorticism (Addison's) disease
- Physiological, i.e. unstressed dog

Increased
- HAC
  - Adrenal-dependent
  - Pituitary-dependent
- Iatrogenic: any exogenous steroids except dexamethasone

UNCOMMON CAUSES

Decreased
- Atypical hypoadrenocorticism (cortisol deficiency)
- Critical illness
- Drugs
  - Chronic androgen use
  - Chronic progestagens or megoestrol acetate

- Secondary hypoadrenocorticism (ACTH deficiency)

Increased
- Severe chronic illness
- Severe stress

ARTEFACT

Decreased
Dexamethasone administration: suppresses cortisol but does not cross-react in cortisol assay

DIAGNOSTIC SIGNIFICANCE

- A basal cortisol $\geq$ 55 nmol/l is not likely to be consistent with hypoadrenocorticism
- A basal cortisol < 55 nmol/l is consistent with hypoadrenocorticism but the diagnosis must be confirmed with an ACTH stimulation test
- Increased cortisol can be caused by HAC or non-adrenal illness and cannot be used to diagnose HAC; dynamic cortisol testing (*q.v.* section 5.3.4) is required

ADJUNCTIVE TESTS

- Adrenal imaging
- Dynamic cortisol tests *q.v.* section 5.3.4
  - ACTH stimulation test
  - Dexamethasone suppression tests
- Endogenous ACTH, *q.v.* section 5.3.4

3.12 CREATINE KINASE

Creatine kinase (CK) is a cytoplasmic enzyme with four main isoenzymes that are found in brain (CK-1), cardiac and skeletal muscle (CK-2 and CK-3) and in mitochondria of many tissues (CK-Mt). Increased serum activities are associated with muscle damage, and the degree of increase is proportional to the degree of muscle damage. Activities can increase rapidly within hours of an insult and decrease rapidly (hours to days) as it has a short half-life.

COMMON CAUSES

Moderate to marked increase
- Inflammatory/infectious myopathy, e.g. immune-mediated, neosporosis, toxoplasmosis
- Inherited/breed-related myopathy/muscular dystrophy
- Muscle damage, e.g. trauma
- Post seizures
- Tremors/shivering

Mild increase
- Endocrinopathy, e.g. hyperadrenocorticism, hypothyroidism
- Exertional rhabdomyolysis
- Intramuscular injection or muscle stick during venepuncture
- Muscle biopsy
- Neuropathy
- Prolonged recumbency
- Puppies: slightly above adult upper reference interval

UNCOMMON CAUSES

Moderate to marked increase
- Anorexia
- Hyperkalaemic myopathy

- Ischaemia/thromboembolic disease
- Malignant hyperthermia/heatstroke
- Neoplasia
- Snakebite
- Toxicity

Mild increase
- Neurological disease
- Nutritional myopathy
- Restraint

ARTEFACT

- Haemolysis
- Inadvertent muscle stick during venepuncture

DIAGNOSTIC SIGNIFICANCE

- CK increases within 4–6 hours of injury, peaks at 12 hours and should return to normal within 24–48 hours
- Increased CK activity should prompt a search for evidence of muscle damage
- May be increased with haemolysis, lipaemia, hyperbilirubinaemia or traumatic sampling
- Persistent elevation is evidence of ongoing injury

ADJUNCTIVE TESTS

- Imaging
- Electrodiagnostics, e.g. electromyogram (EMG), nerve conduction velocity (NCV), muscle/nerve biopsy
- Infectious disease testing, e.g. *Toxoplasma*, *Neospora* serology
- Masticatory muscle testing, i.e. 2M antibody

3.13 CREATININE

Creatinine is produced at a constant rate from normal muscle metabolism and is freely filtered by the glomerulus and excreted unchanged in the urine. Its serum concentration reflects its

LABORATORY ABNORMALITIES

rate of production, which depends on muscle mass, and its rate of excretion, which is a function of GFR. In healthy animals these are quite stable and serum concentrations do not fluctuate significantly.

CAUSES

Decreased
- Reduced muscle mass
  - Severe weight loss
  - Young animals
- Increased GFR
  - Primary polydipsia

Increased
- Azotaemia, *q.v.* section 3.4
- Breeds with proportionately high muscle mass, e.g. sighthounds

DIAGNOSTIC SIGNIFICANCE

- Creatinine is less affected by diet and non-renal factors than urea and is a more accurate reflection of GFR
- Healthy greyhounds often have concentrations above reference range, most likely due to proportion of muscle mass as urea is normal
- Poorly muscled animals produce less creatinine, and so can underestimate azotaemia

3.14 C-REACTIVE PROTEIN (CRP)

CRP is a major acute-phase protein in the dog, produced in the liver in response to inflammatory cytokines. In healthy dogs, concentrations are low (normally < 10 mg/l) but can increase significantly with acute inflammation.
- It is not a specific marker of inflammation.
- The half-life is short and so concentrations drop rapidly with resolution of the inflammation, making serial monitoring useful for assessing response to treatment.

CAUSES

Marked increase
- Inflammation: local or systemic, infectious and non-infectious/immune
  - Bacterial, protozoal, parasitic, vector-borne, viral
  - Immune-mediated, e.g. immune-mediated haemolytic anaemia (IMHA)/thrombocytopenia (IMTP), steroid-responsive meningitis-arteritis (SRMA)
  - Pancreatitis
  - Pyometra
  - Pneumonia
  - Pyelonephritis
- Exercise
- Neoplasia
- Pregnancy

Mild increase
- Congestive heart failure
- Trauma
- Post surgery

ARTEFACT

- There are in-house and reference methodologies available for CRP measurement.
- CRP is stable for up to 14 days at room temperature/refrigerated and in frozen samples. Lipaemia and haemolysis do not appear to affect the assay.

DIAGNOSTIC SIGNIFICANCE

Increased CRP is a more sensitive indicator of inflammation than changes in leukogram or total proteins/globulin.

CRP concentrations are not affected by corticosteroids, non-steroidal anti-inflammatory drugs (NSAIDs) or other treatments affecting neutrophil numbers; however, if an inflammatory process is present and responds to these treatments, the CRP concentration will drop.

ADJUNCTIVE TESTS

- Biochemistry to assess other organs and total proteins/albumin
- Complete haematology for evidence of toxic neutrophils, band neutrophils, mild to moderate anaemia associated with chronic inflammation
- Decreased reticulocyte haemoglobin associated with inflammation (iron deficiency)
- Evaluate for source of inflammation, e.g. thoracic and abdominal imaging, joint imaging, spinal/brain imaging as indicated by physical examination
- Immunological tests, e.g. antinuclear antibody (ANA), Coombs' test, rheumatoid factor
- Infectious disease screening
- Iron profile to assess for iron deficiency
- Synovial fluid analysis and cerebrospinal fluid (CSF) analysis where indicated
- Urinalysis and culture for evidence of urinary tract infection (UTI)

3.15 FOLATE

Folic acid is a dietary vitamin found in green vegetables. It is absorbed via receptors in the proximal SI. Usually measured concurrently with cobalamin, *q.v.* section 3.10.

COMMON CAUSES

Decreased
- Proximal SI disease
  - Antibiotic-induced dysbiosis
  - CIE/IBD

Increased
- Bacterial activity: SI dysbiosis/"SI bacterial overgrowth"
- Dietary excess
- EPI

UNCOMMON CAUSES

Decreased
- Dietary deficiency

Increased
- Dietary supplementation

ARTEFACT

Decreased
- Antibiotics if bioassay used
- Prolonged exposure to light
- Prolonged storage
- Sulfonamides

Increased
- Haemolysis

DIAGNOSTIC SIGNIFICANCE

- Decreased serum folate is a marker for severe/chronic SI diseases
- Increased serum folate may indicate bacterial activity or dietary excess

ADJUNCTIVE TESTS

- cTLI, *q.v.* section 3.28
- Intestinal biopsy
- Intestinal imaging, *q.v.* section 4.1
- Serum cobalamin, *q.v.* section 3.10

3.16 FRUCTOSAMINE

Fructosamine is produced by a non-enzymatic reaction between glucose and amino groups of plasma proteins, especially albumin. The half-life of fructosamine molecules is directly dependent on the half-life of serum proteins, primarily albumin, which is generally 2–3 weeks, making fructosamine an indicator of the blood glucose concentration over a longer period of time than

LABORATORY ABNORMALITIES

a single blood glucose measurement. It is a useful measure of the average glycaemic control in a diabetic over a 2- to 3-week period.

COMMON CAUSES

Decreased
- Insulinoma

Increased
- Diabetes mellitus (DM)

UNCOMMON CAUSES

Decreased
- Chronic insulin overdosing

Increased
- Hypothyroidism, due to reduced turnover of proteins

ARTEFACT

Decreased
- Hypoalbuminaemia

Increased
- Oxytetracyline (increased)
- Severe haemolysis

Diagnostic significance
- Decreased fructosamine is most consistent with insulinoma
- Glycosuria and increased serum frutosamine are consistent with DM; persistent hyperglycaemia confirms the diagnosis
- Useful for monitoring diabetics: increased fructosamine in a managed diabetic indicates poor glycaemic control

ADJUNCTIVE TESTS

Increased fructosamine
- Biochemistry panel
- Blood glucose
- Glycated haemoglobin
- Ketones
- Pancreatic ultrasound
- Urine glucose

Decreased fructosamine: to investigate possible insulinoma
- Computed tomography (CT) of pancreas and liver
- Exploratory laparotomy
- Serum insulin

3.17 GLUCOSE

Glucose is the principal source of energy for mammalian cells and its concentration is maintained in healthy dogs within a quite strict range by hormones which facilitate its entry into or removal from the circulation.
- Insulin enables glucose use and storage and decreases blood glucose concentration.
- Several hormones oppose the action of insulin and increase blood glucose: glucagon, growth hormone, catecholamines, and corticosteroids.

3.17.1 HYPERGLYCAEMIA

Hyperglycaemia is an increase in blood glucose concentration. Increases above the renal threshold (~10 mmol/l) are associated with osmotic diuresis and the consequent clinical signs of DM, i.e. polyuria/polydipsia (PU/PD), polyphagia and weight loss.

COMMON CAUSES

Marked
- DM
- Drugs
  - Corticosteroids
- Naturally occurring insulin resistance in DM
  - HAC

Mild
- Post prandial

UNCOMMON CAUSES

Marked
- Drugs
  - Megoestrol acetate
  - Progestagens
- Naturally occurring insulin resistance in DM
  - Acromegaly
  - Bacterial infection, e.g. pyoderma, UTI
  - Glucagonoma

Mild
- Acromegaly
- Acute pancreatitis
- Drugs
  - Detomidine
  - Ketamine
  - Megoestrol acetate
  - Progestagens
  - Propanolol
  - Xylazine
- Glucose-containing fluids
- HAC
- Physiological
  - Late pregnancy
  - Stress

ARTEFACT

- Rapid separation of serum or plasma from RBCs is necessary to prevent glycolysis and falsely low results.
- Fluoride oxalate tubes to inhibit glycolysis are recommended if separation is likely to be delayed, but haemolysis will release intracellular water and may lower the glucose concentration.

DIAGNOSTIC SIGNIFICANCE

- Failure to control DM adequately with ≤2 units/kg of insulin is indicative of a condition causing insulin resistance
- Glycosuria is not proof of hyperglycaemia, as it can be seen despite euglycaemia
  - Fanconi's syndrome: Basenji
  - Jerky treats
  - Renal glycosuria: Norwegian Elkhound

- Hyperglycaemia > 10 mmol/l in association with glucosuria (and increased fructosamine) is diagnostic of DM.
- Mild increases in serum glucose are not of direct clinical significance.

ADJUNCTIVE TESTS

- Serum fructosamine
- Serum glycosylated haemoglobin
- Urinalysis

3.17.2 HYPOGLYCAEMIA

Hypoglycaemia is a low blood glucose concentration. It can cause clinical signs of neuroglycopenia (weakness, lethargy, seizures, coma) depending both on how low the concentration is and how rapidly it has declined.

COMMON CAUSES

- Hyperinsulinism
  - Insulinoma
  - Insulin overdose in diabetic
- Juvenile hypoglycaemia in toy breeds after fasting
- Xylitol poisoning

UNCOMMON CAUSES

- End-stage liver disease/cirrhosis
- Drugs
  - Propranolol
  - Sulphonylureas, e.g. glipizide
- Hypoadrenocorticism
- Hypopituitarism
- Glycogen storage diseases
  - α 1-4 glucosidase (Pompe disease)
  - Glucose-6-phosphatase (von Gierke's disease)
- Leiomyoma/sarcoma secreting insulin-like peptide
- Neonatal, *q.v.* section 1.35
- Hunting dog hypoglycaemia: may be glucocorticoid-deficient, so consider cortisol testing

- Massive tumour burden
  - Haemangiosarcoma
  - Hepatocellular carcinoma
  - Hepatoma
  - Leukaemia and primary erythrocytosis
  - Other large carcinomas
- Porto-systemic shunt (PSS)
- Pregnancy
- Septicaemia
- Severe, prolonged malnutrition
- Toxins
  - Ethanol
  - Ethylene glycol

ARTEFACT

- Delayed separation of RBCs and serum
- Erythrocytosis
- Failure to use fluoride-oxalate tube

DIAGNOSTIC SIGNIFICANCE

- If samples have been correctly handled, hypo-glycaemia sufficient to cause clinical signs of neuroglycopenia is, in adult dogs, almost exclusively due to insulinoma
- Other causes are rare and usually readily obvious from the history, physical examination or minimum database

ADJUNCTIVE TESTS

- ACTH stimulation test
- Haematology for sepsis, leukaemia
- Serum insulin
- Radiographs and abdominal ultrasound for neoplasia

3.18 IRON PROFILE

- Serum iron is bound to apotransferrin, and the concentration of this transferrin complex can be assayed. However, serum iron concentrations:
  - Fluctuate widely as iron is sequestered in inflammatory diseases
  - Are a poor marker of whole-body iron status as they do not assess iron in RBCs or stored in the liver and bone marrow
- A better, available marker is to measure the total iron-binding capacity (TIBC) concurrently and calculate the percentage saturated with iron.
- Tissue iron is largely stored bound to apoferritin as ferritin. Serum ferritin concentrations are quite stable and are considered a better indicator of total body iron stores (non-haem iron) than serum iron. However, the availability of the assay is very limited and ferritin concentrations can be increased in inflammatory disease.
- Tissue concentrations can also be assessed by liver biopsy and iron quantification, or Prussian blue staining of bone marrow, but these are rarely done.

COMMON CAUSES

Decreased iron, TIBC saturation and ferritin
- External blood loss causing iron deficiency
  - GI tract: gastric ulcer, neoplasia

Decreased iron, but normal or increased TIBC saturation and ferritin
- Chronic inflammatory conditions
- Liver disease

Increased iron and ferritin
- None

UNCOMMON CAUSES

Decreased iron, TIBC saturation and ferritin
- External blood loss causing iron deficiency
  - GI tract: hookworms
  - Severe ectoparasite infestation: fleas, ticks

Increased iron and ferritin
- Dietary excess
- Haematochromatosis
- Massive blood transfusions

ARTEFACT

- Haemolysis (increased)
- EDTA contamination (decreased)

DIAGNOSTIC SIGNIFICANCE

- Decreased serum iron concentration can be due to external blood loss, but is also reduced by chronic inflammatory conditions, and it is the TIBC percentage saturation that is diagnostic
- Iron deficiency is often first suspected by haematological changes as it causes a characteristic microcytic, hypochromic anaemia and indicates chronic, potentially occult, external blood loss

ADJUNCTIVE TESTS

- Faecal occult blood
- Haematology in iron deficiency
  - Anaemia
  - Hypochromasia
  - Decreased mean corpuscular hemoglobin concentration (MCHC)
  - Microcytosis
  - Thrombocytosis
- Imaging to look for source of chronic bleeding

3.19 LIPIDS

3.19.1 HYPERLIPIDAEMIA AND HYPERCHOLESTEROLAEMIA

Increased fasting cholesterol and/or triglycerides
- Lipaemia is an indicator of hypertriglyceridaemia, not hypercholesterolaemia
  - Can indicate inadequate fasting before sampling; this is of no clinical significance, except that lipaemia interferes with other assays and total solids on refractometer
  - Commonly secondary to underlying endocrine or cholestatic disease

COMMON CAUSES

- DM
- Dietary content
- Exogenous glucocorticoid
- HAC
- Hypothyroidism
- Pancreatitis
- Post-prandial lipaemia

UNCOMMMON CAUSES

- Cholestasis/biliary obstruction
- Nephrotic syndrome

- Idiopathic/Breed-related/Primary hyperlipidaemia
  - Hypercholesterolaemia: Briard, Shetland sheepdog
  - Hypertriglyceridaemia: Miniature schnauzer

DIAGNOSTIC SIGNIFICANCE

- Persistent lipaemia after fasting is significant, fast for > 12 hours
- Repeatable finding of hypertriglyceridaemia after a prolonged fast (24 hours), in the absence of other diseases and other abnormalities, suggests primary hyperlipidaemia
- Signs often relate to an underlying cause rather than any hypercholesterolaemia, but hypertriglyceridaemia can be associated with clinical signs
- The secondary consequences of hyperlipidaemia include ocular changes: corneal lipid deposits, lipaemic aqueous humour, lipaemia retinalis, lipid keratopathy

ADJUNCTIVE TESTS

For endocrine/metabolic disease:
- Diagnostic imaging particularly to evaluate adrenals, hepatobiliary system, pancreas

LABORATORY ABNORMALITIES

- Endocrine testing
  - DM: blood glucose and urinalysis to screen for DM ± fructosamine, *q.v.* sections 3.16, 3.17.1 and 3.34.3
  - HAC, *q.v.* section 5.3.4
  - Hypothyroidism, *q.v.* section 5.3.5
- Lipoprotein electrophoresis, ultracentrifugation and precipitation tests
- Testing for pancreatitis: imaging, pancreatic lipase, *q.v.* sections 3.21, 4.1 and 5.1.7
- UPC ratio for protein-losing nephropathy/ nephrotic syndrome, *q.v.* section 3.36

3.19.2 HYPOCHOLESTEROLAEMIA

COMMON CAUSES

- Hypoadrenocorticism
- Intestinal disease, especially protein-losing enteropathy (PLE), causing malabsorption
- Starvation
- Maldigestion/malabsorption
  - Exocrine pancreatic insufficiency
  - Hepatic functional impairment/failure
    - Hepatocellular disease

- PSS
- Lymphangiectasia

UNCOMMON CAUSES

- Dietary deficiency

DIAGNOSTIC SIGNIFICANCE

- No clinical significance *per se*, but a marker for other conditions
- Low serum cholesterol is indicative of low intestinal uptake or impaired hepatic metabolism

ADJUNCTIVE TESTS

- Bile acids for liver function and PSS
- Basal cortisol or ACTH stimulation test for hypoadrenocorticism
- cTLI, B_{12}/folate as indicators of EPI or malabsorption
- Imaging of liver/gastrointestinal tract
- Intestinal biopsy for malabsorption

3.20 LIVER ENZYMES

Increased enzyme activities are markers of either hepatic damage or cholestasis, but do not differentiate primary hepatic disease from reactive hepatic changes secondary to disease elsewhere.

CAUSES

- Primary liver disease
- Secondary (reactive) hepatopathy

ADJUNCTIVE TESTS

- History, physical examination, minimum database and imaging to identify cause of secondary hepatopathy

- Bile acid (or ammonia) to test hepatic function if not jaundiced
- Check CK if aspartate aminotransferase (AST) activity is increased
- Dynamic cortisol testing if ALP activity alone is increased and signs are consistent with HAC
- Liver ultrasound
- Liver biopsy

3.20.1 HEPATOCELLULAR MARKER ENZYMES

DIAGNOSTIC SIGNIFICANCE

- Increased serum hepatocellular enzyme activities are markers of hepatocellular damage but primary cholestatic diseases can cause mild increases as accumulated bile acids damage the hepatocyte cell membrane.

- These tests are not 100% sensitive, and evidence now suggest that measurements of liver-specific microRNAs are more sensitive.
- In acute hepatic injury, the magnitude of the increase correlates to the severity/extent of the damage but is not prognostic and is also increased during the repair process.
- In chronic hepatic injury, the magnitude of the increase does not always correlate to the severity/extent of the damage; in end-stage disease, enzyme activity may be low as few hepatocytes remain.

3.20.1A ALANINE AMINOTRANSFERASE (ALT)

Also known as glutamate pyruvate transaminase (GPT), ALT activity is a sensitive marker of primary hepatocellular damage and repair but is also increased in reactive hepatopathies. Decreased activities are of no clinical significance.

CAUSES

- Isoenzyme induction by:
  - Barbiturates
  - Glucocorticoids
- Primary hepatocellular diseases, q.v. section 5.6
- Primary cholestatic diseases, q.v. section 5.6
- Secondary hepatopathy
  - Any local inflammatory or neoplastic disease
  - Any systemic inflammatory or immune-mediated disease
  - DM
  - HAC
  - Hypoxia
  - IMHA
  - Sepsis

ARTEFACT

- Haemolysis
- Lipaemia

3.20.1B ASPARTATE AMINOTRANSFERASE (AST)

Also known as glutamate oxaloacetate transaminase (GOT), AST activity is a less sensitive marker of hepatic changes than ALT activity but more specific for primary liver disease. However, it is also found in muscle and RBCs, and CK activity should be measured concurrently. Increases suggest more severe damage than if only ALT activity is increased. There is no drug-induced isoenzyme but AST activity is also released by muscle damage and haemolysis.

CAUSES

- Liver damage as for ALT activity
- Haemolysis
- Muscle damage
- No enzyme induction by drugs; any increases are due to hepatocyte or muscle damage

ARTEFACT

- Haemolysis

3.20.1C OTHER HEPATOCELLULAR ENZYMES

A number of other hepatocellular enzyme activities can be assayed:
- Arginase: not liver-specific
- Lactate dehydrogenase (LDH): found in hepatocytes and muscle, like AST
- Glutamate dehydrogenase (GLDH): majority derived from hepatocytes
- Sorbitol dehydrogenase (SDH): liver-specific
They add little to the information provided by ALT and AST activity measurement alone.

3.20.2 CHOLESTATIC MARKER ENZYMES

These enzymes are associated with the biliary canaliculi and bile ducts and serum increases are associated with intra- and extra-hepatic cholestasis, but isoenzymes can also be induced by non-hepatic causes.

3.20.2A ALKALINE PHOSPHATASE (ALP OR ALKP)

Sensitive marker of cholestatic liver disease.

CAUSES

- New bone growth (usually mild and no gamma-glutamyl transferase [GGT] isoenzyme)
  - Bone neoplasia
  - Fractures
  - Osteomyelitis
  - Normal for young growing dog
- Endocrinopathy
  - DM
  - Hyperparathyroidism
- Extrahepatic cholestasis
  - Bile duct obstruction
  - Cholangitis ± cholecystitis
  - Cholelithiasis
  - Pancreatic tumour
  - Pancreatitis
  - Common bile duct or papillary stricture
  - Gall bladder mucocoele
- Intrahepatic cholestasis
  - Cholangitis/cholangiohepatitis
  - Drug-induced cholestasis
  - Nodular hyperplasia
  - Primary hepatocellular disease
    - Sepsis

- Isoenzyme induction by
  - Anticonvulsants
  - Exogenous glucocorticoids
  - HAC
  - Scottish terriers; may be linked to 21-hydroxylase deficiency and adrenal hyperplasia causing progressive increase in ALP enzyme activity with age
    - Asymptomatic
    - Vacuolar hepatopathy progressing to hepatic failure
    - Progression to hepatocellular carcinoma

ARTEFACT

- Haemolysis
- Hyperbilirubinaemia
- Lipaemia

3.20.2B GAMMA-GLUTAMYL TRANSFERASE (GGT)

CAUSES

- As for ALP
- Tends to mirror ALP activity increases but less sensitive and no bone isoenzyme

ARTEFACT

- Lipaemia

3.21 PANCREATIC LIPASE (cPL)

An immunoassay to measure increases in the concentration of the lipase molecule specific to the pancreas as a marker for pancreatitis. As expected, cPL is low in EPI.
- Several testing methodologies are available, including:
  - SNAP cPL®
  - Spec cPL® ELISA
  - Vetscan cPL rapid test

COMMON CAUSES

- Acute pancreatitis (sensitivity and specificity ~80–90%)
- Chronic pancreatitis (unknown sensitivity and specificity)

UNCOMMON CAUSES

- Pancreatic neoplasia

It is unknown whether increased cPL sometimes found in the following conditions is due to concurrent pancreatitis or a false positive.

- CIE/IBD
- IMHA
- Intestinal obstruction
- Intervertebral disc disease (IVDD)
- Potassium bromide administration

DIAGNOSTIC SIGNIFICANCE

- An increased cPL is suggestive of pancreatitis, but the result should be interpreted in conjunction with the history, physical findings, minimum database and ultrasonographic imaging.
- Assay of this pancreas-specific marker facilitates the diagnosis of pancreatitis. Amylase and lipase enzyme activities (*q.v.* section 3.3) and cTLI (*q.v.* section 3.28) are less sensitive

and specific. It is claimed that DGGR lipase activity is as specific as cPL, but this is disputed as DGGR lipase activity is found in EPI.

- Increased cPL is also seen in other conditions, particularly intestinal obstruction, but it is not clear whether there is concurrent pancreatic pathology.
- It is unclear whether the increase in cPL in epileptic dogs on KBr therapy is due to pancreatitis or enzyme leakage related to changes in serum chloride.
- The SpecPL is less sensitive but more specific than the SNAP cPL, whilst a negative SNAP cPL makes a diagnosis of acute pancreatitis less likely.

ADJUNCTIVE TESTS

- Abdominal ultrasound to image pancreas
- Routine haematology and serum biochemistry

3.22 PHOSPHATE

Phosphate is found complexed with calcium in bone, intracellularly and extracellularly. Phosphate is a critical building block of adenosine triphosphate (ATP), the main source of energy for cells and is important in cell membrane structure.

Phosphate is absorbed from the GI tract and excretion is primarily controlled via the kidneys. Regulation of phosphate occurs in combination with calcium via the hormones parathyroid hormone (PTH), calcitriol (the active form of vitamin D), and calcitonin. Insulin and bicarbonate results in intracellular shift of phosphate whereas cellular rupture results in release of phosphate and increase in plasma phosphate.

3.22.1 HYPERPHOSPHATAEMIA

COMMON CAUSES

- Age-related: mild increase normal in growing dogs
- Reduced glomerular fitration *q.v.* section 3.4

- AKI
- CKD
- Hypoadrenocorticism

UNCOMMON CAUSES

- Cell rupture
  - Rhabdomyolysis or osteolysis
  - Snake evenomation
  - Tumour lysis syndrome
  - Thromboembolism
- Hypoparathyroidism
- Nutritional secondary hyperparathyroidism
- Reduced renal excretion
  - Urethral obstruction
  - Uroabdomen
- Vitamin D toxicity (e.g. psoriasis cream)

ARTEFACT

- Haemolysed sample

DIAGNOSTIC SIGNIFICANCE

There are no clinical signs associated directly with hyperphosphataemia.

ADJUNCTIVE TESTS

- Serum biochemistry
- Blood gas analysis
- PTH
- Serum vitamin D panel

3.22.2 HYPOPHOSPHATAEMIA

COMMON CAUSES

- Increased renal excretion
  - Hyperparathyroidism
    - Primary
    - Paraneoplastic secretion of PTH-related protein
  - DM
  - Diuretic use
- Reduced intestinal absorption
  - Vomiting and diarrhoea
- Transcellular shifts
  - Treatment of diabetic ketoacidosis

UNCOMMON CAUSES

- Increased renal excretion
  - Hyperadrenocorticism
  - Hyperaldosteronism
  - Renal tubular defects
- Reduced intestinal absorption
  - Intestinal malabsorption
  - Short bowel syndrome
  - Unbalanced diet, excessive use of phosphate binders
  - Vitamin D deficiency
- Transcellular shifts
  - Re-feeding syndrome

DIAGNOSTIC SIGNIFICANCE

Clinical signs are not observed until severe hypophosphataemia is detected (around < 0.5 mmol/l), where weakness, muscle tremors, and haemolysis (resulting in tachycardia, tachypnoea, dyspnoea, pallor and haemoglobinuria) may be observed.

ADJUNCTIVE TESTS

- Blood gas analysis (acid base)
- PTH and PTHrP
- Serum biochemistry
- Serum vitamin D panel

3.23 POTASSIUM

Potassium is a largely intracellular cation. It is typically assayed at the same time as sodium.

3.23.1 HYPERKALAEMIA

Increased serum potassium occurs if there is failure of intracellular uptake and/or increased leakage, or if there is failure of urinary excretion. Concentrations > 7.5 mmol/l can have a clinical impact, especially on skeletal and cardiac muscle function.

COMMON CAUSES

Marked
- Anuric/oliguric AKI
- Diabetic ketoacidosis, although total body potassium is actually depleted
- Hypoadrenocorticism
- Rupture of urinary tract
- Urinary tract obstruction

Mild
- Acidosis
- CKD

- Dehydration
- Artefact
- Prolonged exposure of serum to clot/delayed separation

UNCOMMON CAUSES

- ACE inhibitors
- Acute tumour lysis
- Ascites
- Chylothorax with repeated thoracocentesis
- Diffuse tissue damage (crush injury)
- Drugs
- GI perforation
- Haemolysis in Akitas and individual dogs with high intracellular potassium
- Hypoaldosteronism
- Iatrogenic
- Potassium-sparing diuretics
- Propranolol
- Pseudo-Addison's, e.g. pregnancy
- Reperfusion injury, e.g. aortic thromboembolism
- Salmonellosis
- *Trichuris* whipworm infestation

ARTEFACT

- Collection in K-EDTA or K-heparin
- Marked leukocytosis or thrombocytosis

DIAGNOSTIC SIGNIFICANCE

- Marked increases are clinically significant causing serious bradyarrhythmia and skeletal muscle weakness
- Mild increases are often artefactual or insignificant

ADJUNCTIVE TESTS

- Abdominal imaging
- Basal cortisol/ACTH stimulation
- Blood gas analysis
- ECG
- Sodium: low in hypoadrenocorticism
- Urea and creatinine for renal and post-renal azotaemia and interpretation of urinalysis

3.23.2 HYPOKALAEMIA

Decreased serum potassium (< 3.5 mmol/l) can be due to inadequate intestinal uptake or increased loss from the extracellular fluid space.

COMMON CAUSES

- Anorexia
- CKD
- Diarrhoea
- Drugs: loop-diuretic therapy, e.g. furosemide
- Insulin therapy
- Potassium-deficient fluid therapy
- Vomiting

UNCOMMON CAUSES

- Alkalosis
- Decreased dietary intake/acidifying diets
- DM
- Fanconi's syndrome
- Hyperadrenocorticism (mild)
- Mineralocorticoid excess
- Post-obstructive diuresis
- Primary hyperaldosteronism
- Renal disease
- Renal tubular acidosis

DIAGNOSTIC SIGNIFICANCE

Recognition of hypokalaemia is important so that correction can be made by potassium supplementation.
- Persistent hypokalaemia despite supplementation indicates a need to check for hypomagnesaemia
- Signs of hypokalaemia include weakness

ADJUNCTIVE TESTS

- Blood gas analysis
- Creatine kinase and AST enzyme activities to evaluate muscle damage
- Creatinine and urea, and urinalysis

- Diagnostic imaging
- Measurement of aldosterone and renin

- Other serum electrolytes
- Urinary fractional excretion

3.24 SODIUM

3.24.1 HYPERNATRAEMIA

Serum sodium concentrations greater than upper reference interval are most often due to water loss rather than solute gain. Clinical signs are typically seen if Na > 170 mmol/l.

COMMON CAUSES

- Dehydration
- Hypotonic water losses
  - Diarrhoea (sodium-poor fluid)
  - HAC (mild)
  - Osmotic diuresis (glucose, mannitol)
    - DM
  - Post-obstructive diuresis
  - Renal disease
- Insensible water loss
  - Fever, hyperthermia
  - Panting
- Restricted intake, especially if associated with polyuria
  - Water withheld accidentally or deliberately
- Salt gain, e.g. sea water ingestion
- Vomiting, especially if intestinal obstruction

UNCOMMON CAUSES

- Hypotonic water losses
  - Diabetes insipidus (DI) (with water restriction)
  - Insensible water loss
  - Burns
  - Third-space effect, e.g. pancreatitis, peritonitis
- Restricted intake
  - Primary hypodipsia or adipsia; reported most often in Miniature schnauzers
  - Central nervous system (CNS) disease: decline in thirst and failure to drink
- Salt gain
  - Activated charcoal
  - Hyperaldosteronism/exogenous mineralo-corticoid excess

- Hypertonic saline
- Increased dietary intake or salt water
- Playdough (home-made) ingestion

DIAGNOSTIC SIGNIFICANCE

- Hypernatraemia is usually secondary to obvious dehydration
- Severe hypernatraemia must be corrected slowly; rapid correction can result in brain oedema
- In some dogs with CNS disease, profound hypernatraemia develops because of adipsia

ADJUNCTIVE TESTS

- Abdominal imaging to assess kidneys, adrenals, intestinal tract
- Brain imaging if an intracranial cause is suspected
- Endocrine function testing
- Potassium may be low
- Proteins may be increased with haemoconcentration and USG is increased
- Urea and creatinine to assess renal function with urinalysis
- Urinalysis to assess for glucosuria and assess USG as indicator of possible causes

3.24.2 HYPONATRAEMIA

In sodium concentrations below lower reference interval, clinical signs become apparent when Na < 132 mmol/l.

COMMON CAUSES

Increased plasma osmolality
- DM

Reduced plasma osmolality
Hypovolaemic
- GI loss (vomiting and diarrhoea, especially if obstruction)
- Hypoadrenocorticism

Normovolaemic
- 5% dextrose infusion

Hypervolaemic
- Congestive heart failure with effusion
- Severe liver disease with ascites

UNCOMMON CAUSES

Increased plasma osmolality
- Mannitol infusion

Reduced plasma osmolality
Hypovolaemic
- Burns
- Third-space effect (peritonitis)

Normovolaemic
- Inappropriate antidiuretic hormone (ADH) release
- Myxoedematous coma in hypothyroidism
- Psychogenic polydipsia

Hypervolaemic
- Advanced kidney disease
- Nephrotic syndrome

ARTEFACT

Pseudohyponatraemia if sodium is measured by flame photometry in lipaemic sample; does not occur with ion-selective electrode.

DIAGNOSTIC SIGNIFICANCE

- If slow onset, signs are related to underlying disease
- Rapid onset is more likely to cause lethargy, depression, vomiting seizures and coma and should be corrected gradually with isotonic saline
- The rate of decrease is more important than the magnitude

ADJUNCTIVE TESTS

- ACTH stimulation testing for hypoadrenocorticism
- Echocardiography
- Glucose
- Imaging
- Potassium
- Thyroid function
- Urea and creatinine, and urinalysis

LABORATORY ABNORMALITIES

3.25 SYMMETRIC DIMETHYLARGININE (SDMA)

SDMA is a product of proteolysis of intracellular proteins and is produced at a steady rate and eliminated predominantly via the kidneys; there is also some enzymatic destruction. It has been shown to be a reliable renal biomarker and correlates well with GFR in humans, dogs and cats. An increased SDMA indicates decreased GFR. This can be due to intrinsic renal disease, pre-renal (dehydration) and post-renal (lower urinary tract obstruction) causes or can reflect other disease processes which secondarily affect the kidneys

It is an earlier indicator of progressive renal dysfunction, often, but not always, increasing before other parameters such as urea and creatinine and before concentrating ability (inappropriately low urine specific gravity) is lost. It is a more reliable indicator than creatinine or urea as it is not influenced by concurrent factors (*q.v.* sections 3.13 and 3.29).

COMMON CAUSES

Kidney disease
- Acute or chronic
- Infection, including pyelonephritis
- Toxicity
- Urinary obstruction/rupture

Non-kidney causes

- Age-related
  - Healthy puppy < 16 µg/dl
  - Healthy adult < 14 µg/dl
- Breed-related, e.g. healthy Greyhound < 20 µg/dL
- Dehydration
- Non-renal neoplasia, e.g. lymphoma due to overexpression of an enzyme involved in SDMA pathway

UNCOMMON CAUSES

Kidney disease

- Amyloidosis
- Congenital kidney disease
- Glomerulopathy

Non-renal causes

- Cardiorenal syndrome
- Hypertension
- Reduced action of enzymatic elimination pathways for SDMA
- Sepsis
- Vector-borne disease

ARTEFACT

- Analytical error
- Haemolysis can falsely decrease SDMA
- Heavy muscling, increasing creatinine > SDMA
- Insignificant trend

DIAGNOSTIC SIGNIFICANCE

- Increased SDMA indicates decreased GFR which may be pre-renal, renal or post-renal in origin. It should not be interpreted as a standalone test, but alongside the history and physical examination, blood tests (particularly urea, creatinine, phosphorus, calcium and potassium), and urinalysis, particularly USG.
- It is also important to understand the critical difference value when looking at trends for monitoring.
  - The critical difference for SDMA is 20%, this means a value should change by ± 20% to be a statistically and clinically significant change in value. In one study the value was as high as 47% when biological and analytical variabilities were taken into account. A rough guide is that a change of 6 µg/dl is required between measurements to be confident a true difference exists.
- SDMA should increase earlier than loss of concentrating ability or increased urea and creatinine.
- Some dogs have increased creatinine with a normal SDMA:
  - Heavily muscled
  - Sample error/artefact could have decreased SDMA, e.g. haemolysis

ADJUNCTIVE TESTS

- Abdominal ultrasound, especially kidneys
- Biochemistry
  - Calcium
  - Creatinine
  - Phosphorus
  - Potassium
  - Urea
- Blood pressure
- Urinalysis
  - Urine culture
  - Urine protein:creatinine (UPC) ratio
- Vector-borne disease screening

3.26 THYROID HORMONE

Assay of T4 is considered a more reliable indicator of thyroid status than triiodothyronine (T3), although T3 is the physiologically active form of thyroxine.

Only the unbound fractions of T3 and T4 are physiologically relevant and total T4 (TT4), i.e. bound plus free, may be decreased in many other illnesses, so-called euthyroid sick syndrome or non-thyroidal illness (NTI). Therefore, whilst a normal TT4 rules out hypothyroidism, a subnormal value requires further analysis by:

- Measurement of endogenous canine-specific thyroid-stimulating hormone (cTSH)
  or
- Free T4 (FT4) by equilibrium dialysis
- Definitive diagnosis by a thyroid-stimulating hormone (TSH) stimulation test is no longer recommended due to cost and potential adverse events with non-medical grade TSH.
- A positive thyroglobulin autoantibody (TGAA) titre indicates lymphocytic thyroiditis but can be present whilst the dog is still euthyroid.
- Measurement of anti-T3 and T4 antibodies is less sensitive than TGAA.
- Free T3 and reverse T3 assays are available but are not used diagnostically.

COMMON CAUSES

Decreased TT4
- Diurnal rhythm
- Euthyroid sick syndrome: normal cTSH
- Normal in sighthounds
- Primary hypothyroidism: decreased fT4, increased cTSH
  - Lymphocytic thyroiditis
- Possible early hypothyroidism: normal cTSH

Increased TT4
- Diurnal rhythm
- Normal in dogs < 3 months of age

UNCOMMON CAUSES

Decreased TT4
- Brachytherapy with I^{131} to treat thyroid tumour
- Drugs
  - Amiodarone
  - Anaesthetics
  - Anti-epileptic drugs except potassium bromide, imepitoin and levetiracetam (Keppra)
  - Anti-thyroid medications: methimazole/thiamazole and other thiouracils and thioureas

- Aspirin
- Carbimazole or methimazole to treat unresectable functional thyroid tumour
- Clomipramine
- Glucocorticoids
- NSAIDs including carprofen
- Sulfonamides
- Hypophysectomy
- Panhypopituitarism
- Secondary hypothyroidism (lack of endogenous TSH)
- Strenuous exercise
- Tertiary hypothyroidism (lack of endogenous thyroid-releasing hormone (TRH))
- Thyroidectomy; unlikely as bilateral glands

Increased TT4
- Accidental ingestion of exogenous thyroid tissue if raw-fed
- Functional thyroid tumour (usually carcinoma)
- Iatrogenic over-supplementation
- Physiological
  - Obesity
  - Pregnancy

ARTEFACT

Decreased
Free T4 measurement must be by equilibrium dialysis due to the potential presence of anti-thyroxine antibodies, but is still prone to error

Increased
T3 and/or T4 autoantibodies may falsely increase T4 unless measuring fT4 by equilibrium dialysis

DIAGNOSTIC SIGNIFICANCE

Decreased
- Decreased fT4 most likely represents primary hypothyroidism, but low TT4 in combination with increased cTSH is diagnostic
- Decreased TT4 alone is caused by both hypothyroidism and euthyroid sick syndrome/NTI
- Decreased TT4 and increased cTSH is indicative of primary hypothyroidism
- Normal TT4 and increased cTSH is suggestive of developing hypothyroidism

LABORATORY ABNORMALITIES

Increased

- A thyroid mass may be palpable
- Hyperthyroidism is rare in dogs, unless on a raw diet

ADJUNCTIVE TESTS

- Haematology: mild normocytic, normochromic anaemia in hypothyroidism

- Biochemistry:
  - Increase in liver enzyme activities in hyperthyroidism
  - Most parameters will be normal in hypothyroidism
  - Serum cholesterol: loose inverse relationship of T4 with cholesterol, i.e. increased in hypothyroidism
- Imaging (CT, ultrasound) in hyperthyroidism and secondary and tertiary hypothyroidism

3.27 TOTAL PROTEIN (ALBUMIN AND GLOBULIN)

Changes in total proteins can be due to changes in albumin or globulin or both.

As albumin is the major colloid osmotic force in plasma, changes in albumin tend to have the most significant effect.

3.27.1 HYPERPROTEINAEMIA

Increased albumin and globulin is almost exclusively caused by dehydration.

3.27.1A HYPERALBUMINAEMIA

CAUSES

Haemoconcentration, i.e. dehydration

ARTEFACT

Lipaemia

3.27.1B HYPERGLOBULINAEMIA

COMMON CAUSES

- Dehydration/haemoconcentration
- Chronic inflammatory/infectious diseases
  - Abscess
  - Hepatitis
  - Immune-mediated disease
  - Nephritis e.g. borreliosis (Lyme disease), leptospirosis
  - Pyoderma

UNCOMMON CAUSES

- Allergy
- Neoplasia
  - Extramedullary plasmacytoma
  - Lymphoma
  - Multiple myeloma (monoclonal)
  - Macroglobulinaemia (IgM myeloma)
- Infectious disease
  - Brucellosis
  - Ehrlichiosis (mono- or polyclonal)
  - Fungal infections
  - Leishmaniasis
  - Neosporosis
  - Toxoplasmosis

DIAGNOSTIC SIGNIFICANCE

- Isolated increases in globulin occur in inflammatory and neoplastic disease and are often associated with a mild/moderate decrease in serum albumin
- Mild increases are most typical of dehydration; typical clinical signs and increased albumin should be noted
- Serum protein electrophoresis
  - Can help classify the cause when hyperglobulinaemia is present in a normally hydrated dog
  - Monoclonal increases indicate multiple myeloma, lymphoma (occasionally) or ehrlichiosis (rarely)

- Polyclonal increases in globulin suggest a chronic inflammatory or neoplastic process

ADJUNCTIVE TESTS

- Infectious disease testing, e.g. *Ehrlichia, Leishmania, Neospora, Toxoplasma*
- Radiographs/CT/imaging for lytic lesions with multiple myeloma or other tumours
- FNA of lymph nodes/masses
- Serum protein electrophoresis
- Urine protein electrophoresis (Bence-Jones proteins)

3.27.2 HYPOPROTEINAEMIA

Hypoproteinaemia can be due to hypoalbuminaemia, hypoglobulinaemia, or decreases in both analytes.

3.27.2A HYPOALBUMINAEMIA

As albumin is the major contributor of colloid osmotic pressure, hypoalbuminaemia < 15 g/l can cause tissue fluid accumulation as ascites (*q.v.* section 2.5) and/or hydrothorax (*q.v.* section 2.21) and/or peripheral oedema (*q.v.* section 2.20).

COMMON CAUSES

- Chronic inflammatory disease (mild)
- External haemorrhage
- Hepatic dysfunction
  - Hepatocellular disease
  - PSS
- Malabsorption/maldigestion/malnutrition
- PLE
  - CIE/IBD
- PLN
  - Glomerulonephritis
- Relative/dilution (mild)
- Sequestration: third-space effect (effusions)

UNCOMMON CAUSES

- Exocrine pancreatic insufficiency (mild)
- Exudative skin disease/burns
- Hypoadrenocorticism
- GI ulceration
- PLE
  - *Ancylostoma* (not in UK)
  - Lymphangiectasia
  - Lymphoma
- Protein-losing nephropathy (PLN)
  - Amyloidosis

DIAGNOSTIC SIGNIFICANCE

- Mild hypoalbuminaemia is seen in most sick dogs as a negative acute phase reaction in response to an increase in globulins
- More severe hypoalbuminaemia is related to increased losses or decreased synthesis or both
- Pattern
  - Liver disease: low albumin, normal–increased globulin
  - PLE: low albumin, low globulin; but globulin can be increased if severe inflammatory disease
  - PLN: low albumin, normal globulin

ADJUNCTIVE TESTS

- B_{12}/folate in suspected intestinal causes
- Imaging to assess intestinal tract, kidneys and liver
- Intestinal biopsy
- Liver function test: bile acids
- Urine protein:creatinine (UPC) ratio to quantify proteinuria

3.27.2B HYPOGLOBULINAEMIA

COMMON CAUSES

- External haemorrhage
- Hepatic insufficiency
- Neonates
- PLE

UNCOMMON CAUSES

- Immunodeficiency
- *q.v.* section 3.27.2B

ADJUNCTIVE TESTS

- Minimum database of haematology and serum biochemistry
- Imaging

3.28 TRYPSIN-LIKE IMMUNOREACTIVITY (TLI)

Canine TLI (cTLI) is an immunoassay to measure decreases in the concentration of the trypsinogen molecule specific to the pancreas; it will also detect free trypsin and so may be increased in pancreatitis.

CAUSES

cTLI < 2.5 µg/l
- Exocrine pancreatic insufficiency (EPI)
  - Pancreatic acinar atrophy
  - Pancreatic hypoplasia
  - End-stage chronic pancreatitis

cTLI < 5.0 but > 2.5 µg/l
- Progression towards EPI
- Protein-losing enteropathy (PLE)
- Subclinical pancreatic disease, e.g. subtotal pancreatic acinar cell destruction secondary to ongoing immune-mediated lymphocytic pancreatitis which may or may not progress to EPI

cTLI > 50.0 µg/l
- Acute pancreatitis (only ~30% sensitive)
- Upper limit of assay; dilution required for absolute result
- In young dogs, sometimes suspected to be due to helminth larval migration

ARTEFACT

- A post-prandial sample may increase the cTLI in a healthy dog, but will not affect the result if EPI is present, although lipaemia makes sample handling more difficult
- Administration of exogenous pancreatic enzymes derived from other species (i.e. bovine or porcine enzyme supplements) orally will not affect the cTLI
- Lipaemia
- Severe haemolysis

DIAGNOSTIC SIGNIFICANCE

- A cTLI < 2.5 ug/l is diagnostic for EPI
- A cTLI between 2.5 and 5 ug/l is equivocal and should be repeated in ~4 weeks whilst treating for EPI in the interim
- An increased cTLI is a poor marker for pancreatitis; cPL is a better test

ADJUNCTIVE TESTS

Serum cobalamin and folate

3.29 UREA

Urea is the final excretory product of the urea cycle and results from the detoxification of ammonia, a product of amino acid (especially glutamine) metabolism and gastrointestinal bacterial fermentation. Hepatocytes are the primary source of urea, which is then freely filtered by the glomerulus and either passively diffuses out of the tubules or is excreted in the urine.

Urea or serum urea is the concentration of the urea molecule in the blood, whereas blood urea nitrogen (BUN) is the concentration of urea nitrogen in the blood. These measurements require conversion to be compared: BUN × 2.14 = Urea.

COMMON CAUSES

Decreased
- Diuresis
  - Iatrogenic, e.g. fluid therapy
  - Primary polydipsia, e.g. psychogenic polydipsia
- Liver dysfunction
  - Acute hepatic failure: toxin, infectious
  - Chronic hepatitis
  - Porto-systemic shunt

Increased
- Decreased GFR
  - Azotaemia, *q.v.* section 3.4
- Catabolic states
- GI haemorrhage
- Post-prandial, especially a high-protein meal
- Yorkshire terriers can have urea slightly above reference range, but normal creatinine

UNCOMMON

Decreased
- Liver dysfunction
- Urea cycle enzyme deficiency
- Nutritional
  - Low-protein diet
  - Malnutrition

DIAGNOSTIC SIGNIFICANCE

- Increased urea contributes to azotaemia, *q.v.* section 3.4
- There are no clinical signs caused directly by a low serum urea concentration, but there may be signs (e.g. PU/PD) due to the underlying cause

ADJUNCTIVE TESTS

Decreased
- Liver enzyme activities
- Markers of hepatic function: albumin, ammonia, bile acids, bilirubin, cholesterol, glucose

Increased
q.v. section 3.4

3B HAEMATOLOGY

3.30 RED BLOOD CELLS (RBCs)

3.30.1 ANAEMIA

Anaemia is the absolute lack of circulating RBCs and results from:
- Decreased RBC production
- Increased RBC destruction (haemolysis)
- Increased RBC loss (haemorrhage)

Anaemia can be classified by
- Degree of anaemia
  - Mild   PCV 30–37%
  - Moderate   PCV 20–29%
  - Severe   PCV 13–19%
  - Very severe   PCV < 13%
- Regenerative response or lack of it
  - Non-regenerative anaemia
    - Acute or chronic
    - RBC parameters
      - Lack of reticulocytosis
      - RBC size can be microcytic, normocytic or macrocytic
      - RBC may be hypochromic or normochromic

- Reticulocyte haemoglobin decreased with iron deficiency
- Tend to develop more slowly as RBC survival time is 100–120 days, thus giving the dog time to compensate with clinical signs only occurring at a lower haematocrit
- Pre-regenerative anaemia
  - Appear to be non-regenerative initially, as it takes 3–7 days for a regenerative response to develop after an acute insult
- Regenerative anaemia: haemolysis or haemorrhage
  - Acute RBC loss
  - RBC parameters, (Figure 3.1)
    - Anisocytosis
    - Decreased reticulocyte haemoglobin (NB: can be increased as an artefact with severe haemolysis)
    - Polychromasia
    - Reticulocytosis
      - It takes 72 hours after the onset of anaemia until an increase in reticulocytes is seen

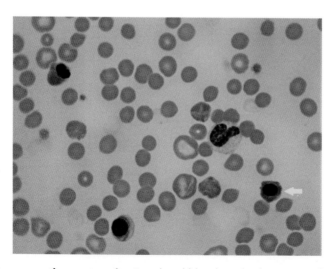

Figure 3.1 Regenerative anaemia. Peripheral blood smear showing marked red blood cell (RBC) regeneration, with nucleated RBCs (yellow arrow), polychromasia (multi-coloured RBCs) and anisocytosis (variably sized RBCs).

- It takes 5–7 days for peak reticulocytosis to occur
- Nucleated RBCs in the absence of reticulocytosis do *not* indicate regeneration.
- The degree of reticulocytosis in haemolysis tends to be greater than with haemorrhage because the iron is available for reuse.
- When blood loss is insufficient to cause hypovolaemic shock, the severity of clinical signs due to the anaemia depends not only on the absolute haematocrit but also its rate of decline.

COMMON CAUSES

REGENERATIVE ANAEMIA

Blood loss/haemorrhage
Bleeding disorders
- Anticoagulant intoxication: vitamin K antagonists, e.g. warfarin and derivatives
- Thrombocytopenia

Gastrointestinal blood loss
- Gastric ulcers
- Ulcerated neoplasia

Neoplasia
- Intracavitary bleeding, e.g. haemangiosarcoma

Trauma
- External blood loss
- Internal blood loss

Haemolysis
Immune-mediated disease
- Primary (idiopathic) IMHA
- Secondary to another disease process e.g. lymphoma, infections

Mechanical fragmentation
- DIC
- Neoplasia, e.g. haemangiosarcoma

NON-REGENERATIVE ANAEMIA
Immune-mediated disease
- Precursor-targeted immune mediated anaemia (PIMA)

Iron deficiency
- Chronic, often occult, GI bleeding: initially regenerative, i.e. reticulocytosis, but later hypochromasia and microcytosis, indicating poor regeneration
  - Gastric ulcers
  - Ulcerated neoplasm

Secondary to extra-marrow factors
- Anaemia of chronic disease: infection, inflammation, neoplasia
- Chronic liver disease
- Chronic renal disease
- Hypoadrenocorticism: may appear normal during acute crisis due to volume depletion and concentration of remaining RBCs; will become apparent after return of normal circulating volume
- Hypothyroidism: physiological response to reduced basal metabolic rate

UNCOMMON CAUSES

REGENERATIVE ANAEMIA

Blood loss/haemorrhage
Bleeding disorders
- Congenital coagulation factor deficiency (haemophilia)
- Disseminated intravascular coagulation (DIC)

Blood-sucking ectoparasites
- Fleas and ticks

Gastrointestinal blood loss
- Alimentary lymphoma
- *Ancylostoma* hookworms (not in UK)
- CIE/IBD
- Duodenal ulcers
- Secondary to other disease, e.g. pancreatitis

Neoplasia
External bleeding

Urinary tract bleeding
- Haemorrhagic cystitis
- Idiopathic renal haematuria
- Neoplasia

LABORATORY ABNORMALITIES

Haemolysis

Blood parasites/infectious diseases (most not endemic in UK)
- Babesia
- *Dirofilaria*: caval syndrome
- *Ehrlichia*
- *Leptospira*
- *Mycoplasma haemocanis*: only if splenectomised

Chemical or toxic injury
- Heinz body anaemia: oxidant damage
- Hypophosphataemia, e.g. correction of diabetic ketoacidosis
- Kale
- Lead poisoning
- Onion/garlic intoxication
- Snake or bee venom toxicity
- Urinary antiseptics containing methylene blue
- Vitamin K1
- Zinc toxicity

Immune-mediated disease
- Isoimmune haemolytic disease of neonates
- Secondary to another disease process, e.g. lymphocytic leukaemia, bacterial/fungal/viral infections, granulomatous disease, SLE
- Secondary to drug administration, e.g. cephalosporins, potentiated sulphonamides, modified live virus vaccines, potentially any drug
- Transfusion reaction

Intracorpuscular problem
- Hereditary non-spherocytic anaemia: Beagles and Poodles
- Hereditary stomatocytosis: Alaskan malamute, Drentse patrijshonds, Miniature schnauzers
- Phosphofructokinase deficiency: American Cocker spaniel, English Springer spaniel
- Predisposition to oxidant injury, e.g. high potassium concentrations and low glutathione concentrations in RBCs: Akita
- Pyruvate kinase deficiency: Basenji, WHWT

Mechanical fragmentation
- Dirofilariasis
- Splenic disease, e.g. torsion
- Haemolytic uraemic syndrome
- Vasculitis

NON-REGENERATIVE ANAEMIA

Iron deficiency
- Chronic external blood loss: initially regenerative, i.e. reticulocytosis, but later hypochromasia and microcytosi indicating poor regeneration
  - Chronic bleeding from skin lesions, e.g. neoplasia
  - Chronic often occult GI bleeding: CIE/IBD
  - Ectoparasite infestation: fleas, ticks
- Repeated phlebotomy

Nutritional deficiencies
- Folic acid
- Iron
- Vitamin B$_{12}$

Inherited selected cobalamin deficiency (Imerslund-Gräsbeck syndrome), *q.v.* sections 3.10, 5.7.1.2C

Anaemia with other cytopenias or pancytopenia
- Alkylating chemotherapy agents
- Bone marrow neoplasia
  - Lymphoproliferative
  - Myeloproliferative
  - Metastatic
- Drugs
  - Chloramphenicol
  - Griseofulvin
  - Phenylbutazone
  - Trimethoprim-sulfa
- Ehrlichiosis
- Idiopathic
- Ionizing radiation
- Myelophthisis: myelodysplasia, myelofibrosis, neoplasia
- Parvovirus
- Toxins
  - Oestrogen
  - Snake venom

DIAGNOSTIC SIGNIFICANCE

For any anaemia to cause clinical signs it must be of sufficient severity and/or develop at a such a rate that compensatory mechanisms become insufficient.

- Moderate to severe anaemias require investigation and the first step is to distinguish regenerative from pre-regenerative and non-regenerative
- Mild, chronic/stable anaemias are most likely secondary to chronic disease elsewhere and do not need investigating *per se*.

ADJUNCTIVE TESTS

- ACTH stimulation test for hypoadrenocorticism
- Antinuclear antibody (ANA) test for evidence of immune-mediated disease but of limited value
- Bone marrow aspirate/core biopsy in non-regenerative anaemias with no other cause identified
- Clotting assessment if considering toxic access to anticoagulants or DIC
- Coombs' test for evidence of IMHA or PIMA
- C-reactive protein as a marker for systemic infection
- Exploratory laparotomy for assessment/biopsy of spleen
- Faecal occult blood loss (limited use)
- Faecal parasitological examination
- Genetic tests where appropriate
- Hepatic/renal biopsy if suggested as cause of anaemia
- Infectious disease tests, e.g. serology/PCR for *Babesia*, *Ehrlichia*, *Leptospirosis*, *Leishmania*, fungal diseases, etc.
- Iron profile in non-regenerative anaemia
- Oestradiol in non-regenerative anaemia
- Thyroid hormone assessment for hypothyroidism in non-regenerative anaemia
- Urinalysis to identify source of blood loss

3.30.2 ERYTHROCYTOSIS

An increase in the red cell numbers.

COMMON CAUSES

- Breed-related, e.g. sighthounds, some Dachshunds
- Relative erythrocytosis: dehydration/haemoconcentration
- Splenic contraction

UNCOMMON CAUSES

- Absolute erythrocytosis
  - Endocrine
    - Acromegaly
    - HAC
    - Hyperthyroidism
  - Primary erythrocytosis (previously polycythaemia vera)
  - Secondary due to hypoxia
    - BOAS
    - Chronic pulmonary disease
    - Congenital heart disease with right to left shunt
    - High altitude
  - Inappropriate erythropoietin secretion by renal and nonrenal tumours, e.g. leiomyoma
  - Methaemoglobinaemia

DIAGNOSTIC SIGNIFICANCE

Use breed-specific reference intervals.
- Bone marrow aspiration: does not help differentiate primary and secondary absolute erythrocytosis
- Brachycephalic breeds tend to have a higher PCV, as do sighthounds (50–65%) and some Dachshunds
- Clinical signs are uncommon until the PCV is greater than 60%
- Splenic contraction causes mild increase, typically < 60%
- Total proteins increased with relative erythrocytosis and are often normal with absolute erythrocytosis

ADJUNCTIVE TESTS

- Bone marrow aspiration or biopsy is unhelpful.
- Complete haematological evaluation, i.e. platelets and WBCs.
- Erythropoietin concentration: if increased consistent with secondary absolute erythrocytosis but if normal does not exclude it. In patients with primary erythrocytosis, results are typically low/normal.

- Imaging e.g. thoracic radiography/CT, echocardiography, abdominal ultrasound to exclude other causes.
- Pulse oximetry/blood gas analysis to identify hypoxia, e.g. $SPO_2 < 90\%$ indicates severe hypoxia.
- Serum biochemistry to assess for indicators of relative erythrocytosis, i.e. dehydration–increased protein, urea and interpret with urinalysis and specific gravity.

3.31 PLATELETS

3.31.1 THROMBOCYTOPENIA

Thrombocytopenia is a decrease in the blood platelet count below $150 \times 10^9/l$.

It is most commonly caused by immune-mediated thrombocytopenia (IMTP), where the platelet count is usually $< 10 \times 10^9/l$.

COMMON CAUSES

Decreased platelet production
- Bone marrow infiltration/neoplastic proliferation
- Myelosuppressive drugs

Increased platelet consumption/use
- Diffuse bleeding
- DIC
- Neoplasia: adherence to tumour endothelium due to abnormal endothelial development

Increased platelet destruction
Immune-mediated thrombocytopenia (IMTP)
- Primary/autoimmune
- Secondary
  - Associated with neoplasia
  - Drugs adsorbed to platelets
  - Systemic infectious agents

- Viral infections, e.g. distemper, infectious canine hepatitis (ICH), herpesvirus, parvovirus

UNCOMMON CAUSES

Decreased platelet production
- Aplasia/hypoplasia bone marrow
- Ineffective platelet production
- Myelosuppressive drugs
- Rickettsial organisms (*Ehrlichia*) (not common in UK)

Increased platelet consumption/use
- Sequestration
- Splenic torsion
- Severe vasculitis

Increased platelet destruction
- Direct damage to platelets by bacterial toxins
- Secondary immune-mediated thrombocytopenia (IMTP)
  - Bacterial infections: leptospirosis, salmonellosis, bacteraemia
  - Fungal disease
  - Protozoal/*Babesia* infections
  - Rickettsial infections: ehrlichiosis, Rocky Mountain spotted fever

ARTEFACTS

- Undetected clot in sample (check tube)
- Macrothrombocytes in CKCSs are not counted by automated analyser

DIAGNOSTIC SIGNIFICANCE

Smear assessment is essential to estimate platelet count and evaluate for platelet clumps or macrothrombocytes.

- Platelet count between 50 and $150 \times 10^9/l$ does not typically cause bleeding unless platelet function is abnormal, but it is a potential marker of consumption by an underlying disease
- Spontaneous bleeding is not usually seen until platelets $< 50 \times 10^9/l$
- The platelet count in IMTP is often $< 10 \times 10^9/l$

ADJUNCTIVE TESTS

- Assess for hepatosplenomegaly, internal lymphadenopathy and any other abnormalities
- Bone marrow biopsy where there is concern about primary bone marrow disease
- Coagulation screen for DIC/other haemostatic defects
- Coombs' test, ANA to evaluate for immune-mediated disease if other cell lines affected
- Infectious disease testing e.g., culture, serology, PCR
- Platelet antibody tests not reliable for IMTP
- Platelet factor 3 (PF3) release test not reliable for IMTP
- Thoracic and abdominal radiographs to identify any internal abnormalities not detected on physical examination
- Ultrasound of liver and spleen

3.31.2 THROMBOCYTOSIS

Thrombocytosis is an increase in the blood platelet count above $500 \times 10^9/l$ and of clinical importance requiring investigation if persistently $> 1,000 \times 10^9/l$.

COMMON CAUSES

- Secondary (reactive) thrombocytosis
  - Drugs
    - Glucocorticoids
    - Vincristine
  - Underlying disease
    - Iron-deficiency anaemia
- Transient
  - Splenic contraction

UNCOMMON CAUSES

- Primary (essential) thrombocytosis
- Secondary (reactive) thrombocytosis
  - Chronic inflammation/infection
  - DIC
  - Gastrointestinal disease
  - HAC
  - Haemolytic anaemia
  - Haemorrhagic anaemia
  - Metabolic disease
  - Neoplasia
  - Trauma

DIAGNOSTIC SIGNIFICANCE

- If the thrombocytosis is repeatable and $> 1,000 \times 10^9/l$ this could indicate primary thrombocytosis and may be accompanied by other cytopenias or leukocytosis; however, milder thrombocytosis is most commonly secondary/reactive and so a search for these underlying causes should be pursued
- Platelet morphology is usually normal, regardless of cause

ADJUNCTIVE TESTS
- Bone marrow aspirate/core biopsy
- Coagulation profile
- Imaging to rule out other causes
- Search for underlying disease as indicated by signs/laboratory abnormalities

LABORATORY ABNORMALITIES

3.32 WHITE BLOOD CELLS (WBCs)

3.32.1 LEUKOCYTOSIS

An increase in the total circulating WBC count.

The most common cause is an increase in the total number of neutrophils (neutrophilia) and is often, partly, a stress response, as well as an inflammatory response.

COMMON CAUSES

Eosinophilia
Hypersensitivity/immune-mediated reactions
- Atopy
- Flea allergy

Parasitism, e.g.
- *Angiostrongylus vasorum*
- *Dirofilaria* in endemic areas
- *Trichuris vulpis*

Lymphocytosis
- Age-related: young animals > adults
- Other
  - Chronic infections (particularly those which elicit antibody response)
  - Hypoadrenocorticism ± eosinophilia
  - Physiological
  - Response to exercise, excitement or forceful handling
- Puppy vaccination

Monocytosis
- Glucocorticoid therapy
- HAC
- Inflammatory disease, especially pyogranulomatous/suppurative/necrotic inflammatory disease
- Immune-mediated disease
- Neoplasms with necrotic centres

Neutrophilia
- Physiological
  - Adrenaline release

- Stress (endogenous or exogenous corticosteroids)
- Reactive
  - Acute inflammation
  - Chronic inflammation
- Infectious
  - Localised
    - Abscess
    - Pyometra
  - Systemic
- Non-infectious/inflammatory
  - Acute pancreatitis
  - Haemorrhage/haemolysis
  - Immune-mediated disease
  - Tissue necrosis

UNCOMMON CAUSES

Eosinophilia
- Hypersensitivity/immune-mediated reactions
- Food allergy
- Eosinophilic bronchopneumopathy: previously called pulmonary infiltrate with eosinophils)
- Eosinophilic gastroenteritis
- Eosinophilic myositis
- Panosteitis (GSD)
- Eosinophilic leukaemia
- Hypoadrenocorticism
- Oestrus in some female dogs
- Parasitism
  - *Ancylostoma caninum* (not endemic in UK)
  - *Dirofilaria* (not endemic in UK); can have concurrent basophilia
  - *Filaroides hirthii* (infection from foxes)
  - *Oslerus osleri* (rarely)
  - *Toxocara* (common infection, but rarely causes eosinophilia)
  - *Uncinaria stenocephala*

Lymphocytosis
- Neoplasia
- Acute lymphoblastic leukaemia
- Chronic lymphocytic leukaemia
- Lymphoma

Monocytosis
- Monocytic/myelomonocytic leukaemia

Neutrophilia
- Early oestrogen toxicity
- Myeloproliferative disorder
- Neoplasia: large necrotic tumour
- Non-infectious/inflammatory
- Surgery

DIAGNOSTIC SIGNIFICANCE

The WBC response is defined both by independent changes in individual cell lines, and by the pattern of changes in all cell lines, e.g. a stress leukogram is defined as neutrophilia, lymphopenia and eosinopenia.

ADJUNCTIVE TESTS

Depending on which cell line is increased:
- Allergy testing/parasite treatment with eosinophilia
- Aspiration/biopsy of lymph nodes/liver/spleen if abnormal/enlarged
- Bone marrow analysis if leukaemia is suspected
- Parasite treatment and diet trial for patients with eosinophilia
- Imaging for source of inflammation/infection or possible malignancy
- Infectious disease testing, e.g. culture, serology, PCR

3.32.2 LEUKOPENIA

A decrease in the total circulating WBC count caused by a decrease in one or all the white cell lines.
- A stress leukogram overall causes leukocytosis (neutrophilia, monocytosis) but there may a decrease in other WBC lines i.e. eosinopenia and lymphopenia
- Lack of neutrophils means that the classical signs of infection may not be evident, e.g. lack of pus formation

- Neutropenia is usually followed by rebound neutrophilia with left shift due to release of cells from maturation and storage pools

COMMON CAUSES

Eosinopenia
- Acute inflammation and infection (endogenous corticosteroid release)
- HAC
- Exogenous steroid
- Part of stress leukogram

Lymphopenia
- Impaired production
  - Prolonged corticosteroid use
- Loss of lymph containing lymphocytes
  - Intestinal lymphangiectasia
- Neoplasia
- Part of stress leukogram
- Viral disease
  - Parvovirus

Neutropenia
- Anaesthesia
- Excessive demand/consumption
  - Infectious diseases
  - Sepsis
- Reduced production
  - Bone marrow disease
  - Parvovirus
- Neoplasia
- Sequestration in marginating pool
- Toxic and drug reactions
  - Chemotherapy
  - Oestrogen
  - Phenobarbitone

UNCOMMON CAUSES

Eosinopenia
Tissue inflammation with production of eosinophilic chemotactic substances leading to eosinopenia

Lymphopenia
- Impaired production
  - Chemotherapy

- Inherited selected cobalamin deficiency (Imerslund-Gräsbeck syndrome), *q.v.* sections 3.10, 5.7.1.2C
- Irradiation
- Loss of lymph
  - Repeated drainage of chylothorax
- Septicaemia/endotoxaemia
- Sequestration in marginating pool
  - Anaesthesia
- Viral disease
  - Distemper
  - Infectious hepatitis

Neutropenia
- Excessive demand/consumption
  - Drug-induced
  - Hypersplenism
  - Immune-mediated neutropenia
- Paraneoplastic
- Ineffective production
  - May result from myeloid leukaemia or myelodysplasia
  - Myelodysplasia often has anaemia, neutropenia and thrombocytopenia associated to varying degrees often associated with maturation arrest
- Reduced production: bone marrow disease
  - Cyclic haematopoiesis neutropenia in grey collie; also called cyclic neutropenia as most affected because of shortest half-life

- Trapped neutrophil syndrome in Border collies
- Sequestration in marginating pool
  - Anaphylactic shock
  - Endotoxic shock

DIAGNOSTIC SIGNIFICANCE

The WBC response is defined both by changes in individual cell lines and by the overall pattern of the independent changes in all cell lines. Percentages of each cell type within the WBC count should only be used to calculate absolute numbers of each cell line.

ADJUNCTIVE TESTS

Depending on which cell line is decreased:
- Anti-neutrophil antibody testing if available for immune-mediated neutropenia
- Blood culture
- Bone marrow evaluation
- Imaging for source of consumption/overwhelming inflammation/infection
- Infectious disease testing, e.g. serology, PCR, culture
- Urinalysis and urine culture

3.33 PANCYTOPENIA

Decrease in all blood cell lines, i.e. anaemia, thrombocytopenia and leukopenia.

UNCOMMON CAUSES

Pancytopenia is uncommon; therefore all causes are categorised as uncommon.
- Neoplasia
- Immune-mediated disease
- Infectious diseases, e.g. ehrlichiosis, leishmaniosis, parvovirosis
- Toxin/drug, e.g., oestrogen, chemotherapeutic drugs, phenobarbitone, sulfa drugs, irradiation

DIAGNOSTIC SIGNIFICANCE

- In endemic areas, infectious diseases are the most common cause of pancytopenia
- Hypoproteinaemia with parvovirus compared to hyperproteinaemia with ehrlichiosis or leishmaniosis
- Leukopenia is more severe with parvovirus and ehrlichiosis
- Oestrogen toxicity should be considered in entire females and males (functional Sertoli cell tumour) or in dogs receiving exogenous oestrogen *q.v.* section 5.9.6
- Thrombocytopenia is more severe with ehrlichiosis

ADJUNCTIVE TESTS

- As per anaemia/thrombocytopenia or leukopenia as individual entities, e.g., imaging, infectious disease tests, immune function tests
- Bone marrow cytology/histology

3C URINALYSIS

Urinalysis is a critical step in the investigation of many medical disorders and is particularly informative when assessing for urinary tract disorders (renal, including tubular and glomerular disease and lower urinary tract disease) and systemic diseases such as endocrinopathies (DM, HAC, DI).

3.34 BIOCHEMICAL ANALYSIS

Urine dipstick analysis is a simple patient-side test that provides semi-quantitative results by colour change, interpreted as concentration of each analyte.

Available dipsticks may include pH, leucocytes, nitrite and urobilinogen; these results are disregarded in veterinary medicine as they are either not validated or accurate.

3.34.1 PROTEIN

The protein pad on a urine dipstick is most sensitive for albumin, and poorly sensitive for globulins (e.g. Bence-Jones proteins). The result must be interpreted in light of the urine concentration; a small amount (trace) of protein may be normal in concentrated urine (even higher results may be detected in very concentrated urine), whereas the same result in dilute urine may be of more significance. Alkaline urine (pH > 8) and presence of detergents can result in false positive reactions.

Urine protein:creatinine (UPC) ratio is a more accurate assessment for proteinuria and should be performed in cases where proteinuria is a consideration, based on clinical suspicion or dipstick. Causes of proteinuria, *q.v.* section 3.36.

3.34.2 BILIRUBIN

The bilirubin pad detects conjugated bilirubin. Dogs have a low renal threshold, therefore 1+ bilirubin in concentrated urine may be a normal finding. Male dogs are able to conjugate bilirubin from resorbed haemoglobin, therefore this is more commonly detected in healthy male than female dogs.

CAUSES

- Cholestatic liver disease
- Haemolysis, *q.v.* section 3.30.1
- Physiological: normal in concentrated urine, especially in male dogs

3.34.3 GLUCOSE

Glucosuria occurs when the renal threshold for glucose is exceeded in the blood (10 mmol/l) or due to a failure to resorb filtered glucose by the renal tubules. False positives may be observed on dipsticks when urine is contaminated (e.g. by NSAIDs).

CAUSES

- Hyperglycaemia glucosuria – diabetes mellitus, may observe transiently in systemic disorders (uncommon in dogs; due to stress or pancreatitis)
- Normoglycaemia glucosuria
  - Copper-associated hepatitis in Labrador retrievers

- Fanconi syndrome
- Tubular injury
  - Jerky treat ingestion
  - Leptospirosis
  - Pyelonephritis

3.34.4 HAEM

The blood pad detects peroxidase-like activity as found in haemoglobin:
- Haematuria
- Haemoglobinuria
- Myoglobinuria
  Haematuria may be discriminated from haemoglobinuria/pigmenturia by spinning the urine and observing for a red blood cell precipitate following centrifugation.

CAUSES

- Haematuria
  - Iatrogenic (due to collection technique)
  - Pathological
    - Haemostatic disorders
    - Idiopathic renal haemorrhage
    - Neoplasia
    - Urinary tract inflammation
    - Sterile haemorrhagic cystitis
    - Urolithiasis
    - Urinary tract infection

- Haemoglobinuria
  - Due to lysed RBCs (storage artefact)
  - Due to haemolysis
    - Intravascular IMHA
    - Haemolytic transfusion reaction
- Myoglobinuria
  - Severe muscle injury
    - Inherited myopathy
    - Massive crush injury
    - Thromboembolism
    - Snake evenomation

ARTEFACT

- False positives due to presence of bacterial peroxidases

3.34.5 KETONES

The ketone pad mainly detects acetoacetic acid and acetone, with poor sensitivity for beta hydroxybutyrate. False positives may be observed with strongly coloured urine.

CAUSES

- Uncontrolled fat metabolism
  - Uncontrolled DM
  - Starvation, especially in young dogs

3.35 SEDIMENT

3.35.1 RED BLOOD CELLS

Sediment analysis will aid discrimination between haematuria and haemoglobinuria. (See above for causes of increase numbers.)

3.35.2 WHITE BLOOD CELLS

Presence of < 5 WBCs per high-powered field is generally considered within normal limits.

CAUSES

- Blood contamination from urine collection method, especially cystocentesis
- Neoplasia
- Sterile inflammation
  - Sterile haemorrhagic cystitis
  - Urolithiasis
- Urinary tract infection

3.35.3 EPITHELIAL CELLS

- Neoplastic cells
  - Transitional cell carcinoma cells may slough and be detected in the urine
- Renal tubular epithelial cells
  - Large numbers may be detected in renal tubular injury
- Squamous epithelial cells
  - May be detected in prostatic squamous metaplasia
  - May be contaminants especially in voided or catheterised samples

3.35.4 CRYSTALS

- Ammonium biurate
  - May be detected in breeds (Dalmatian, English bulldog, Black Russian terrier), or due to high blood ammonia as seen in particular in congenital porto-systemic shunts and other porto-vascular anomalies
- Bilirubin
  - Cholestatic liver disease
  - Concentrated urine, as with bilirubinuria
  - RBC destruction
- Calcium oxalate
  - Ethylene glycol toxicity
  - Genetic tendency to calciuresis: Miniature schnauzers
  - Hypercalcaemia
  - Normal finding
  - Storage artefact

- Cystine
  - Observed due to inborn error of metabolism
  - Sex-linked in some breeds and in these cases observed only in male entire dogs
- Struvite
  - May be seen in clinically normal dogs
  - Presence more likely in alkaline urine but can be seen at any pH
  - Urease-positive urinary tract infections promote formation

3.35.5 TUBULAR CASTS

- Fatty casts
  - Thought to represent tubular degeneration
- Granular casts
  - Should be interpreted in the context of the patient's presenting problems; small numbers may be of uncertain significance, or may reflect tubular injury
- Hyaline casts
  - Small amounts are normal in concentrated urine; increased numbers may be seen in the presence of proteinuria

3.35.6 WAXY CAST

Final stage of cast degeneration, indicates a more chronic tubular injury, and always of pathological significance.

3.36 URINE PROTEIN: CREATININE (UPC) RATIO

Proteinuria may be pre-renal, renal or post-renal in origin, and is defined as an increase in the urine protein:creatinine (UPC) ratio > 0.2.

The UPC ratio provides a quantified result for the degree of protein loss in urine. It is more accurate than urine dipstick analysis as it is not affected by urine dilution or concentration. The degree of increase is useful in terms of guiding need for further investigations and/or monitoring treatment.

- In azotaemic dogs, borderline proteinuria (0.2–0.5) is considered of greater significance and intervention may be considered
- In contrast, borderline proteinuria in non-azotaemic dogs would be considered equivocal
- Proteinuria > 0.5 is overt proteinuria
  - UPC > 2 is considered likely to be glomerular in origin (provided the sample is not macroscopically blood-tinged)
  - UPC > 3.5 is considered high-magnitude proteinuria

CAUSES

Pre-renal proteinuria
- Overload proteinuria: excessive filtration of protein overwhelming reabsorption capacity (haemoglobinuria, myoglobinuria, Bence-Jones proteinuria)
- Physiologic proteinuria
  - Transient causes: pyrexia, seizures, strenuous exercise
  - Hypertension, hyperadrenocorticism

Renal proteinuria
- Pathological proteinuria
  - Glomerular disorders (glomerulonephropathies)
    - Amyloidosis
    - Glomerulonephritis
    - Primary
    - Immune complex deposition
  - Interstitial disorders
    - Leptospirosis

- Pyelonephritis
- Renal neoplasia
- Uroliths
- Tubular disorders
  - AKI
  - Fanconi's syndrome
  - Inherited selected cobalamin deficiency (Imerslund-Gräsbeck syndrome), *q.v.* sections 3.10, 5.7.1.2C
- Physiologic proteinuria
  - HAC
  - Hypertension

Post-renal proteinuria
- Urinary tract haemorrhage
- Urinary tract infection
  - Cystitis
  - Prostatitis
  - Vaginitis
- Urinary tract inflammation
  - Sterile haemorrhagic cystitis
  - Urethritis
  - Urolithiasis

3.37 URINE SPECIFIC GRAVITY (USG)

In a healthy dog the USG should be appropriate for its hydration status, i.e. a dehydrated dog should produce a concentrated urine.

- DI
- DM
- Renal dysfunction

USG > 1.030 – HYPERSTHENURIA

If patient is azotaemic this increases suspicion of prerenal causes

USG < 1.030

- In the presence of dehydration, prior to intravenous fluid therapy, this implies inappropriate urine concentration ability and may occur for many causes

USG 1.008–1.012 – ISOSTHENURIA

This may increase suspicion of renal dysfunction

USG < 1.008 – HYPOSTHENURIA

Active dilution of urine by renal tubules, if the dog is dehydrated on examination in the presence of hyposthenuria this should increase suspicion of DI

SECTION 4
IMAGING PATTERNS

In this section, differential diagnoses for specific plain radiographic and ultrasonographic patterns and appearances are listed. Relevant further imaging modalities (contrast radiography, cross-sectional imaging, i.e. CT and MRI, scintigraphy) are suggested.

4.1 ABDOMEN

4.1.1 RADIOGRAPHY

Generalised changes seen on plain abdominal radiographs are listed.

q.v. section 5 for organ-specific changes.

4.1.1A ABDOMINAL ENLARGEMENT AND MASS(ES)

Figure 4.1.1

COMMON CAUSES

Cranial abdomen
- Hepatomegaly, *q.v.* section 2.8, Figure 4.1.1a
- Mesenteric lymphadenomegaly

Mid-abdomen
- Small intestine (SI)
  - Foreign body
  - Intussusception
- Spleen
  - *q.v.* section 2.28, Figure 4.1.1b

Caudal abdomen
- Bladder distension
- Prostatomegaly, *q.v.* section 2.23, Figure 4.1.1c
- Pregnancy, Figure 4.1.1d
- Pyometra, *q.v.* section 5.9.5

UNCOMMON CAUSES

Cranial abdomen
- Adrenal mass
- Gastric distension/mass
- Hepatic neoplasia
- Pancreas
  - Chronic fibrosing pancreatitis
  - Pancreatic adenocarcinoma

Mid-abdomen
SI
- Neoplasia
  - Adenocarcinoma

- Lymphoma
- Gastrointestinal (GI) stromal tumour
- Leiomyoma/leiomyosarcoma

Spleen
- *q.v.* section 2.28

Caudal abdomen
- Cryptorchidism
- Colonic or caecal mass
- Sublumbar lymphadenopathy

4.1.1B CALCIFICATION (BONE/MINERAL DENSITY)

Figure 4.1.2

COMMON CAUSES

- Alimentary tract
  - Foreign body, Figure 4.1.2a
  - Ingesta, including some medications, Figure 4.1.2b
- Genital tract
  - Pregnancy, Figure 4.1.2c
- Liver
  - Cholelithiasis
- Peritoneal cavity
  - Artefact: coat contamination
- Urinary tract
  - Nephrocalcinosis, *q.v.* section 5.12
    - Hyperadrenocorticism (HAC)
    - Hypercalcaemia
  - Urolithiasis, *q.v.* Figure 4.1.2d

UNCOMMON CAUSES

- Adrenal glands
  - Idiopathic
  - Neoplasia
- Genital tract
  - Chronic prostatitis
  - Fetal mummification
  - Ovarian neoplasia

IMAGING PATTERNS

Notes on Canine Internal Medicine, Fourth Edition. Victoria L. Black, Kathryn F. Murphy, Jessie Rose Payne, and Edward J. Hall.
© 2022 John Wiley & Sons Ltd. Published 2022 by John Wiley & Sons Ltd.

(a)

(b)

(c)

(d)

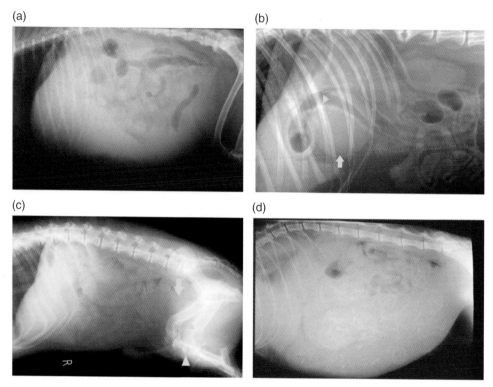

Figure 4.1.1 Abdominal enlargement and masses

4.1.1a Hepatomegaly

Right lateral plain radiograph showing an enlarged abdomen due to cranial abdominal organo-megaly, and loss of peritoneal detail. Subsequent ultrasonographic imaging demonstrated an enlarged liver extending caudally beyond the costal arch due to multiple metastatic nodules from a primary intestinal tumour (not visible on the radiograph) and a small volume of free fluid.

4.1.1b Splenic mass

Left lateral plain abdominal radiograph showing a circular abdominal mass effect (arrow) with the gas-filled duodenum looping over it (arrow head). An encapsulated splenic haematoma was found at laparotomy, but in a right lateral view this could have could been mistaken for a fluid-filled gastric antrum or gastric foreign body.

4.1.1c Prostatic mass and hypertrophic osteopathy

Right lateral plain abdominal radiograph showing a caudal abdominal mass (arrow). Contrast urography or ultrasound confirmed a prostatic mass and a cranially displaced bladder. In addi-tion, palisaded periosteal new bone (arrow heads) is visible on the long bones of the hind limbs due to hypertrophic osteopathy (HO, Marie's disease). Although more commonly associated with thoracic masses, HO can be a consequence of abdominal masses. (*Image courtesy of Chris Warren-Smith, Langford Vets.*)

4.1.1d Pregnancy

Right lateral abdominal radiograph of a 7-week-pregnant bitch. Marked abdominal enlargement is associated with a soft tissue density in the ventral abdomen containing multiple fetal skeletons. (*Image courtesy of Margaret Costello, Vision Diagnostic Imaging.*)

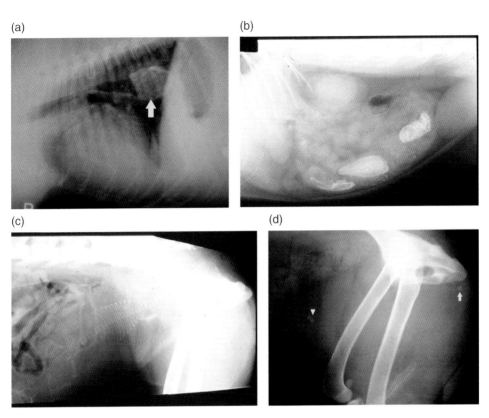

Figure 4.1.2 Calcification

4.1.2a Oesophageal foreign body
Although not an abdominal problem, this right lateral plain thoracic radiograph clearly demonstrates a mineral density in the distal oesophagus (arrow). Plain radiographs should always be taken before any contrast studies, which may mask such a bony foreign body.

4.1.2b Chronic obstruction
Right abdominal radiograph showing a gravel sign with mineralised material accumulating in the small intestine proximal to a chronic partial obstruction. (*Image courtesy of Margaret Costello, Vision Diagnostic Imaging.*)

4.1.2c Pregnancy
Right lateral abdominal radiograph showing a mineralised fetal skeleton within the caudal abdomen and pelvic canal in a pregnant bitch. (*Image courtesy of Margaret Costello, Vision Diagnostic Imaging.*)

4.1.2d Urolithiasis
Right lateral radiograph of the caudal abdomen demonstrating multiple small, calcified cystoliths (arrow head). The hindlegs have been pulled forward to visualise a urolith in the urethra (arrow). (*Image courtesy of Chris Warren-Smith, Langford Vets.*)

- Prostatic neoplasia
- Prostatic/paraprostatic cyst
- GI tract
  - Gravel sign with obstruction
  - Uraemic gastritis
- Liver
  - Abscess
  - Chronic cholecystitis
- Cyst/granuloma/haematoma
- Hepatic neoplasia
- Incidental biliary calcification
- Limy bile
- Mesenteric and/or sublumbar lymph nodes
  - Neoplasia
- Pancreas
  - Chronic pancreatitis

- Neoplasia
- Peripancreatic fat necrosis
- Pseudocyst
- Peritoneal cavity
  - Abdominal fat
    - Bates bodies: clinically insignificant, idiopathic, dystrophic fat calcification
    - Pansteatitis
  - Arterial calcification in HAC
  - Calcinosis cutis
  - Ectopic pregnancy
  - Mammary gland neoplasia
  - Myositis ossificans
- Spleen
  - Abscess
  - Haematoma
  - Histoplasmosis
- Urinary tract
  - Chronic cystitis
  - Neoplasia
  - Nephrocalcinosis
  - Nephrotoxins

4.1.1C EXTRA-INTESTINAL GAS

COMMON CAUSES

- Pneumoperitoneum

- GI tract perforation, Figure 4.1.3a
  - Linear foreign body
  - Non-steroidal anti-inflammatory drug (NSAID)-induced ulcer; more likely if concurrent steroids
  - Post-surgical dehiscence
  - Sharp/penetrating GI foreign body
- Post-exploratory laparotomy: takes 1–2 weeks to fully resolve, Figure 4.1.3b

UNCOMMON CAUSES

- Abdominal wall perforation
- Emphysematous cholecystitis
- Emphysematous cystitis
- Gastric
  Aerophagia
  - Dyspnoea
  - Dysphagia
- Pneumobilia
  - Congenital abnormality
  - Incompetent sphincter of Oddi
    - Passage of large gallstone
    - Scarring related to chronic pancreatitis
- Infection by gas-forming organisms, e.g. emphysematous cholecystitis
- Surgical biliary procedure

(a)

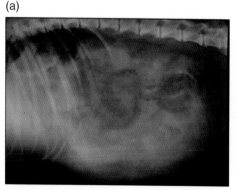

(b)

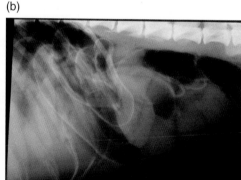

Figure 4.1.3 Pneumoperitoneum
4.1.3a Gastrointestinal perforation
Right abdominal radiograph showing accumulation of free gas within the peritoneal cavity due to a GI perforation. Gas is particularly noticeable dorsally caudal to the diaphragm and a loss of serosal detail in the ventral abdomen is suggestive of free fluid and possible peritonitis. (*Image courtesy of Margaret Costello, Vision Diagnostic Imaging.*)
4.1.3b Post-laparotomy
Right abdominal radiograph showing free gas within the peritoneal cavity following a laparotomy. Serosal surfaces of the intestinal loops are outlined due to the volume of free gas present. There is severe diffuse ileus present post operatively. (*Image courtesy of Margaret Costello, Vision Diagnostic Imaging.*)

- Pneumatosis intestinalis (pneumatosis coli if restricted to colon)
  - Intramural bowel gas due to mucosal ulceration
    - Necrotising enterocolitis
    - Respiratory causes of increased intra-abdominal pressure (hypothetical)
- Pneumoperitoneum
  - GI tract perforation
    - Eosinophilic gastroenteritis
    - Remote mast cell tumour
    - Intestinal adenocarcinoma
  - Penetrating wound through abdominal wall
- Pneumoretroperitoneum
  - Infection with gas-forming organisms, usually caused by tracking a foreign body (FB)
  - Gas-tracking from pneumomediastinum

4.1.1D   GAS DILATION OF GI TRACT

The presence of some gas in the intestine is normal, but accumulations causing dilation or with odd distribution may be abnormal. A rule of thumb is that any SI dilation > 1.5 times the height of the body of L5 is likely to indicate obstruction.

COMMON CAUSES

Gastric
- Aerophagia
  - Greedy eating
- Gastric dilatation-volvulus (GDV), Figure 4.1.4a

Small intestinal
Lumenal diameter < 1.5× the height of the L5 body
- Aerophagia
- Enteritis
- Generalised or focal ileus
  - Electrolyte imbalances, e.g. hypokalaemia
  - Enteritis
  - Recent abdominal surgery
- Normal

Lumenal diameter > 1.5× the height of the L5 body
- Error
  - Mistaking colon for SI
- Intestinal obstruction, Figure 4.1.4b
  - Foreign body
  - Intussusception

Bunching with comma-shaped gas bubbles
- Linear foreign body

(a)

(b)

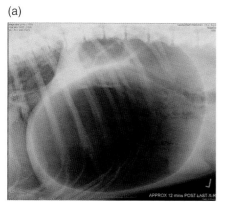
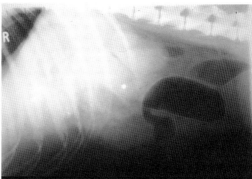

Figure 4.1.4 Gas dilation of GI tract
4.1.4a Gastric dilatation-volvulus
Right lateral plain cranial abdominal radiograph showing massive gas dilation of the stomach with compartmentalisation consistent with gastric dilatation-volvulus. (*Image courtesy of Chris Warren-Smith, Langford Vets.*)
4.1.4b Intestinal obstruction
Right lateral plain abdominal radiograph showing marked dilation of two small intestinal loops consistent with an intestinal obstruction.

Large intestine
Normal

UNCOMMON CAUSES

Gastric
- Aerophagia
  - Dysphagia
  - Dyspnoea

Small intestine
Lumenal diameter < 1.5× the height of the L5 body
Normal or
- Adhesions
- Enteritis
- Generalised or focal ileus
- Hypokalaemia
- Peritonitis

Lumenal diameter > 1.5× the height of the L5 body
- Intestinal obstruction
  - Adhesions
  - Entrapment in ruptured diaphragm
  - Incarceration in internal hernia
  - Incarceration in inguinal or umbilical hernia
  - Neoplasia
  - Volvulus
- Generalised, severe ileus
  - Dysautonomia
  - Visceral myopathy: leiomyositis
  - Visceral neuropathy: mesenteric ganglionitis

4.1.1E   LOSS OF CONTRAST/ PERITONEAL DETAIL/SEROSAL DETAIL

COMMON CAUSES

- Artefact
  - Superimposed material, e.g. wet hair, ultrasound gel
  - Underexposure
- Ascites, *q.v.* section 2.5, Figure 4.1.1a
  - Low-protein transudate
  - Exudate

- Septic abdomen
- GI perforation
- High-protein modified transudate
- Other fluids
  - Blood
    - Ruptured splenic or hepatic haemangiosarcoma
    - Trauma
- Lack of intra-abdominal fat
  - Severe weight loss
  - Young dog (also has predominantly brown fat with a soft-tissue density)

UNCOMMON CAUSES

- Ascites, *q.v.* section 2.5
  - Exudate
  - Other fluids
    - Bile
    - Chyle
    - Urine
- Carcinomatosis: may cause ill-defined granular/nodular pattern
- Peritonitis
  - Pansteatitis
  - Pancreatitis: may cause ill-defined granular/nodular pattern
  - Septic abdomen
    - *Nocardia* infection
    - Ruptured pyometra
    - Tuberculosis

4.1.1F   METAL DENSITIES

COMMON CAUSES

- Contrast media
- Gunshot/BB pellets
- Ingested metal FBs, e.g. battery, coin, fish hook, needle/pin, tinsel (Figure 4.1.5)

UNCOMMON CAUSES

- Heavy metal poisoning: ingested lead paint
- Penetrating FB
- Vascular clips or Ameroid constrictor

(a)   (b)

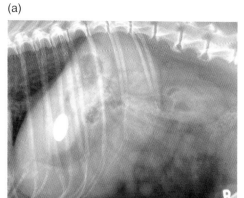
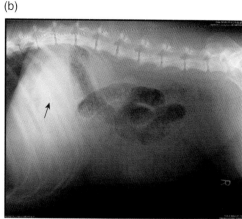

Figure 4.1.5 Metal FB
Whilst metal fragments in the GI tract may be incidental findings, large or sharp objects should be removed.
4.1.5a Coin in the stomach (*Image courtesy of Chris Warren-Smith, Langford Vets.*)
4.1.5b Fish hook in the stomach (*Image courtesy of Chris Warren-Smith, Langford Vets.*)

4.1.1G   ORGAN DISPLACEMENT

Figure 4.1.6

COMMON CAUSES

- Abdominal masses, *q.v.* section 2.2, Figure 4.1.1
- Enlarged bladder
- GDV
- Linear foreign body causing bunching of SI
- Microhepatica, Figure 4.1.6a
- Organomegaly, *q.v.* section 2.2
- Ruptured diaphragm, Figure 4.1.6b

UNCOMMON CAUSES

- Abdominal wall muscle weakness or rupture
- Adhesions
- Carcinomatosis
- Inguinal or umbilical hernia
- Massive ascites
- Overinflation of lungs
- Peritoneo-pericardial diaphragmatic hernia (PPDH)
- Retroperitoneal expansile lesion
  - Abscess (tracking FB)

- Haemangiosarcoma
- Haematoma
  - Anticoagulant poisoning
  - Trauma
  - Ruptured kidney or ureter(s)
- Sclerosing peritonitis

4.1.1H   ORGANOMEGALY OR CHANGE IN SHAPE

- Endocrine
- Haemopoietic (spleen)
- Hepatobiliary
- Reproductive
- Urinary
q.v. sections 2.2, 4.1.1A, 5, Figure 4.1.1a
- Intra-abdominal/mesenteric lymph nodes
  - Inflammation
    - Secondary to infection/inflammation within peritoneal cavity or abdominal organs
    - Sterile (steroid-responsive) lymphadenitis
    - Neutrophilic lymphadenitis
    - Pyogranulomatous lymphadenitis
  - Neoplasia
    - Alimentary lymphoma
    - Multicentric lymphoma
    - Metastatic disease

(a)

(b)

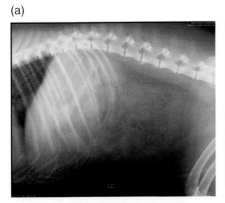
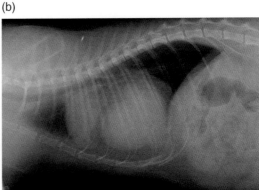

Figure 4.1.6 Organ displacement
4.1.6a Microhepatica
Right lateral plain abdominal radiograph with a small liver due to a congenital porto-systemic shunt identified by the cranial tilting of the gastric axis (solid line).
4.1.6b Ruptured diaphragm
Plain left lateral radiograph of the thorax and cranial abdomen in a dog with a ruptured diaphragm. The abdominal contents have been shifted cranially and viscera are visible in the caudal thorax. (*Image courtesy of Chris Warren-Smith, Langford Vets.*)

4.1.2 ULTRASOUND

Only generalised and non-organ changes are listed. Changes in specific organ size (decreased or increased), shape and echogenicity are detailed in section 5.

4.1.2A FREE ABDOMINAL FLUID

COMMON CAUSES

- Ascites, *q.v.* 2.5
  - Low-protein transudate
  - High-protein modified transudate
  - Other
    - Blood
- Neoplasia (Figure 4.1.7)
- Normal: sliver of fluid, especially in young animals
- Peritonitis
  - Pancreatitis: may cause ill-defined granular/nodular pattern
  - Septic abdomen
    - GI perforation

UNCOMMON CAUSES

- Ascites, *q.v.* 2.5
  - Other
    - Bile
    - Chyle
    - Urine
  - Carcinomatosis
  - Immune-mediated haemolytic anaemia (IMHA): small volume occasionally seen
  - Peritonitis
  - Pansteatitis
  - Septic abdomen
    - *Nocardia* infection
    - Ruptured pyometra
    - Tuberculosis
- Post-laparotomy

4.1.2B LYMPHADENOPATHY – MESENTERIC/INGUINAL/ SUBLUMBAR

Figure 4.1.8
- Inflammation
  - Secondary to infection/inflammation within peritoneal cavity or abdominal organs

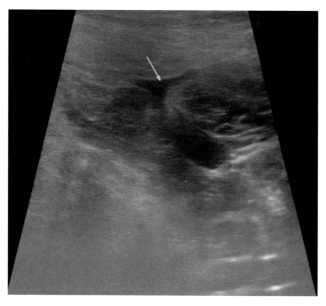

Figure 4.1.7 Free fluid (splenic mass)
Ultrasound image showing a heterogeneous splenic mass with a small volume of free fluid (arrow) around it. (*Image courtesy of Chris Warren-Smith, Langford Vets.*)

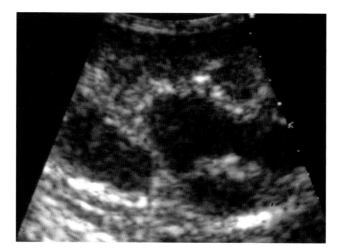

Figure 4.1.8 Mesenteric lymph node ultrasound
Ultrasound image of mesenteric lymph nodes.

- Sterile (steroid-responsive) lymphadenitis
  - Neutrophilic lymphadenitis
  - Pyogranulomatous lymphadenitis
- Neoplasia
  - Alimentary lymphoma
  - Multicentric lymphoma
  - Metastatic disease

IMAGING PATTERNS

4.2 BONE

Refer to orthopaedic textbooks for further information on the diagnosis and treatment of orthopaedic conditions.

4.2.1 BONE DEFORMITIES

Bone deformities describe abnormalities in the curvature and shape of bones which may result in abnormal congruity of joints and therefore abnormal limb function and joint disease. In young dogs abnormal limb angulation should be detected and addressed early to improve likelihood of joint congruity and reducing risk of subluxation.

Chondrodystrophic dogs will have abnormal limb length as a result of their genetic background which may result in significant orthopaedic disease in some dogs. Mediolateral abnormalities (valgus and varus) are more likely to have significant impact on weightbearing of the limb than craniocaudal abnormalities due to the inability to adapt to abnormalities in the mediolateral plane.

Diet has been linked with development of angular limb deformities in dogs, especially giant breeds. Diets must be carefully formulated for growing giant-breed dogs, in particular calorie, calcium and phosphorus content.

COMMON CAUSES

- Developmental angular limb deformities, e.g. breed-related
- Traumatic angular deformities, e.g. synostosis due to fracture healing in young dogs

UNCOMMON CAUSES

- Congenital abnormalities (abnormalities developing during gestation)
  - Dysmelia
    - Amelia: lack of a limb
    - Hemimelia agenesis of a limb bone, e.g. radial or tibial
  - Phocomelia

- Dactyly
  - Ectrodactyly: split paw
  - Polydactyly: supernumerary digits
  - Syndactyly: fused digits
- Congenital hypothyroidism: short broad skulls, shortened vertebral bodies, epiphyseal dysgenesis and delayed maturation
- Osteogenesis imperfecta: a defect in collagen resulting in fragile bones, radiographically normal with evidence of multiple fractures
- Rickets (hypovitaminosis D), *q.v.* section 4.2.2A
- Renal osteodystrophy (rubber jaw), *q.v.* section 4.2.2A
- Rottweiler dogs can have abnormalities in sesamoid bones; this can result in lameness in some dogs but may be subclinical in others

4.2.2 BONE DENSITY CHANGES

4.2.2A DECREASED BONE DENSITY (OSTEOPENIA)

Generalised decreased bone density or osteopenia may be detected during investigations into fractures or lameness, or as an incidental finding. It is recognised by comparing the radiographic density of bone to adjacent soft tissue. It is a rare finding, and its significance will depend on the underlying aetiology.

CAUSES

Hypovitaminosis D (rickets)
- Animals may present with lameness, constipation, pathological fractures and lateral bowing of long bones, and, in some cases, signs of hypocalcaemia (tremors, facial pruritus, seizures).
- Hypocalcaemia is typically present; with increased parathyroid hormone in most cases (aside from hypoparathyroidism), calcidiol and calcitriol may be useful; calcitriol is low in most cases, aside from hereditary vitamin D receptor defects.

- In young growing dogs the pathology is most apparent at the metaphyses of the long bones with lack of mineralisation and widened physes, bowing of long bones and enlarged costochondral junctions alongside generalised osteopenia. There may also be evidence of previous or current pathological fractures.
- In adult dogs in addition to generalised osteopenia the jaw is preferentially affected in some cases, mimicking changes in renal hyperparathyroidism.
- Occurs due to nutritional deficiency (nutritional hyperparathyroidism, most commonly all meat boneless diets), impaired intestinal absorption, hypoparathyroidism or hereditary disorders (vitamin D receptor or metabolism defects).

Mucopolysaccharidosis
- Affected dogs may present with joint laxity, corneal opacity, and facial deformities
- A range of genetic mutations in glycosaminoglycan catabolism, resulting in very rare lysosomal storage diseases
- Diagnosis
  - A urine Berry MPS spot test can be used in some disorders
  - Inclusion bodies may be detected on blood smear evaluation
  - Genetic tests are available for a limited number of mucopolysaccharidosis disorders
- Radiological findings include bowing of long bones, soft tissue swelling of joints, angular limb deformities and reduced bone density

Renal hyperparathyroidism
- Animals may present with signs related the renal disease (inappetence, oral ulceration polyuria/polydipsia [PU/PD], weight loss, vomiting), or due to the bone disorder (pathological fractures, jaw swelling, tooth loss).
- Diagnosis is typically achieved with serum biochemistry (renal parameters), urinalysis, renal imaging and radiological findings. Parathyroid hormone (PTH) concentrations and calcidiol and calcitriol may be useful.
- Occurs in renal disease due to excessive phosphorus, FGF 23, and decreased calcium and calcitriol (1,25 hydroxy-vitamin D) levels with resultant increased parathyroid hormone.

- Radiological findings include diffuse decreased opacity of the skull with thinning of the cortices, resulting in opaque teeth surrounded by soft tissue opacity.
- Young dogs are more commonly affected. This is thought to be due to the increased sensitivity of their bones to the action of PTH; the condition also appears to preferentially affect the bones of skull and the jaw.

4.2.2B INCREASED BONE DENSITY

Increased bone density may be detected after taking radiographs to investigate lameness or bone pain, or as an incidental finding. It is a rare finding, and its significance will depend on the underlying aetiology.

CAUSES

Calvarial hyperostosis
- Bone density of the flat bones of the skull is increased, with irregular bony proliferation.
- Dogs typically present with head swelling, pain, lymphadenopathy, and sometimes lameness; pyrexia may be detected.
- Episodes end once skeletal maturity is reached. In some dogs permanent swelling may remain.
- First noted in male Bullmastiffs, now reported in other breeds and female dogs: American Staffordshire bull terrier, English Springer spaniel, Weimaraner.
- Supportive management is the treatment of choice, with acute flare-ups typically self-limiting.

Craniomandibular osteopathy, Figure 4.2.1
- An increased bone density of mandibles and tympanic bullae with symmetric periosteal and subperiosteal new bone formation.
- Dogs typically present with reluctance to eat, pain, and enlarged mandibles on palpation; pyrexia may be detected.
- Episodes end once skeletal maturity is reached but some dogs have a permanently reduced range of jaw motion.

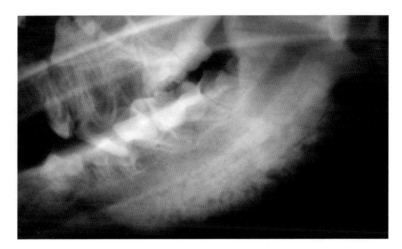

Figure 4.2.1 Craniomandibular osteopathy
Radiograph of the mandibular area of a WHWT with craniomandibular osteopathy, showing excessive new bone that could be mistaken for osteomyelitis or a bone tumour. (*Image courtesy of Frances Barr.*)

- Occurs most commonly in young Cairn terriers, Scottish terriers and WHWT.
- Supportive management is the treatment of choice, with acute flare-ups typically self-limiting.

Osteopetrosis
- A hereditary increased bone density, rarely reported in dogs
- Associated with inability to stand in puppies, shifting lameness, severe anaemia and neurological deficits (vestibular disease) in young dogs
- Occurs due to osteoclast impairment and deficient bone remodelling
- There is not an available specific treatment; in people the disorder results in progressive anaemia and ultimately premature death

Panosteitis
- Dogs typically present with lameness, which can be shifting, and pain on direct palpation of long bones; dogs may also have pyrexia and inappetance
- Most commonly affected are young (< 2 years) large-breed dogs; there appears to be predisposition for male dogs
- Radiological findings include radiopaque patchy sclerosis within the medullary canals but these findings may lag behind clinical signs (2–3 weeks later)

- Changes are thought to be due to a combination of genetic factors and diet, resulting in oedema with resultant compression of intra-osseous blood vessels and ischaemia

4.2.3 BONE LUCENCIES AND PROLIFERATIVE LESIONS

Focal areas of bone lucency or bone destruction may be detected during investigations of lameness or pain, screening for neoplasia, or incidentally. Lucencies and bone destruction may have distinct margins, or may have a lack of clear demarcation, and may be in combination with proliferative lesions, which are detected as periosteal reactions.

CAUSES

Avascular necrosis of the femoral head (Legg-Calve-Perthes-disease)
- Dogs typically present with insidious onset progressive pelvic limb pain with pain on hip extension.
- Occurs in young (3–13 months) toy- and small-breed dogs (e.g. Yorkshire terriers, West Highland white terriers, toy poodles and pugs) and is thought to be heritable.

- Radiological findings initially may be detected as focal or increased opacity in the lateral proximal femoral epiphysis. Later there may be collapse of the subchondral bone of the femoral head and secondary degenerative joint disease.
- Sensitivity of radiographs is limited and contrast-enhanced MRI may be required.

Bone cysts

- Bone cysts, unlike tumours, result radiologically in well-marginated lytic lesions with minimal periosteal reaction, unless there is a pathological fracture with healing
- Dogs may present with lameness, in particular if there is a pathological fracture, or the lesion may be detected as an incidental finding
- Primary bone cysts
  - Most common, with aneurysmal bone cysts less commonly detected
  - Typically occur in the diaphysis or metaphysis
  - Typically occur in young dogs, although may be asymptomatic and therefore detected at any age
- Rare aneurysmal bone cysts
  - Are located eccentrically within the metaphysis
  - May be detected at any age
  - May be a precursor for neoplastic transformation
- The diagnosis is typically tentative: CT and MRI may be beneficial, and surgical biopsies may be collected during curettage if the dog is displaying clinical signs

Bone tumours (primary or metastatic)

- Osteosarcoma, Figure 4.2.2a
  - Dogs typically present with progressive severe lameness; the distal radius and femur, and proximal humerus are the most common sites.
  - Most common bone tumour in dogs.
  - Most common in older, large-breed dogs: Rottweilers, Labradors, Bernese mountain dogs.
  - Radiologically, cortical lysis is a typical finding, and is often poorly marginated with associated periosteal new bone formation and palisading new bone

formation in the surrounding soft tissue. Pathological fractures may be detected, in particular where lysis is severe.
- Rarer bone tumours
  - Chondrosarcoma
  - Haemangiosarcoma
  - Lymphoma
  - Metastatic neoplasia
  - Plasma cell tumours (multiple myeloma)
- A tentative diagnosis is typically reached, unless fungal disease is a consideration, where biopsy for histopathology should be performed

Hypertrophic osteopathy (HO) (Figure 4.1.1c)

- A paraneoplastic syndrome (Marie's disease) most commonly associated with intrathoracic neoplasia, although it has been reported in non-intrathoracic neoplasia (e.g. bladder) and non-neoplastic disorders (e.g. bronchial foreign body, dirofilariasis, pneumonia)
- Dogs may present due to the primary disease (e.g. cough, lethargy, weight loss), or related to the HO (lameness, swollen feet with pain on palpation)
- Radiological findings are characterised by symmetrical periosteal new bone formation (palisading); this can affect any bone but particularly affects distal limbs including the metatarsal, metacarpal bones and phalanges
- Further investigations are focused on identifying the proposed trigger via imaging, etc.

Metaphyseal osteopathy

- Sometimes called hypertrophic osteodystrophy, but not to be confused with HO (Marie's disease).
- Affects young dogs (typically 3–4 months); Weimaraner.
- Dogs typically present with severe limb pain, pyrexia, lethargy, and may be non-ambulatory (sometimes misinterpreted as neurological disease); severely affected dogs may have concurrent systemic signs, i.e. GI, respiratory.
- Radiological findings are characteristically detected as a radiolucent line in the metaphysis proximal and parallel to a zone of increased radiodensity adjacent to the physis. The tibia, radius and ulna are most commonly affected and radiographic changes may lag 3–5 days behind clinical signs, Figure 4.2.2b.

IMAGING PATTERNS

(a)   (b)   (c)

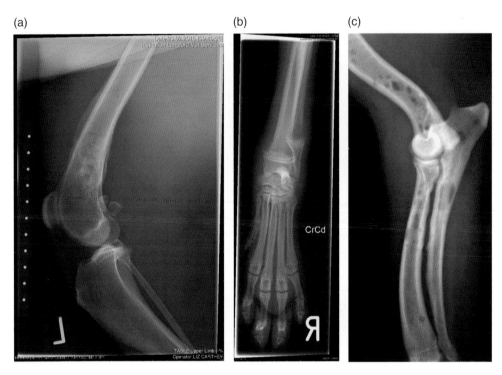

Figure 4.2.2 Lucencies and proliferative lesions
4.2.2a Osteosarcoma
Mottled lytic lesion in the distal femur, with reactive periosteal new bone. (*Image courtesy of Chris Warren-Smith, Langford Vets.*)
4.2.2b Metaphyseal osteopathy
Dorso-palmar radiograph of the right distal forelimb showing radiolucent line in the metaphysis proximal and parallel to a zone of increased radiodensity adjacent to the physis in the growth plate regions of the ulna and radius of a young dog. (*Image courtesy of Chris Warren-Smith, Langford Vets.*)
4.2.2c Multiple myeloma
Lateral radiograph of the forelimb showing multiple lytic lesions in all long bones, due to multiple myeloma. (*Image courtesy of Frances Barr.*)

- The diagnosis can only be confirmed by biopsy, although this is rarely performed as a presumptive diagnosis is based on signs and radiological changes.
- There may be a temporal association with vaccination; however, this could be due to the age of onset of signs.

Multiple myeloma
- Dogs present with signs related to hypercalcaemia (polyuria and polydipsia), hyperviscosity due to hyperglobulinaemia (polyuria, polydipsia, blindness, bleeding diathesis, seizures, and immunodeficiency) or bone pain and lameness

- Diagnosis is achieved with a combination of osteolytic bone lesions, serum protein electrophoresis, presence of Bence-Jones proteinuria, and demonstration of excessive plasma cells in the bone marrow
- Radiologically characterised by lytic bone lesions. These may be detected in the axial skeleton (vertebrae, ribs) or long bones, Figure 4.2.2c. There may also be diffuse osteopenia
- Radiographic changes are not always detected (~50% of cases)

Osteomyelitis
- Bacterial infection occurs secondary to:
  - Dental disease

- Haematogenous spread, e.g. metaphyseal osteomyelitis in Border collies with the congenital immunodeficiency, trapped neutrophil syndrome, *q.v.* section 5.7.1.2E
- Implant-related infections
- Open fractures
- Wounds, e.g. bites, foreign bodies
- Dogs typically present with lameness, pain, pyrexia and soft tissue swelling; draining tracts may be found
- Fungal and protozoal infection is less common
Aspergillosis in the spine has been reported in immunocompromised German shepherd dogs (GSDs)

- Radiological findings include periosteal new bone formation, medullary lysis and increased density, cortical thinning and resorption and presence of bone sequestra; findings may lag behind clinical signs
- The sensitivity of radiographs may be inadequate to detect lesions and a diagnosis may have to be made by
  - Culture and sensitivity
  - CT imaging
  - Nuclear scintigraphy
  - Serology when fungal or protozoal infection is suspected

4.3 THORAX

4.3.1 ALVEOLAR PATTERN

An alveolar pattern is characterised by soft tissue opacity within the lung fields due to presence of fluid (blood, oedema, pus) or cellular infiltrates. Pulmonary vasculature within the soft tissue density region is obscured; in contrast, bronchial structures may remain air-filled, resulting in air bronchograms. The margins of regions of alveolar lung patterns may be indistinct, or, if a single lung lobe is affected, there may be a sharp demarcation (lobar sign) (Figure 4.3.1).

Alveolar lung patterns may be detected in dogs with tachypnoea, dyspnoea, cough, or a combination of clinical signs, *q.v.* sections 1.13, 1.18. Clinical history and physical examination are vital in interpreting findings.

COMMON CAUSES

- Atelectasis: collapse of lung lobes due to a reduced volume, and resultant mediastinal shift
  - Artefact seen especially in anaesthetised dogs, in particular if time spent in lateral recumbency
  - Bronchial obstruction
  - External compression of lung, e.g. pneumothorax
- Aspiration pneumonia: typically right middle lung lobe, Figure 4.3.1a

- Bronchial foreign body: most often right caudal lung lobe
- Cardiogenic oedema: occurs in combination with pulmonary vasculature distension
- Lungworm (*Angiostrongylus vasorum*): typically patchy, peripheral distribution

UNCOMMON CAUSES

- Infectious bronchopneumonia: bacterial, viral
- Non-cardiogenic oedema: typically caudodorsal but can be more diffuse, no pulmonary vasculature change
- Pulmonary haemorrhage: typically diffuse, Figure 4.3.1b
- Lung lobe torsion: single lung lobe, often in the presence of pleural effusion
- Neoplasia: rarely, carcinoma and round cell infiltrate result in alveolar pattern

4.3.2 BRONCHIAL PATTERN

A bronchial pattern is characterised by an increased opacity surrounding the bronchial tree and occurs due to infiltration of the bronchi or peribronchial area with fluid, cellular infiltrates or hyperplasia, fibrosis, or smooth muscle hypertrophy. A bronchial pattern is detected as the presence of bronchi in the periphery of the lung, thickened end-on bronchi

(a)

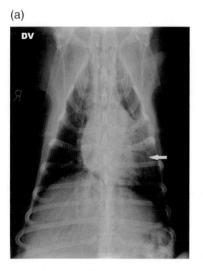

(b)

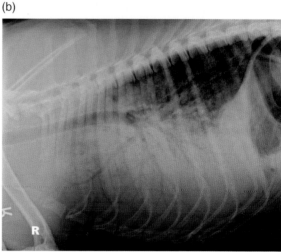

Figure 4.3.1 Alveolar pattern
4.3.1a Alveolar – aspiration pneumonia
Dorso-ventral thoracic radiograph showing consolidation of the left middle lung field with air bronchograms (arrow) consistent with aspiration pneumonia. (*Image courtesy of Chris Warren-Smith, Langford Vets.*)
4.3.1b Alveolar – haemorrhage
Right lateral thoracic radiograph showing consolidation of the ventral lung fields with multiple air bronchograms due to pulmonary haemorrhage. (*Image courtesy of Chris Warren-Smith, Langford Vets.*)

('doughnuts') and thickened longitudinal bronchi ('tramlines'), Figure 4.3.2.

Acute bronchial disease may not be apparent on radiographs which are poorly sensitive for bronchial disorders in dogs. Bronchial patterns are most commonly seen in dogs with a chronic cough.

Bronchiectasis is observed as abnormally dilated bronchi with loss of normal tapering as bronchi travel to the periphery of the lung. This reflects chronic bronchial disease (or, rarely, congenital) and is expected to be irreversible.

COMMON CAUSES

- Chronic bronchitis
- Chronic inflammation: most commonly causes a bronchointerstitial or alveolar lung pattern
  - Bronchopneumonia: bacterial, viral
  - Microaspiration, i.e. secondary to gastroesophageal reflux disease/aerodigestive syndrome
- Eosinophilic bronchopneumopathy: may also have pulmonary nodules and lymphadenopathy

UNCOMMON CAUSES

- Infiltrative neoplasia, e.g. lymphoma but more commonly causes alveolar or interstitial lung pattern
- Parasitic infection

4.3.3   CHANGES IN CARDIAC OUTLINE AND PULMONARY VASCULATURE

Changes in cardiac outline may be detected on radiography performed as part of investigation of cardiothoracic or systemic disease or, in some cases, can be observed as an incidental finding. Changes may reflect generalised cardiomegaly, specific chamber or vessel enlargement, or a small cardiac silhouette, *q.v.* section 5.2.

On the lateral projection the cardiac silhouette is divided into four chambers delineated horizontally by the widest point of the heart and vertically from apex to mid-base. Clockwise from 12 o'clock the chambers are the left atrium, left ventricle, right ventricle and right atrium, respectively, Figure 4.3.3.

(a)   (b)

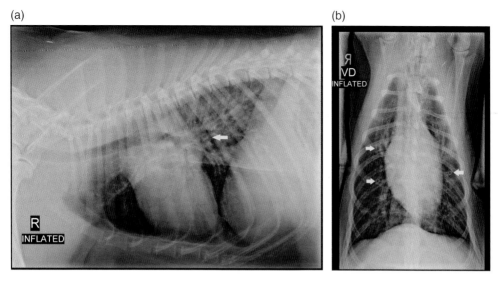

Figure 4.3.2 Bronchial pattern
Lateral (4.3.2a) and ventro-dorsal (4.3.2b) radiographs demonstrating a marked bronchial pattern in a dog with a chronic cough. Thickened bronchial walls in cross-section have the appearance of 'ring doughnuts' (arrows).

(a)   (b)

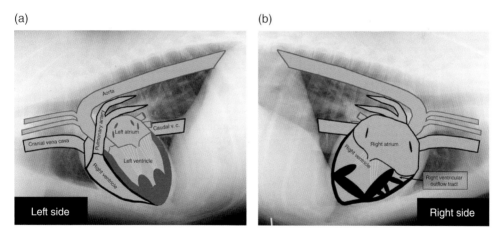

Figure 4.3.3 Cardiac outline
4.3.3a Left side
Outline of normal heart and major vessels superimposed on a lateral radiograph of the thorax.
4.3.3b Right side
Outline of normal heart and major vessels superimposed on a lateral radiograph of the thorax.

On the dorsoventral projection the heart structures can be divided similarly to a clock face:
- 12–1 o'clock: aorta
- 2 o'clock: pulmonary artery
- 2–3 o'clock: left auricular appendage
- 3–6 o'clock: left ventricle
- 6–9 o'clock: right ventricle
- 9–11 o'clock: right atrium

Potential changes in cardiac outline with left- and right-sided heart failure are shown in Figures 4.3.4. Pulmonary oedema in left-sided and congestive heart failure may obscure the cardiac outline, Figure 4.3.5.

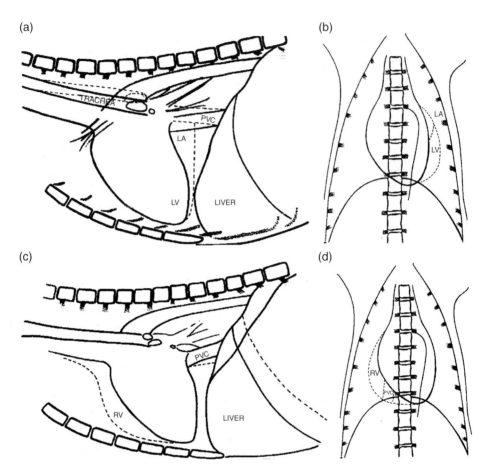

Figure 4.3.4 Changes in cardiac outline ------ indicates displacement of outline
LA, left atrial enlargement; LV, left ventricular enlargement; PVC, posterior (caudal) vena cava;
RV, right ventricular enlargement
4.3.4a Left-sided cardiac failure
Line diagram of a lateral thoracic view, showing changes found in left-sided cardiac failure.
4.3.4b Left-sided cardiac failure
Line diagram of a dorso-ventral thoracic view, showing changes found in left-sided cardiac failure.
4.3.4c Right-sided cardiac failure
Line diagram of a lateral thoracic view, showing changes found in right-sided cardiac failure, with
an enlarged posterior (caudal) vena cava.
4.3.4d Right-sided cardiac failure
Line diagram of a dorso-ventral thoracic view, showing changes found in right-sided cardiac failure, with an enlarged posterior (caudal) vena cava.

Cardiomegaly is suspected when the heart is wider than 60% of the width of the thorax at the maximal location on the dorsoventral projection and spanning more than three rib spaces on the lateral projection. A vertebral heart score (VHS) can be calculated from a right lateral projection; this is calculated as the length of the heart (carina to apex) plus the width of the heart (perpendicular to the widest point) and measured as the number of vertebrae starting from thoracic vertebrae 4. A normal dog VHS is 9.7 ± 0.5, although breed variations are noted.

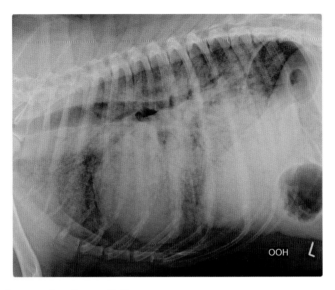

Figure 4.3.5 Congestive heart failure
Left lateral thoracic radiograph of a dog in congestive heart failure. A marked interstitial-alveolar pattern with prominent air bronchograms is consistent with severe pulmonary oedema, with an air-filled stomach suggestive of dyspnoea. The pulmonary changes mask many of the changes in the cardiac silhouette including likely right heart enlargement and the splitting of the caudal main-stem bronchi suggestive of left atrial enlargement.

Pulmonary vasculature assessment is critical, in particular when considering suspicion of congestive heart failure, and can be assessed on dorsoventral and lateral radiographic projections. Pulmonary veins on these views are, respectively, medial and ventral to the pulmonary artery, both of which run parallel to the bronchus. The vein and artery are of roughly equal size; on the lateral projection the vessels should be no greater in diameter than the proximal third of the third rib. On the dorsoventral view the caudal pulmonary vessel should be no greater in width than the width of the ninth rib where they intersect.

COMMON CAUSES

Cardiomegaly
- Generalised
  - Dilated cardiomyopathy (DCM)
  - Pericardial effusion: a crisp outline of the heart may be visible due to lack of movement blur
- Left-sided
  - Degenerative mitral valve disease
  - Subaortic stenosis

- Right-sided
  - Degenerative valve disease
  - Pulmonic stenosis

Microcardia
- Distributive shock
- Hypovolaemic shock

Pulmonary venous enlargement
- Left-sided congestive heart failure

UNCOMMON CAUSES

Aortic enlargement
- Systemic hypertension
- Dilation of aortic arch with subaortic stenosis
- Proximal descending aorta enlargement with patent ductus arteriosus

Cardiomegaly
- Generalised
  - Peritoneal-pericardial diaphragmatic hernia
- Left-sided
  - Patent ductus arteriosus causing left-to-right shunt

- Mitral valve dysplasia
- Endocarditis
- Right-sided
- Pulmonary hypertension
- Tricuspid valve dysplasia

Microcardia

- Hypoadrenocorticism
- Obstructive shock: lack of venous return due compression of the caudal vena cava, e.g. GDV

Pulmonary vessels

- Pulmonary artery enlargement
  - *Dirofilaria* infection: peripheral 'pruning' of the arteries may also be seen
  - Pulmonary thromboembolism
  - Pulmonary hypertension
- Pulmonary trunk enlargement
  - Pulmonary hypertension
  - Pulmonic stenosis
- Pulmonary venous enlargement
  - Left atrial obstruction (e.g. thrombus, neoplasia)

- Pulmonary vessel size
  - Increased
    - Hypervolaemia (fluid overload)
    - Left-to-right shunt
  - Decreased
    - Hypovolaemia
    - Right-to-left shunt

4.3.4 INTERSTITIAL PATTERN

An interstitial pattern is characterised by a hazy increase in lung opacity and occurs due to the increased presence of fluid or cellular infiltrate within the interstitial tissue, Figure 4.3.6a.

An interstitial lung pattern can be

- Structured (also called nodular), representing an aggregation of cells within the supporting interstitium, ranging from many micronodular lesions as in a miliary lung pattern, Figure 4.3.6b, to large solitary lesions

or

(a)

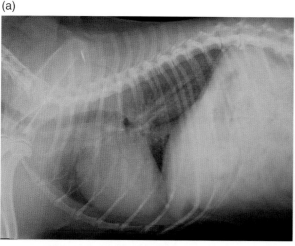

(b)

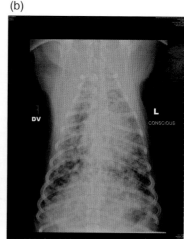

Figure 4.3.6 Interstitial pattern
4.3.6a Diffuse

Lateral thoracic radiograph showing increased lung density that follows the pattern of the pulmonary vasculature in a dog with idiopathic pulmonary fibrosis. (Image courtesy of Chris Warren-Smith, Langford Vets.)

4.3.6b Miliary

Dorso-ventral thoracic radiograph showing a miliary interstitial pattern due to multiple metastases. (Image courtesy of Chris Warren-Smith, Langford Vets.)

IMAGING PATTERNS

- Unstructured which appears as reduced definition of the normal pulmonary anatomy, Figure 4.3.6a

Interstitial lung patterns may be detected in dogs with dyspnoea/tachypnoea, exercise intolerance, cyanosis (*q.v.* sections 1.18, 1.22, 2.6), or a combination of clinical signs, or as part of staging when neoplastic disease is detected remote from the lungs. Pulmonary hypertension should be a consideration in cases with significant interstitial lung disease.

COMMON CAUSES

- Artefact due to hypoinflation of lung
- Early cardiogenic or non-cardiogenic pulmonary oedema
- Lungworm (*Angiostrongylus*): typically patchy peripheral
- Pulmonary osteomata: benign interstitial mineralisations around 1–2 mm in size
- Pulmonary neoplasia, Figure 4.3.6b
  - Metastatic, e.g. carcinoma, round-cell neoplasia, sarcoma
  - Primary, e.g. bronchoalveolar carcinoma, bronchogenic carcinoma, histiocytic sarcoma

UNCOMMON CAUSES

- Pulmonary fibrosis
- Infectious disease
  - Bacterial pneumonia, e.g. *Mycobacterium*
  - Fungal pneumonia, e.g. *Cryptococcus, Blastomycosis*
  - Parasitic pneumonia, e.g. *Pneumocytsis*
  - Viral pneumonia, e.g. Herpes virus
- Pulmonary granulomas
  - Eosinophilic granulomas
  - FB reaction
  - Lymphomatoid granulomatosis
  - *Mycobacterium*
- Pulmonary haemorrhage
- Pulmonary hypertension
- Uraemic pneumonitis

4.3.5 LOSS OF DETAIL

Loss of detail within the thoracic cavity is characterised by a lack of the usual pulmonary lung pattern (with visible vasculature and bronchi) and should be discriminated from atelectasis or consolidation (*q.v.* section 4.3.1). Large pulmonary and mediastinal masses may also result in loss of normal pulmonary architecture on thoracic radiography.

Pleural space disease (pleural effusion, pneumothorax) should be diagnostically and therapeutically sampled in order to aid investigations (*q.v.* sections 2.21, 2.22). Mediastinal masses may be very large and can obscure normal lung; sampling via fine needle aspiration and/or Tru-cut biopsy under ultrasound guidance may be considered where safe to do so.

COMMON CAUSES

- Excessive body condition (excessive intrathoracic fat may cause a fat opacity change within the thoracic cavity and must be discriminated from pleural effusion which is soft tissue opacity)
- Mediastinal mass
  - Lymphoma
  - Thymoma
- Pleural effusion, *q.v.* section 2.21
  - Modified transudate (right-sided congestive heart failure)
  - Pyothorax
  - Transudate; hypoalbuminaemia, *q.v.* section 3.27.2B
- Pneumothorax, *q.v.* section 2.22
  - Spontaneous
  - Traumatic
- Pulmonary neoplasia

UNCOMMON CAUSES

- Mediastinal mass
  - Lymphadenomegaly (e.g. due to infectious disease such as *Mycobacterium spp.*)

- Pleural effusion, *q.v.* section 2.21
  - Chylothorax, e.g. idiopathic, neoplastic
  - Haemorrhage, e.g. anticoagulant rodenticide toxicity, neoplasia
  - Modified transudate (vasculitis)
- Transudate (low oncotic pressure; protein-losing enteropathy or nephropathy)
- Pulmonary mass
  - Granuloma (foreign body reaction)

SECTION 5

ORGAN SYSTEMS

The relevant clinical presentations and physical, laboratory and imaging abnormalities (identified in sections 1–4, respectively) are given for each major internal organ system. Then the diagnostic approach and the methods of investigation of each organ system are briefly explained. Finally, the more common diseases of each system are covered alphabetically. For each, its aetiology, predisposition, historical clues, clinical signs, laboratory test results, treatment and monitoring, sequelae and prognosis are given in note form.

ORGAN SYSTEMS

5.1 ALIMENTARY SYSTEM

Problems

Presenting complaints
q.v. section 1
1.5 Anorexia/hyporexia/inappetence
1.11 Constipation
1.15 Diarrhoea
1.16 Drooling
1.17 Dysphagia
1.18 Dyspnoea
1.23 Faecal incontinence
1.24 Flatulence/borborygmi
1.25 Haematemesis
1.26 Haematochezia
1.29 Halitosis
1.31 Melaena
1.36 Polyphagia
1.41 Regurgitation
1.45 Stunting/failure to grow
1.46 Tenesmus and dyschezia
1.49 Vomiting
1.53 Weight loss

Physical abnormalities
q.v. section 2
2.1 Abdominal enlargement
2.2 Abdominal masses
2.17.1 Abdominal pain
2.5 Ascites
2.16 Oral masses
2.29 Stomatitis

Laboratory abnormalities
q.v. section 3
3.3 Amylase and lipase
3.10 Cobalamin
3.15 Folate
3.18 Iron status
3.21 Pancreatic lipase
3.23 Potassium
3.24 Sodium
3.27 Total protein/albumin
3.28 Trypsin-like immunoreactivity (TLI)

Diagnostic Approach

In general, signs of gastrointestinal (GI) disease reflect the anatomical region affected:

• Constipation	= Large intestine (LI)
• Diarrhoea	= Small intestine (SI) or large intestine or both Pancreas
• Haematochezia	= LI
• Malabsorption	= SI
• Melaena	= Stomach and/or SI
• PLE	= SI ± stomach and/or colon
• Regurgitation	= Oesophagus
• Vomiting ± haematemesis	= Stomach SI

- GI diseases can affect more than one part of the GI tract simultaneously
- Diarrhoea can usually be localised to the SI or LI by the nature of diarrhoea and defecation but can also be due to concurrent SI and LI disease ('mixed pattern diarrhoea')
- Non-GI diseases can cause typical GI signs
- The overall diagnostic approach is to rule out non-GI causes of GI signs first, before specific investigations

Malabsorption
- Failure of digestion and assimilation of one or more nutrients
- Clinical signs
  - Diarrhoea
  - Polyphagia
  - Weight loss

Protein-losing enteropathy (PLE)
- Severe, diffuse intestinal diseases causing hypoalbuminaemia and often, but not invariably, hypoglobulinaemia; ascites can develop when serum albumin < 15 g/l

ORGAN SYSTEMS

Notes on Canine Internal Medicine, Fourth Edition. Victoria L. Black, Kathryn F. Murphy, Jessie Rose Payne, and Edward J. Hall.

- Alimentary lymphoma (AL)
- Chronic inflammatory enteropathy (CIE)/ inflammatory bowel disease (IBD)
- Fungal enteritis (pythiosis) (not in UK)
- Lymphangiectasia
- Poor prognosis: ~50% dead within 6 months of diagnosis
  - Failure to respond to treatment
  - Thromboembolism

Diagnostic Methods
History
Presenting signs reflect somewhat the anatomical region affected listed in the table above

Clinical examination
- Dehydration in acute disease
- Weight loss in chronic disease
- Specific signs for individual diseases listed below

Laboratory findings
- No pathognomonic haematological or biochemical changes in GI disease
- Identification of dehydration
- Identification of GI bleeding
- Identification of PLE
- Normal results help rule out non-GI causes of GI signs
- Faecal examination
  - Parasitological examination may give specific diagnosis
  - Stool culture unhelpful as potential pathogens also isolated from clinically healthy dogs
- PLE
  - Hypoalbuminaemia
  - Hypocalcaemia
  - Hypoglobulinaemia typical but not invariably present

Imaging
q.v section 4.1

Plain radiographs
- Abnormal distension of GI organs
- Abdominal masses
- Foreign bodies
- Gas patterns
  - Free peritoneal gas
  - Intestinal gas pattern

- Loss of intra-peritoneal detail
- Mineralisation
- Organ displacement

Contrast radiographs
- Highlight structural abnormalities
- Investigate GI motility

Ultrasound examination
- Investigate organ structure
  - Position and size
  - GI wall thickness
    - Thickening in some cases of CIE/IBD and AL, Figure 5.1.1a
  - Wall layering, Figure 5.1.1b
    - Loss of layers suggestive of neoplasia, Figure 5.1.1a
    - Normal: lumen-mucosa-submucosa-muscularis-serosa
    - More than the normal five layers: intussusception, Figure 5.1.1c
    - Mucosal speckling or striations consistent with inflammation or lymphangiectasia, Figure 5.1.1d

Empirical treatment
- Scientifically unsatisfactory method of diagnosis but CIEs can be characterised on response to antibacterials, diet and immunosuppressants
  - Antibiotic responsive diarrhoea (ARD)
  - Food-responsive enteropathy (FRE)
  - Non-responsive enteropathy (NRE)
  - Steroid-responsive enteropathy (SRE) or immunosuppressant-responsive enteropathy (IRE)

Special investigative techniques
- Cobalamin and folate, *q.v.* sections 3.15, 3.10 respectively
- C-reactive protein, *q.v.* section 3.14
- Faecal markers
  - Alpha$_1$-protease inhibitor as a marker for a PLE (not available outside North America)
  - Calprotectin as a marker of inflammation
- Intestinal inspection and biopsy
  - Endoscopy
    - Anaesthetic risk
    - Ileum difficult to access via colonoscopy
    - Jejunum largely inaccessible

ORGAN SYSTEMS

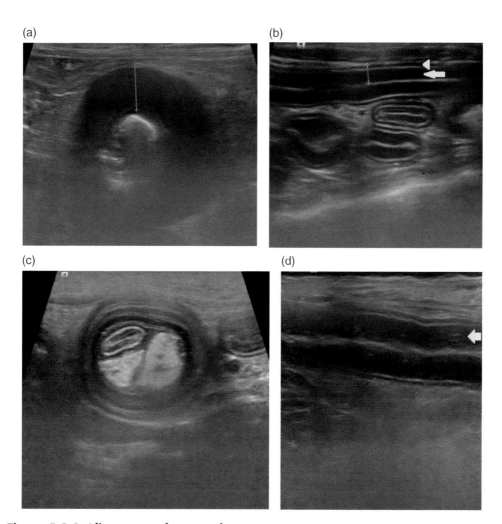

(a)

(b)

(c)

(d)

Figure 5.1.1 Alimentary ultrasound

5.1.1a Alimentary lymphoma

Transverse image of a very thickened small bowel loop (1.2 cm) with complete loss of layering consistent with alimentary lymphoma.

5.1.1b Normal intestinal layers

Longitudinal section of small bowel showing normal layering: the hyperechoic layers of serosa, submucosa and lumen are separated by the hypoechoic layers of the muscularis (arrow head) and thicker mucosa (arrow).

5.1.1c Ultrasound: intussusception

Cross-sectional image of an intussusception showing more than the normal five ultrasonographic layers.

5.1.1d Ultrasound: mucosal speckling

Longitudinal section of small bowel with the normal five ultrasonographic layers, but with diffuse speckling in the normally hypoechoic mucosal layer consistent with a chronic enteropathy. (*All images courtesy of Chris Warren-Smith, Langford Vets.*)

- Minimally invasive
- No wound healing or convalescence
- Small biopsies

NB: Endoscopic biopsies should always be taken, even if GI tract looks grossly normal.

- Exploratory laparotomy
  - Anaesthetic risk
  - Can biopsy all levels of SI
  - Can inspect/biopsy extra-intestinal organs
  - Full-thickness biopsies
  - Surgical risk
  - Wound healing and convalescence
- Pancreas-specific enzymes, *q.v.* sections 3.3, 3.21, 3.28, 5.1.7

5.1.1   OROPHARYNX

The mouth and its associated structures are responsible for prehending, chewing and swallowing food.

Presenting complaints
q.v. section 1
- Anorexia/hyporexia/inappetence
- Bleeding
- Drooling
- Dysphagia
- Halitosis
- Nasal discharge
- Regurgitation

Physical abnormalities
q.v. section 2
- Mandibular lymphadenopathy
- Oral mass
- Pain
- Stomatitis

Laboratory abnormalities
q.v. section 3
- Azotaemia in uraemia
- Otherwise generally unremarkable

Diagnostic Approach
- Complete oral examination; may require sedation or GA
- Cranial nerve examination before sedation for neuromuscular causes of dysphagia

- Laboratory testing for underlying systemic disease; crucial if uraemia is suspected
- Remove any obvious cause, e.g. foreign body
- Radiograph teeth and tooth roots to diagnose dental disease
- Radiograph skull if suspected bone involvement
- Take fine needle aspirates (FNAs) or incisional or excisional biopsies of any suspect lesions
- Treat dental disease if no other cause detected

Diagnostic Methods
History
- See presenting complaints above
- Nasal discharge if oro-nasal fistula

Clinical examination
- Observe eating and drinking if dysphagia reported
- See physical abnormalities above

Laboratory findings
- Azotaemia in uraemia
- Usually no directly significant abnormalities

Imaging
Plain radiographs
- Look for dental disease
- Look for bone involvement: abscess/osteomyelitis, tumour

Special investigative techniques
- Neurological examination
- Electromyogram (EMG) of temporal muscles
- Fluoroscopic assessment of swallowing motion
- 2M antibody for temporal myositis

5.1.1A   CRANIOMANDIBULAR OSTEOPATHY

Aetiology
- Rare inherited condition; mutation of SLC37A2 gene

Major signs
- Dysphagia

ORGAN SYSTEMS

Minor signs
- Cycles of pain, hyporexia and pyrexia

Potential sequelae
- Inability to open jaw

Predisposition, Historical clues
- Affects young, growing West Highland White terriers (WHWTs) and other small terrier breeds

Clinical examination, Laboratory findings
  q.v. section 1.17

Imaging
- Excessive growth of jaw bones, almost resembling neoplasia, *q.v.* Figure 4.2.1

Special investigations
- DNA test

Treatment
- Analgesia
- No specific treatment but signs may ameliorate when growth finishes unless the jaw is permanently locked

Prognosis
- Guarded: cycles of pain are a welfare issue and complete locking of the jaw may require euthanasia

5.1.1B CRICOPHARYNEAL ACHALASIA

Aetiology
- Rare disease caused by either increased tone in cricopharyngeus muscle or asynchrony between pharyngeal contraction delivering a bolus and relaxation of the cricopharyngeus

Major signs
- Dysphagia

Minor signs
- Coughing
- Reflux rhinitis
- Weight loss

Potential sequelae
- Inhalation pneumonia
- Euthanasia

Predisposition and historical clues
- Cocker spaniels in UK are predisposed
- Dachshunds are predisposed in North America

Clinical examination/laboratory findings
  q.v. section 1.17

Imaging
- Fluoroscopy required to make a diagnosis

Special investigations
- EMG

Treatment
- Botox injections into cricopharyngeus may provide temporary relief
- Cricopharyngeal myotomy may be curative if muscle tone is increased but may worsen signs if there is asynchrony

Prognosis
- Guarded

5.1.1C MASTICATORY MYOSITIS

Aetiology
- Immune-mediated
- Eosinophilic infiltrate, followed by muscle atrophy and fibrous tissue formation

Major signs
- Dysphagia
- Initially, painful, swollen temporal muscles
- Temporal muscle atrophy and inability to open mouth later

Minor signs
- Drooling
- Weight loss through inability to eat

Potential sequelae
- Permanent closure of jaw

Predisposition, Historical clues
- No known predispositions
- Gradual onset of signs
- Dog drops food during prehension

Clinical examination
- Temporal muscle swelling initially, which may be painful
- Ultimately atrophy and fibrosis, so it is physically impossible to open the mouth

Laboratory findings
Haematology
Eosinophilia in some but not all cases

Serum biochemistry
Usually unremarkable except increased creatine kinase

Imaging
Skull radiographs
- Unremarkable
- Rule out temporomandibular joint disease

Special investigations
- EMG
- Temporal muscle biopsy: do not biopsy the frontalis muscle as not affected
- 2M antibody

Treatment
- Prednisolone at up to 2 mg/kg/day, then weaning whilst monitoring jaw opening
- Breaking down of fibrous tissue under general anaesthesia (GA) in severe cases but risk of jaw fracture
- Tube feeding if dog can't eat

Monitoring
- Measure size of oral bite

Prognosis
- Guarded
- Some cases need prolonged steroid therapy

5.1.1D   ORAL NEOPLASIA

q.v. section 2.16

Aetiology
- Spontaneous tumour: benign/malignant, odontogenic/non-odontogenic

Major signs
- Drooling, *q.v.* section 1.16
- Dysphagia, *q.v.* section 1.17

Minor signs
- Bleeding
- Halitosis
- Pain

Potential sequelae
- Metastatic spread
- Recurrence after surgical excision
- Uncontrollable haemorrhage

Predisposition, Historical clues, Clinical examination
q.v. section 2.16

Laboratory findings
- Anaemia if profuse, prolonged haemorrhage
- Usually unremarkable

Imaging, Special investigations
q.v. sections 2.16, 4.2

Treatment
- Radical excision for rostral tumours
- Surgery plus chemotherapy for malignant melanoma
- Surgery plus radiotherapy for squamous cell carcinoma

Monitoring
- Visual inspection
- FNA of mandibular lymph nodes
- Chest radiographs or CT

Prognosis
- Good for benign lesions
- Guarded for malignant lesions

Odontogenic fibroma (epulides)
Good following excision, but recurrence likely

Papilloma

- Spontaneous resolution in most cases
- Azithromycin reported to speed up resolution

Fibrosarcoma

- Depends on whether radical excision can achieve wide margins

Squamous cell carcinoma

- May respond to radiation therapy
- Potentially curable if wide margin of excision

Osteosarcoma, malignant melanoma

- Guarded to grave due to high metastatic potential

5.1.1E STOMATITIS

Aetiology

q.v. section 2.29

- Inflammation of the oral mucosa most commonly caused by bacteria, and usually associated with dental and periodontal disease

Major signs

- Drooling
- Halitosis

Minor signs

- Blood-stained saliva
- Dysphagia with pain on attempting to eat

Potential sequelae

- Gingival recession
- Loss of teeth

Predisposition, Historical clues, Clinical examination, Laboratory findings

q.v. section 2.29

Imaging

- Usually unremarkable unless significant dental disease

Special investigations

q.v. section 2.29

Treatment

- Remove inciting cause, e.g. foreign body
- Remove diseased teeth
- Scaling and polishing teeth
- Antibacterials
  - Chlorhexidine mouth wash
  - Metronidazole and spiramycin for anaerobes

Monitoring

- Visual inspection

Prognosis

- Good, but preventative measures must be taken to prevent recurrence of dental disease

5.1.2 SALIVARY GLANDS

- The salivary glands [mandibular, orbital (zygomatic), parotid and sublingual] produce saliva
- A sialocoele is a ruptured salivary duct and is treated surgically
  - A ranula is a sialocoele that occurs on the base of the mouth under the tongue
- Medical conditions of the salivary gland are rare
  - Adenocarcinoma
  - Hypersialosis
  - Salivary gland infarction
  - Sialoadenitis

Presenting complaints

q.v. section 1

- Anorexia/hyporexia/inappetence
- Drooling
- Dysphagia
- Vomiting

Physical abnormalities

q.v. section 2

- Lymphadenopathy (mandibular)
- Pain
- Pyrexia
- Stridor
- Swollen salivary gland

Laboratory abnormalities

q.v. section 3

- Azotaemia (pre-renal)
- Leukocytosis

Diagnostic approach
- Examine salivary glands by palpation
- FNA or biopsy
- Imaging is generally unrewarding; sialography is technically difficult

History, Clinical examination, Laboratory findings, Imaging
- See specific diseases below

Special investigative techniques
- FNA
- Biopsy

5.1.2A HYPERSIALOSIS/ SALIVARY GLAND INFARCTION/ SIALOADENITIS

Aetiology
Idiopathic but may be a spectrum of the same condition, as all have been reported to improve with phenobarbitone.

Hypersialosis
- Hypertrophy and increased saliva production possibly due to overstimulation by CNS

Salivary gland infarction
- Spontaneous infarction of gland

Sialoadenitis
- Inflammation of the salivary gland
  - Commonly spontaneous, possibly immune-mediated
  - Occasionally caused by paramyxovirus (mumps)

Major signs
- Dysphagia
- Drooling
- Pain on palpation
- Vomiting: may be persistent and relatively resistant to anti-emetics

Minor signs
- Halitosis

Potential sequelae
- Death in severe cases
  - Euthanasia may be necessary if pain cannot be controlled

Predisposition
- Salivary gland infarction reported in Jack Russell terrier
- Historical clues
- Sudden onset of clinical signs

Clinical examination
- Drooling saliva
- Dull and depressed
- Swollen painful salivary glands
- Pyrexia

Laboratory findings
- Leukocytosis not invariably present, especially with sialoadenosis

Imaging
- Generally unhelpful

Special investigations
- FNA and/or biopsy

Treatment
- Antibiotics in case of infection probably not needed
- Immunosuppression with prednisolone
- Phenobarbitone at anti-epileptic doses

Monitoring
- Clinical response
- Salivary gland size

Prognosis
- Guarded

5.1.3 OESOPHAGUS

Presenting complaints
q.v. section 1
- Cardinal sign is regurgitation
- Minor signs
  - Anorexia/hyporexia/inappetence
  - Drooling

- Dysphagia
- Polyphagia (re-eats regurgitated food)
- Secondary respiratory signs may develop from inhalation of inadequately swallowed food
  - Cough
  - Dyspnoea
  - Halitosis
  - Nasal discharge
- Weight loss

Physical abnormalities
q.v. section 2
- Dilated cervical oesophagus sometimes present in megaoesophagus
- Palpable foreign body (FB) only if in cervical oesophagus
- Pyrexia secondary to inhalation pneumonia

Laboratory abnormalities
q.v. section 3
- Leukocytosis if inhalation pneumonia
- Pre renal azotaemia if unable to swallow water
- Otherwise generally unremarkable

Diagnostic approach
- Distinguish regurgitation from vomiting
- Investigate first by:
  - plain radiographs and/or
  - endoscopy
- Barium swallow
  - Plain film after barium mixed with food to detect stricture or vascular ring anomaly
  - Fluoroscopic assessment of swallowing

Diagnostic methods
History
- *q.v.* Presenting complaints listed above

Clinical examination
- *q.v.* Physical abnormalities listed above
- Auscultate thorax
- Palpate cervical oesophagus

Laboratory findings
- Usually no significant abnormalities

Imaging
Plain radiographs
- Oesophagus normally not visible
- Some air in the oesophagus may be seen with sedation or GA, especially if difficulty during intubation
- Air-filled oesophagus in megaoesophagus, *q.v.* Figure 5.1.2
  - Tracheal stripe
  - Visible dorsal and ventral borders on lateral view
- Gravel sign sometimes present with obstruction
- Radiodense foreign bodies

Contrast radiographs
- Fluoroscopic assessment of swallowing motion
- Radiolucent foreign bodies
- Partial obstructions: strictures and vascular ring anomalies

Special investigative techniques
- Endoscopy
- Manometry (not available in practice)
- Megaoesophagus causes
  - ACTH stimulation tests
  - Serum acetylcholine receptor antibody
  - Thyroid status

5.1.3A FOREIGN BODY

Aetiology
Accidental ingestion
- Stick injury

Deliberate ingestion
- Bones and chews
- Fish hooks
- Others

Major signs
- Regurgitation
  - May still be able to swallow liquids if irregular FB
  - Solids regurgitated immediately

Minor signs
- Agitation if FB causes discomfort
  - Odynophagia (pain on swallowing)

ORGAN SYSTEMS

- Retching/gulping
- Depression from dehydration, perforation
- Drooling saliva

Potential sequelae
- Oesophagitis
- Oesophageal stricture
- Perforation of oesophageal wall
  - Broncho-oesophageal fistula (rare)
    - Chronic cough
  - Mediastinitis
  - Pleural effusion

Predisposition
- More common in young and greedy dogs
- WHWTs are vastly over-represented

Historical clues
- Acute onset in previously healthy animal
- Ingestion may have been observed

Clinical examination
- Outwardly unremarkable in most cases
- Occasionally FB will be palpable in pharynx or cervical oesophagus

Laboratory findings
- No significant changes
- Leukocytosis if perforation and subsequent mediastinitis
- Pre-renal azotaemia if ingestion of fluids impaired

Imaging
Radiographs
Plain
- Radiodense FB
- If perforated
  - Mediastinitis
  - Pneumothorax or pleural effusion
  - Subcutaneous emphysema

Contrast
- Should *not* be given *before* plain radiographs, as radiodense FB will be obscured
- Use iodinated contrast if perforation is suspected
  - Identify radiolucent FB
- Rule out other differential diagnoses

Special investigations
- Oesophagoscopy
  - Identification of FB
  - Possible removal of FB
  - Evaluation of post-traumatic oesophagitis, perforation

Treatment
Removal of FB
- Endoscopically
- Rigid forceps under fluoroscopic guidance
- Surgical removal if:
  - Significant perforation
  - Stick injury requiring exploration of soft tissues
  - Other removal methods unsuccessful
- Treat oesophagitis, *q.v.* section 5.1.3C

Monitoring
- Check for clinical signs of persistent oesophagitis or stricture formation
- Repeat endoscopy if signs persist

Prognosis
- Excellent if FB removed quickly with no perforation
- Guarded if severe circumferential oesophageal ulceration as stricture may occur
- Guarded if surgical removal is required
- Poor if perforation and mediastinitis and pyothorax develop

5.1.3B MEGAOESOPHAGUS (MO)

Aetiology
Primary
- Acquired-idiopathic MO
- Congenital-idiopathic MO
- Myasthenia gravis (MG), *q.v.* section 5.8.10
  - Congenital MG
  - Focal MG, affecting just oesophagus ± pharynx
  - Generalised MG with concurrent skeletal muscle weakness

Secondary
NB: Signs of underlying disease are usually as important as regurgitation.

ORGAN SYSTEMS

Achalasia
- Increased tone of lower oesophageal sphincter

Myopathies
- Dermatomyositis
- Dystrophin deficiency
- Polymyositis
- Systemic lupus erythematosus (SLE)
- Toxoplasmosis

Neuropathies/junctionopathies
- Bilateral vagal damage
- Botulism
- Brain stem disease
  - Hydrocephalus
  - Meningoencephalitis
- Giant axonal neuropathy
- Polyradiculoneuritis
- Tick paralysis

Toxins
- Anticholinesterase
- Acrylamide
- Food-related peripheral neuropathy
- Lead
- Thallium

Miscellaneous
- Distemper
- Glycogen storage disease Type II
- Hypoadrenocorticism
- Hypothyroidism (association but no proof of causation)
- Thymoma

Localised
A dilated, dysfunctional segment oesophagus
   NB: Not true megaoesophagus as distal oesophagus is normal.
- Diverticulum
- Persistent right aortic arch or other congenital vascular anomalies
- Stricture
- Tumour

Major signs
- Regurgitation
- Inhalation pneumonia
  - Coughing
  - Dyspnoea/tachypnoea
  - Pyrexia

Minor signs
- Appetite
  - Initially increased; may re-eat regurgitated food
  - Later, decreased if pneumonia develops
- Ballooning of cervical oesophagus
- Halitosis
- Lethargy
- Nasal discharge
- Weight loss

Potential sequelae
- Cachexia
- Severe inhalation pneumonia leading to death

Predisposition
- Idiopathic megaoesophagus
  - Congenital and acquired MO are most common in large- and giant-breed dogs, especially German shepherd dog (GSD), Great Dane, Irish setter, Irish Wolfhound
  NB: Persistent right aortic arch (PRAA) also seen in GSD and Irish setter

Historical clues
- Regurgitation is the major sign, but is sometimes mistaken for vomiting
- Acquired MO most common 5–7 years
- Congenital MO causes signs at weaning (as does PRAA)
- Coughing is a common sign
- Epidemics caused by food-related peripheral neuropathy
- Lethargy/weakness if generalised MG

Clinical examination
Visual inspection
- Ballooning of cervical oesophagus (rare)
- Depressed and dyspnoeic
- Halitosis
- Nasal discharge and coughing
- Weight loss

Auscultation
- Moist lung sounds if inhalation pneumonia
- 'Slopping' sounds from fluid in oesophagus

Palpation
Gag reflex may be absent if pharynx is also affected

ORGAN SYSTEMS

Laboratory findings

Haematology

Low-grade inflammatory leukogram if inhalation pneumonia

Serum biochemistry
- Usually unremarkable
- Pre-renal azotaemia if ingestion of fluids impaired

Imaging

Plain radiographs
- Entire oesophagus dilated and gas-filled from neck extending to diaphragm, Figure 5.1.2
  NB: Beware of over-interpretation of passive dilatation under GA.

Barium swallow
- Usually not required for diagnosis
- Assess oesophageal dysmotilty – dilated, hypomotile
- Danger of inhalation

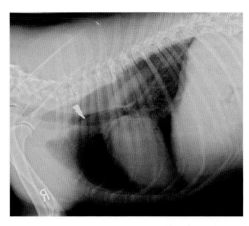

Figure 5.1.2 Megaoesophagus. Right lateral thoracic radiograph of a dog with idiopathic megaoesophagus. An air-filled oesophagus lies dorsal to the heart and its ventral border can be seen crossing the trachea (the so-called tracheal stripe, yellow marker) at the level of the second to fourth rib. Inhalation pneumonia in the ventral middle lung fields is not easy to visualise as it overlies the cardiac silhouette. (*Image courtesy of Chris Warren-Smith, Langford Vets.*)

Special investigations

Manometry

Not available in practice

Oesophagoscopy
- Dilated oesophagus often difficult to assess endoscopically
- Pooling of swallowed and refluxed material
- Danger of aspiration on induction of and recovery from GA

Focal myasthenia gravis (MG)
- Acetylcholine receptor antibody titre
- Edrophonium ('Tensilon') response test ineffective as any response is too weak/transient to detect

Generalised MG
- Acetylcholine receptor antibody titre, but negative in congenital MG
- Edrophonium response test

Hypothyroidism

Thyroid function tests

Polymyositis and polyneuropathy
- Creatine kinase
- EMG

Systemic lupus erythematosus
- Anti-nuclear antibody
- Evidence of multi-organ disease

Treatment

Idiopathic megaoesophagus

No specific therapy
- Postural feeding with head elevated above stomach using gravity to deliver food to stomach
  - Bailey chair may aid positioning
  - Empirically try different food textures, e.g. gruel, kibble, meatballs

- Antibiotics for inhalation pneumonia
  - Need to be given parenterally as oral delivery impaired
- Gastrostomy tube feeding
  - Maintains nutritional intake
  - Not recommended as it does not stop inhalation of saliva
- Prokinetics
  - Cisapride and metoclopramide may worsen signs
  - No evidence that bethanechol helps
- Sildenafil (1 mg/kg q8–12h) in congenital MO, and may help acquired MO if secondary to achalasia

Myasthenia gravis
q.v. section 5.8.10
- Anticholinesterase inhibitors
  - Neostigmine parenterally initially to restore swallowing
  - Pyridostigmine @ 1–3 mg/kg PO BID
  - Atropine may be needed to reduce salivation
  - Avoid over-dosing, causing cholinergic crisis
- Immunosuppression
Danger of immunosuppression when pneumonia present, and may be unnecessary as spontaneous recovery possible
- Prednisolone
  - Start at low dose and increase to avoid muscle weakness
  - Ultimately give @ 2 mg/kg/day
- Azathioprine
  - Give @ 2 mg/kg PO SID
  - Monitor haematology
- Mycophenolate mofetil
  - Give @ 5–10 mg/kg PO BID

Monitoring
- Anti-acetylcholine receptor antibody titre
  - Stop immunosuppression when titre becomes negative, usually in about 6 months
- **Clinical response**

Prognosis
- Guarded to poor

- Congenital disease sometimes resolves spontaneously or can be treated successfully with sildenafil
- Idiopathic disease potentially manageable but not curable
- MG potentially curable or spontaneous recovery
- Death from inhalation pneumonia and malnutrition common

5.1.3C OESOPHAGITIS

Aetiology
Gastric reflux of acid, pepsin and digestive enzymes
- Acute and persistent vomiting
- During anaesthesia
- Hiatal hernia
- Spontaneous reflux oesophagitis

Ingestion
- Foreign bodies
  - Bones, chews, etc.
- Caustics, e.g accidental administration of sodium hydroxide (caustic soda) rather than sodium carbonate (washing soda) to induce emesis
- Drugs acting locally if not swallowed fully
  - Doxycycline tablets (only reported in cats so far)
  - NSAIDs
- Hot liquids and food, e.g. baked potato, meatballs, causing thermal injury

Major signs
- Anorexia
- Drooling and gulping
- Odynophagia
- Regurgitation is less common than in other oesophageal disorders

Minor signs
- Blood in regurgitated material
- Lethargy
- Weight loss

Potential sequelae
- Stricture formation, *q.v.* section 5.1.3E

Predisposition
- No age or sex predisposition
- Oesophageal FB in WHWT
- Reflux under GA more likely if:
  - Not fasted
  - Obesity
  - Operating table tilted head-down
  - Prolonged recovery, e.g. after ovariohyster-ectomy for pyometra

Historical clues
- A recent history of:
  - Ingestion of caustics
  - FB removal
  - GA (with known or presumed reflux)
- Because of pain, the dog may appear uncomfortable and 'regurgitate actively'

Clinical examination
- Dull/depressed/anxious

Laboratory findings
- No significant changes

Imaging
- Usually no significant findings on plain or static contrast studies
- Dysmotility and/or spontaneous reflux may be seen if fluoroscopy is available

Special investigations
- Oesophagoscopy
  - Bleeding
  - Inflammation
  - Erosions
  - Mucosa very friable on contact with endoscope
  - Ulcers

Treatment
Prevent perpetuation of damage by further gastric reflux
- Cisapride (preferably) or metoclopramide to increase tone in lower oesophageal sphincter
- Acid blockade with twice daily proton pump inhibitor, *q.v.* section 5.1.4F

Rest oesophagus
- Soft, liquidised food
- Gastrostomy tube feeding or postural feeding

Treat oesophageal inflammation
- Sucralfate
  - To coat ulcers
  - Give @ 5–10 ml PO up to six times daily
- Local anaesthetic gels to aid swallowing
- Prednisolone? (no evidence)

Monitoring
- Clinical response
- Repeat oesophagoscopy

Prognosis
- Good if treated aggressively
- Guarded to poor if stricture develops

5.1.3D SLIDING HIATAL HERNIA

Aetiology
- Hiatal hernia permitted by weak phrenico-oesophageal ligaments and enlarged oesophageal hiatus; may be a congenital defect in some brachycephalic dogs
- Sliding of the hernia is more likely with increased intra-abdominal pressure
  - Abdominal organomegaly
  - Obesity
  - Tenesmus
- Sliding of the hernia is provoked by upper airway obstruction
  - Brachycephalic obstructive airway syndrome (BOAS)
  - Laryngeal paralysis

Major signs
- Regurgitation

Minor signs
- Decreased appetite
- Gulping, lip-licking
- Vomiting

Potential sequelae
- Oesophagitis

Predisposition
- Brachycephalic breeds with BOAS
- Laryngeal paralysis in old, large-breed dogs, especially Labradors

ORGAN SYSTEMS

Historical clues

- Although regurgitation is the major sign, affected dogs may also vomit, confusing the history
- Predisposition in small brachycephalics, especially Boston terrier, French bulldog and Pug

Clinical examination/laboratory findings

- Usually unremarkable

Imaging

Thoracic radiographs

Plain

- Often unremarkable as sliding hernia is intermittent; if lucky, gas in stomach is seen cranial to the line of the diaphragm

Contrast

- Fluoroscopy is required to observe herniated stomach sliding cranial to the diaphragm, and may require abdominal compression with paddles

Special investigations

Oesophagoscopy

- Evidence of distal oesophagitis, sometimes with a crease around the lower oesophageal sphincter
- Gastric cardia cranial to edge of diaphragmatic hiatus in retroflexed view
- Herniation can be provoked whilst observing the sphincter
  - Abdominal compression
  - Three spontaneous breaths with the endotracheal tube temporarily occluded

Treatment

Reduce precipitating factors

- BOAS surgery
- Divided meals
- Weight reduction

Medical management

- Cisapride
- Proton pump inhibitor

Surgical management

- Fundic gastropexy

- Fundoplication
- Phrenoplasty

Prognosis

- Fair with medical management
- Reduction of signs with surgery: surgical expertise dependent, and complete resolution unlikely

5.1.3E   STRICTURE

Aetiology

- Healing of severe ulceration by fibrosis
- Follows severe oesophagitis, or FB removal

Major signs

- Regurgitation
- Other signs of oesophagitis

Minor signs

- Lethargy
- Weight loss

Potential sequelae

- Inhalation pneumonia
- Cachexia
- Euthanasia if treatment is unsuccessful

Predisposition

- See oesophagitis above
- Stricture usually develops within 1–2 weeks of severe oesophagitis

Historical clues

- Progressively smaller pieces of food can be swallowed
- Small volumes of liquids can still be swallowed

Clinical examination

- Outwardly unremarkable initially
- Weight loss, and ultimately cachexia with time

Laboratory findings

- Unremarkable

ORGAN SYSTEMS

Imaging
Radiographs
Plain
- Unremarkable unless gravel sign from remnants of trapped food

Contrast
- Liquid barium suspension may pass stricture
- Barium mixed with food (barium meal) will highlight obstruction

Special investigations
- Oesophagoscopy
  - Observation of stricture
  - Proximal oesophagitis
  - Treatment by dilation

Treatment
Dilate stricture
- May need to be done twice weekly for between 1 and 20 times before stricture is abolished
- Endoscopic injection of triamcinolone into stricture before dilation may be helpful
- Fluoroscopic assessment during dilation may help ensure complete stretching

Bougienage
- Progressively larger diameter, conical, rubber-tipped probes (e.g. Savary-Gilliard dilators) passed
- Danger of tearing from shear forces

Balloon dilatation
- Balloon catheter passed alongside or through endoscope
- Radial stretching force produces less tearing

Treat resultant oesophagitis
- As above
- Gastrostomy tube feeding to rest the oesophagus if severe oesophagitis
- No evidence that oral prednisolone or colchicine prevent stricture from re-forming

Monitoring
- Clinical response
- Repeat oesophagoscopy

Prognosis
- Guarded
  - Danger of oesophageal tearing
  - Stricture tends to re-form

5.1.4   STOMACH

Problems
Presenting complaints
q.v. section 1
- Anorexia
- Drooling
- Haematemesis
- Halitosis
- Melaena
- Vomiting
- Weight loss

Physical abnormalities
q.v. section 2
- Abdominal discomfort/pain
- Abdominal enlargement

Laboratory abnormalities
q.v. section 3
- Anaemia if gastric ulceration
- Azotaemia from dehydration
- Usually unremarkable

Diagnostic approach
- The cardinal sign of gastric disease is vomiting but:
  - Non-GI diseases can cause vomiting
  - Intestinal and pancreatic diseases can cause vomiting
- Thus the overall diagnostic approach is to:
  - First rule out non-GI causes of vomiting
  - Investigate stomach and intestine

Diagnostic methods
History
- The cardinal sign is vomiting
- Haematemesis (fresh blood or 'coffee grounds'-type material in vomitus) is most commonly due to gastric ulceration, *q.v.* section 1.25

Clinical examination
- Often unremarkable
- Cranial abdominal discomfort if ulcerative disease
- Cranial abdominal mass if large tumour
- Tympany with gastric dilatation-volvulus (GDV)

Laboratory findings
- Frequently normal, but helps rule out non-GI diseases
- No pathognomonic changes
- Anaemia, *q.v.* section 3.30.1
  - Anaemia of chronic disease
  - Iron deficiency anaemia
  - Pre-regenerative or regenerative anaemia with acute blood loss
- Secondary electrolyte abnormalities
  - Dehydration and hypochloraemic metabolic alkalosis if loss of gastric acid
  - Dehydration and metabolic acidosis if vomiting of intestinal and gastric contents
- Hypoglycaemia in young animals not eating

Imaging
Plain radiographs
- Identification of gastric wall thickening is unreliable
- Free abdominal gas (gastric perforation)
- GDV
  - Reverse of gas pattern
  - Compartmentalisation of stomach
- Gastric mass
- Normal right lateral
  - Gas fills fundus
  - Fluid in antrum – do not mistake for circular FB
- Normal left lateral
  - Gas in antrum
  - Fundus-antral axis is a marker of hepatic size
- Radiopaque FB

Contrast radiographs
- Low yield if vomiting and diarrhoea
  - Only indicated if unremarkable plain films with unhelpful laboratory results and endoscopy unavailable

- Fluoroscopic assessment of gastric emptying
  - Monitor gastric motility and delayed emptying
  - Pyloric obstruction
- Irregular mucosa/rugal folds/masses
- Radiolucent FB

Ultrasound examination
- Abnormal gastric wall layering and thickness
  - Gastric tumour
  - Gastric ulcer
- FB

Special investigative techniques
- Gastroscopy
  - Inspection
  - Biopsy
  - FB removal
- Serum pepsinogen
  - Test for gastric damage
  - Not commercially available
- Sucrose permeability
  - Not commercially available
- Exploratory laparotomy

5.1.4A ACUTE GASTRITIS

Aetiology
q.v. section 1.49 for non-gastric causes of acute vomiting
- Acute haemorrhagic diarrhoea syndrome (AHDS)/haemorrhagic gastroenteritis (HGE)
  - Diarrhoea is major concurrent sign and despite the vomiting there is no gastritis histologically
- Dietary indiscretion (change in diet, overindulgence)
- Drugs causing gastric ulceration
  - Cytotoxics
  - High doses of glucocorticoids
  - NSAIDs
- Gastric foreign body
- Parvovirus infection *q.v.* section 5.1.5.1D
- Toxins

Major signs
- Vomiting
  - Bile

ORGAN SYSTEMS

- Blood
- Foreign material
- Mucus and swallowed saliva

Minor signs
- Bloating
- Eructation
- Lethargy/anorexia/depression
- Polydipsia
- Pyrexia

Potential sequelae
- Dehydration
- Hypochloraemic metabolic alkalosis if pyloric obstruction
- Metabolic acidosis if intestinal contents refluxed and vomited as well

Predisposition
- AHDS/HGE in toy breeds
- Parvovirus in unvaccinated dogs
- Young dogs are more likely to scavenge or contract infections

Historical clues
- Exposure to toxins, drugs, scavenging
- Sudden onset of vomiting in previously healthy dog
- Concurrent diarrhoea if generalised GI inflammation

Clinical examination
- Unremarkable in mild cases
- Anorexia/lethargy/depression in severe cases
- Cranial abdominal discomfort
- Dehydration

Laboratory findings
Largely to rule out non-GI diseases, especially hypoadrenocorticism

Haematology
- Haemoconcentration
- Rarely an inflammatory leukogram

Serum biochemistry
- Pre-renal azotaemia
- Increased serum protein concentrations

Urinalysis
- Hypersthenuria is appropriate if dehydrated
- Isosthenuria indicates renal component for any azotaemia

Imaging
Radiographs
Plain
- Usually unremarkable
- FB

Contrast
Rarely indicated in acute disease

Ultrasound examination
- FB
- Gastric ulceration sometimes visible
  - Disruption of surface ± gas within the wall
  - Thickened oedematous wall

Special investigations
- ACTH stimulation test if suspicion of hypoadrenocorticism

Treatment
Usually self-limiting with symptomatic support
- Parenteral fluid therapy most important
- Antibiotics not normally indicated
- Acid blockade (H_2 antagonist or PPi)
- Anti-emetic: only *after* obstruction ruled out
  - Maropitant @ 1 mg/kg SC or slow IV SID and/or
  - Metoclopramide @ 0.5 mg/kg PO TID and/or
  - Ondansetron @ 0.5 mg/kg IV initially then 0.2 mg/kg SC TID
- Sucralfate only indicated if gastric ulceration and haematemesis, *q.v.* section 5.1.4F

Monitoring
- Clinical response
- Hydration status

Prognosis
- Excellent for complete recovery

5.1.4B   CHRONIC GASTRITIS

Aetiology
- Chronic gastritis of unknown aetiology
  - Autoimmune response to self antigen?
  - Food allergy
  - Giant hypertrophic gastritis (incorrectly termed Ménétrier's disease)
  - Helicobacter infection – not proven in dogs
  - Part of idiopathic CIE/IBD syndrome
    - Eosinophilic gastritis
    - Hypertrophic gastritis
    - Lympho-plasmacytic gastritis most common
- Chronic FB
- Drugs
  - Corticosteroids: probably don't cause gastritis but impair healing of any damage to the gastric mucosal barrier
  - NSAIDs: major cause of gastric ulceration
- Increased HCl production
  - Gastrinoma (very rare)
  - Mast cell tumour
- *Physaloptera* spp. infection (not in UK)
- Uraemia; gastric mineralisation rather than inflammation

Major signs
- Chronic vomiting
  - Bile
  - Blood
  - Food

Minor signs
- Abdominal discomfort
- Borborygmi
- Diarrhoea if part of CIE/IBD or gastrinoma
- Inappetence
- Lethargy/depression
- Weight loss

Potential sequelae
- Gastric ulceration
- Progression to gastric carcinoma, as in man, has not been described in dogs

Predisposition
- None

Historical clues
- Chronic vomiting, with little progression of signs
- Eating grass
- Often vomit bile in the morning, and seem better if fed early

Clinical examination
- Usually unremarkable
- May be dull and have lost weight

Laboratory findings
Haematology
- Often unremarkable
- Occasional blood loss anaemia

Serum biochemistry
- Often unremarkable
- Normal results help rule out extra-intestinal diseases
- Occasional hypoproteinaemia through blood loss

Imaging
Radiographs
Plain
- Usually unremarkable
- FB

Contrast
- Irregular mucosa sometimes
- Rule out outflow obstruction if fluoroscopy available

Ultrasound examination
Thickening of gastric wall possible, but wide variation in thickness normally

Special investigations
Gastroscopy
- Biopsies always taken even if grossly normal
- Incomplete emptying of the stomach
- Irregular friable mucosa
- Occasional spontaneous haemorrhages
- Superficial ulceration

Histology
- Eosinophilic gastritis
- Hypertrophic gastritis
- Lympho-plasmacytic gastritis

ORGAN SYSTEMS

Treatment

Acid blockade

q.v. section 5.1.4F

- H_2 antagonists at least TID, but may be unsuccessful as tolerance develops quickly
- Proton pump inhibitors BID

Anti-emetics

- Maropitant
- Metoclopramide

Dietary modification

- Exclusion diet trial in case gastritis is a dietary sensitivity
- Low-fat, highly digestible food speeds gastric emptying

Immunosuppression

- Judicious use of steroid as it may impair the mucosal barrier
  - Prednisolone @ 1–2 mg/kg/day PO
- Mycophenolate or cytotoxic agent if steroid side effects are unacceptable

Triple therapy

- To treat *Helicobacter* infection
- Combination of two antibiotics (e.g. amoxycillin and metronidazole) plus a proton pump inhibitor (PPI)
- No evidence that *Helicobacter* are pathogenic in dogs and that triple therapy is indicated

Monitoring

- Clinical response
- Repeat gastroscopy and biopsy

Prognosis

- Guarded – often manageable but not curable

5.1.4C GASTRIC CARCINOMA

Aetiology

- No evidence to incriminate *Helicobacter*, unlike in man
- Gastric dysplasia has been identified as a prequel in Tervuren Belgian shepherd
- Spontaneous neoplasia

Major signs

- Anorexia
- Haematemesis
- Vomiting
- Weight loss

Minor signs

- Drooling saliva
- Dull/depressed

Potential sequelae

- Anaemia
- Cachexia
- Metabolic alkalosis
- Death

Predisposition

- 7–10 years of age
- Belgian shepherd, Bull terrier, Chow Chow, Collies (especially Rough collie)

Historical clues

- Insidious onset of chronic vomiting
- Fresh or changed blood in vomitus
- Gradual decline in appetite

Clinical examination

- Pale mucous membranes if anaemic
- Rarely, a palpable abdominal mass
- Tachycardia if active bleeding

Laboratory findings

Haematology

- Anaemia from blood loss and chronic illness
  - Regenerative or non-regenerative
  - Microcytic iron deficiency anaemia if prolonged course

Serum biochemistry

- Hypoproteinaemia from blood loss

Imaging

Radiographs

Plain

- Cranial abdominal mass occasionally obvious
- Interpretation of thickening of gastric wall notoriously unreliable
- Chest radiographs should be taken, but visible lung metastasis unusual

Contrast
- Delayed gastric emptying
- Irregular mucosal outline
- Poorly distensible stomach

Ultrasound examination
- Gastric and hepatic lymph node enlargement
- Gastric ulceration
- Liver metastasis
- Loss of normal layering
- Mass lesion or thickening of gastric wall

CT
- Most sensitive indirect imaging technique

Special investigations
Endoscopy and biopsy
- Ulcerated mass visible, typically arising on the lesser curvature
- Biopsies may be too superficial to reach a diagnosis

Exploratory laparotomy and biopsy
- Full-thickness biopsies more diagnostic
- Opportunity for resection

Treatment
- Surgical resection, but often not resectable
- Chemotherapy not shown to be effective

Monitoring
- Clinical response
- Repeat endoscopy

Prognosis
- Grave
- Most cases are euthanased because of advanced disease at time of diagnosis

5.1.4D GASTRIC DILATATION-VOLVULUS (GDV)

Aetiology
- Accumulation of gas and frothy ingesta, combined with inability to eructate, causes dilatation of stomach
- Dilatation causes torsion of stomach around its long axis, usually 360° in a clockwise direction (pylorus lies left-dorsal)

- Endotoxins and inflammatory mediators cause cardiac arrhythmias
- Obstruction of caudal vena cava and venous return from viscera causes hypovolaemic shock
- Splenic torsion may also occur
- Stretching of gastric wall ± tearing of short gastric arteries causes gastric ischaemia and ultimately gastric wall necrosis
- Unknown cause, but numerous epidemiological risk factors identified

Major signs
- Abdominal discomfort
- Bloating
- Retching and unproductive attempts to vomit
- Weakness/collapse

Minor signs
- Dyspnoea
- Pale mucous membranes with prolonged capillary refill time (CRT)
- Tachycardia

Potential sequelae
- Gastric rupture and septic peritonitis
- Shock
- Ventricular tachycardia
- Disseminated intravascular coagulation
- Death

Predisposition
- Large-/giant-, deep-chested-breed dogs: Great Dane, GSD, Irish setter
- Potential risk factors
  - Anxious personality
  - Following excitement, car ride
  - Feeding single variety of food
  - Feeding from raised bowl
  - Possible association with weather/season
- No association with:
  - Dry food
  - Exercise

Historical clues
- Sudden onset of unproductive retching and bloating, sometimes following excitement/car journey

Clinical examination
- Distended cranial abdomen
- Tachypnoea
- Tympany on percussion
- Weak thready pulses and tachycardia
- Weak/collapsed

Laboratory findings
Haematology
- May not be performed as presumptive diagnosis is made on clinical signs ± imaging
- Haemoconcentration

Serum biochemistry
- May not be performed as presumptive diagnosis is made on clinical signs
- Hyperlactataemia may be prognostic
- Pre-renal azotaemia

Imaging
Plain radiographs
- Dilated stomach
- GDV is a continuum, and presence or absence of volvulus on radiographs is irrelevant to treatment
- Volvulus (Figure 4.1.4a) confirmed by:
  - Reverse of normal gas pattern
  - Compartmentalisation of stomach

Special investigations
ECG
- Ventricular premature contractions (VPCs) or ventricular tachycardia

Treatment
Surgical intervention, either acutely to correct a torsion, or later to perform an elective gastropexy, is always indicated.

Emergency stabilisation
Correction of shock
 Aggressive fluid therapy
  - Balanced electroyte
  - Colloid
  - Hypertonic saline

Gastric decompression
- Orogastric tube
- Needle gastrocentesis

- Temporary flank gastrostomy if stomach tubing not possible even after needle decompression

Surgery
- Gastric derotation
- Removal of devitalised fundic wall if necessary
  - Inversion: quicker and safer
  - Partial gastrectomy
- Antral gastropexy
  - Belt-loop: strongest gastropexy
  - Circumcostal: risk of pneumothorax
  - Incisional: currently the most preferred technique
  - Incorporation of stomach in abdominal wall closure (not commonly practised in UK)
  - Tube gastrostomy: allows post-operative decompression

Supportive
- Anti-arrhythmics: lidocaine for significant ventricular tachycardia *q.v.* section 5.2.4.2C
- Antibiotic cover
- Correction of electrolyte abnormalities

Monitoring
- ECG
- Haematemesis indicating gastric necrosis
- Signs of bloating
- Temperature, pulse and respiration (TPR) for signs of sepsis

Prognosis
- Variable (full recovery or death) depending on:
  - Need for partial gastrectomy
  - Speed of treatment
  - Ventricular arrhythmias
- Recurrence rate is significantly decreased if gastropexy performed

5.1.4E DELAYED GASTRIC EMPTYING

Aetiology
- Delayed gastric emptying and vomiting of gastric contents is caused by:

ORGAN SYSTEMS

- Alterations in gastric motility, i.e. no outflow obstruction
- Physical obstruction of pylorus

Altered motility
- Acidosis
- Diabetic neuropathy
- Dysautonomia
- Gastritis/gastric ulceration
- Hypoadrenocorticism
- Hypokalaemia
- Idiopathic gastric hypomotility
- Malabsorption causing physiological delay in gastric emptying
- Neoplastic infiltration
- Opioid administration
- Pain
- Pancreatitis
- Peritonitis
- Uraemia

Anatomical obstruction
- Chronic hypertrophic pylorogastropathy (CHPG), also known as antral mucosal hypertrophy
- FB acting as a 'ball-valve'
- Giant hypertrophic gastritis
- Neoplasia
  - Antral polyp
  - Carcinoma
  - Lymphoma
  - Leiomyoma/sarcoma
- Pyloric stenosis: congenital muscular hypertrophy

Major signs
- Vomiting delayed after eating

Minor signs
- Abdominal distension
- Reduced appetite
- Weight loss

Potential sequelae
- Dehydration
- Hypochloraemic metabolic alkalosis

Predisposition
- CHPG in male, toy-breed dogs, especially Lhasa Apso, Pekingese, Shih Tzu

- Congenital pyloric stenosis in brachycephalic dogs
- Giant hyperophic gastritis in Basenji and Boxer

Historical clues
- Vomiting of food occurs hours/days after eating
- Known ingestion of FB

Clinical examination
- Usually unremarkable except mild dehydration and weight loss
- Distended stomach sometimes palpable

Laboratory findings
Haematology
- Usually unremarkable
- Haemoconcentration if dehydrated

Serum biochemistry
- Usually unremarkable
- Increased serum protein concentration and pre-renal azotaemia if dehydrated

Imaging
Radiographs
Plain
- Distended stomach
- Radiodense FB
- Stomach contains mixture of gas ngesta

Contrast
- Delayed gastric emptying
  - Normal emptying begins within 2 and is complete by 8 hours
    - Dependent on nature of contrast agent: time for iodine < barium suspension < barium meal
    - Great individual variation depending on stress
- Persistent 'beak' of contrast at pylorus consistent with stenosis or CHPG
- Radiolucent FB

Ultrasound examination
- Gas and ingesta in stomach
- Thickening of pyloric muscle or mucosa

Special investigations
- Endoscopy
- Exploratory laparotomy

Treatment
Altered motility
- Correct underlying cause, e.g. potassium supplementation, weaning of opioids
- Dietary modification; low-fat diet empties more rapidly
- Prokinetics
  - Cisapride @ 0.5 mg/kg TID/QID
  - Erythromycin @ 1–2 mg/kg TID
  - Metoclopramide @ 0.5 mg/kg TID/QID
  - Ranitidine: also blocks acid secretion but currently unavailable
  - Nizatidine: also blocks acid secretion but currently unavailable

Anatomical obstruction
- Removal of FB
- Fredet-Ramstedt pyloromyotomy
- Heineke-Mikulicz pyloroplasty
- Y-U pyloroplasty best option for CHPG

Monitoring
- Clinical response

Prognosis
- Excellent if FB removed
- Good for CHPG and congenital pyloric stenosis if pyloroplasty is successful

5.1.4F GASTRIC ULCER

Aetiology
- Ulcer(s) extending through the epithelium
- Potentially caused by anything damaging the gastric mucosal barrier
  - NSAIDs: most important cause in dogs
  - Abrasive gastric foreign body
  - Acute and chronic gastritis, *q.v.* sections 5.1.4A, 5.1.4B
  - Acute neurological disease or trauma
  - Gastric carcinoma, *q.v.* section 5.1.4C
  - Gastric leiomyoma/sarcoma
  - Gastric lymphoma
  - Gastrinoma
  - Histamine release from mast cell tumour
  - Portal hypertension in end-stage liver disease
  - Uraemic gastritis

Major signs
- Vomiting
- Haematemesis

Minor signs
- Abdominal pain/discomfort
- Anorexia
- Melaena
- Weight loss

Potential sequelae
- Anaemia
- Gastric perforation and septic peritonitis
- Death from blood loss if gastric artery eroded

Predisposition
- Gastric carcinoma, *q.v.* section 5.1.4C
- NSAIDs more commonly used to treat osteoarthritis in older dogs
- Renal and liver failure more common in older dogs

Historical clues
- Administration of NSAIDs
- Cutaneous mast cell tumour
- Icterus and other signs of liver failure
- Polyuria/polydipsia (PU/PD) and other signs of renal failure

Clinical examination
- Cranial abdominal pain
- Dull/depressed
- Pale mucous membranes
- Tachycardia

Laboratory findings
Haematology
q.v. section 3.30.1
- Microcytic anaemia if chronic bleeding
- Regenerative anaemia

Serum biochemistry
- Hypoproteinaemia

Imaging
Radiographs
Plain
- Usually unremarkable
- Pneumoperitoneum if gastric perforation

Contrast
- Occasionally ulcerated mucosa is highlighted
- Leakage of contrast indicates perforation

Ultrasound examination
- Irregular mucosa
- Minimal thickening, *cf.* neoplasia
- Sometimes loss of layering

Special investigations
- Endoscopy
- Exploratory laparotomy if perforated or major haemorrhage

Treatment
Remove underlying cause
- Stop NSAIDs

Chemical diffusion barrier
- Sucralfate
  - Complex of aluminium and sucrose octasulphate
  - Binds ulcerated tissue and prevents acid attack
  - Give @ 500 mg to 1 g per dog PO q6-8h

Acid blocker
Antacids
- Aluminium, magnesium hydroxide or carbonate
- Need to be given at least six times daily

H_2 antagonists
- Block histamine-mediated acid secretion and not very effective as tolerance quickly develops
- Cimetidine @ 5 mg/kg QID
- Famotidine @ 1 mg/kg SID
- Nizatidine @ 1 mg/kg BID: currently unavailable
- Ranitidine @ 2mg/kg ID/TID: currently unavailable

Proton pump inhibitor (PPI)
- Completely block gastric epithelial pump that secretes hydrogen ions
- Omeprazole @ 0.7 mg/kg BID or esomeprazole

Surgery
Resection and repair perforating ulcer

Monitoring
- Clinical response
- Haematology
- Repeat gastroscopy

Prognosis
- Good if underlying cause can be removed and treatment started before perforation

5.1.5   SMALL INTESTINE

Problems
Presenting complaints
q.v. section 1
- Abdominal discomfort/pain
- Abdominal enlargement: mass or ascites
- Anorexia
- Diarrhoea
- Haematemesis
- Haematochezia (more commonly large intestinal)
- Halitosis
- Melaena
- Polyphagia
- Pruritus
- Vomiting
- Weight loss

Physical abnormalities
q.v. section 2
- Abdominal enlargement
- Anaemia
- PLE
  - Ascites
  - Peripheral oedema
  - Pleural effusion
- Pyrexia

Laboratory abnormalities
q.v. section 1
- Amylase
- Hypocalcaemia in PLEs
- Hypocholesterolaemia due to malabsorption
- Hypokalaemia
- Hyponatraemia
- Hypoproteinaemia (hypoalbuminaemia)
- Leukocytosis
- Leukopenia
- Total protein

Diagnostic Approach
- Diarrhoea
  - Can be caused by extra-intestinal diseases
  - Is the cardinal sign of SI disease, *q.v.* section 1.15
  - Is usually a diffuse problem affecting both the SI and LI causing 'mixed pattern diarrhoea' but primary SI disease can occur and can be distinguished by:
    - Clinical signs
      - Frequency < 3 times per day
      - No tenesmus
      - Weight loss
    - Faecal characteristics
      - Large volume
      - ± Melaena
      - ± Steatorrhoea
      - Watery
- Thus the overall diagnostic approach is to rule out the extra-intestinal causes first
- The extent of investigations and the rapidity with which they are performed depends on:
  - How acute or chronic the problem is
  - How severe the problem is

Diagnostic Methods
- Depends on whether acute or chronic SI disease

5.1.5.1 ACUTE SMALL INTESTINAL DISEASES

Diagnostic Approach
- Acute diarrhoea is most often self-limiting, but can be life-threatening, and has many causes, *q.v.* section 1.15.1
- It is often not restricted to the SI, but affects the whole GI tract, *q.v.* section 5.1.4A
- Differentiate primary (GI) and secondary (non-GI) disease by history, physical examination and laboratory findings
- If primary GI disease present, determine whether the patient requires:
  - Symptomatic support only
  - Intensive medical therapy

- Surgical intervention

Diagnostic Methods
History
- Borborygmi
- Diarrhoea, *q.v.* section 1.15
  - ± Haemorrhagic
  - Varies from soft to profuse and watery
- Vomiting, *q.v.* section 1.49
- Weight loss is not a feature

Clinical examination
- Dehydration
- Palpation for pain, FB, masses or intussusception

Laboratory findings
Haematology
- Often unremarkable except for haemoconcentration

Serum biochemistry
- Often unremarkable except for dehydration-related changes
  - Pre-renal azotaemia
  - Increased total protein
- Normal results help rule out non-GI causes

Urinalysis
- Hypersthenuria in the face of dehydration is appropriate

Faecal examination
- Identify parasites

Imaging
- Identify
  - Pancreatitis
  - Surgical conditions, e.g. intussusception, FB

Special investigative techniques
q.v. section 1.15
- Endoscopy is rarely indicated in acute disease
- Exploratory laparotomy if intussusception
- Spec cPL if pancreatitis is suspected

5.1.5.1A   ACUTE ENTERITIS

Aetiology
Dietary
- Dietary indiscretion
  - Change in diet
  - Overindulgence
  - Scavenging
  - Food intolerance or allergy
- Toxins, especially mycotoxins in garbage and mouldy food

Bacterial infection
q.v. section 5.1.5.1C
- *Campylobacter*
- *Clostridium*
- *E. coli*

Viral infection
- Coronavirus (mild)
- Parvovirus, *q.v.* section 5.1.5.1D

Partial obstruction (surgical)
- Intussusception
- Linear FB

Major signs
- Diarrhoea
  - ± Blood
  - Large volume, watery
- Vomiting

Minor signs
- Abdominal discomfort
- Borborygmi
- Dull/depressed/lethargic
- Tenesmus if concurrent acute colitis
- Tremors if scavenged mouldy food, due to tremorgenic mycotoxins

Potential sequelae
- Dehydration
- Hypovolaemic shock if severe
- Sepsis
- Death if hypoadrenocorticism or uncorrected surgical disease

Predisposition
- Raw feeding
- Sudden change in diet
- Young dogs are more likely to be susceptible to infections
- Young dogs are more likely to scavenge

Historical clues
- Contact with possible infection sources
- Known access to inappropriate diet
- Lack of parvovirus vaccination
- Opportunity to scavenge

Clinical examination
- Unremarkable in mild cases
- Dehydration
- Dull/depressed
- Mild abdominal discomfort
- No abnormality on abdominal palpation if non-surgical

Laboratory findings
Haematology
- Often unremarkable except for haemoconcentration

Serum biochemistry
- Often unremarkable except for dehydration
  - Pre-renal azotaemia
  - Increased serum protein
- Hypoglycaemia in puppies and toy-breed dogs
- Rule out non-GI causes

Urinalysis
- Hypersthenuria in face of dehydration is appropriate

Faecal examination
- Stool culture unreliable
- To identify parasites

Imaging
Radiographs
Plain
- Bunching of bowel with linear foreign body
- Mild ileus quite common with inflammatory/infectious diseases
- No sign of obstructive disease

Contrast
No intestinal obstruction

ORGAN SYSTEMS

Ultrasound examination
- No evidence of obstruction/intussusception
- Large volume of liquid intestinal contents

Special investigations
- ACTH stimulation test
- Exploratory laparotomy if a surgical condition is identified

Treatment
- *Nil per os* – except in young and toy-breed dogs at risk of hypoglycaemia
- Parenteral fluid therapy
- Symptomatic treatment

Antibiotics
- Indicated if AHDS/HGE or parvovirosis *and* the dog is systemically unwell
- Not necessary in uncomplicated acute enteritis

Anti-emetics
- Only *after* obstruction is ruled out
  - Maropitant @ 1.0 mg/kg SC or slow IV, 2 mg/kg PO SID
  - Metoclopramide @ 0.5 mg/kg PO TID
  - Ondansetron @ 0.5 mg/kg IV initially then 0.2 mg/kg SC TID

Anti-diarrhoeals
- Opioid motility modifying and antisecretory drugs if infective or surgical causes are ruled out
  - Diphenoxylate @ 0.05 mg//kg PO TID if available
  - Loperamide @ 0.1 mg//kg PO TID: will cause drowsiness in Collies, etc. with MDR-1 mutation
- Antimuscarinics: not the best choice as they cause ileus
  - Butylscopolamine (Buscopan) ± metamizole @ 0.1 ml/kg IV or IM
- Protectants – act by absorbing free water and bacterial toxins
  - Bismuth
  - Kaolin
  - Pectin

Monitoring
- Clinical response
- Packed cell volume (PCV)/total protein (TP) and other markers of dehydration

- If the dog is not improving after 48–72 hours of symptomatic therapy, the case must be re-assessed

Prognosis
- Excellent for full recovery as long as fluid therapy is adequate

5.1.5.1B   ACUTE HAEMORRHAGIC DIARRHOEA SYNDROME (AHDS)/ HAEMORRHAGIC GASTROENTERITIS (HGE)

AHDS is now considered a more correct term than HGE, as gastritis is not present.

Aetiology
- Uncertain
  - Suspected enterotoxaemia
    - *Clostridium perfringens* Type A netF toxin incriminated

Major signs
- Haemorrhagic diarrhoea
- Vomiting

Minor signs
- Abdominal discomfort
- Dull/depressed

Potential sequelae
- Hypovolaemic shock
- Death

Predisposition
- Tends to recur in individuals
- Toy-breed dogs but can be seen in large-breed dogs
  - Miniature schnauzer, Maltese and Yorkshire terriers

Historical clues
- Owner may recognise some precipitating 'stress'
- Sudden onset of signs in previously healthy dog

Clinical examination

- Dull/depressed
- Skin turgor often relatively normal because of rapid loss of plasma does not allow for equilibration from intracellular fluid
- 'Raspberry jam'-like faeces on rectal thermometer
- Slow CRT
- Tachycardia

Laboratory findings

Haematology
- Marked haemoconcentration
- PCV >60, and >80 in very severe cases
- No abnormal WBC response

Serum biochemistry
- Often unremarkable initially
- Hypoproteinaemia after fluid therapy

Urinalysis
- Hypersthenuria

Faecal parasitology
- Any endoparasites will add to morbidity

Imaging

- Unremarkable

Special investigations

- Endoscopy would find normal stomach but SI mucosal ulceration, but is not clinically justified
- Stool cultures and measurement of C. perfringens enterotoxin are unhelpful as it can be a normal commensal

Treatment

- Resuscitative fluid therapy at shock doses
  - i.e. 10–20 ml/kg IV boluses
  - Then rate reduction when PCV below 55
- Antibiotics may not be necessary
- Antidiarrhoeals
- Nil per os
- Plasma transfusion if hypoproteinaemic

Monitoring

- Clinical response
- PCV: keep below ~55% by adjusting fluid rate

Prognosis

- Mortality is low if resuscitative fluid therapy is used
- Tendency to recur in individual dogs

5.1.5.1C BACTERIAL ENTERITIS

Bacterial infection is often believed to be the cause of acute gastroenteritis but is probably rarer than suspected; viral diseases are probably more common. As healthy dogs can also carry potential bacterial pathogens, empirical antibiotic use is not indicated in acute gastroenteritis. Most infections are self-limiting, and the dangers of inducing antibacterial resistance and a carrier state outweigh the perceived benefits.

Aetiology

- *Campylobacter* spp.
  - *C. jejuni* is considered pathogenic
  - *C. upsaliensis* is the more common isolate and may not be pathogenic in dogs
- *Clostridium* spp.
  - *Clostridium difficile*
    - Important nosocomial pathogen in humans
    - Rarely identified as a pathogen in dogs
  - *Clostridium perfringens*
    - *C. perfringens* Type A *netF* toxin incriminated in AHDS/HGE, *q.v.* section 5.1.5.1B
    - *C. perfringens* enterotoxin incriminated in stress-related diarrhoea, but not proven
- *E. coli*
  Often a *commensal*, with pathogenicity depending on the expression of virulence factors:
    - Adherent and invading (AIEC): cause of granulomatous colitis, *q.v.* section 5.1.6D
    - Enterohaemorrhagic (EHEC): release of a range of cytotoxins that kill enterocytes
    - Enteroinvasive (EIEC): can invade the mucosa and cause bloody diarrhoea
    - Enteropathic (EPEC): cause microvillar damage and pedestal formation on enterocytes; may persist and cause chronic disease
    - Enterotoxigenic (ETEC): release of a range of toxins that stimulate secretory diarrhoea

- *Salmonella* spp.
  - Can cause haemorrhagic diarrhoea, but also found in stool of healthy dogs, especially if fed raw meat
  - Septicaemia is a rare complication
  - Antibacterial treatment not recommended unless there is evidence of sepsis

Major signs
- Acute, sometimes bloody diarrhoea
- Vomiting

Minor signs
- Abdominal discomfort
- Dull/depressed

Potential sequelae
- Dehydration
- Death

Predisposition
- Roaming and scavenging
- Unsanitary housing

Historical clues
- Owner may recognise some precipitating 'stress'
- Sudden onset of signs in previously healthy dog

Clinical examination
- Signs of dehydration

Laboratory findings
Haematology
- Haemoconcentration
- ± Inflammatory leukogram

Serum biochemistry
- Changes related to dehydration

Urinalysis
- Hypersthenuria

Faecal culture
- Problematic, as the same organisms can often be isolated from the stool of clinically healthy dogs, and therefore isolation does not prove causation

Faecal parasitology
- Any endoparasites will add to morbidity

Imaging
- Ileus wth intraluminal gas, but not consistent with obstruction, *q.v.* sections 4.1.1D, 5.1.5.1E

Special investigations
- Endoscopy is not clinically justified
- Stool cultures are unhelpful as isolate can be a normal commensal

Treatment
- Empirical use of antibiotics is *not* recommended
- Intravenous fluid therapy as required
- Antidiarrhoeals (kaolin, pectin, bismuth, etc.)
- *Nil per os*
- Probiotics: may not be efficacious but safer than giving antibiotics

Monitoring
- Clinical signs
- PCV/total solids (TS)

Prognosis
- Good for complete recovery

5.1.5.1D   PARVOVIROSIS

Aetiology
- Canine parvovirus (CPV2); current strains in UK are 2a and 2b; 2c is present in some countries
- Attacks rapidly dividing tissue
  - Bone marrow, causing leukopenia (neutropenia and/or lymphopenia) with consequent immunosuppression
  - Intestinal crypts, causing haemorrhagic diarrhoea
  - Myocardium in unprotected neonate causing sudden death or cardiomyopathy; uncommon now because vaccination or exposure of bitch usually provides maternally derived antibody cover

Major signs
- Diarrhoea: haemorrhagic in ~60% of severe cases
- Vomiting

Minor signs
- Dull/weak/lethargic
- Pyrexia

Potential sequelae
- Death from endotoxaemia and/or sepsis

Predisposition
- Young (unvaccinated) dogs

Historical clues
- Acute course after 5–10 days' incubation
  - Day 1 – Off-colour, pyrexia
  - Day 2 – Vomiting
  - Day 3 – Diarrhoea
- Exposure to potential infection
- Unvaccinated

Clinical examination
- Dull/depressed
- Dehydration
- Moderate abdominal discomfort
- Haemorrhagic diarrhoea on thermometer

Laboratory findings
Haematology
- Haemoconcentration
- Leukopenia, especially neutropenia, in about 50% of cases requiring hospitalisation
- Regenerative left shift appears during early recovery as bone marrow starts to release immature cells

Serum biochemistry
- Pre-renal azotaemia
- Increased liver enzymes secondary to intestinal inflammation
- Hypoproteinaemia after fluid therapy

Urinalysis
- Hypersthenuria

Faecal examination
- Any endoparasites will add to morbidity

Imaging
Radiographs
Plain and contrast
- Generalised ileus often present
- No specific obstruction

Ultrasound
- Complete lack of peristalsis in ~75% of cases

Special investigations
- Serology (haemagglutination inhibition)
  - Positive IgM titre
  - Rising IgG titre necessary, as single titre merely indicates exposure or vaccination
- Identification of parvo antigen in faeces
  - Electron microscopy: rarely available
  - SNAP® test: most useful in practice
  - ELISA
  - PCR: may be too sensitive and detect environmental virus

Treatment
- Fluid therapy
- Intravenous antibiotic cover
- Metoclopramide constant rate infusion and/or maropitant
- ω-Interferon has been shown to shorten the recovery phase

Monitoring
- Clinical response
- Hydration status
- WBC count

Prognosis
- Initially guarded, as end result is variable
  - Death if overwhelming endotoxaemia/sepsis
  - Full recovery
- Prognosis depends on:
  - Age
  - Leukopenia
  - Vaccination status

ORGAN SYSTEMS

5.1.5.1E SMALL INTESTINAL OBSTRUCTION

Aetiology
- FB
- Incarceration
  - External hernia
    - Inguinal
    - Umbilical
  - Internal hernia
    - Through mesenteric defect
- Intussusception
- Neoplasia
  - Adenocarcinoma most common
  - GI stromal tumour (GIST)
  - Lymphoma
  - Leiomyoma/sarcoma
  - Mast cell tumour
- Post-surgical stricture
- Volvulus

Major signs
- Vomiting
  - Faecal-like material if low obstruction
  - Large volume of bilious fluid if high obstruction

Minor signs
- Abdominal discomfort
- Anorexia
- Depression/lethargy
- Diarrhoea
- Haematochezia
- Melaena

Potential sequelae
- Dehydration
- Perforation and peritonitis
  - Death from sepsis and hypovolaemic shock

Predisposition
- Intussusception in puppies
- FBs more likely in younger dogs
- Tumours in older dogs
- Volvulus in dogs with EPI

Historical clues
- Acute onset of vomiting
- Intussusception often preceded by diarrhoea

- Known scavenging or dog's favourite toy missing

Clinical examination
- Dehydration
- Dull and depressed
- Palpation of mass or FB
- Rarely, ileo-colic intussusception protrudes from anus

Laboratory findings
Haematology
Inflammatory leukogram if severe localised inflammation or perforation

Serum biochemistry
- Hyponatraemia and hypokalaemia in prolonged cases
- Pre-renal azotaemia

Urinalysis
- Hypersthenuria is appropriate

Imaging
q.v. section 4.1

Radiographs
Plain
- FB
- Gravel sign: accumulation of material proximal to obstruction, Figure 4.1.2b
- Ileus
  - Bowel loop dilatation (Figure 4.1.1b) generally indicates obstruction when greater than:
    - Twice the width of the tenth rib
    - 1.5 x the height of the L5 vertebral body
  - Mass
- Pneumoperitoneum if perforated

Contrast
- Radiolucent FB
- Use iodinated contrast if perforation suspected

Ultrasound examination
- Multiple layered structure of intussusception, Figure 5.1.1c
- FB
- Mass: thickened and loss of layering

Special investigations
- Exploratory laparotomy

Treatment
- Masitinib or toceranib for unresectable GISTs
- Surgical removal of FB, correction of intussusception, or excision of tumour

Monitoring
- Signs of sepsis and peritonitis
  - Abdominal discomfort
  - Abdominal effusion
  - Brick red mucous membrane colour
  - Hypovolaemia
  - Persistence of vomiting
  - TPR

Prognosis
- Guarded to good, depending on:
  - Duration of obstruction
  - Water/electrolyte disturbances
  - Perforation and sepsis
  - Vascular compromise of SI, e.g. infarction in volvulus is grave
- Neoplasia
  - Good for leiomyoma
  - Guarded for GIST and leiomyosarcoma
  - Poor for adenocarcinoma unless complete resection after early diagnosis

5.1.5.2 CHRONIC SMALL INTESTINAL DISEASES

Diagnostic Approach
Having ruled out non-GI causes by history, physical examination and minimum database, and localised signs to the SI by history and faecal characteristics:

1 Rule out simple causes, such as diet-related and parasitism
2 Perform canine trypsin-like immunoreactivity (cTLI) test to rule out EPI *before* further investigations
3 Suspect PLE if hypoalbuminaemia
4 Faecal culture often unhelpful
5 Folate and cobalamin to screen for infiltrative bowel disease, *q.v.* sections 3.15, 3.10 respectively

6 Radiographs to screen for masses, partial obstruction
7 Ultrasound examination to examine bowel wall thickness and structure, and identify masses
8 Endoscopy: biopsy should always be performed, even if no gross abnormalities are found
9 Exploratory laparotomy and biopsy if endoscopy unavailable or non-diagnostic, or focal disease found on imaging

Diagnostic Methods
History
- Diarrhoea
  - Infrequent, large volume watery diarrhoea is suggestive of SI disease, but mixed pattern diarrhoea is often present due to more diffuse disease
  - Melaena may indicate upper GI haemorrhage, and in association with diarrhoea suggests SI bleeding
- Increased appetite with malabsorption
- Vomiting
  - SI disease can reflexly inhibit gastric emptying
  - SI disease can stimulate vomiting directly
- Weight loss

Clinical examination
- Ascites occurs if a PLE causes significant hypoalbuminaemia (< 15 g/l), *q.v.* sections 2.5, 3.27.2A
- Borborygmi
- Polyphagia in the presence of diarrhoea is suggestive of malabsorption
- Weight loss is characteristic of SI disease

Laboratory findings
Haematology
- Commonly unremarkable in primary, chronic GI disease

Serum biochemistry
- Commonly unremarkable in primary, chronic GI disease
- Panhypoproteinaemia is suggestive of PLE, but hypoalbuminaemia is key finding

ORGAN SYSTEMS

Urinalysis
- Commonly unremarkable

Faecal examination
- Identify parasites

Imaging
q.v. section 4.1

Special investigative techniques
- Faecal α_1-protease inhibitor (α_1-PI) – not available outside the United States
  - Endogenous serum protein that is lost into faeces if PLE is present
  - It parallels albumin loss but is not readily biodegradable in faeces and so persists and can be assayed by ELISA
  - Marker of PLE even before significant hypoproteinaemia has developed
- Folate and cobalamin
  - Principle, *q.v.* sections 3.15, 3.10 respectively
  - Interpretation
    - Decreased folate suggests proximal SI damage
    - Decreased cobalamin suggests distal SI damage
    - Decreased folate and cobalamin suggests generalised SI damage and diffuse malabsorption
    - Increased folate or decreased cobalamin may indicate bacterial dysbiosis
    - Increased folate plus decreased cobalamin is suggestive of ARD
  - Low sensitivity and specificity because results affected by
    - Anorexia
    - Dietary vitamin content
    - Nature, severity and duration of SI disease
- cTLI, *q.v.* section 3.28
- Intestinal biopsy

5.1.5.2A ALIMENTARY LYMPHOMA (AL)

Aetiology
- Spontaneous, but hypothesised that it may be a progression from lymphocytic-plasmacytic enteritis (LPE)

- Most commonly large cell (lymphoblastic); small cell lymphoma uncommon in dogs
- Variable anatomical distribution
  - Usually restricted to GI tract but may involve mesenteric lymph nodes (LNs)
  - Can be part of multicentric lymphoma
  - Sometimes restricted to stomach or rectum
  - Usually diffuse involvement of SI, but focal masses can occur

Major signs
- Anorexia
- Ascites if albumin < 15 g/l, i.e. PLE
- Chronic diarrhoea
- Weight loss

Minor signs
- Lethargy
- Generalised SC oedema
- Dyspnoea if hydrothorax or pulmonary thromboembolism (PTE)

Potential sequelae
- PLE
- Thromboembolism: PTE, renal infarcts
- Severe cachexia
- Death

Predisposition
- No age, sex or breed predisposition

Historical clues
- Intractable wasting disease causing diarrhoea ± melaena or haematochezia
- Often depressed with anorexia

Clinical examination
- Mesenteric lymphadenomegaly
- Palpable thickening of bowel loops very subjective

Laboratory findings
Haematology
- Anaemia of chronic disease or GI bleeding
- Lymphocytosis not common
- Paraneoplastic eosinophilia occasionally

Serum biochemistry
- Hypoalbuminaemia consistent with a PLE
- Hyperglobulinaemia rarely

Imaging
Radiographs
- Often unremarkable
- Loss of peritoneal detail if ascitic and/or cachexic

Ultrasound examination
- Bowel wall thickening
- Loss of layering very suggestive of neoplasia (Figure 5.1.1a) but not invariably present

Special investigations
- FNA of mesenteric LN and, potentially, of thickened SI wall
- Biopsy
  - Endoscopic: may miss affected area
  - Surgical: more reliable diagnostically, but risk of dehiscence
- Special histopathological techniques
  - Immunohistochemistry of intestinal biopsy
  - PCR for antigen receptor rearrangement (PARR): may be unreliable in the GI tract
  - Histology-guided mass spectroscopy (HGMS): not yet available in the UK
- MicroRNA not commercially available

Treatment
- Multi-agent chemotherapy with cyclophosphamide-vincristine-prednisolone (COP) or cyclophosphamide-doxorubicin-vincristine-prednisolone (CHOP) protocols
- Prednisolone and chlorambucil for small-cell lymphoma

Monitoring
- Clinical remission
- Serum albumin if PLE
- WBC

Prognosis
- Poor for large-cell lymphoma
  - Failure to gain remission
  - Intestinal perforation
- Small cell lymphoma and rectal lymphoma have a better prognosis

5.1.5.2B ANTIBIOTIC-RESPONSIVE DIARRHOEA (ARD)

Aetiology
- Dysbiosis is a disturbance of the normal intestinal microbiome but can be:
  - Primary
    - ARD
    - Specific bacterial infection
  - Secondary to:
    - Antibiotic therapy
    - Any chronic enteropathy
    - Diet change
    - PPI administration
- The cause of ARD can be:
  - Primary
    - Idiopathic in young, large-breed dogs
    - Formerly known, incorrectly, as small intestinal bacterial overgrowth (SIBO)
    - SIBO was originally described as an increase in the number of bacteria in the upper SI during the inter-digestive phase and defined by the number of bacteria cultured from duodenal juice
    - Normal $< 10^5$ total or $< 10^4$ anaerobic colony-forming units/ml
    - These figures are erroneous, because the technique has great variability even in an individual dog, and greater numbers have been found in healthy dogs
  - Secondary
    - Exocrine pancreatic insufficiency (EPI)
    - Partial intestinal obstruction
    - Redundant, 'blind-loop' of bowel
- Dysbiosis may cause malabsorption and diarrhoea by:
  - Brush border biochemical changes
  - Cobalamin sequestration, leading to malabsorption and deficiency
  - Competition for nutrients
  - Deconjugation of bile salts causing fat malabsorption
  - Deconjugated bile salts and hydroxylated fatty acids from bacterial fermentation stimulate colonic secretion
  - Failure of microbiome to convert primary to secondary bile acids

Major signs
- Chronic diarrhoea
  - Continuous or intermittent
  - Varying from soft to very watery
- Coprophagia
- Polyphagia
- Stunting or weight loss

Minor signs
- Borborygmi and flatus
- Greasy hair coat
- Occasionally anorexia
- Occasionally, secondary colitis-like diarrhoea
- Vomiting

Potential sequelae
- Cobalamin deficiency
- Ill-thrift
- Permanent stunting
- Transformation to LPE hypothesised but not proven

Predisposition
- Large/giant breeds
- Young dogs < 2 years

Historical clues
- Antibiotic-responsive
  - ARD appearing in older dog suggests development secondary to an underlying cause, e.g. partial obstruction due to neoplasia
- Coprophagia is most characteristic of SIBO or EPI
- Some response to dietary manipulation
- Suggestive clinical signs in young dog of predisposed breed, especially GSD

Clinical examination
- Thin
- Stunted
- Poor hair coat

Laboratory findings
Haematology
- Usually unremarkable

Serum biochemistry
- Usually unremarkable

Faecal examination
- Parasitology should be performed to eliminate complicating infections

Imaging
Radiographs
- Unremarkable in idiopathic SIBO
- Gravel sign if underlying partial obstruction

Ultrasound examination
- Unremarkable

Special investigations
- cTLI: EPI should be ruled out before other investigations, as predisposition and signs are very similar
- Antibiotic trial
  - Not generally recommended except in predisposed dogs (e.g. young GSD), and only after empirical parasite treatment and diet trial
- Duodenal juice culture
  - Claimed 'gold standard'
  - Very difficult to do in practice and unreliable results
- Folate and cobalamin
  - Classic increased folate, decreased cobalamin is only seen in 5% of dogs with culture proven SIBO
  - Using just increased folate or decreased cobalamin as a marker improves sensitivity but decreases specificity
- Intestinal biopsy
  - Normal or subtle/mild inflammatory changes

Treatment
Antibacterials
- SIBO is partly defined as 'antibiotic-responsive diarrhoea'
- Use broad-spectrum, low-cost, safe antibiotics
  - Oxytetracycline @ 10–20 mg/kg PO TID
  - Metronidazole @ 10–15 mg/kg PO BID
  - Tylosin @ 20 mg/kg PO BID; can treat relapses with 5 mg/kg PO
- Some dogs require continuous antibiotics, but may be controlled by lower doses
- Some dogs need single course or intermittent administration of antibiotics

Diet
- Fat restriction reduces volume of diarrhoea
- Prebiotics (e.g. fructo-oligosaccharides) may modulate the SI microbiome and/or the mucosal immune response

Probiotics
Logical choice, but no reports of success with current preparations

Faecal microbiota transplantation
Hypothetically may be useful, but no controlled studies so far

Vitamins
Vitamin B_{12} supplementation if dog is cobalamin-deficient

Monitoring
- Clinical response
- Serum cobalamin

Prognosis
- Guarded to good
  - May 'grow out of' the condition
  - May only need intermittent antibiotics
  - May need continuous antibiotics to control signs

5.1.5.2C CHRONIC INFLAMMATORY ENTEROPATHY (CIE)

Formerly known as inflammatory bowel disease (IBD)

Aetiology
- There are numerous potential causes of intestinal inflammation
  - Dietary sensitivity/food-responsive enteropathy (FRE)
  - Idiopathic
  - Various infections
- Suspected immune dysregulation leading to loss of tolerance to bacteria
- Variety of histological types (*most common type)

- Eosinophilic enteritis (EE) or gastro enteritis (EGE)
- Immunoproliferative small intestinal disease (IPSID)
- Lympho-plasmacytic enteritis (LPE)* (and/or colitis)
- Mixed lymphoplasmacytic-eosinophilic

Major signs
- Diarrhoea
  - Infrequent (< 3 times per day) unless concurrent colonic involvement
  - Large volume
  - Watery
- Vomiting
- Weight loss

Minor signs
- Abdominal discomfort
- Altered appetite
  - Anorexia if severe inflammation
  - Polyphagia if malabsorption
- Borborygmi
- Melaena and occult bleeding more common with EGE
- Poor hair coat secondary to malabsorption

Potential sequelae
- Protein-losing enteropathy (PLE)
  - Ascites/oedema
  - Hypoproteinaemia
- Lymphoma: hypothesised that LPE undergoes neoplastic transformation
- Thromboembolism

Predisposition
- All forms of CIE/IBD are rare in dogs < 1 year
- EGE in GSDs
- LPE in GSDs, Shar peis
- IPSID rare and only documented in Basenji

Historical clues
- Acute initiating event in some cases, e.g. following scavenging or viral enteritis
- Chronic intermittent signs for a long period
- Waxing-waning problem that is gradually getting worse or more frequent

ORGAN SYSTEMS

Clinical examination
- Variable body condition from normal (or even overweight) to cachexic
- Dull/depressed in severe CIE/IBD
- Ascites/oedema if PLE
- Thickened bowel loops sometimes palpable, but interpretation is subjective

Laboratory findings
Haematology
- Often unremarkable
- Anaemia of chronic disease, or blood loss
- Sometimes a mild/moderate neutrophilia
- Eosinophilia is an unreliable marker of EGE, and parasitism should be considered first

Serum biochemistry
- Often unremarkable
- Panhypoproteinaemia is typical in PLE, although severe inflammatory disease may cause increased globulins
- Hypocalcaemia in PLEs, largely reflecting hypoalbuminaemia, but ionised hypocalcaemia (and hypomagnesaemia) can occur due to calcium and vitamin D malabsorption
- Hypocholesterolaemia suggestive of malabsorption
- Hypocobalaminaemia
- Hypovitaminosis D
- Increased liver enzymes, secondary to intestinal inflammation

Urinalysis
- Proteinuria if secondary immune-complex glomerulonephritis

Faecal examination
- Identification of parasites or pathogenic bacteria may suggest cause of intestinal inflammation, rather than idiopathic CIE/IBD

Imaging
Radiographs
Plain
- Usually unremarkable
- Thickening of bowel wall difficult to assess on plain films

Contrast
- Irregular mucosal surface consistent with infiltration (i.e. CIE/IBD or AL)

Ultrasound
- Increased intestinal wall thickness is seen sometimes but may be due to tissue oedema rather than inflammatory infiltrate if a PLE
- Layering of intestinal wall should be present
- Mesenteric lymphadenopathy is present sometimes
- Speckling of normally hypoechoic mucosal layer (Figure 5.1.1d)

Special investigations
- Faecal α_1-PI as a marker for a PLE; only available in North America
- Folate and cobalamin
  - Decreases suggestive of infiltrative disease (CIE/IBD or lymphoma)
  - Indication for ileal biopsies
  - Subnormal serum concentrations indicate need for supplementation
- Intestinal biopsy after diet trial, or if:
  - 'Criteria of concern', i.e.:
    - Anorexia
    - Abnormal abdominal palpation or imaging
    - Haematemesis or melaena
    - Persistent, frequent vomiting
    - PLE
    - Severe weight loss/cachexia
  - or if:
    - Anorexia makes a diet trial impossible
    - Steroid or antibiotic trials are considered inappropriate
    - There is a suspicion of neoplasia or lymphangiectasia
  - Endoscopic biopsy preferred to surgical, as no convalescence before starting steroids
    - Retained food in stomach due to delayed gastric emptying
    - Irregular mucosa
    - Erosions, ulceration, bleeding
  - Surgical biopsy is more likely to be representative of disease
    - Duodenal biopsies and ideally ileal biopsies, especially if hypocobalaminaemia
    - Histological classification applied to CIE/IBD
    - However, an underlying cause for the inflammation must be ruled out before confirming idiopathic disease

Treatment

Antibiotics
- May reduce the antigenic burden on the mucosal immune system but no evidence to support their use

Metronidazole
- Debated whether it modulates immune response
- 10–15 mg/kg PO BID

Oxytetracycline
- May be anti-inflammatory
- 10 mg/kg PO TID

Diet
- Easily digestible, restricted fat, gluten-free diet has symptomatic benefits
- Response to an exclusion diet suggests FRE

Faecal microbiota transplantation
- No published evidence of efficacy and safety

Immunosuppression
Prednisolone
- First-choice immunosuppressant for IBD
- Start at 2–4 mg/kg PO SID
- Reduce after 2–3 weeks to 1–2 mg/kg PO SID
- Then taper every few weeks to find minimum effective dose
- Increase dose again if relapse and consider alternative immunosuppressants for their steroid-sparing effect

Azathioprine
- Adjunctive immunosuppressant
- 2 mg/kg/day initially, reducing to every other day after 4–6 weeks
- Potentially bone marrow suppressive, so monitor haematology
- Toxicity in individuals is related to activity of the degradatory thiopurine s-methyltransferase (TPMT) enzyme

Chlorambucil
- Effective in one study of CIE/IBD

Ciclosporin (Cyclosporin)
- Limited evidence of efficacy in steroid-resistant CIE/IBD

- Serum concentrations not related to efficacy as it undergoes enterohepatic recycling

Probiotics
- Limited evidence of benefit

Vitamin supplements
- Oral folic acid
- Vitamin B_{12} by weekly SC injection (250–1,000 µg) or daily oral dosing (500–2,000 µg)

Monitoring
- Clinical response
- Serum albumin concentration
- Side effects of steroids
- Repeat intestinal biopsy

Prognosis
- Guarded
- Potential individual outcomes
  - Weaned off all medication completely
  - Need low-dose continuous therapy
  - Only respond to high-dose therapy
  - Failure to respond
  - Possible transformation to lymphoma – not proven

5.1.5.2D DIETARY SENSITIVITY

Aetiology
- Food allergy is an adverse food reaction due to immunological causes
  - Food hypersensitivity is an adverse food reaction due to a Type I (IgE-mediated) reaction
  - Most GI food allergies are probably Type IV
  - The characterization of some cases of CIE/IBD as 'food-responsive enteropathies (FREs)' blurs the distinction between them and a true allergy
- Food intolerance is an adverse food reaction due to non-immunological causes
  - Foods causing histamine release via non-immunological mechanisms
  - Food containing non-digestible, osmotically active substance
  - Food containing pharmacologically active substance

Major signs
- Cutaneous signs are the most common mani-festation of food allergy
  - Pruritus
  - Secondary lesions due to self-trauma
- GI signs are non-specific
  - Diarrhoea
  - Vomiting

Minor signs
- Other signs of GI dysfunction

Potential sequelae
- Anaphylaxis and urticaria

Predisposition
- Allergic food disease possibly more common in WHWT and retrievers
- None for food intolerance, although specific individuals may have an idiosyncratic reaction

Historical clues
- Combination of GI signs and pruritus
- Positive response to an exclusion diet
- Signs associated with particular foodstuffs

Clinical examination
- Signs of self-trauma: erythema, excoriation, scaling, etc.

Laboratory findings
Haematology
- No specific changes noted
- Eosinophilia is not pathognomonic for die-tary sensitivity

Serum biochemistry
- No specific changes noted

Imaging
- Unremarkable

Special investigations
- Allergy testing
  - Serology for food-specific antibodies is unreliable
  - Gastroscopic food sensitivity testing is technically demanding, and can only iden-tify Type 1 hypersensitivity reactions

- Endoscopic biopsy
Any inflammatory changes in the SI are non-specific and must still be followed by a diet trial
- Exclusion diet trial, ideally performed before biopsy if the dog is systemically well
  - Remission on exclusion diet
    - Fed as sole food for trial period of at least 3 weeks, until remission achieved
    - Hydrolysed diet preferred
    - Single novel protein diet if hydrolysed diet refused
  - Relapse when challenged with original diet
  - Rescue by exclusion diet

Treatment
- Avoidance of allergen

Monitoring
- Clinical response

Prognosis
- Excellent if offending foodstuff can be elimi-nated from diet

5.1.5.2E   INTESTINAL PARASITISM

Aetiology
- Intestinal parasitism is common and regular anthelmintic administration is standard practice
- Infections can be via transplacental or trans-mammary routes, contact with infected fae-ces or a contaminated environment, or eating raw offal
- The severity of signs can vary from asympto-matic to potentially fatal depending on:
  - Age of dog
  - Numbers of the infective agent
  - Nutritional and immune status of the dog
  - Species of parasite
  - Treatment history

Cestodes (Tapeworms)
- *Dipylidium caninum*
  - Asymptomatic infection but passage of proglottids may be observed
  - Fleas are the intermediate host

- *Echinococcus granulosus*
  - Dog is definitive host and infection is asymptomatic
  - Infection of sheep and humans causes hydatid disease
- *Echinococcus multilocularis*
  - Dogs, foxes and beavers are definitive hosts
  - Endemic in Central and Eastern Europe, but not yet present in UK
  - Serious zoonotic infection
- *Mesocestoides* spp.
  - Dogs and cats are definitive hosts
  - Geographically widespread (Europe and North America) but not endemic in UK
  - Intestinal tapeworms usually cause no signs; ill-thrift may occur with heavy burden and co-infections
  - Larval migration can cause cystic tetrathyridiosis, with proliferation within the peritoneal cavity and infection of organs including the liver
  - Cystic tetrathyridiosis may be asymptomatic or cause peritonitis
- *Taenia* spp.
  - Asymptomatic infection
  - Rabbits, rodents and ruminants are intermediate hosts
  - Infection by ingestion of meat containing intermediate life-stage (cysticercus or coenurus)

Nematodes (Helminths)
Ascarids (Roundworms)
- *Toxocara canis* very common
- *Toxascaris leonina* less common
- Trans-placental, trans-mammary and environmental routes of infection
- Rarely cause clinical signs except in puppies
  - Diarrhoea
  - Ill-thrift
  - Pot-belly
- Intestinal obstruction can occur in puppies with massive worm burden
- Zoonotic, causing ocular or visceral *larva migrans*

Hookworms
- *Ancylostoma caninum*
  - Potential to cause death through GI blood loss
  - Has not been found in the UK

- *Uncinaria stenocephala*
  - Sporadic infections in UK
  - Can cause significant GI signs
  - Larval migration through the skin can cause interdigital dermatitis

Spiruroidea
- *Spirocerca lupi*
  - Prevalent in South Africa and eastern Mediterranean countries; not endemic in UK
  - Induces oesophageal granulomas causing signs of oesophageal disease
  - May transform to oesophageal osteosarcoma

Threadworms
- *Strongyloides stercoralis*
  - Uncommon parasite
  - Can be asymptomatic but severe hyperinfection reported

Whipworms
- *Trichuris vulpis*
  - Predilection for caecum and LI, causing colitis-like signs

Trematodes (flukes/flatworms)
Alaria alata
- Most prevalent in Eastern Europe; not recorded in UK
- Usually asymptomatic

Heterobilharzia americanum
- Endemic in southeastern United States, causing canine schistosomiasis
- Infection by:
  - Ingestion of snail intermediate host or penetration of the skin by cercariae while dogs are swimming/wading in contaminated water
  - Cercariae migrate through the lungs and to the liver; adults then move via the portal veins to the mesenteric veins to mate and deposit eggs which produce proteolytic enzymes allowing penetration through the mesenteric veins and intestinal mucosa to enter the intestine
- Granulomatous enteritis ± liver disease
  - Can be fatal
  - Typical chronic GI signs of vomiting and diarrhoea, weight loss, etc.

ORGAN SYSTEMS

Major signs
- Diarrhoea
- Haematochezia
- Weight loss

Minor signs
- Pot belly
- Pruritus at sites of skin penetration, e.g. *Heterobilharzia*, *Uncinaria*
- Visible parasites in vomit or stool
- Vomiting

Potential sequelae
- Infections may be asymptomatic but treatment is justified by the zoonotic risk
- Death from severe hookworm or *Heterobilharzia* infection

Predisposition
- Young animals

Historical clues
- Known infection of in-contact dogs
- Lack of worming history

Clinical examination
- Ranges from normal to emaciation

Laboratory findings
Haematology
- Often unremarkable
- Anaemia (regenerative or iron deficiency) with blood-sucking parasites
- Eosinophilia more common with parasites that embed in the mucosa, e.g. hookworm, whipworm, or are within blood vessels, e.g. *Heterobilharzia*

Serum biochemistry
- Often unremarkable
- Mild/moderate hypoproteinaemia if blood loss
- Increased liver enzymes caused by larval migration

Faecal examination
- Baermann technique for *Strongyloides* larvae
- Faecal antigen tests for helminths and cestodes

- Identification of cestode, nematode and trematode ova
  - Formalin-ether most reliable for most ova
  - Sugar or salt flotation and sedimentation methods less suitable due to faecal fat content
  - Salt sedimentation for *Heterobilharzia*

Imaging
Radiographs and ultrasound
- Often unremarkable

Special investigations
- *Heterobilharzia*
  - Faecal PCR
  - Intestinal biopsy

Treatment
NB: There is geographical variation in availability and licensing of anthelmintics.
- Cestodes
  - Bunamidine
  - Epsiprantel
  - Praziquantel
- Helminths
  - Emodepside
  - Fenbendazole
  - Febantel
  - Macrocyclic lactones: ivermectin, selamectin, moxidectin, and milbemycin oxime
    - Ivermectin not safe in breeds with MDR1 mutation, i.e. Collies, etc.
    - Ivermectin recommended for *Strongyloides*, but other macrocyclic lactones not tested
  - Nitroscanate
  - Piperazine for roundworms
  - Pyrantel; not effective against *Trichuris*
- Trematodes
  - Combined praziquantel and fenbendazole
  - High-dose praziquantel
  - Prolonged fenbendazole course

Monitoring
- Routine faecal flotation or periodic empirical deworming

Prognosis
- Excellent with appropriate treatment

ORGAN SYSTEMS

5.1.5.2F INTESTINAL PROTOZOAL INFECTIONS

Aetiology
Protozoal organisms can cause intestinal infections with signs of diarrhoea, etc. Infection is typically acquired from ingestion of contaminated water.
- Amoebiasis
  - *Entamoeba histolytica* is a rare canine infection causing colitis
  - Reverse zoonosis in sub-tropical and tropical countries
- Coccidiosis
  - *Cryptosporidium*
    - Rare infection in dogs and often asymptomatic
  - *Cystoisospora* (formerly *Isospora*):
    - *Four species: C. canis, C. ohioensis, C. neorivolta and C. burrowsi*
    - Coccidia infection is only considered significant in puppies
    - Any infection in adult is likely secondary to an underlying enteropathy
  - *Hammondia* and *Sarcocystis* coccidia are rarely diagnosed
- Giardiasis
  - *Giardia* infection is common in dogs: up to 40% of puppies
  - Assemblages (genotypes) C and D differ from human infections, but A and B assemblages infecting humans have been found in canine faeces
  - Pathogenicity is debated as infection is reported to cause:
    - Asymptomatic self-limiting infection
    - Asymptomatic carrier status
    - Acute self-limiting gastroenteritis
    - Chronic enteritis
  - Re-infection is possible
- Other motile protozoa
  - *Tritrichomonas* is an infection of cats but has been reported once in symptomatic dogs
  - Other ciliated or flagellated, motile protozoa (*Balantidium, Pentatrichomonas*) are considered commensals

Major signs
- Diarrhoea

Minor signs
- Colitis-like signs
- Weight loss

Potential sequelae
- Chronic infection
- Self-limiting infection

Predisposition
- Co-infection or underlying enteropathy
- Young animals
  - After stresses, such as weaning
  - Poor nutrition, poor sanitation, or overcrowding

Historical clues
- Access to infected hosts or contaminated environment

Clinical examination
- Ranging from normal to poor body condition

Laboratory findings
Haematology and serum biochemistry
- Usually unremarkable
- Rarely hypoproteinaemia
- Faecal examination
  - Coccidia
    - Acid-fast stain for *Cryptosporidium*
    - ELISA
    - Faecal flotation
    - Immunofluorescence
  - *Giardia*
    - Antigen testing: ELISA or SNAP® test
      - More sensitive than zinc sulphate flotation of single sample
      - May remain positive for some time after treatment
    - Immunofluorescence
    - Wet preparation and direct microscopy insensitive

- Zinc sulphate flotation
  - Oocysts difficult to recognise if inexperienced
  - Testing three samples is 95% sensitive
  - Pooled samples collected over three days may be adequate if well-mixed

Imaging
- Usually unremarkable

Special investigations
- Search for co-infections

Treatment
NB. Geographical variation in availability and licensing of anti-protozoals
- *Cryptosporidium*
  - Nitazoxanide most likely to be effective
  - Azithromycin and tylosin have been recommended; paromomycin has been recommended but is toxic
- *Cystoisospora*
  - Amprolium
  - Sulfonamides or trimethoprim-sulfa
  - Toltrazuril: 10–30 mg/kg PO q24h for 1–3 days
    - Diclazuril or ponazuril are alternatives in some countries
- *Giardia*
  - Combination of praziquantel, pyrantel and febantel
  - Fenbendazole: 50 mg/kg PO q24h for 3–5 days
  - Metronidazole: 25 mg/kg PO q 12h for 5–7 days
    - High dose required and close to neurotoxic dose
  - Environmental decontamination
    - Prevent access to contaminated water source
    - Treat asymptomatic animals in the household
    - Wash coat to remove oocysts

Monitoring
- Clinical signs
- Repeat faecal examination, but antigen test may remain positive for some time and possibly infection is only ever suppressed not eliminated

Prognosis
- Most infections are either self-limiting or can be effectively treated
- Resistance is sometimes suspected
  - Combination of fenbendazole and metronidazole suggested
  - Prevent re-infection

5.1.5.2G   LYMPHANGIECTASIA

Aetiology
- Abnormal dilatation of the intestinal lymphatics leading to:
  - Fat malabsorption
  - Protein-losing enteropathy (PLE) from lipoprotein loss
- Causes
  - Congenital malformation
  - Idiopathic
    - May have associated lymphangitis and lipogranulomas
    - Occasionally there is concurrent chylothorax
  - Secondary obstruction
    - Neoplastic infiltration
    - Pericardial disease
    - Right heart failure

Major signs
- Chronic diarrhoea: may occur later in disease after ascites develops
- Weight loss

Minor signs
- Ascites and/or generalised subcutaneous oedema and/or hydrothorax if PLE
- Polyphagia in early stages

Potential sequelae
- PLE
- Thromboembolism
- Severe cachexia

Predisposition
- Breed associations
  - Maltese terrier
  - Norwegian Lundehund
  - Rottweiler

- Soft-coated Wheaten terrier
  - May have concurrent protein-losing nephropathy (PLN)
  - May not be a true lymphangiectasia but CIE/IBD and secondary lymphatic dilation
- Yorkshire terrier

Historical clues
- Intractable wasting disease

Clinical examination
- Ascites/generalised subcutaneous oedema/muffled heart sounds with pleural effusion secondary to PLE
- Poor body condition

Laboratory findings
Haematology
- Lymphopenia

Serum biochemistry
- Panhypoproteinaemia typical of PLE
- Hypocalcaemia, reflecting hypoalbuminaemia
- Hypocholesterolaemia suggestive of fat malabsorption
- Serum folate and cobalamin can be normal as they are not absorbed via the lymphatics

Imaging
Radiographs
- Often unremarkable

Ultrasound examination
- Bowel wall thickening may be due to tissue oedema
- Hyperechoic striations in mucosa representing dilated lacteals

Special investigations
- Faecal α_1-PI: only available in North America
  - May detect PLE before hypoproteinaemia develops
  - Potential screening test in predisposed breeds
- Folate and cobalamin, *q.v.* sections 3.15, 3.10 respectively
  - Unchanged, as water-, not fat-, soluble

- Intestinal biopsy
  - Diagnosis is by histological appearance but disease may be patchy
  - Grossly dilated lymphatics seen on endoscopy if duodenum is affected
  - Full-thickness surgical biopsies from several levels of the SI may be needed for an accurate diagnosis
  - Presence of lipogranulomas (multiple, small white spots) on mesentery at laparotomy is very suggestive

Treatment
- Prednisolone (up to 1 mg/kg/day) may reduce associated inflammation and produce a clinical improvement
- Low-fat diet reduces fat malabsorption and amount of diarrhoea
  - A reduced-fat, highly digestible diet is indicated
  - A low-fat, weight-reducing diet is contra-indicated
  - Successful treatment with ultra-low-fat diet reported
- Positive response to ciclosporin reported anecdotally

Monitoring
- Clinical response
- Serum proteins

Prognosis
- Guarded
  - Can cause intractable diarrhoea and weight loss
  - Can respond to steroids
  - Can resolve spontaneously

5.1.6 LARGE INTESTINE

Problems
Presenting complaints
q.v. section 1
- Faecal incontinence
- Flatulence
- Haematochezia
- Tenesmus and dyschezia
- Vomiting

Physical abnormalities
q.v. section 2
- Abdominal discomfort/pain
- Abdominal enlargement

Laboratory abnormalities
q.v. section 3
- Anaemia
- Hyperkalaemia
- Hyponatraemia
- Leukocytosis

Diagnostic Approach
- Constipation causing tenesmus should be distinguished from diarrhoea by history and physical examination.
- Diarrhoea is usually a diffuse problem affecting both the SI and LI causing 'mixed pattern diarrhoea'. However, primary LI disease can occur and can be localised to the LI by the nature of diarrhoea and defecation distinguished by:
  - Clinical signs
    - Increased frequency
    - No weight loss
    - Tenesmus
  - Faecal characteristics
    - Haematochezia
    - Mucoid
    - Small volume
- Extent of investigations and the rapidity with which they are performed depends on:
  - How acute or chronic the problem is
  - How severe the problem is
- In chronic disease colonoscopy is indicated if dietary therapy fails.

Diagnostic Methods
History
- Deformation of stool shape by pelvic mass
- Haematochezia with diarrhoea suggests colitis
- Haematochezia without diarrhoea suggests focal bleeding, especially neoplastic disease
- Tenesmus before passing any faeces suggests constipation
- Tenesmus after diarrhoea suggests colitis
- Weight loss is not a feature unless advanced neoplasia or repeated withholding of food

Clinical examination
Abdominal palpation for constipation or mass

Rectal examination
- Constipation
- Diarrhoea
- Haematochezia
- Rectal mass
- Rule out perineal hernia as cause of tenesmus

Laboratory findings
- Usually unremarkable
- Hyponatraemia and hyperkalaemia reported with whipworm infection

Imaging
Radiographs
- Abdominal mass
- Accumulated faecal material in constipation
- Often unremarkable

Ultrasound
- Thickened wall and loss of layering with neoplastic diseases
- Often unremarkable

Special investigative techniques
- Colonoscopy

5.1.6A ACUTE COLITIS

Aetiology
Dietary
- Dietary indiscretion
- Change in diet
  - Overindulgence
  - Scavenging
  - Sudden change in diet
- Food allergy
- Food intolerance
- Toxins, especially garbage

Infection – Bacterial
- *Campylobacter*
- *Clostridium*
- *E. coli*

Infection – Parasitic
- *Giardia*; infects SI, but can cause colitis-like signs
- *Trichuris* whipworms

Infection – Viral
- Parvovirus

Inflammatory
- CIE/IBD

Traumatic
- Abrasions from bone fragments

Major signs
- Diarrhoea
  - ± Haematochezia
  - Mucus
  - Small volume
- Tenesmus

Minor signs
- Abdominal discomfort

Potential sequelae
- Progression to chronic colitis

Predisposition
- Young dogs are more likely to scavenge

Historical clues
- Contact with possible sources of infection
- Known access to inappropriate diet
- Opportunity to scavenge

Clinical examination
- Unremarkable in mild cases
- Dull/depressed
- Mild mid-caudal abdominal discomfort
- No other abnormality on abdominal palpation

Laboratory findings
- Often unremarkable

Faecal examination
- *Giardia* oocysts
- *Trichuris* ova
- Stool culture can be misleading

Imaging
Radiographs
- Unremarkable

Special investigations
- ACTH stimulation test if abnormal electrolytes

Treatment
Symptomatic treatment
- *Nil per os*
- Parenteral fluid therapy as necessary

Antibiotics
May be needed in haemorrhagic diarrhoea if dog is sytemically unwell

Anti-diarrhoeals
- Opioid motility modifiers
  - Loperamide @ 0.1 mg//kg PO TID
- Dietary fibre: acts by absorbing free water and providing colonocyte nutrients
- A short course of sulfasalazine may be effective, *q.v.* section 5.1.6B

Monitoring
- Clinical response: signs are likely to be self limiting
- If the dog is not improving after 72 hours of symptomatic therapy, the case should be re-assessed

Prognosis
Good for complete recovery

5.1.6B   CHRONIC COLITIS

Aetiology
- CIE/IBD
  - Eosinophilic colitis (or gastro-enterocolitis)
  - Lympho-plasmacytic colitis (and enteritis): most common
- Colonic infection
  - *Clostridium difficile*
  - *Clostridium perfringens*
  - *Histoplasma capsulatum*: fungal infection found in Mississippi, Missouri, and Ohio River valleys in United States; along the

southern Great Lakes and the St. Lawrence Seaway in Canada; not in UK
- *Trichuris* whipworms
- Food allergy
- Granulomatous (histiocytic ulcerative) colitis, *q.v.* section 5.1.6D

Major signs
- Diarrhoea
  - Haematochezia
  - Mucus
  - Small volume
- Tenesmus
- Weight loss is not a feature

Minor signs
- Abdominal discomfort

Potential sequelae
- Persistence of problem

Predisposition
- Granulomatous (histiocytic ulcerative) colitis in young Boxers and French bulldogs
- Idiopathic lympho-plasmacytic colitis: GSD

Historical clues
- Clinical signs
- No weight loss unless food is withheld

Clinical examination
- Usually unremarkable

Rectal examination
- Blood and mucus
- Thickened irregular mucosa

Laboratory findings
Haematology and serum biochemistry
- Usually unremarkable
- Blood loss anaemia is uncommon

Faecal examination
- *Trichuris* ova

Imaging
Radiographs
Plain
- Unremarkable

Contrast
- Not very helpful
- Thickened, irregular, ulcerated mucosa

Special investigations
- Colonoscopy and biopsy
- Folate and cobalamin, *q.v.* sections 3.15, 3.10 respectively
  - If abnormal, indicates concurrent SI disease

Treatment
A diet trial is recommended before any drug therapy.

Antibacterials
- May reduce the antigenic burden on the mucosal immune system, but not shown to be of benefit in combination with immunosuppressants
  - Metronidazole @ 10–15 mg/kg PO BID/TID
    - Active against colonic anaerobes
    - Limited evidence of immune modulatory effect
    - Risk of neurotoxicity with chronic use

Anti-inflammatories
- Prednisolone
- Sulfasalazine @ 10–20 mg/kg PO BID
  - 5-Aminosalicylic acid derivative, released in colon with direct anti-inflammatory effect
  - Contra-indicated if concurrent SI inflammation is present
  - Keratoconjunctivitis is a serious side effect: perform periodic Schirmer tear tests

Diet
- Response to exclusion diet suggests food allergy, not idiopathic CIE/IBD
- Easily digestible, hypoallergenic is helpful
- Fibre
  - Moderately fermentable for colonocyte nutrition
    e.g. ispaghula, beet pulp, chicory
  - Non-fermentable to regulate motility and bind water
    e.g. wheat bran
- Response to exclusion diet suggests foood-responsive enteropathy or allergy, and not idiopathic CIE/IBD

Easily digestible
- Prednisolone/azathioprine/chlorambucil, *q.v.* section 5.1.5.2C

Monitoring
- Clinical response
- Periodic Schirmer tear test if using sulfasalazine
- Repeat colonoscopy

Prognosis
- Excellent for parasitic colitis
- Good for control of lymphoplasmacytic colitis

5.1.6C   CONSTIPATION

Aetiology
- *q.v.* section 1.11

Major signs
- Dyschezia
- Failure to pass faeces or small, hard, dry faeces
- Haematochezia if intraluminal cause
- Tenesmus

Minor signs
- Anorexia
- Lethargy
- Paradoxical diarrhoea: scant liquid faeces passed around the sides of constipated mass
- Vomiting

Potential sequelae
- Progressively worsening constipation leading to:
  - Obstipation
    - Disruption of colonic musculature and development of megacolon

Predisposition, Historical clues, Clinical examination, Laboratory findings, Imaging, Special investigations
- *q.v.* section 1.11

Treatment
Correct underlying cause
- Rehydration
- Castration for prostatomegaly
- Stop drugs
- Surgery for perineal disease

Dietary modification
- Non-fermentable fibre, e.g. wheat bran
- Moderately fermentable fibre, e.g. ispaghula, psyllium, sterculia

Laxatives
- For treatment and ongoing prevention
- Osmotic
  - Lactulose
  - Polyethylene glycol (PEG 3350)
- Lubricant
  - Liquid paraffin (mineral oil); beware of inhalation
  - Paraffin paste
- Surfactant
  - Docusate
  - Sodium citrate
- Stimulant
  - Castor oil
  - Danthron/poloxamer
- Glycerol

Enemas
- Docusate
- Phosphate; not in toy breeds
- Warm soapy water

Monitoring
- Ability to pass faeces naturally

Prognosis
- Good for mild constipation if underlying cause can be addressed
- Poor if severe obstipation or uncorrectable underlying cause

ORGAN SYSTEMS

5.1.6D GRANULOMATOUS (HISTIOCYTIC ULCERATIVE) COLITIS

Aetiology
- Intracellular infection in the colon by attaching and invading *E. coli* (AIEC)
- Predisposition for Boxers and French bulldogs related to mutation(s) in neutrophil or macrophage bacteriocidal activity

Major signs
- Colitis
  - Diarrhoea
  - Haematochezia
  - Tenesmus

Minor signs
- Weight loss

Potential sequelae
- Antibacterial resistance
- Iron deficiency anaemia

Predisposition
- Young dogs
- Boxers and French bulldogs almost exclusively, but also reported in Alaskan malamute

Historical clues
- Young dog with severe colitis
- Poor response to immunosuppression

Clinical examination
- Poor body condition

Rectal examination
- Digital rectal examination
- Fresh blood and mucus
- Diarrhoea
- Thickened, irregular mucosa

Laboratory findings
- Usually unremarkable

Imaging
Radiographs
Plain
- Unremarkable

Contrast
- Not very helpful
- Thickened, irregular, ulcerated mucosa

Special investigations
- Colonoscopy and biopsy
- Culture and sensitivity testing of *E. coli* isolated from tissue
- Staining of periodic acid schiff (PAS)-positive macrophages in biopsies
- Fluorescent *in-situ* hybridisation (FISH) localisation of AIEC

Treatment
- Fluoroquinolones for 4–6 weeks can be curative, but development of antibiotic resistance is a problem
- Ideally based on culture and sensitivity performed before treatment
- Poor response to immunosuppressants

Monitoring
- Clinical response
- Repeat colonoscopy and biopsy

Prognosis
- Guarded, as antibiotic resistance may develop

5.1.6E LARGE INTESTINAL NEOPLASIA

Aetiology
- Spontaneous tumour; clear mutation pathway in humans not yet demonstrated
  - Adenocarcinoma most commonly affecting rectum or caecum
  - Benign polyps usually in rectum
  - Lymphoma

Major signs
- Constipation
- Haematochezia
- Tenesmus

Minor signs
- Deformation of stool
- Diarrhoea
- Dyschezia

- Dysuria
- Weight loss in advanced disease

Potential sequelae
Adenocarcinoma
- Metastasis to sublumbar LN, liver, lungs
- Obstruction of colon

Benign polyps
- May theoretically undergo malignant transformation

Lymphoma
- May be part of diffuse disease or restricted to rectum and distal colon, *q.v.* section 5.1.5.2A

Predisposition
- More common in older dogs

Historical clues
- Presence of fresh blood on stool of normal consistency is suggestive of a bleeding mass and not colitis

Clinical examination
- Mass or constipation on abdominal palpation

Rectal examination
- Haematochezia
- Mass

Laboratory findings
- Usually unremarkable

Imaging
Radiographs
Plain
- Caudal abdominal mass
- Sublumbar lymphadenopathy
- Pulmonary metastasis

Contrast
- Barium enema may identify mass, but superseded by colonoscopy

Ultrasound examination
- Caudal abdominal mass
- Sublumbar lymphadenopathy

Special investigations
- Colonoscopy and biopsy

Treatment
- Removal of polyp
  - Eversion of rectum and submucosal resection is curative
  - Traction and avulsion often result in recurrence
- Surgical resection of carcinoma, but often inoperable

Monitoring
- Recurrence of constipation and/or haematochezia

Prognosis
- Excellent for polyp, although recurrence can occur if not complete excision
- Grave for carcinoma

5.1.7 PANCREAS

Problems
Presenting complaints
q.v. section 1
- Anorexia or polyphagia
- Diarrhoea
- Haematemesis
- Haematochezia
- Melaena
- Polyuria/polydipsia (PU/PD)
- Vomiting
- Weight loss

Physical abnormalities
q.v. section 2
- Abdominal discomfort/pain
- Pyrexia
- Icterus/jaundice

Laboratory abnormalities
q.v. section 3
- Amylase and lipase
- Azotaemia
- Bile acids
- Bilirubin
- Hypocalcaemia

ORGAN SYSTEMS

ORGAN SYSTEMS

- Hyperglycaemia
- Hyperlipidaemia/hypercholesterolaemia
- Hypokalaemia
- Hyperglobulinaemia
- Liver enzyme alterations
- Leukocytosis
- Leukopenia
- Canine pancreatic lipase (cPL)
- Canine trypsin-like immunoreactivity (cTLI)

Diagnostic Methods
History
- Malabsorption (polyphagia, diarrhoea, weight loss) with EPI
- Vomiting with pancreatitis

Clinical examination
- Abdominal palpation for masses and pain

Laboratory findings
- *q.v.* specific conditions below

Serum amylase, lipase and DGGR lipase
- Not highly specific
- Hyperlipasaemia noted in Boxers

Serum trypsin-like immunoreactivity (cTLI)
- Assay measures circulating trypsinogen and trypsin
  - Decreased in EPI
  - Increased in pancreatitis

Serum pancreatic lipase (cPL)
- Assay measures circulating pancreatic lipase
  - Decreased in EPI
  - Increased in pancreatitis

Imaging
Radiographs
q.v. specific conditions below

Ultrasound
- Abnormalities of size and echogenicity in pancreas

Special investigative techniques
- Pancreatic biopsy

5.1.7A   ACUTE PANCREATITIS

Aetiology
- Spontaneous inflammation of pancreas
  - Activation of proteases and phospholipases within pancreas initiate autodigestion
  - Inflammation spreads to cause localised peritonitis and fat necrosis
  - Systemic release of proteases eventually overwhelms circulating anti-proteases and reticulo-endothelial system and then causes systemic problems
- Severity of the condition varies from mild, oedematous pancreatitis to severe necrotising pancreatitis
- Specific cause not known, but risk factors identified
  - High-fat diet/dietary indiscretion
  - Obesity
  - Hyperlipidaemia
    - Hyperadrenocorticism (HAC)
    - Primary hyperlipidaemia
  - Inherited mutation of trypsinogen or pancreatic secretory inhibitor not proven in dogs
  - Pancreatic ischaemia
    - Anaesthesia
    - GDV
    - Hypovolaemia
  - Trauma
  - Drugs
    - Azathioprine
    - L-asparaginase
    - Potassium bromide
  - NB: Corticosteroids are *not* now considered a risk factor.

Major signs
- Abdominal pain
  - May adopt the 'prayer' position but not pathognomonic and often absent
- Diarrhoea
- Icterus if bile duct obstructed by pancreatic inflammation (extrahepatic bile duct obstruction, EHBDO)
- Vomiting

Minor signs
- Anorexia
- Depression
- Haematochezia
- Melaena
- Pyrexia

Potential sequelae
Local
- Pancreatic abscess
- Pseudocyst
- Recurrent episodes

Systemic
- Acute renal failure
- Cardiac arrhythmias
- Pleural effusion

Leading to:
- Shock
- DIC
- Death

Predisposition
- Obese, middle-aged females
- Hyperlipidaemia: Miniature schnauzer
- Toy breeds, but may be environmental factors (diet, lack of exercise, etc.)

Historical clues
- Sudden onset of GI signs
- Abdominal pain in 60% of cases
- Diarrhoea in 33% of cases
- Vomiting in 90% of cases
- Episode of dietary indiscretion

Clinical examination
- Dull and depressed
- Cranial abdominal discomfort or pain

Laboratory findings
Haematology
- Leukocytosis with neutrophilia and left shift

Serum biochemistry
- Transient hyperglycaemia
- Hyperlipidaemia
- Occasional hypocalcaemia
- Increased liver enzymes
- Hyperbilirubinaemia if EHBDO
- Increased amylase, *q.v.* section 3.3
  - Low sensitivity and specificity (62 and 71%, respectively)
- Increased lipase, *q.v.* section 3.3
  - Greater sensitivity but lower specificity (73 and 55%, respectively)
  - DGGR-lipase more specific but probably not as specific as cPL

Urinalysis
- Hypersthenuria is appropriate

Imaging
Plain radiographs
- Classic radiographic changes are unreliable and non-specific
  - Lateral displacement of duodenum by pancreatic mass seen on ventro-dorsal (VD) view
  - Localised peritonitis giving loss of detail in right cranial quadrant
  - Ileus of adjacent duodenum and transverse colon

Ultrasound examination
- Sensitivity of pancreatic ultrasound is operator-dependent
  - Abscess or pseudocyst rare
  - Free fluid around pancreas
  - Hyperechoic fat
  - Mottled echogenicity
  - Pain when pressure applied with probe
  - Thickened

Special investigations
- Increased cTLI, *q.v.* section 3.28
  - Assay range is for low values to diagnose EPI; dilutions may be needed to quantify increases
  - Low sensitivity and moderate specificity (33 and 65%, respectively)
  - Transient rise early in the disease, then normalises or goes subnormal
- Increased cPL, *q.v.* section 3.21
  - Good sensitivity and high specificity (80 and >95%, respectively)
- Pancreatic biopsy

- Definitive diagnosis but risk of hypotension during anaesthesia and handling of pancreas may make pancreatitis worse

Treatment
- Establish food intake as soon as possible, once vomiting is controlled
- Parenteral fluids
- Plasma transfusion to replace circulating anti-proteases
- Analgesia: choice depends on severity
  - Buprenorphine or methadone
  - Fentanyl epidural
  - Intraperitoneal bupivacaine
  - Morphine-lidocaine-ketamine (MLK infusion)
- Antibiotic cover debatable
- Corticosteroids generally considered contra-indicated but one unblinded study showed benefit
- Fuzapladib blocks activation of adhesion molecules (integrin) expressed on the inflammatory cell surface to prevent inflammatory cells from adhering to vascular endothelial cells and infiltrating tissue thereby control exacerbation of pancreatitis. Currently only marketed in Japan.
- Ultrasound-guided drainage or partial pancreatectomy for pseudocyst or abscess
- Convalescence on fat-restricted diet

Monitoring
- Clinical response
- Repeat ultrasound examination may not distinguish active from inactive disease

Prognosis
- Good with mild pancreatitis
- Potentially fatal with necrotising pancreatitis

5.1.7B   CHRONIC PANCREATITIS

Aetiology
- Possible autoimmune pancreatitis in Cocker spaniels
- Repeated attacks of acute pancreatitis or smouldering low-grade inflammation

- Replacement of acinar tissue with fibrous tissue eventually; may form fibrotic mass

Major signs
- Abdominal discomfort
- Vomiting

Minor signs
- Abdominal mass if excessive fibrosis
- Diarrhoea
- Jaundice from EHBDO
- Weight loss

Potential sequelae
- Diabetes mellitus (DM)
- EHBDO
- EPI

Predisposition
- As for acute pancreatitis

Historical clues
- Repeated episodes of GI signs

Clinical examination
- Cranial abdominal discomfort
- Occasionally pancreatic mass is palpable

Laboratory findings
Haematology
- Mild inflammatory leukogram

Serum biochemistry
- Amylase and lipase even less sensitive than in acute pancreatitis
- Increased ALP activity; tends to be >ALT activity increase
- Hyperbilirubinaemia if EHBDO
- Hyperglycaemia if DM develops

Imaging
Radiographs
Plain
- Same non-specific changes as for acute pancreatitis
- Cranial abdominal mass
- Mass may be calcified

Ultrasound examination
• Abnormal pancreatic mass

Special investigations
• Pancreatic biopsy
• Sensitivity and specificity of cTLI, cPL is unknown

Treatment
• Supportive care as for acute pancreatitis
• Maintenance on fat-restricted diet
• Controlled weight loss
• Oral pancreatic enzymes have not been shown to be beneficial
• Biliary diversion (e.g. cholecystoduodenos-tomy) for EHBDO

Monitoring
• Clinical response
• If weight loss occurs
  • Blood and urine glucose for development of DM
  • cTLI for development of EPI

Prognosis
• Guarded for short-term alleviation
• Poor for long-term success; repeated episodes and progression likely

5.1.7C EXOCRINE PANCREATIC INSUFFICIENCY (EPI)

Aetiology
• Malabsorption from failure of digestion as a consequence of a lack of pancreatic enzymes
• Congenital pancreatic hypoplasia
  • Rare
  • May have concurrent DM
• End-stage chronic pancreatitis
• Pancreatic acinar atrophy
  • Heritable trait proven in GSD and Rough collie
  • May be auto-immune, as preceding lym-phocytic pancreatitis reported
  • Most common cause of EPI

Major signs
• Diarrhoea
  • Large volume
  • Steatorrhoea
  • Variable consistency ('cow-pat' to watery)
• Polyphagia, including coprophagia
• Weight loss

Minor signs
• Occasional tenesmus
• Poor, greasy coat
• Polydipsia – 'eating water'
• Vomiting

Potential sequelae
• Cachexia
• DM if hypoplasia or chronic pancreatitis
• Intestinal volvulus

Predisposition
Chronic pancreatitis
• Older dogs
• Miniature schnauzer
• Cocker spaniel

Pancreatic acinar atrophy
• 6 months–6 years of age
• GSDs represent two-thirds of cases
• Collies, Chow Chow, CKC spaniel, small terriers

Historical clues
• Signs of malabsorption
  i.e. Diarrhoea and weight loss despite an increased/ravenous appetite

Clinical examination
• Bright and alert
• Poor body condition
• Poor greasy coat

Laboratory findings
Haematology
• Usually unremarkable

Serum biochemistry
• Usually unremarkable
• Hypocholesterolaemia

Urinalysis
• May have low urine specific gravity (USG) if polydipsic

Imaging
Radiographs
Unremarkable, except for poor abdominal detail due to loss of fat

Ultrasound examination
• Pancreas cannot be identified, but it is not always visible in normal dogs

Special investigations
• Folate and cobalamin
  • Increased folate and decreased cobalamin are common because of secondary SIBO, and lack of pancreatic intrinsic factor
• cTLI
  • Subnormal cTLI (0.1–2.5 µg/l; normal 5.0–35 µg/l) is diagnostic
  • Very high sensitivity and specificity

Treatment
Exogenous enzyme supplementation
• Fresh pancreas (100–200 g per meal) works best
• Dried, powdered extract can be effective
• Enteric coated preparations are least effective

Diet
• Highly digestible
• Fat restriction is controversial as it reduces secondary bacterial fermentation and hence diarrhoea, but it restricts the calorie intake so the dog can't gain weight
• Feed two to three meals per day; more frequent meals require more enzyme, which is expensive
• Feed more than maintenance calories for the dog's ideal body weight so that it gains weight

Antibiotics
• Secondary SIBO complicates EPI
• Give 10 mg/kg oxytetracycline PO with each meal

Vitamins
• Vitamin B$_{12}$
  • By injection or, despite the lack of intrinsic factor from the pancreas, oral supplementation
  • Monitoring
• Stool consistency
• Weight gain

Prognosis
• Good for control
• Life-long condition

5.2 CARDIOVASCULAR SYSTEM

Problems
Presenting complaints
q.v. section 1
1.5 Anorexia
1.13 Coughing
1.18 Dyspnoea and tachypnoea
1.22 Exercise intolerance
1.51 Weakness, collapse and syncope
1.53 Weight loss

Physical abnormalities
q.v. section 2
2.1 Abdominal enlargement
2.3 Abnormal lung sounds
2.4 Arrhythmias
2.5 Ascites
2.6 Cyanosis
2.8 Hepatomegaly
2.15 Murmur
2.20 Peripheral oedema

Laboratory abnormalities
q.v. section 3
3.4 Azotaemia (pre-renal)
3.8 Cardiac biomarkers
3.30.2 Erythrocytosis (polycythaemia)

Diagnostic Approach
1 Suspect cardiac disease from clinical signs and physical examination
   - Auscultation
   - Capillary refill
   - Palpation of pulses
   - Percussion
2 ECG
3 Blood pressure (BP)
4 Echocardiography
5 Radiography
6 Cardiac catheterisation in some cases

Diagnostic Methods
History
- May be minimal history if cardiac disease is compensated
- Likely presenting complaints and physical abnormalities listed above

Clinical examination
Visual inspection
- Body condition may be poor with severe congestive heart failure (CHF) due to loss of muscle mass
- Cachexia is more common with right-sided CHF

Physical examination
- Mucous membrane colour/capillary refill time (CRT)
  - Cyanosis, *q.v.* section 2.6
    - Assess cranial and caudal mucous membranes as differential cyanosis can occur
  - Pallor suggests poor peripheral circulation with vasoconstriction or reduced haemoglobin: check PCV to differentiate
  - Prolonged CRT implies reduced perfusion, e.g. cardiogenic shock, hypovolaemic shock
- Jugular veins
  - Hepatojugular reflux: apply firm pressure to the cranial abdomen for 1 minute, which will displace blood from congested liver into the caudal vena cava and therefore increase return to the right atrium; this will cause jugular filling if the right atrium is unable to accommodate the increased venous return
  - Jugular distension and pulsation is an indicator of increased right atrial pressures
- Palpation
  - Abdomen
    - Ascites; if there is also jugular distension: suggests right-sided CHF
    - Hepatomegaly due to congestion
  - Apex beat
    - Apex beat can be displaced to the right with ventricular enlargement or masses
    - Less obvious in obese, barrel-chested animals or with pericardial or pleural effusions
    - Prominent in thin-skinned and narrow-chested dogs

ORGAN SYSTEMS

Notes on Canine Internal Medicine, Fourth Edition. Victoria L. Black, Kathryn F. Murphy, Jessie Rose Payne, and Edward J. Hall.
© 2022 John Wiley & Sons Ltd. Published 2022 by John Wiley & Sons Ltd.

- Prominent with increased sympathetic tone: post-exercise and in hyperkinetic conditions, e.g. anaemia
- Extremities
  - Cold periphery suggests poor cardiac output and peripheral circulatory shut down
- Precordial thrill
  - Vibrations of a heart murmur (Grade V/VI or higher) can be felt; helps to identify point of maximal intensity of murmurs that radiate widely
- Pulse
  - Palpate femoral pulse at same time as auscultation of the heart
  - Note pulse deficits ('dropped' beats), i.e. heart sounds but no pulse
  - Pulse quality affected by:
    - Difference between systolic and diastolic BP, i.e. pulse pressure: determined by heart rate, stroke volume (SV) and peripheral vascular resistance
    - Palpability: varies with conformation of hindlimbs and physical condition of dog
- Pulse character
  - Absent: iliac thrombosis, neoplasia, cardiac arrest/severe hypotension
  - Hyperkinetic: sometimes described as 'water hammer pulse' due to increased SV or reduced peripheral vascular resistance (PVR), e.g. aortic insufficiency, anaemia, bradycardia (large SV), patent ductus arteriosus (PDA)
  - Hypokinetic: reduced SV and increased PVR, e.g. cardiac tamponade, dilated cardiomyopathy (DCM), hypoadrenocorticism, tachyarrhythmias
  - *Pulsus paradoxus*: exaggerated fall in pressure with inspiration and increase in pressure with expiration; can be found in pericardial effusions
  - *Pulsus alternans* can occur with severe myocardial failure: the pulse alternates in strength despite normal sinus rhythm, reflecting an alternation in the strength of left ventricular contraction
  - Variable: usually associated with arrhythmias
- Percussion
  - Abdominal percussion (ballottement) to detect fluid thrill with ascites
  - Horizontal line of dullness in the ventral thorax with pleural effusion

Cardiac examination
Auscultation
- Ideally perform with animal standing

(a)

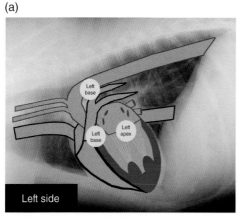

(b)

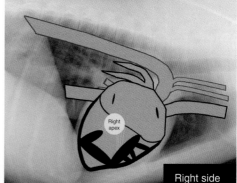

Figure 5.2.1 Auscultation
5.2.1a Left-side auscultation
Outline of normal heart superimposed on a lateral radiograph of the thorax indicating sites for auscultation of murmurs audible on the left side.
5.2.1b Right-side auscultation
Outline of normal heart superimposed on a lateral radiograph of the thorax indicating the site for auscultation of murmurs audible on the right side.

- Auscultate left and right sides over all valve areas, Figure 5.2.1
  - Begin with palpation and feel for apex beat: place stethoscope there to listen over mitral valve (left apex) and assess heart rate, rhythm and for any abnormalities in auscultation, e.g. murmur, gallop, etc.
  - Move forward one rib space at a time and reassess any abnormalities until stethoscope head is fully under the triceps muscles (left base) and cannot be moved further cranially
  - Stethoscope may need to be moved cranially and caudally several times before left-sided auscultation is complete
  - Repeat on the right side of the chest
- Normal heart sounds: only two are heard
  - S1: first sound 'lub', associated with closure of mitral/tricuspid valves and heard loudest over the apex
  - S2: second sound 'dub', associated with closure of aortic/pulmonic valves and heard loudest over the heart base
- Audibility
  - Decreased by pleural effusion, mediastinal mass, pericardial effusion, obesity
  - Increased by cardiomegaly, anaemia, thin body condition, pneumothorax
  - Intrathoracic mass may displace sounds
- Heart rate
  - Normal 70–140 beats per minute
  - Decreased
    - Bradyarrhythmia
    - Fit, healthy, relaxed patient often accompanied with sinus arrhythmia
    - Increased vagal tone, e.g. brachycephalic conformation, central nervous system (CNS) depression, gastrointestinal (GI) disease often accompanied by sinus arrhythmia
  - Increased
    - CHF
    - Fear, exercise, excitement, fever, pain
    - Tachyarrhythmia
- Rhythm
  - Assess for regularity, equality with pulse and pattern of rhythm, Figure 5.2.2a
  - Sinus arrhythmia: normal rhythm in which the rhythm speeds up and slows down in a regular pattern often, but not always associated with breathing, i.e. respiratory sinus arrhythmia speeds up with inspiration and slows with expiration Figure 5.2.2b
- Abnormal rhythms
  - Premature beats (often heard as the pause that occurs after the premature beat): isolated irregularities in rhythm can be supraventricular or ventricular in origin
  - Runs of tachycardia: can be supraventricular or ventricular in origin
  - Sustained pauses: bradyarrhythmias
  - Chaotic, irregular rhythm with no predictability: atrial fibrillation most likely
- Abnormal sounds
  - Abnormal respiratory noises, e.g. crackles with pulmonary oedema, decreased audibility ventrally with pleural effusion
  - Friction sounds due to pericardial or pleural effusions
  - Gallop sounds often indicate increased risk of CHF
    - S3: passive filling of the ventricles in early diastole – only heard in dogs with diastolic ventricular overload (e.g. DCM, PDA, etc.)
    - S4: filling of the ventricles due to atrial contraction in late diastole – only heard in dogs with high filling pressures, third-degree atrioventricular (AV) block
  - Split S2: Delayed closure of pulmonic valve (due to pulmonary hypertension, heartworm) or aortic valve (due to severe aortic stenosis) causes duplication of second heart sound
- Murmurs: vibrations due to turbulence of blood
  - Grade
    - I: Very quiet murmur not heard immediately on auscultation or in noisy surroundings
    - II: Murmur quieter than the heart sounds, often only heard at the point of maximal intensity
    - III: Murmur of similar intensity to heart sounds; prominent and immediately audible but not loud
    - IV: Murmur louder than heart sounds, often audible over large area, but no precordial thrill
    - V: Murmur louder than heart sounds with a precordial thrill

- VI: Murmur very loud with precordial thrill – can be heard with the stethoscope off the chest wall and sometimes heard without the need for a stethoscope
- Phase of cardiac cycle
  - Continuous: occurs in both systole and diastole, often with varying intensities throughout the cardiac cycle, e.g. PDA
  - Diastolic: rare and often accompanies systolic murmur (e.g. aortic endocarditis)
  - Systolic: the most common type of murmur (e.g. aortic/pulmonic stenosis, mitral/tricuspid valve regurgitation, ventricular septal defect)
- Profile
  - Crescendo-decrescendo: a murmur that gets louder and quieter, commonly due to blood being ejected from a ventricle into a blood vessel, e.g. aortic/pulmonic stenosis
  - Band shaped: a murmur that doesn't change in intensity, commonly due to blood being pushed from a high-pressure chamber to a low-pressure chamber, e.g. mitral/tricuspid regurgitation, ventricular septal defect
  - Decrescendo: a murmur that gets quieter in intensity, commonly due to blood leaking back into a ventricle from a blood vessel, e.g. aortic/pulmonic insufficiency
- Point of maximal intensity, Figure 5.2.1a
  - Left apex: mitral valve
  - Left base: aortic valve/pulmonic valve/PDA (higher up on chest compared to aortic/pulmonic valves)
  - Right apex: tricuspid valve, Figure 5.2.1b
- Radiation
  - Widely radiating murmurs are more often associated with clinically significant lesions than localised murmur
  - Depends on direction of flow of stenotic or regurgitant jet and the energy of the blood flow
  - Murmurs can radiate up the neck; auscultate this area
- Differentials for murmurs
  - Left apex
    - Systolic
      - Myxomatous mitral valve disease

- Dilated cardiomyopathy
- Mitral valve dysplasia (regurgitation): rare
- Mitral endocarditis: rare
  - Diastolic
    - Mitral valve dysplasia (stenosis): rare
- Left base
  - Systolic
    - Anaemia
    - Aortic stenosis
    - Flow murmur (up to grade III/VI)
    - Pulmonic stenosis
  - Diastolic
    - Aortic endocarditis: rare
  - Continuous
    - Patent ductus arteriosus
- Right apex - systolic
  - Ventricular septal defect
  - Tricuspid valve dysplasia: rare

Laboratory findings
- Generally unremarkable

Haematology
- Adaptive erythrocytosis in right to left shunts
- Mild anaemia and leukocytosis may be seen in CHF
- Neutrophilia and left shift may be found in endocarditis

Serum biochemistry
- ALT: slight increase is common with reduced cardiac output
- NTproBNP will increase with severity of acquired disease; less information is available about the use in congenital disease
- Plasma proteins tend to fall in CHF
- Troponin I is more likely to be increased with advanced acquired disease; less information is available about the use in congenital disease
- Urea: slight increase is common in CHF, i.e. pre-renal azotaemia

Imaging
Plain radiographs
q.v. section 4.3
- Views

- Right lateral and dorsoventral of thorax as a minimum; may not be possible in dyspnoeic patients
- Ideally both laterals and dorsoventral
- Heart size
  - Assess for generalised cardiomegaly as well as specific chamber enlargements; patients with CHF should have cardiac enlargement, Figure 4.3.5
  - Increased heart size more likely to be significant if present in both lateral and DV radiographs
  - Normal heart size does not exclude cardiac disease, but may make heart disease less likely to be the cause of clinical signs
- Vessels
  - Caudal vena caval distension suggests increased risk of developing right-sided CHF
  - Post-stenotic dilation of the aorta may be seen in cases of aortic stenosis
  - Post-stenotic dilation of the pulmonary artery may be seen in cases of pulmonic stenosis
  - Pulmonary arterial distension compatible with pulmonary hypertension
  - Pulmonary hypovascularity with hypovolaemia with right to left shunts, haemorrhagic shock and hypoadrenocorticism
  - Pulmonary venous distension suggests increased risk of developing left-sided CHF
- Pulmonary pattern
  - Interstitial to alveolar pattern with pulmonary oedema; this generally starts in the perihilar region but may be more generalised with more severe oedema, Figure 4.3.5
- Other
  - Pleural effusion, ascites and hepatomegaly may be seen with right-sided CHF

Special investigative techniques
- Angiography
  - Selective by cardiac catheterisation to identify intracardiac or vascular lesions
  - Use iodine solutions
- BP measurement

- Cardiac catheterisation
  - Assess central venous pressure in patients with suspected CHF
  - Measure chamber pressures
  - Obtain samples for blood gas analysis to help identify shunts
- Echocardiography
  - Useful information on structure and function of heart
    - Aids the diagnosis of congenital and acquired abnormalities
    - Bubble echocardiography provides contrast
- Electrocardiography (ECG)
  - Part of minimum data base for suspected cardiac disease
  - Usually recorded in right lateral recumbency in dogs
  - Artefacts are common with gross movement, fine movement (muscle tremor), respiration, alternating current (A/C) interference, poor baseline definition, poor electrode contact
  - Assess
    - Heart rate
    - Regularity of rhythm
    - P for every QRS
    - QRS for every P
    - P and QRS reasonably and consistently related
    - Morphology of complexes
  May indicate
    - Altered myocardial metabolism, e.g. electrolyte imbalance/hypoxia
    - Evidence of chamber enlargement/hypertrophy but not very sensitive or specific
- Real-time ECG monitoring
  - 24-hour Holter monitor
  - Telemetry (in-hospital)
  - Implantable loop recorders: prolonged recording (2–3 years of battery life) but only 'events' are saved for review
- MRI
  - Gold standard for cardiac assessment in humans; rarely used in veterinary medicine

ORGAN SYSTEMS

(a)

(b)

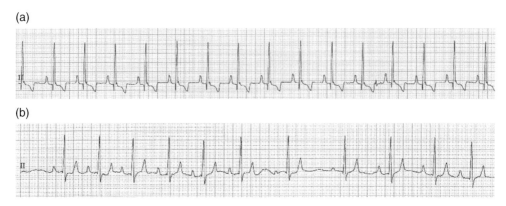

Figure 5.2.2 Normal ECG
5.2.2a Sinus rhythm
Lead II ECG showing normal sinus rhythm with regular R-R intervals (50 mm/s, 10 mm/mV).
5.2.2b Sinus arrhythmia
Lead II ECG showing variable R-R intervals between complexes due to elevated vagal tone causing sinus arrhythmia (50 mm/s, 10 mm/mV).

5.2.1 ACQUIRED CARDIAC DISEASES

Cardiac dysfunction can develop with age because of:
- Myocardial disease ± acquired arrhythmias
- Pulmonary hypertension
- Valvular insufficiency

Management
Many of these conditions lead to CHF, *q.v.* section 5.2.3 for generic management options

5.2.1A ARRHYTHMOGENIC RIGHT VENTRICULAR CARDIOMYOPATHY (ARVC)

Aetiology
- Also known as Boxer cardiomyopathy, although other breeds can be affected
- Fibro-fatty infiltration of the right ventricular myocardium resulting in ventricular arrhythmias and, in some cases, right ventricular dilation with systolic dysfunction which can lead to right-sided CHF

Major signs
- Ascites
- Asymptomatic

- Dyspnoea
- Lethargy/weakness
- Reduced exercise tolerance
- Syncope

Minor signs
- Weight loss/cachexia

Potential sequelae
- Syncopal episodes
- Development of right-sided CHF
- Sudden death

Predisposition
- Boxers
- Usually middle-aged to older dogs

Historical clues
- May be asymptomatic
- Syncopal episodes

Physical examination
- May be unremarkable
- Arrhythmias

Laboratory findings
- May be unremarkable
- Pre-renal azotaemia and increased ALT activity with very poor cardiac output

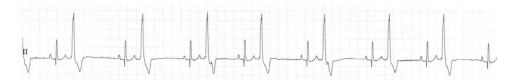

Figure 5.2.3 ARVC. Lead II ECG in a Boxer with arrhythmogenic right ventricular cardiomyopathy, showing right ventricular origin ventricular arrhythmias (50 mm/s, 10 mm/mV).

Imaging
Plain radiographs
q.v. section 4.3
- Usually normal
- May see right-sided cardiomegaly
- Pleural effusion/ascites if concurrent right-sided CHF

Echocardiography
- 2D and M-mode
  - Usually unremarkable
  - May see right heart dilation, either generalised or an outpocketing in the right ventricular outflow tract
  - May have generalised systolic dysfunction secondary to sustained arrhythmias; this often improves once the arrhythmias are controlled
- Colour Doppler and pulsed wave/continuous wave Doppler are often unremarkable

Special investigations
Electrocardiography
- May be normal due to the intermittent nature of the arrhythmias
- Right ventricular origin ventricular arrhythmias (Figure 5.2.3)

ECG Holter monitor
- Identify paroxysmal arrhythmias in cases if not detected on routine ECG
- Collect baseline for arrhythmia complexity prior to starting anti-arrhythmics (if considered safe to do so)

Treatment
- Management of ventricular arrhythmias
  - Anti-arrhythmics: choice depends on clinical signs and echocardiographic appearance; may require lidocaine, mexiletine, sotalol or amiodarone

Monitoring
- Echocardiography
- ECG Holter monitoring

Prognosis
- Many patients die suddenly but the time to death can be very variable, with some dogs living several years from diagnosis

5.2.1B   DILATED CARDIOMYOPATHY (DCM)

Aetiology
- DCM is a primary myocardial disease, manifesting as left ventricular dilation with systolic dysfunction
- The reduction in cardiac output leads to compensatory mechanisms being activated
  - Sympathetic stimulation causing tachycardia and vasoconstriction
  - Renin-angiotensin-aldosterone system (RAAS) activation to retain sodium and water, to maintain systemic BP
  - These result in increased circulating volumes and therefore increased intra-cardiac pressures, leading to further left atrial and left ventricular enlargement and eventually left-sided CHF
- Many patients develop arrhythmias, both ventricular and supraventricular, and sustained arrhythmias can lead to the development of right-sided CHF
- Some patients: left atrial and left ventricular dilation leads to stretch of the mitral annulus, leading to mitral regurgitation

- Variety of causes
  - Boutique, exotic or grain-free (BEG) diets: association not fully understood
  - Genetic defects
  - Myocarditis
  - Taurine deficiency: American Cocker spaniels
- Ventricular arrhythmias in the absence of echocardiographic abnormalities are considered a manifestation of dilated cardiomyopathy in certain predisposed breeds

Major signs
- Ascites
- Asymptomatic
- Dyspnoea
- Lethargy/weakness
- Reduced exercise tolerance
- Syncope

Minor signs
- Cough
- Weight loss/cachexia

Potential sequelae
- Development of left-sided CHF
- Development of arrhythmias (ventricular and supraventricular) leading to syncopal episodes and reduced exercise tolerance
- Sudden death is possible in all cases

Predisposition
- Boxer, Cocker spaniel, Dobermann, Great Dane, Irish wolfhound, Newfoundland, Saint Bernard
- Middle-aged to older dogs, except Portuguese Water dogs diagnosed at less than 6 months

Historical clues
- May be asymptomatic
- Syncopal episodes
- Development of murmur in susceptible breed
- Development of CHF in susceptible breed

Physical examination
- Soft band profile left apical systolic murmur secondary to valvular incompetence; not present in every case
- Arrhythmia: supraventricular and ventricular

- Gallop sounds may be detected on auscultation
- Hypokinetic pulse (poor stroke volume)
- Weight loss

Laboratory findings
- May be unremarkable
- Cardiac biomarkers (NT-proBNP and troponin I) can be used as part of screening for DCM in predisposed breeds but beware of significant breed differences in normal NT-proBNP when interpreting results, *q.v.* section 3.8
- Pre-renal azotaemia and increased ALT activity with very poor cardiac output
- Markedly increased troponin I in cases caused by myocarditis
- Reduced whole blood taurine concentrations in some American Cocker spaniels

Imaging
Plain radiographs
q.v. section 4.3
- May be normal if primarily arrhythmic manifestation
- Interstitial or alveolar pattern with left-sided CHF
- Progressive left-sided (or global) cardiomegaly
- Pulmonary venous congestion
- Pleural effusion/ascites if concurrent right-sided CHF

Echocardiography
- 2D and M-mode, Figure 5.2.4
  - Left ventricular dilation with measures of systolic function (fractional shortening, ejection fraction) reduced
  - Secondary left atrial dilation
- Colour Doppler may show mitral regurgitation into the left atrium, often with a single jet taking a central course
- Pulsed wave/continuous wave Doppler
  - Mitral regurgitation velocities are normally 5–6 m/s

Special investigations
BP
- May be normal

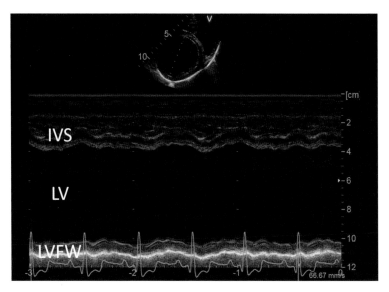

Figure 5.2.4 Dilated cardiomyopathy. M-mode echocardiogram of a dog with dilated cardiomyopathy showing a dilated left ventricle and reduced systolic function. IVS - interventricular septum; LV - left ventricle, LVFW - left ventricular free wall.

- Some patients have output failure and so are systemically hypotensive

Electrocardiography
- May be normal
- Sinus complexes may show wide P waves and tall R waves
- Arrhythmias – particularly ventricular arrhythmias and atrial fibrillation

ECG Holter monitor
- Identify paroxysmal arrhythmias in syncopal cases if not detected on routine ECG
- Collect baseline for arrhythmia complexity prior to starting anti-arrhythmics (if considered safe to do so)

Treatment
- Pre-clinical
  - Pimobendan has been shown to delay the onset of CHF
- Management of CHF
  1 Diuretics (furosemide, spironolactone)
  2 Pimobendan
  3 Angiotensin converting enzyme (ACE) inhibitors; avoid in cases of systemic hypotension
- Management of arrhythmias

- Anti-arrhythmics – depends on the ECG diagnosis, clinical signs and echocardiographic appearance
  - Atrial fibrillation: may require diltiazem, digoxin
  - Ventricular arrhythmias: may require lidocaine, mexiletine, sotalol, amiodarone
- Other
  - Diet change for those on a BEG diet
  - Taurine supplementation for those with documented deficiency

Monitoring
- Echocardiography
- ECG Holter monitoring

Prognosis
- Prognosis varies according to breed and severity of disease at presentation
  - Cocker spaniels seem to have a long course of disease
  - Dobermanns have a high incidence of sudden death with a short clinical course
  - Giant breeds identified because of arrhythmia may remain clinically silent for years
- Can survive several years with careful management
- Outlook is poor once CHF develops

ORGAN SYSTEMS

ORGAN SYSTEMS

5.2.1C HEARTWORM DISEASE/ DIROFILARIASIS

Aetiology

Canine heartworm disease is caused by a filarial nematode, *Dirofilaria immitis*, and is transmitted by mosquitos. Although it is called 'heartworm', its main effect is to cause pulmonary hypertension and thromboembolic pulmonary disease.

Another form of dirofilariosis, caused by *Dirofilaria repens*, can cause subcutaneous nodules containing larvae. It rarely causes serious disease but is potentially zoonotic.

NB: *Angiostrongylus vasorum* is known variably as a 'heartworm' or a 'lungworm', but should not be confused with *Dirofilaria* or other, rarer lungworms, e.g. *Crenosoma vulpis* (fox lungworm), *Eucoleus aerophilus* (formally *Capillaria aerophilus*), *Eucoleus boehmi*, *Filaroides hirthi*, and *Oslerus osleri* (formally *Filaroides osleri*).

Angiostrongylus causes disease when larvae migrate into the airways or through an acquired bleeding diathesis.

Major signs

High worm burden/strenuous exercise can provoke signs
- Asymptomatic often for many months to years
- Congestive heart disease (right-sided)
- Cough
- Dyspnoea
- Exercise intolerance
- Syncope

Minor signs (serious but less common)
- Caval syndrome
  - Dyspnoea
  - Haemoglobinuria
  - Heart murmur

Potential sequelae
- Adult heartworms in pulmonary vessels cause *cor pulmonale* and pulmonary hypertension
- Immune-complex glomerular disease with proteinuria

- Migration of worms into the caudal vena cava can cause hepatic and renal disease, and femoral artery occlusion
- Occasionally, severe worm burdens cause life-threatening caval syndrome
- Pulmonary thromboembolism (PTE) can develop from worm fragments and dead adult worms during treatment

Predisposition
- None

Historical clues
- Adult worms can live up to 7 years and clinical signs can present years after exposure
- Travel/movement in infected and endemic areas: North America, Mediterranean countries

Physical examination
- Often normal
- Abnormal respiratory sounds
- Dyspnoea/tachypnoea
- Pyrexia with acute PTE
- Signs of right-sided congestive heart failure: ascites, hepatomegaly, jugular venous distension
- Split heart sounds with severe pulmonary hypertension
- Weight loss

Laboratory findings
Haematology
- Often no specific changes
- Eosinophilia and basophilia
- Non-regenerative anaemia with severe disease
- Regenerative anaemia and hyperbilirubinaemia with caval syndrome

Serum biochemistry
- Increased globulins possible
- Increased liver enzymes with right-sided congestive failure
- Microfilariae may be seen on blood smear examination or blood-contaminated cytology samples
- Proteinuria ± azotaemia

Imaging
Thoracic radiographs
- Initially, normal after infection

- Interstitial pattern due to perivascular inflammation
- Enlarged right ventricle and right pulmonary artery
- Pulmonary arteries
  - Enlarged, greater than the diameter of pulmonary veins
  - Tortuous, stopping abruptly ('pruning')

Echocardiography
- Pulmonary hypertension
  - Right ventricle hypertrophy/dilation
  - Pulmonary artery dilation and increased flow velocity
  - High velocity tricuspid regurgitation
- Worms may be seen as double-lined structures in pulmonary arteries

Special investigations
Antigen and microfilariae will not be detected until at least 5–6 months post-infection, therefore generally wait 7 months post-exposure before testing
- Antigen test to detect antigen from adult females: sensitive and specific
  - Can get false negative
    - Low worm burden
    - Male-only infection
    - Macrocylic lactones preventative treatment
  - Consider checking result with a different antigen test
  - Consider heat treatment of sample
- Knott's test to detect microfilaria: can have false negative if occult infection and in dogs treated with macrocyclic lactones; always use antigen test concurrently
- PCR to detect microfilarial DNA: highly specific but less sensitive than Knott's test. Can differentiate species; use in addition to antigen test.
- Microscopic blood film: low sensitivity

Treatment
Refer to the American Heartworm Society website where an individualised treatment plan can be created.
- May need to treat with other drugs before adulticide, e.g. steroids, diuretics, vasodilators, inotropes, fluids

- Adulticide treatment with melarsomine:
  - Effective against worms > 4 months old
  - Pre-treat with doxycycline 10 mg/kg q24h for 30 days to reduce *Wolbachia* numbers (bacteria living with *Dirofilaria*) and possibly also suppress microfilaraemia. Treating *Wolbachia* spp. seems to reduce some of the pathology (pulmonary and renal inflammation) associated with filarial disease.
  - Give macrocyclic lactone (ivermectin, milbemycin, moxidectin or selamectin) on Day 1 and then ongoing monthly
    - If high levels of microfilariae, pre-treat with anti-histamines and prednisolone
    - Some suggest monthly administration for 3 months before using adulticide treatment
  - Melarsomine is given at 2.5 mg/kg by deep IM injection on day 30, day 60 and day 61
  - Coughing dogs are given prednisolone at anti-inflammatory doses till effective: 0.5 mg/kg BID 7 days, then 0.5 mg/kg SID for 7 days then 0.5 mg/kg EOD for 7–14 days
  - Dying heartworms cause significant pathology
    - Risk of pulmonary thromboembolism during treatment
    - Signs include low-grade fever, cough, haemoptysis, worsening of right CHF
    - Usually evident within 7–10 days (occasionally up to 4 weeks)
  - Strict restriction of exercise is important to reduce risk
    - Restricted exercise until at least 1 month after last adulticide injection to reduce risk of thromboembolism
  - No clear evidence for aspirin helping to reduce risk
- Alternative schedules exist if needed
- Surgical, trans-venous removal of worms recommended with caval syndrome

Monitoring
- Clinical assessment ± repeat cardiac evaluation
- Antigen testing from 6 months post-adulticide ± microfilarial test

Prevention

- Clinical improvement is possible without complete elimination of adult heartworms so preventative measures are vital
- Screen all dogs for infection before starting preventatives, i.e. ensure healthy dogs
- Annual retesting in endemic areas
- Heartworm prevention medication from 6–8 weeks of age either year-round or 1 month either side of mosquito season
  - Macrocylic lactone: ivermectin, milbemycin, moxidectin, selamectin
    - If started > 8 weeks of age, perform antigen test at 6 months after initial dose
    - If > 7 months of age when starting, test before treating
    - Test annually
    - Consider year-round use
- Keep dogs indoors during mosquito feeding time
- Use mosquito repellent and reduce mosquito habitats

Prognosis

- Good with asymptomatic infection
- Guarded with symptomatic infection
- Poor with caval syndrome

5.2.1D MYXOMATOUS MITRAL VALVE DISEASE

Aetiology

- Also known as: endocardiosis, degenerative mitral valve disease, chronic valvular disease
- Progressive myxomatous degeneration of the AV valves and chordae tendinae, resulting in thickening of the valve leaflets, stretching and, later, rupture of the chordae tendinae, which leads to prolapse of the valve (bulging of the valve into the atrium during systole)
- Responsible for more than 75% of all acquired cardiac disease in dogs
- Alterations to valvular apparatus lead to incompetence of the valve and so regurgitation occurs
  - Small volumes of mitral regurgitation are not haemodynamically significant

- Large volumes of mitral regurgitation result in reduced cardiac output and therefore compensatory mechanisms are activated, including sympathetic stimulation of vasoconstriction and RAAS activation to retain sodium and water, to maintain systemic BP; these result in:
  - Increased circulating volumes
  - Leading to increased intra-cardiac pressures
  - Leading to left atrial and left ventricular enlargement and eventually left-sided CHF
- The mitral valve is most commonly and most severely affected; many cases also have tricuspid valve changes, although right-sided enlargement and CHF is a rare consequence
- American College of Veterinary Internal Medicine (ACVIM) consensus staging system:
  - A: At-risk breed but no evidence of disease
  - B: Disease present but without clinical signs
    - B1: No evidence of cardiac enlargement
    - B2: Evidence of cardiac enlargement
  - C: Congestive heart failure
  - D: Refractory CHF

Major signs

- Asymptomatic
- Coughing
- Dyspnoea
- Exercise intolerance
- Lethargy

Minor signs

- Syncope
- Weight loss

Potential sequelae

- Development of left-sided CHF
- Development of pulmonary hypertension secondary to elevated left atrial pressures can result in syncope and right-sided CHF
- Rupture of chordae tendinae can lead to acute decompensation
- Rupture of left atrium can result in development of pericardial effusion; this is often, but not always, fatal

Predisposition

- Increased prevalence in small- to medium-breed dogs: CKCS, Chihuahua, Dachshund, Miniature poodle, Miniature pinscher, Whippet
- Males tend to develop the disease at a younger age than females
- Middle-aged to old dogs but can be diagnosed in young dogs (aged 1–2 years) in predisposed breeds
- Multifactorial, polygenic threshold trait in CKCS

Historical clues

- Can be asymptomatic for a prolonged period of time – may never develop clinical signs
- Loss of sinus arrhythmia and development of tachycardia over time indicate progressive cardiac remodeling is likely
- Murmur is often present for several years, getting gradually louder, before clinical signs develop

Physical examination

- Murmur
  - Band-shaped systolic murmur with point of maximal intensity at the left apex
  - Murmur grade related to severity of stenosis
  - Murmur may radiate widely with more severe disease
- Presence of sinus arrhythmia (parasympathetic vagal tone) indicates unlikely to be at high risk for developing CHF in the near future
- Signs of left-sided CHF
  - Dyspnoea
  - Pulmonary crackles
  - Tachycardia

Laboratory findings

- Usually unremarkable
- Cardiac biomarkers (NT-proBNP and troponin I) correlated with severity of disease, *q.v.* section 3.8

Imaging

Plain radiographs
- May be normal in early disease
- Progressive left-sided (or global) cardiomegaly

- Pulmonary venous congestion
- Interstitial or alveolar pattern with left-sided CHF, Figure 4.3.5

Echocardiography

- 2D and M-mode
  - Mitral valve thickening and prolapse: degree varies from breed to breed
  - Secondary left atrial and left ventricular dilation in advanced cases (stage B2 and beyond)
- Colour Doppler will show mitral regurgitation into the left atrium, often with multiple jets taking eccentric courses
- Pulsed wave/continuous wave Doppler
  - Mitral regurgitation velocities are normally 5–6 m/s

Special investigations

- Electrocardiography
  - Often normal
  - Wide P waves
  - Tall R waves
  - Arrhythmias (usually supraventricular) in advanced cases

Treatment

- Stage B2:
  - Pimobendan has been shown to delay the onset of CHF
- Stage C: management of left-sided CHF
  1. Diuretics (furosemide, spironolactone)
  2. Pimobendan
  3. ACE inhibitors
  4. Anti-arrhythmic therapy based on ECG diagnosis and clinical signs
- Surgical valve repair or replacement – limited availability

Monitoring

- Auscultation
- Clinical response
- Imaging (X-ray or echocardiography) in patients without clinical signs to identify progression from stage B1 to stage B2

ORGAN SYSTEMS

Prognosis
- Fair to guarded – some patients live with a normal life expectancy while others progress rapidly, despite medical management

5.2.2 CONGENITAL CARDIAC DISEASES

The most common congenital abnormalities identified in dogs are:
- Aortic stenosis
- Patent ductus arteriosus
- Pulmonic stenosis

Although these conditions are congenital, clinical signs may not manifest until later in life when heart failure or arrhythmias develop.

5.2.2A AORTIC STENOSIS

Aetiology
- Different forms of congenital stenosis are seen:
  - Aortic hypoplasia: aorta narrower than normal, may be seen in conjunction with valvular stenosis
  - Sub-valvular stenosis (most common form): fibro-muscular ring of tissue in the sub-valvular region that develops over the first year of life
  - Valvular stenosis: fusion of the valve leaflets
- Stenosis can range from mild to severe; with more severe stenoses, increased afterload results in left ventricular hypertrophy and can eventually lead to left atrial enlargement and left-sided CHF as well as ventricular arrhythmias

Major signs
- Asymptomatic
- Exercise intolerance
- Syncope

Minor signs
- Dyspnoea
- Hind-limb weakness
- Stunted growth

Potential sequelae
- Likelihood of clinical signs (CHF, syncope, sudden death) developing related to severity of stenosis
- Patients with subaortic stenosis at increased risk of developing aortic valve endocarditis, unrelated to severity of stenosis

Predisposition
- Aortic hypoplasia: can be considered normal in Boxers
- Sub-aortic stenosis: Newfoundland, Boxer, GSD, Golden retriever, Rottweiler, German Short-haired pointer, Great Dane, Samoyed
- Valvular stenosis: Bull terrier

Historical clues
- May be asymptomatic for some time
- Syncopal episodes usually occur when the dog has sudden bursts of exercise or excitement
- Murmur; grade may increase in the first year of life with sub-aortic stenosis

Physical examination
- Hypokinetic and delayed pulses
- Murmur
  - Crescendo-decrescendo systolic murmur with point of maximal intensity at the left base
  - Murmur radiates to thoracic inlet and right base
  - Murmur grade related to severity of stenosis
- Left-sided CHF: dyspnoea and adventitious lung sounds
- Prominent apex beat

Laboratory findings
Usually unremarkable

Imaging
Plain radiographs
q.v. section 4.3
- Normal
- Left ventricular enlargement may be seen
- ± Left atrial dilation
- ± Post stenotic dilation of ascending and descending aorta

Echocardiography
- 2D and M-mode
  - Depending on the type of stenosis, may see ridge of tissue in the sub-valvular region, aortic valve leaflet fusion or an aorta that is hypoplastic (compared to pulmonary artery, should be roughly the same diameter)
  - May see no overt abnormalities in mild cases
  - Concentric left ventricular hypertrophy in more severe cases
  - Left atrial dilation in severe cases
  - Post-stenotic dilation of ascending aorta in moderate to severe cases
- Colour Doppler will show aliasing at the level of the stenosis, consistent with the step up in velocity
- Pulsed wave/continuous wave Doppler
  - Measured from a sub-costal view
  - Most patients have velocities of 1.0–1.5 m/s but up to 2.2 m/s is normal in some breeds
  - Mild stenosis < 3.5 m/s (< 50 mmHg)
  - Moderate 3.5–4.5 m/s (50–80 mmHg)
  - Severe > 4.5 m/s (> 80 mmHg)

Special investigations
Cardiac catheterisation
Will demonstrate the stenosis, left ventricular hypertrophy and post-stenotic dilation of the aorta

Electrocardiography
- May be unremarkable
- Ideally including 24-hour ECG Holter monitoring
- Left ventricular ectopics due to myocardial hypoxia/ischaemia
- Tall R waves
- ± ST segment depression (hypoxic change)
- ± notched QRS complex

Treatment
- Cases with sub-aortic stenosis, irrespective of severity of stenosis, require prophylactic treatment with antibiotics prior to any procedure in which bacteraemia is anticipated
- Mild cases usually do not require any other treatment

- Severe cases
  - Medical management
    - Avoid extreme exertion, particularly sudden bursts of excitement or exertion
    - Ventricular arrhythmias controlled with anti-arrhythmics (often β-blockers or sotalol)
    - If concentric left ventricular hypertrophy use β-blockers to improve diastolic filling and decrease myocardial oxygen consumption; no effect on survival but can improve clinical signs
  - Balloon valvuloplasty
    - No evidence of improved survival times but can improve clinical signs, although re-stenosis can occur
    - High-risk procedure and so only performed if patient's clinical signs are having a significant impact on quality of life and life expectancy
    - Sub-aortic stenosis: requires cutting balloon to cut into the muscular ridge before a high-pressure balloon is used to further tear muscle and reduce obstruction
    - Valvular stenosis: a balloon can treat open fused leaflets but significant aortic insufficiency can occur, pushing the patient into left-sided CHF
  - Surgical correction
    - A high-risk procedure with improvement in clinical signs but no improvement in survival times and re-stenosis can occur

Monitoring
- Clinical signs
- Regular repeated echocardiography and 24-hour ECG Holter monitor

Prognosis
- Excellent for mild cases
- Poor for severe cases

5.2.2B MITRAL VALVE DYSPLASIA

Aetiology
- A congenital defect in mitral valve: absent, abnormal or fused valve leaflets

ORGAN SYSTEMS

- Can have mitral stenosis, regurgitation or a combination of both; regurgitation is the more common manifestation
- Increase in left atrial pressures from either stenosis or chronic large volume of regurgitation can result in left atrial dilation and left-sided CHF

Major signs
- Coughing (left atrial enlargement and bronchial compression)
- Dyspnoea
- Exercise intolerance

Minor signs
- Haemoptysis
- Syncope or acute development of dyspnoea can occur following a period of sudden excitement/exertion if mitral stenosis is a major component of the dysplasia

Potential sequelae
- Development of left-sided CHF
- Development of supraventricular arrhythmias

Predisposition
- Bull terrier (stenosis and regurgitation), Dalmatian, GSD, Golden retriever, Great Dane, Mastiff, Newfoundland

Historical clues
- Can be asymptomatic for some time
- Episodes of collapse or respiratory distress after periods of exertion/excitement

Physical examination
- Left apical murmur: either band-shaped systolic (regurgitation) or decrescendo diastolic (stenosis)
  - As diastolic murmur is not always audible, murmur grade does not correlate with severity
  - Systolic murmur can radiate extensively, and grade can be variable
- Adventitious lung sounds if in left-sided CHF
- Arrhythmia may be auscultated/palpated, e.g. atrial fibrillation due to severe left atrial enlargement

Laboratory findings
- Usually unremarkable

Imaging
Plain radiographs
q.v. section 4.3
- Left atrial and left ventricular enlargement
- Pulmonary venous congestion ± pulmonary oedema

Echocardiography
- 2D and M-mode
  - Abnormal appearance and movement of the mitral valve
  - Left atrial and left ventricular dilation
- Colour Doppler will show jets of mitral regurgitation and will also show aliasing of blood on inflow if there is significant mitral stenosis
- Pulsed wave/continuous wave Doppler
  - Mitral regurgitation (expect velocities of 5–6 m/s due to pressure gradient from left ventricle to left atrium)
  - Stenosis will be evident as increased mitral E–wave velocities with prolonged pressure half time

Special investigations
Electrocardiography
- May be normal
- ± wide P waves
- ± tall R waves
- ± arrhythmias – supraventricular arrhythmias, including atrial fibrillation, are the most common arrhythmias

Treatment
- Medical management of arrhythmias
  - Diltiazem and/or digoxin commonly used to control atrial fibrillation rate
- Medical management of left-sided CHF
  1. Diuretics (furosemide, spironolactone)
  2. Pimobendan
  3. ACE inhibitors
- Balloon valvuloplasty of severe mitral stenosis is possible but there is limited information about long-term outcome
- Surgical repair under cardio-pulmonary bypass has been performed but there is limited availability

Monitoring

- Clinical signs
- Echocardiography
- 24-hour ECG Holter monitoring if there are arrhythmias

Prognosis

- Good to guarded, depending on degree of mitral regurgitation/stenosis

5.2.2C PATENT DUCTUS ARTERIOSUS

Aetiology

- The *ductus arteriosus* is a fetal link between the aorta and pulmonary artery and allows blood to bypass the lungs during fetal life; it should close within the first few days after birth, becoming the *ligamentum arteriosum*
- Dogs with a patent *ductus arteriosus* (PDA) have incomplete closure (varying degrees) of the *ductus arteriosus* and so flow persists through the ductus arteriosus after birth
- The amount of blood that shunts through a PDA is dependent on how much the vessel closes down in early life
  - If the PDA doesn't close at all, which is rare, large volumes of blood enter the pulmonary artery, causing pulmonary hypertension; this leads to reversal of flow across the PDA ('right to left' PDA, 'reverse' PDA) and can cause caudal cyanosis and erythrocytosis. The development of a reverse PDA can occur at any stage, but it is often prior to the first vaccination appointment
  - The more common scenario is that the PDA partially closes down so there is flow through the PDA from aorta to pulmonary artery ('left to right' PDA); this results in over-circulation of the lungs, left atrial and left ventricular dilation and eventually left-sided CHF

Major signs

- Asymptomatic
- Dyspnoea

Minor signs

- Differential cyanosis (cyanotic caudally) with reverse PDA, *q.v.* section 2.6
- Hindlimb weakness or collapse with reverse PDA
- Seizures (due to erythrocytosis) with reverse PDA

Potential sequelae

- Left-sided CHF
- Death

Predisposition

- Sex predisposition females:males = 3:1
- Cocker spaniel, Chihuahua, Collie, English Springer spaniel, GSD, Pomeranian, Poodle, Shetland sheepdog, Welsh Corgi, Yorkshire terrier

Historical clues

- May be asymptomatic for some time
- Murmur should be detectable from first veterinary assessment

Physical examination

- Murmur
  - Continuous, usually high-grade, 'machinery' murmur high up at the left base
  - It can radiate widely to right base and thoracic inlet or can be very localised to high left base
  - Waxes in systole and wanes through diastole
- Excessive blood flow through the lungs can result in tachypnoea in the absence of CHF
- Hyperdynamic peripheral pulses ('water hammer' pulses) due to a large difference between systolic and diastolic pressures (systolic pressure slightly increased and diastolic pressure significantly reduced due to runoff of blood into the PDA during diastole)
- Left sided CHF: dyspnoea and adventitious lung sounds
- Reverse PDA (very rare) – differential cyanosis (i.e. cyanosis of caudal but not cranial mucous membranes) and absence of classic PDA murmur

Laboratory findings
- Usually unremarkable
- Erythrocytosis with some reverse PDAs

Imaging
Plain radiographs
q.v. section 4.3
- Dilated pulmonary trunk
- Dilated descending aorta
- Left atrial and left ventricular enlargement
- Pulmonary over-circulation
- ± Pulmonary oedema
- Right heart enlargement with pulmonary under-circulation with reverse PDA

Echocardiography
- 2D and M-mode
  - Left atrial and left ventricular dilation
  - Hyperkinetic left ventricle (may develop systolic dysfunction if left untreated)
  - Ductus visualised entering the left pulmonary artery
  - Pulmonary artery dilation
  - Right ventricular hypertrophy with reverse PDA
- Colour Doppler
  - Continuous blood flow into the left pulmonary artery across the ductus (not present with reverse PDA)
  - Mitral regurgitation due to left heart dilation and stretch of the mitral annulus
  - Tricuspid regurgitation due to right heart dilation with reverse PDA
- Pulsed wave/continuous wave Doppler
  - Continuous flow across PDA (systolic velocities around 5 m/s)
  - Tricuspid regurgitation velocities can be used to estimate probability of pulmonary hypertension being present

Special investigations
Cardiac catheterisation and angiography
- Visualise the PDA, assess pressures and determine direction of flow through the PDA

Electrocardiography
- May be normal
- Deep Q waves in leads I, II, III and aVF ± right axis deviation with reverse PDAs
- Tall R waves

- Wide P waves (P mitrale)
- Various arrhythmias, particularly atrial fibrillation

Treatment
- If CHF and arrhythmias are present, these should be treated before occlusion
- Management of CHF
  1 Diuretics (furosemide, spironolactone)
  2 Pimobendan
  3 ACE inhibitors
- Occlusion of the PDA
  - Minimally invasive transcatheter procedures
    - Amplatz Canine Ductal Occluder
    - Vascular coils
    - Vascular plugs
  - Surgical ligation
- Reverse PDAs often can't be closed safely
  - Sildenafil to reduce pulmonary pressures
  - Phlebotomy or hydroxyurea to maintain PCV 55–65%

Monitoring
- Clinical signs
- PCV monitoring with reverse PDA

Prognosis
- 64% die by 1 year old without intervention
- Normal or near normal lifespan if PDA is the only congenital abnormality and is closed before the development of significant chamber dilation and dysfunction
- Surgery in older dogs carries a higher risk as the ductus and dilated pulmonary arteries are friable

5.2.2D   PULMONIC STENOSIS

Aetiology
- Congenital stenosis is usually valvular, although two forms are seen:
  - Type A – pulmonic valve leaflets normal (thin) but partially fused together
  - Type B – hypoplastic pulmonary annulus with thickened valve leaflets
  - Some patients will have a mixed type, with components of type A and type B
- Stenosis can range from mild to severe; with more severe stenoses, increased afterload

results in right ventricular hypertrophy and can eventually lead to right atrial enlargement and right-sided CHF as well as ventricular arrhythmias

Major signs
- Asymptomatic
- Exercise intolerance
- Syncope

Minor signs
- Ascites
- Dyspnoea
- Prominent jugular pulse
- Stunted growth

Potential sequelae
- Likelihood of clinical signs (CHF, syncope, sudden death) developing related to severity of stenosis

Predisposition
- Boxer, Chihuahua, Cocker spaniel, English bulldog, French bulldog, Miniature schnauzer, terrier breeds

Historical clues
- May be asymptomatic for some time
- Murmur should be detectable from first veterinary assessment
- Syncopal episodes usually occur when the dog has sudden bursts of exercise or excitement

Physical examination
- Apex beat may be more prominent on right due to right ventricular hypertrophy
- Murmur
  - Crescendo-decrescendo systolic murmur with point of maximal intensity at the left base
  - Murmur grade related to severity of stenosis
  - Murmur radiates dorsally
- Pulse quality good
- Right sided CHF: jugular distension, hepatomegaly, ascites, hepatojugular reflux, dyspnoea

Laboratory findings
- Usually unremarkable

Imaging
Plain radiographs
q.v. section 4.3
- Normal if mild case
- Post stenotic dilation of pulmonary trunk
- Right ventricular enlargement

Echocardiography
- 2D and M-mode
  - Concentric right ventricular hypertrophy in more severe cases
  - Fusion of pulmonic valve leaflets and/or hypoplasia of the pulmonary artery with abnormal pulmonic valves
  - May see no overt abnormalities in mild cases
  - Pressure overload of the right ventricle can lead to flattening of the interventricular septum or paradoxical motion of the interventricular septum
  - Post-stenotic dilation of pulmonary artery in moderate to severe cases
  - Right atrial dilation in severe cases
- Colour Doppler will show aliasing at the level of the stenosis, consistent with the step up in velocity
- Pulsed wave/continuous wave Doppler
  - Most patients have velocities of around 1.0 m/s
  - Mild stenosis < 3.5 m/s (< 50 mmHg)
  - Moderate 3.5–4.5 m/s (50–80 mmHg)
  - Severe > 4.5 m/s (> 80 mmHg)

Special investigations
Cardiac catheterisation
- Will demonstrate the stenosis, right ventricular hypertrophy and post-stenotic dilation of the pulmonary artery

Electrocardiography
- Deep S waves in leads I, II, III and aVF
- Right axis deviation
- ± Right ventricular origin ventricular ectopics

Treatment
- Mild cases do not require treatment

- Severe cases should be assessed for suitability for balloon valvuloplasty – works best for those with thin, fused pulmonic valve leaflets
  - Success is considered a 50% reduction in pressure gradient
- Alternatives for those where balloon valvuloplasty has failed or isn't considered appropriate, e.g. hypoplastic pulmonary arteries:
  - Pulmonic stent – relatively new procedure, limited availability
  - Surgical options (limited availability):
    - Patch graft but requires cardiac bypass
    - Right ventricular to pulmonary artery conduit surgery performed under inflow occlusion

Monitoring
- Clinical signs
- Regular repeated echocardiography ± 24-hour ECG Holter monitor if arrhythmias identified

Prognosis
- Mild to moderate disease may have no effect on life expectancy
- Patients with severe stenosis (either that do not undergo an interventional procedure or who are left with severe stenosis after an interventional procedure) are at increased risk of developing arrhythmias, CHF and sudden death
- Severe cases: depends on results of balloon valvuloplasty (or other surgical intervention)

5.2.2E   TETRALOGY OF FALLOT

Aetiology
- Congenital abnormality in the division of the *truncus arteriosus* during the formation of the aorta and pulmonary artery – uneven division of the *truncus arteriosus* leads to a large aorta and small pulmonary artery and therefore an inability of the dividing septum to fuse to the interventricular septum – this creates a ventricular septal defect and leaves the right ventricle exposed to systemic pressures as well as the increased afterload created by the pulmonary hypoplasia, and consequent right ventricular hypertrophy

- The four abnormalities are:
  - Over-riding aorta
  - Pulmonic stenosis
  - Right ventricular hypertrophy
  - Ventricular septal defect
- Blood tends to shunt right to left, mixing deoxygenated blood into the systemic circulation; erythrocytosis develops secondary to the hypoxaemia

Major signs
- Cyanosis
- Gasping for breath during periods of exertion/excitement
- Severe exercise intolerance
- Stunted growth
- Syncope

Potential sequelae
- Right-sided CHF: rare outcome
- Seizures/obtundation due to erythrocytosis
- Sudden death

Predisposition
- Autosomal dominant mode of inheritance with variable penetrance: English bulldog, Keeshond

Historical clues
- Ill-thrift from early age

Physical examination
- Mucous membranes are cyanosed most obviously after exercise/excitement due to drop in peripheral vascular resistance and worsening right to left shunting
- Murmur
  - Pulmonic stenosis often the most obvious component of the murmur: left basilar crescendo-decrescendo systolic murmur that radiates dorsally and to the left apex
  - Right apical band-shaped systolic murmur due to tricuspid regurgitation may also be heard
- Pulse quality usually normal

Laboratory findings
- Erythrocytosis/polycythaemia

Imaging

Plain radiographs

q.v. section 4.3

- Right ventricular enlargement
- Hypovascular lung fields

Echocardiography

- 2D and M-mode
  - Flat or paradoxical motion of interventricular septum
  - Hypoplastic pulmonary trunk
  - Over-riding aorta (overlying the ventricular septal defect)
  - Right ventricular hypertrophy
  - Ventricular septal defect
- Colour Doppler will show aliasing at the level of the pulmonic stenosis and shunting across the ventricular septal defect
- Pulsed wave/continuous wave Doppler
  - Assess pressure gradient across the pulmonic stenosis
  - Assess velocity of shunting across the ventricular septal defect

Special investigations

Bubble study

- Confirm right to left shunting across the ventricular septal defect

Electrocardiography

- Deep S waves in leads I, II, III and aVF
- Right axis deviation

Treatment

- Acute crisis
  - Complete rest
  - Intravenous fluid therapy (IVFT)
  - Oxygen
  - Sodium bicarbonate if acidosis present
- Medical management
  - Avoid agents that cause systemic vasodilation, e.g. acepromazine
  - Non-specific β-blockers (propranolol) may reduce shunting
  - Phlebotomy or hydroxyurea to control erythrocytosis
- Surgical management
  - Closure of ventricular septal defect and creating a bypass of the pulmonic stenosis; requires cardiopulmonary bypass so rarely performed
  - Creation of a subclavian artery to pulmonary artery shunt (modified Blalock-Thomas-Taussig shunt) to increase pulmonary blood flow and oxygenation
  - Pulmonary artery stent placement can increase pulmonary blood flow

Monitoring

- PCV
- Clinical signs

Prognosis

- Death generally occurs in young adult dogs
- Sudden death is common
- Some patients can tolerate the defect for some time if pulmonary blood flow is maintained and hyperviscosity controlled

5.2.2F   TRICUSPID DYSPLASIA

Aetiology

- Congenital defect in tricuspid valve: absent, abnormal or fused valve leaflets
- Can have tricuspid stenosis, regurgitation or a combination of both – regurgitation is the more common manifestation but there is a wide spectrum of disease
- Increase in right atrial pressures from either stenosis or chronic large volume of regurgitation can result in right atrial dilation and right-sided CHF
- Association with tricupsid valve dysplasia and a particular congenital supraventricular tachycardia (orthodromic atrioventricular reciprocating tachycardia)

Major signs

- Dyspnoea (pleural effusion)
- Ascites
- Exercise intolerance

Minor signs

- Cardiac cachexia with right-sided CHF

Potential sequelae

- Development of right-sided CHF
- Development of supraventricular arrhythmias

Predisposition
- Labrador Retriever, Boxer, GSD, English bulldog, Bullmastiff

Historical clues
- May be asymptomatic for some time
- Murmur not always heard at first veterinary assessment but may be detected at subsequent visits as the disease progresses

Physical examination
- Right apical band-shaped systolic murmur due to tricuspid regurgitation – not always correlated with severity
- Decrescendo diastolic murmur due to stenosis – rare to hear
- Arrhythmia may be auscultated/palpated – e.g. atrial fibrillation due to severe right atrial enlargement
- Jugular distension, dull lung sounds with pleural effusion, and hepatomegaly and abdominal distension with ascites if in right-sided CHF
- Reduced body condition often present when in CHF

Laboratory findings
- Usually unremarkable

Imaging
Plain radiographs
q.v. section 4.3
- Right atrial and right ventricular enlargement
- Caudal vena caval distension ± pleural effusion/ascites

Echocardiography
- 2D and M-mode
  - Abnormal appearance and movement of the tricuspid valve
  - Flattening of the interventricular septum in diastole due to right ventricular volume overload
  - Right atrial and right ventricular dilation
- Colour Doppler will show jets of tricuspid regurgitation and will also show aliasing of blood on inflows if there is significant tricuspid stenosis
- Pulsed wave/continuous wave Doppler

- Stenosis will be evident as increased tricuspid E-wave velocities with prolonged pressure half time
- Tricuspid regurgitation: expect velocities of 2–3 m/s due to pressure gradient from right ventricle to right atrium

Special investigations
Electrocardiography
- May be normal
- ± Splintered QRS complexes
- ± Deep S waves in II, III, aVF
- ± Tall P waves
- ± Arrhythmias: supraventricular arrhythmias, including atrial fibrillation, are the most common arrhythmias

Treatment
- Medical management of right-sided CHF
  1. Diuretics (furosemide, spironolactone)
  2. Pimobendan
  3. ACE inhibitors
- Medical management of arrhythmias
  - Diltiazem and/or digoxin commonly used to control atrial fibrillation rate
- Surgical options for repair under cardiopulmonary bypass have been performed but there is limited availability
- Balloon valvuloplasty of severe tricuspid stenosis is possible but there is limited information about long term outcome

Monitoring
- Clinical signs
- Echocardiography
- 24-hour ECG Holter monitoring if there are arrhythmias

Prognosis
- Good to guarded, depending of degree of tricuspid regurgitation/stenosis

5.2.2G VENTRICULAR SEPTAL DEFECT

Aetiology
- Congenital failure of closure of ventricular septum

- Blood shunts from high-pressure left ventricle to lower-pressured right ventricle, resulting in additional blood going to the lungs and back to the left heart
- Size of defect influences potential outcome
  - Large defect: large volume of blood shunting from left ventricle to right ventricle – large volume of blood travelling through the lungs to the left heart leading to either:
    - Left-sided CHF
    - or
    - Pulmonary hypertension: right to left shunting occurs and can result in right-sided CHF or erythrocytosis secondary to systemic hypoxia
  - Small defect (most common): small volume of blood shunting from left ventricle to right ventricle with minimal haemodynamic consequences

Major signs
- Asymptomatic
- Dyspnoea

Minor signs
- Cyanosis and weakness with right to left shunting VSD
- Seizures (due to erythrocytosis) with right to left shunting VSD

Potential sequelae
- Left-sided CHF
- Pulmonary hypertension, resulting in right-sided CHF, syncope and erythrocytosis
- Some VSDs appear to close, seen as aneurysmal dilation of the interventricular septum; it is not always clear how this occurs but it may be due to adherence of a tricuspid valve leaflet

Predisposition
- Predisposed breeds: English bulldog, English Springer spaniel, WHWT; known genetic basis in Keeshond

Historical clues
- Asymptomatic – murmur identified at routine examination
- Exercise intolerance

Physical examination
- Band-shaped systolic murmur with point of maximal intensity over right craniosternal area
- Grade of murmur is inversely correlated with the size of the defect
- Hyperkinetic pulse if significant left to right shunting
- A separate murmur of pulmonic stenosis (relative) may be heard due to increased blood flow across a normal valve

Laboratory findings
- Unremarkable
- Erythrocytosis may be present if right to left shunting

Imaging
Plain radiographs
q.v. section 4.3
- Left atrial and left ventricular enlargement
- Pulmonary over-circulation
- ± Pulmonary oedema
- Right heart enlargement with pulmonary under-circulation with right to left shunting VSD
  Echocardiography
- 2D and M–mode
  - Left atrial and left ventricular dilation with larger defects
  - Right ventricular hypertrophy with right to left shunting VSDs
  - Septal defect most commonly identified in the membranous region of the interventricular septum just below the aortic valve but can be present anywhere along the interventricular septum
  - Small defects can be difficult to visualise and the heart may be otherwise unremarkable; larger defects are more obvious with more secondary consequences being seen
- Colour Doppler
  - Mitral regurgitation due to left heart dilation and stretch of the mitral annulus
  - Systolic blood flow from left ventricle to right ventricle: most common VSD location has blood travelling from just below the aortic valve in the left ventricle to just below the tricuspid valve in the right ventricle
  - Tricuspid regurgitation due to right heart dilation with right-to-left VSDs

ORGAN SYSTEMS

- Pulsed wave/continuous wave Doppler
  - Systolic flow across VSD (expect velocities around 5 m/s)
  - Tricuspid regurgitation velocities can be used to estimate probability of pulmonary hypertension being present

Special investigations
Electrocardiography
- May be unremarkable
- Tall R waves
- ± Wide P waves
- Deep Q waves in leads I, II, III and aVF ± right axis deviation with right to left shunting

Treatment
- Often not needed
- Management of left-sided CHF
  1 Diuretics (furosemide, spironolactone)
  2 Pimobendan
  3 ACE inhibitors
- Phlebotomy if severe erythrocytosis
- Minimally invasive, thoracotomy and hybrid techniques reported for VSD closure – limited availability
- Pulmonary artery banding
  - Palliative to protect the pulmonary vascular bed but only cases considered at high risk for left-sided CHF

Monitoring
- Clinical signs
- Echocardiography

Prognosis
- High-velocity gradients but with small defects may be well tolerated with minimal signs
- Guarded with large VSD or if pulmonary hypertension develops

5.2.3 CONGESTIVE HEART FAILURE (CHF)

Aetiology
- The clinical signs that occur due to the retention of sodium and water leading to congestion and oedema, secondary to abnormal cardiac function as a result of:

- Acquired heart disease
- Arrhythmias
- Congenital heart disease
- Pericardial disease
- Depending on the underlying condition, left-sided or right-sided CHF may develop and, in some conditions, both left- and right-sided CHF may occur
- Left-sided CHF is characterised by pulmonary oedema (Figure 4.3.5) whereas right-sided CHF is characterised by pleural effusion, ascites, occasionally pericardial effusion and, in extreme cases, peripheral oedema

Treatment
If possible, treat the underlying cause
- Drain pericardial effusion
  - Often don't then need to treat the secondary right-sided CHF as it will resolve within 24–48 hours
- Medical management/pacemaker as appropriate for underlying arrhythmia
  - May require temporary management of CHF signs but may not need long-term treatment, depending on presence of structural heart disease
    - Arrhythmias such as atrial fibrillation and some ventricular arrhythmias are secondary to structural heart disease and so may still require management of CHF and in some cases, the management of the CHF signs must take priority in the first few hours to days over the management of the arrhythmia (e.g. rate control for atrial fibrillation may be delayed until CHF is controlled)
    - Arrhythmias such as AV block and some ventricular arrhythmias are not associated with structural cardiac disease and so usually don't require long-term CHF once management for arrhythmia is instituted

Acute CHF treatment
- Oxygen supplementation
  - Flow-by
  - Oxygen cage
  - Nasal cannulas
- Diuretics
  - Furosemide

- Potent diuretic acting on $Na^+/K^+/2Cl^-$ co-transporter in thick ascending limb of loop of Henle
- 2 mg/kg initially with top-ups of 1–2 mg/kg every 1–2 hours until respiratory rate and effort normalising
- IV is ideal route of administration but can be given IM or SC if difficult to achieve IV access
- Can cause hypotension, azotaemia, hyponatraemia, hypochloraemia and hypokalaemia
- Can be given as a continuous rate infusion (0.5 mg/kg/hour) in severe cases
- Sedation for anxious patients
  - Butorphanol @ 0.2–0.4 mg/kg IM or IV
  - Addition of low dose of acepromazine (2–10 µg/kg) or midazolam (0.2–0.3 mg/kg) to butorphanol for particularly anxious patients
- Thoracocentesis/abdominocentesis if required
  - Drain fluid from chest as much as possible
  - Drain fluid from abdomen only if it is so distended that it is limiting breathing
    - If need to drain, only remove enough fluid to make the abdomen soft; do not drain abdomen fully as there will be a loss of proteins and electrolytes in the fluid
  - Therapeutic but will also provide diagnostic samples
- Positive inotropic support
  - Pimobendan
    - Phosphodiesterase III inhibitor (positive inotrope) and calcium sensitiser (vasodilation)
    - Licensed for use in CHF secondary to myxomatous mitral valve disease and dilated cardiomyopathy but used in CHF secondary to many other conditions
    - 0.15 mg/kg BID IV or 0.25–0.3 mg/kg BID oral, ideally 1 hour before food
      - Oral is generally preferred unless the patient is incapable of taking oral medication (e.g. extremely oxygen-dependent, on a ventilator, vomiting frequently) or if it is considered that

gut absorption is likely to be poor due to significantly reduced cardiac output or GI wall oedema
- Should not be used in clinical conditions where augmenting cardiac output is not possible for functional or anatomical reasons e.g. aortic stenosis, pulmonic stenosis
- Side effects limited but occasional diarrhoea and vomiting seen
  - Dobutamine
    - Beta-1 agonist given as a continuous rate intravenous infusion at 5–20 µg/kg/minute (start at the low end and increase incrementally)
    - Only used if significant systemic hypotension and low output signs, despite pimobendan therapy
    - Requires continuous ECG monitoring as can cause tachyarrhythmias
    - May also see nausea, vomiting and seizures
    - Down-regulation of beta receptors means that it is only effective for approximately 48 hours of infusion
- Vasodilators
  - Sodium nitroprusside
    - Mimics nitric oxide to cause arterial and venous vasodilation
    - Arteriodilation: reduces afterload and therefore improves cardiac output
    - Venodilation: increases venous capacitance and therefore reduces the amount of blood returning to the heart (preload)
    - Rapid onset of action with short half-life – start at 1 µg/kg/minute and increase in 1 µg/kg/minute increments to a maximum dose of 5 µg/kg/minute
    - Continuous infusion given with an aim of maintaining systolic BP at 90–100 mmHg to help manage acute, severe, life-threatening pulmonary oedema
    - Requires near-continuous BP monitoring (either arterial catheter or non-invasive BP monitoring every 15–30 minutes) due to risk of systemic hypotension
    - Drug is light-sensitive and so the syringe/giving set must be wrapped

- Cyanide toxicity occurs with prolonged use, particularly at higher dose rates, and so it is rarely used for more than 24 hours
- Discontinue drug gradually

Chronic CHF treatment

- Diuretics
  - Furosemide
    - 1–2 mg/kg PO BID or TID, and titrate to lowest effective dose
    - Dose will likely be increased over time following relapses of CHF
  - Spironolactone
    - Competitive antagonist of aldosterone binding to the Na⁺/K⁺ ATPase pump in the distal convoluted tubule
    - Potassium-sparing diuretic – weak diuretic but helpful in sequential nephron blockade
    - Potential anti-remodelling effects via inhibition of aldosterone receptors – reduced myocardial fibrosis and endothelial dysfunction
    - 2–4 mg/kg PO SID – ideally given with food
  - Torasemide
    - Binds to the same receptors as furosemide (Na⁺/K⁺/2Cl⁻ co-transporter in thick ascending limb of loop of Henle) but more potent and therefore potentially more renal side effects
    - Used in cases of furosemide resistance (giving 10–12 mg/kg/day of furosemide with continuing clinical signs of CHF and no evidence of azotaemia or decreased electrolytes)
    - Dose based on the last effective furosemide dose – total daily furosemide dose calculated and divided by 10 to give the total daily torasemide dose – this dose should then be divided into two equal doses and given twice daily
- Pimobendan
  - 0.25–0.3 mg/kg BID – ideally 1 hour before food
- ACE inhibitors
  - Inhibit angiotensin converting enzyme, blocking angiotensin II production, resulting in vasodilation, decreasing sodium and water retention and potentially reducing some of the aldosterone-induced remodelling
  - Should be avoided in cases of systemic hypotension – may be avoided for first 7–10 days if there was significant systemic hypotension during initial presentation
  - Enalapril 0.5 mg/kg PO SID-BID
  - Benazepril 0.25–0.5 mg/kg PO SID

Monitoring

Acute CHF

- Respiratory rate and effort
- Renal values and electrolytes
  - Ideally collect as baseline and then every 24 hours during hospitalisation – more frequently may be required if intense treatment required (continuous-rate infusions)
- Patient demeanour

Chronic CHF

- Clinical side effects, e.g. frequent urination at night/accidents in the house, may prompt a reduction in furosemide dose
- Patient compliance with medication: consider combi-pills if owners are struggling with giving all medications (e.g. benazepril plus spironolactone such as Cardalis®)
- Respiratory rate and effort
- Renal values and electrolytes
  - 7–10 days after initial hospitalisation and any furosemide dose increase
  - Every 3–6 months long-term if otherwise doing well

5.2.3A LEFT-SIDED CONGESTIVE HEART FAILURE

Major signs

- Coughing
  - Bronchial compression from left atrial enlargement
  - Pulmonary oedema itself rarely causes coughing
- Exercise intolerance or lethargy
- Dyspnoea/tachypnoea/orthopnoea

Minor signs

- Anorexia
- Nocturnal restlessness

ORGAN SYSTEMS

- Syncopal episodes (forward failure of cardiac output)
- Sudden death
- Weight loss

Potential sequelae
- Death due to respiratory fatigue

Predisposition
- Acquired heart disease
  - Myxomatous mitral valve disease
  - Dilated cardiomyopathy
- Arrhythmias
  - Any sustained bradyarrhythmia or tachyarrhythmia
- Congenital heart disease
  - Aortic stenosis
  - Mitral valve dysplasia
  - Patent ductus arteriosus
  - Ventricular septal defect

Historical clues
- Evidence of advanced structural cardiac disease
- Progressive increase in respiratory rate and effort over time can be detected if the owner is monitoring for this, although sudden development of signs of left-sided CHF can occur in some conditions (myxomatous mitral valve disease due to chordal rupture)

Physical examination
- Pale mucous membranes
- Pulmonary crackles: pulmonary oedema vs primary lung disease
- Tachycardia/absence of sinus arrhythmia
- Tachypnoea/dyspnoea
- Signs which may be present, depending on the underlying reason:
  - Abnormal cardiac rate and rhythm
  - Changes in pulse quality
  - Gallop sounds
  - Murmur
  - Prominent or displaced apex beat

Laboratory findings
- Generally unremarkable
- If possible, collect baseline biochemistry to assess the effect of treatment on renal function and electrolytes

- May have evidence of decreased organ perfusion: azotaemia, increased ALT

Imaging
Plain radiographs
q.v. section 4.3
- Cardiomegaly
- Pulmonary venous distension
- Interstitial/alveolar pattern – initially perihilar but can be generalised if severe, Figure 4.3.5

Echocardiography
- B lines on lung ultrasound
- Evidence of left atrial enlargement and underlying structural heart disease

Special investigations
BP
- To assess for systemic hypotension

ECG
- To assess for rhythm disturbances
Treatment and monitoring,
q.v. section 5.2.3

5.2.3B   RIGHT-SIDED CONGESTIVE HEART FAILURE

Major signs
- Ascites
- Dyspnoea (pleural effusion)
- Exercise intolerance

Minor signs
- Gastrointestinal signs (diarrhoea, vomiting)
- Inappetence
- Nocturnal restlessness
- Subcutaneous oedema
- Syncope
- Weight loss/cachexia

Potential sequelae
- Death due to respiratory fatigue due to pleural effusion is possible

Predisposition
- Acquired heart disease
- Dilated cardiomyopathy

ORGAN SYSTEMS

ORGAN SYSTEMS

- Arrhythmias
  - Any sustained bradyarrhythmia or tachyarrhythmia
- Congenital heart disease
  - Pulmonic stenosis
  - Tricuspid valve dysplasia
- Pericardial disease
  - Pericardial effusions where pericardial pressures exceed right atrial pressures

Historical clues
- Evidence of advanced structural cardiac disease
- Progressive increase in respiratory effort (although not necessarily respiratory rate) over time can be detected if the owner is monitoring for this
- Apparent weight gain despite no alterations in diet (ascites)
- Alterations in sleeping positions/pattern (either sleeping less or sleeping in sternal recumbency with head propped up) is often reported

Physical examination
- Ascites
- Hepatojugular reflux
- Hepatomegaly
- Jugular venous distension ± jugular pulse
- Pleural effusion (dullness on percussion ventrally, reduced heart sounds)
- Subcutaneous oedema

Laboratory findings
- Generally unremarkable
- May have evidence of decreased organ perfusion (azotaemia, increase in ALT activity)
- If possible, collect baseline biochemistry to assess the effect of treatment on renal function and electrolytes

Imaging
q.v. section 4.3
Plain radiographs
- Cardiomegaly
- Pleural effusion (if this is suspected clinically, it is safer not to lie the patient in lateral recumbency for radiographs – instead consider ultrasound to rule in/out pleural effusion)

- Ascites

Echocardiography
- Pleural effusion on thoracic ultrasound and/or ascites on abdominal ultrasound
- Evidence of right atrial enlargement and underlying structural heart disease
- May identify pericardial effusion

Special investigations
- BP to assess for systemic hypotension
- ECG to assess for rhythm disturbances
- Fluid analysis of pleural/abdominal fluid to rule out other causes of fluid accumulation

5.2.4 ARRHYTHMIAS

Arrhythmias can cause clinical signs and ultimately lead to CHF, but must be distinguished from normal rhythms on clinical examination and ECG.

SINUS RHYTHMS

ECG changes
- Normal PQRST in regular rhythm, Figure 5.2.2a

Aetiology
- Normal activation of the atria and, via the conduction system, the ventricles by the pacemaker (sinus node) at a normal rate of 70–140 beats per minute (bpm)

Major signs
- None

Further investigations and treatment
- None required

SINUS ARRHYTHMIA

ECG changes
Normal PQRST with regular phasic acceleration and deceleration in heart rate, often synchronous with respiration, Figure 5.2.2b

Aetiology
- Common in normal, fit, relaxed dogs
- Often associated with increased vagal tone so the heart rate tends to be at the lower end of normal range
- Accentuated in diseases with increased vagal tone, e.g. airway obstruction/respiratory disease, GI disease, increased intra-cranial pressure, mediastinal disease,
- Even if cardiac disease is present, patients are generally well -compensated and not at imminent risk of CHF

Major signs
- None due to rhythm, but may have signs of underlying disease causing high vagal tone

Further investigations and treatment
- None required for arrhythmia but may need to investigate and treat underlying disease causing high vagal tone

5.2.4.1   BRADYARRHYTHMIAS

Rhythm disturbances associated with a slow heart rate.

5.2.4.1A   ATRIAL STANDSTILL

ECG changes
- Absence of P waves
- Regular slow escape rhythm < 60/minute: QRS complexes often normal shape but can be of prolonged duration

Aetiology
- Absence of any atrial activity: sinoatrial node still fires but does not depolarise the atrium and impulses are conducted by internodal pathways from SA node to AV node
- Temporary atrial standstill with hyperkalaemia or digoxin toxicity
- Terminal atrial standstill with a 'dying' heart

Major signs
- Right-sided CHF
- Weakness, lethargy, syncope

Predisposition
- Persistent atrial standstill most commonly reported in English Springer spaniels

Further investigations
- Echocardiography to assess for infiltrative disease causing arrhythmia
- Measure serum potassium concentration
- Rule out digoxin toxicity by measuring serum concentrations
- Investigations for significant, life-limiting systemic disease (haematology, biochemistry, urinalysis, ± thoracic imaging, ± abdominal imaging) prior to pacemaker implantation

Treatment
- Treat primary cause if identified
- Pacemaker implantation for persistent atrial standstill but due to costs of implantation and strict rest requirements for 4-week recovery, discuss cost/benefit with owners

Prognosis
- Good if successful implantation and capture
- Seroma and infection are most common complications after implantation
- Periodic pacemaker checks required to control rate and check battery life
- Potential for breakage or movement of leads
- Some patients have progression of disease leading to worsening right-sided CHF despite pacemaker implantation

5.2.4.1B   ATRIOVENTRICULAR (AV) BLOCK

ECG changes
- AV block is a failure to conduct impulses normally through the AV node
- First-degree heart block
  - May be seen in the context of sinus arrhythmia (Figure 5.2.2b)
  - P and QRS waves are normal in conformation but the PR interval is prolonged
- Second-degree heart block
  - P wave is normal, but there is an occasional or frequent failure of conduction through

(a)

(b)

(c)

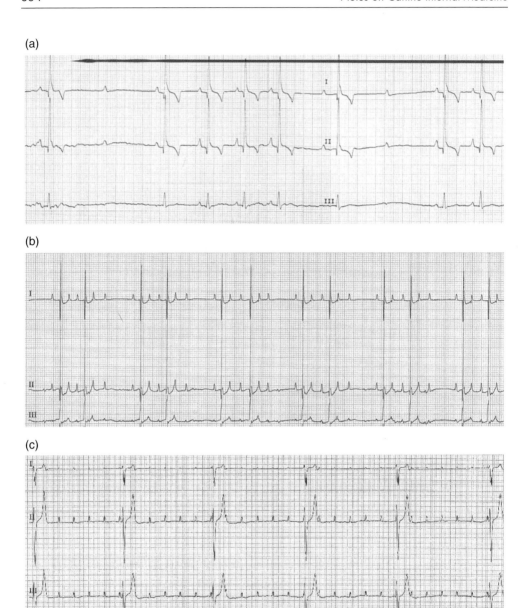

Figure 5.2.5 Atrioventricular block

5.2.5a Second-degree Mobitz type I

Leads I, II and III ECG showing Mobitz type I second-degree atrioventricular block: the P wave is normal, but the PR interval becomes prolonged with progressive complexes until it eventually blocks (50 mm/s, 10 mm/mV).

5.2.5b Second-degree Mobitz type II

Leads I, II and III ECG showing Mobitz type 2 second-degree atrioventricular block: there is no alteration in PR interval in the complexes preceding a blocked P wave (25 mm/s, 20 mm/mV).

5.2.5c Third-degree AV block

Leads I, II and III ECG showing third-degree atrioventricular block: complete dissociation between the P waves and the QRS complexes which are wide and bizarre (25 mm/s, 10 mm/mV).

ORGAN SYSTEMS

the AV node, resulting in an absence of the associated QRS complex

- Mobitz type I (Figure 5.2.5a)
  - May be seen in the context of sinus arrhythmia
  - PR interval becomes more prolonged with progressive complexes until it eventually blocks
  - This can be very subtle and often requires 50 mm/s paper speed to visualise
- Mobitz type II (Figure 5.2.5b)
  - No alteration in PR interval in the complexes preceding a blocked P wave
- Third-degree heart block (Figure 5.2.5c)
  - Complete dissociation between the P waves and the QRS complexes
  - P waves often faster than normal sinus rhythm
  - QRS complexes are ventricular in origin (escape complexes) and so are often wide and bizarre, as well as being at low rates (60–70 bpm if originating from junctional cells high up in the bundle of His, 20–40 bpm if originating from Purkinje fibres)

Aetiology

- First-degree AV block and Mobitz type I second-degree AV block imply vagal control of the rhythm
  - Fit, healthy patients: physiological increase in vagal tone
  - Drugs, e.g. beta-blockers, calcium channel blockers, digoxin
  - Hyperkalaemia
  - Pathological increase in vagal tone: GI disease, increased intra-cranial pressure, mediastinal disease, respiratory disease/airway obstruction
- Mobitz type II second-degree AV block and third-degree AV block
  - AV nodal fibrosis in older dogs
  - Drugs, e.g. beta-blockers, calcium channel blockers, digoxin
  - Myocarditis/endocarditis
  - Neoplastic infiltration of nodal tissue
  - Trauma to AV node

Major signs

- First-degree AV block and Mobitz type I second-degree AV block usually have no clinical signs related to rhythm
- Mobitz type 2 second-degree AV block and third-degree AV block
  - May have weakness, lethargy, syncope or signs of CHF; right-sided CHF more common than left-sided CHF
  - With very slow escape rhythms, peripheral pulses will be hyperdynamic

Further investigations

- First-degree AV block and Mobitz type I second-degree AV block
  - Assess whether increase in vagal tone is physiological or pathological
- Mobitz type II second-degree AV block and third-degree AV block
  - Assess for myocarditis (troponin I), access to drugs, and use echocardiography to assess for overt neoplastic infiltration, endocarditis and presence of cardiomegaly secondary to bradycardia, q.v. section 3.8
  - Investigations for significant, life-limiting systemic disease (haematology, biochemistry, urinalysis, ± thoracic imaging, ± abdominal imaging) prior to considering pacemaker implantation

NB: There may not be time to perform extensive investigations in a patient with unstable third-degree AV block prior to pacemaker implantation.

Treatment

- First-degree AV block and Mobitz type I second-degree AV block
  - If underlying conditions increasing vagal tone are present, treatment should be aimed at these; no treatment for rhythm required
- Mobitz type II second-degree AV block
  - May not require treatment if not causing clinical signs but patient should be monitored for progression of arrhythmia
  - Can consider positive chronotropic drugs (terbutaline, theophylline) but may not be successful
  - May require pacemaker implantation if causing clinical signs

ORGAN SYSTEMS

- Third-degree AV block
  - Highly likely to require pacemaker implantation
  - The lower the heart rate, the more an emergency
  - Due to costs of implantation and strict rest requirements for 4-week recovery, discuss cost/benefit with owners
  - Positive chronotropic drugs very unlikely to be successful

5.2.4.1C SINUS BRADYCARDIA

ECG changes

Normal PQRST but at lower than normal heart rates (< 60–70 bpm)

Aetiology

- Normal in some fit dogs, giant-breed dogs
- May be seen in diseases with elevated vagal tone, e.g. GI disease, increased intra-cranial pressure, mediastinal disease, respiratory disease/airway obstruction
- Drugs, e.g. sedatives
- Hypothermia
- Hypothyroidism

Major signs

- None due to rhythm, but may have signs of underlying disease causing high vagal tone

Further investigations

- Investigate for underlying diseases

Treatment

- Treat the underlying condition – the rhythm itself rarely needs specific anti-arrhythmic therapy
- Activity test to determine if vagally mediated: take dog for run and re-listen/re-ECG immediately after exercise; increase in heart rate implies vagally mediated
- Atropine response test to determine if vagally mediated: 0.04 atropine mg/kg SC and repeat ECG 30 minutes later; increased rate suggests vagally mediated bradycardia

5.2.4.1D SINUS ARREST

ECG changes

- Unexpected pause in rhythm with no QRS complex
  - Pause is more than 2 RR intervals
  - The length of the pause is not normally a multiple of the RR interval (impossible to assess in the context of sinus arrhythmia)
- Pause may be interrupted by an atrial or ventricular escape complex

Aetiology

- Common, normal variation in brachycephalics
- Abnormal increase in vagal tone
- Atrial pathology
- Sinus-node dysfunction – may be seen in context of sick sinus syndrome
- Drugs (beta blockers, calcium channel blockers)
- Electrolyte imbalances (hyperkalaemia)

Major signs

- If prolonged can cause syncope

Further investigations

- Rule out treatable causes (drug overdose, electrolyte imbalances, etc.)

Treatment

- Atropine/exercise may abolish disturbance if due to excessive vagal tone
- Treat underlying cause – if seen in context of sick sinus syndrome, may require pacemaker implantation

5.2.4.1E SICK SINUS SYNDROME

Also known as 'brady-tachy syndrome.'

ECG changes

- Collection of arrhythmias, including some or all of sinus arrest, sinus bradycardia, AV blocks and supraventricular tachycardia, often with abrupt changes in rhythm (Figure 5.2.6)

ORGAN SYSTEMS

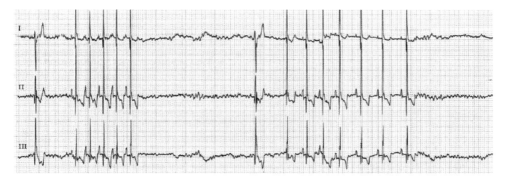

Figure 5.2.6 Sick sinus syndrome. Leads I, II and III ECG from a dog with sick sinus syndrome, showing a range of arrhythmias, including sinus arrest, atrioventricular block and supraventricular tachycardia, with abrupt changes in rhythm (25 mm/s, 10 mm/mV).

Aetiology
- Unknown, suspected to be idiopathic

Predisposition
- Reported most commonly in Miniature schnauzers, WHWT
- > 6 years old

Major signs
- May have no clinical signs
- Clinical signs of syncope and weakness

Special investigations
- Echocardiography to assess for infiltrative disease causing arrhythmias
- Rule out digoxin toxicity as this may mimic sick sinus syndrome
- 24-hour ECG Holter monitoring to assess cause of collapse (sinus arrest vs episodes of supraventricular tachycardia)
- Investigations for significant, life-limiting systemic disease (haematology, biochemistry, urinalysis, ± thoracic imaging, ± abdominal imaging) prior to pacemaker implantation

Treatment
- Positive chronotropic drugs (terbutaline, theophylline) may be used to control clinical signs but are not successful in all cases and some patients may only respond initially and then require pacemaker implantation
- Treatment of choice is pacemaker implantation
- Due to costs of implantation and strict rest requirements for 4-week recovery, discuss cost/benefit with owners

5.2.4.2 TACHYARRHYTHMIAS

Rhythm disturbances associated with an increased heart rate, with complexes having an origin that is:
- Supraventricular
  - From the sinoatrial node

  or
  - From anywhere above the AV node
- Ventricular
  - An ectopic focus within the ventricle

5.2.4.2A SINUS TACHYCARDIA

ECG changes
- Normal PQRST with regular rhythm at rates of 150–200 bpm

Aetiology
- Appropriate response to anaemia, exercise, fear and stresses, hypovolaemia, pyrexia
- Patients with advanced cardiac disease develop sinus tachycardia in response to sympathetic stimulation trying to maintain cardiac output

Major signs
- None due to rhythm but may have signs of underlying disease

Further investigations and treatment
- None required for rhythm – may need to investigate and treat underlying disease

5.2.4.2B SUPRAVENTRICULAR TACHYARRHYTHMIAS

ECG changes
- Complexes originating from anywhere above the AV node other than the sinoatrial node
- Electrical activity travels through the AV node and uses the His-Purkinje system; therefore, normal narrow QRS complexes
- Different types of supraventricular arrhythmia (SVT) result in different appearances:
  - Focal atrial tachycardia
    - Originates from an ectopic focus within the atrium
    - P wave is present but may have a different appearance to a sinus P wave, i.e. may be negative, positive or biphasic
    - May have single atrial premature complexes or sustained runs of SVT; careful examination may show that the rate speeds up slightly at the beginning of the run and slows down slightly at the end of the run

- Orthodromic atrioventricular reciprocating tachycardia (OAVRT)
  - Abrupt onset/offset of the SVT
  - Bypass tract connecting the atrium and ventricle
  - In certain circumstances, electrical activity cycles rapidly down through the AV node, through the ventricle, up the bypass tract, through the atrium and back down through the AV node
  - May see delta waves on sinus complexes: slurring of the PR interval as some of the electrical activity travels down the bypass tract to reach the ventricle before the majority of the electrical activity gets through the AV node to the ventricle
  - P waves usually negative during the run of SVT
- Atrial fibrillation (AF) (Figure 5.2.7)
  - No coordinated atrial activity: atrium fibrillating in uncoordinated manner
  - No evidence of P waves: may see fibrillation waves but ECG settings can mean that these are filtered out
  - Irregular rhythm: QRS occurs when sufficient fibrillation activity depolarises the AV node at the same time
  - Once present, unlikely to revert to sinus rhythm

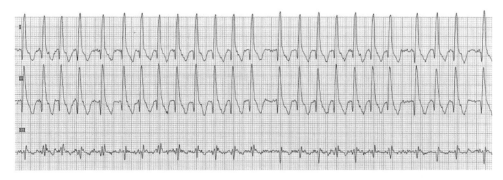

Figure 5.2.7 Atrial fibrillation. Leads I, II and III ECG showing atrial fibrillation; there is no evidence of P waves with fibrillation waves and an irregular rhythm of the QRS occurring when the fibrillation depolarises the AV node (50 mm/s, 5 mm/mV).

Aetiology
- Any disease that results in atrial enlargement, e.g. DCM, mitral valve disease
- Autonomic imbalance
- Digoxin toxicity
- Structural atrial disease (myocardial disease, infiltrative disease, myocarditis)
- OAVRT is a congenital bypass tract
- Large-breed dogs can develop AF without cardiac disease ('lone' AF), often at normal heart rates rather than tachycardic

Major signs
- May hear single premature beats and feel associated pulse deficits
- Sudden-onset tachycardia and weak peripheral pulses with focal atrial tachycardia or OAVRT
- Irregular rhythm with weak pulses with AF; pulse rate often lower than heart rate
- Usually no clinical signs for single premature beats
- Weakness, lethargy, syncope with sustained supraventricular arrhythmias – severity of signs depends on the heart rate
- Sustained arrhythmias can cause myocardial failure and result in CHF; right-sided more common that left-sided
- May have sudden death with sustained arrhythmias

Predisposition
- Lone AF: large-breed dogs
- OAVRT: Boxer, Labradors

Further investigations
- Echocardiography to assess for structural cardiac disease: may be difficult to assess if patient is very tachycardic as persistent tachycardia will cause systolic dysfunction and chamber dilation that may be reversible once the rhythm is controlled
- Troponin I to assess for myocarditis, *q.v* section 3.8.2
- 24-hour ECG Holter monitoring to assess for frequency and complexity of rhythm
- In young patients with suspected OAVRT, electrophysiological studies to identify the location of the bypass tract

Treatment
- Single premature beats do not require treatment
- Treatment aims
  - Focal atrial tachycardia or OAVRT: return to sinus rhythm with limited runs of supraventricular tachycardia
  - Atrial fibrillation (AF)
    - Reduce average heart to around 100–120 bpm on 24-hour ECG Holter monitor
    - Cardioversion to sinus rhythm if no evidence of structural heart disease
- Vagal manoeuvre (ocular or carotid sinus massage) in sustained focal atrial tachycardia/OAVRT may terminate the rhythm
- Drugs to block the AV node in symptomatic sustained focal atrial tachycardia or OAVRT:
  - These are both short acting drugs and are therefore used to 'break' the rhythm back to sinus rhythm rather than acting as a permanent fix; this approach is rarely taken with AF as the aim of AF treatment is not normally to return to sinus rhythm but instead control the rate and so chronic oral therapy is used instead
  - Diltiazem
    - First choice if size/function of heart is unknown
    - 0.1–0.25 mg/kg IV over 1–2 minutes; can repeat up to a total dose of 0.75 mg/kg
  - Esmolol
    - 0.05–0.50 mg/kg IV over 5 minutes
    - May avoid if in CHF/considered at high risk for CHF
- Oral therapy for ongoing management of supraventricular arrhythmias
  - Diltiazem
    - First choice for supraventricular arrhythmias if there is significant structural disease present
    - 2–3 mg/kg BID-TID
    - Lots of different preparations available with different release formulas (modified release, sustained release, etc.) – these are not interchangeable and so a single brand should be used whenever possible
  - Digoxin
    - Often added to treatment with diltiazem for AF patients

ORGAN SYSTEMS

- 3–5 µg/kg BID
  - Variable response with variable degrees of side effects, most commonly gastrointestinal
- Atenolol
  - Often start with low dose and wean up over a week or two
  - 0.5–2.0 mg/kg BID
  - Negative inotrope and negative chronotrope so use with caution if echocardiography shows poor systolic function or left atrial enlargement
- With any anti-arrhythmic, a repeat 24-hour ECG Holter monitor should be performed 7–14 days after treatment with anti-arrhythmic – make sure good control of arrhythmias and no pro-arrhythmic effect
- Electrical cardioversion to sinus rhythm for lone AF not always successful and may revert to atrial fibrillation after the procedure
- Ablation of bypass tract after physiological mapping can be a cure for OAVRT

5.2.4.2C VENTRICULAR TACHYARRHYTHMIAS

ECG changes

- Complexes originating from an ectopic focus within the ventricles and therefore not following the His-Purkinje conduction system
- Usually have wide and bizarre appearance and are not preceded by a P wave (Figure 5.2.8)
- Different shapes depend on where in the ventricle the complex originates from
- Can be premature complexes or escape complexes:
  - Premature complex: earlier than the next expected sinus complex
  - Escape complex: occur due to lack of signal to ventricular myocardium and so occur later than the next expected sinus complex, seen in context of third-degree AV block and sinus arrest
- Terminology:
  - Single ventricular premature complex: single ventricular beat occurring earlier than expected

- Bigeminy: repeating pattern of two beats (one ventricular premature complex and one sinus complex)
- Trigeminy: repeating pattern of three beats (two sinus complexes followed by one ventricular premature complex)
- Couplet: two ventricular premature complexes in a row (Figure 5.2.8a)
- Triplet: three ventricular premature complexes in a row (Figure 5.2.8a)
- Accelerated idioventricular rhythm: run of ventricular beats at a rate similar to underlying sinus rhythm (generally up to 160 bpm)
- Ventricular tachycardia: run of four or more ventricular premature complexes at rates of > 180 bpm (Figure 5.2.8b)
- Ventricular fibrillation: no coordinated activity in the ventricles – irregular and bizarre movement with no recognizable waveforms or complexes
- Monomorphic: all ventricular beats have the same appearance, implying their origin is the same ventricular ectopic focus
- Pleomorphic: more than one appearance to the ventricular beats (often two) but not changing from beat to beat, implying more than one ventricular ectopic focus
- Polymorphic: ventricular beats vary in appearance from beat to beat, implying multiple unstable ventricular ectopic foci

Aetiology

- Structural cardiac disease in which there is fibrosis or damage to the ventricular myocardium:
  - Aortic/pulmonic stenosis
  - ARVC
  - DCM
- Cardiac neoplasia
- Drugs e.g. digoxin, anaesthetic agents
- Myocarditis/endocarditis
- Primary arrhythmias, i.e. no evidence of primary structural changes
  - ARVC
  - DCM
  - Inherited ventricular arrhythmias in GSDs
- Systemic disease
  - Abdominal disease

(a)

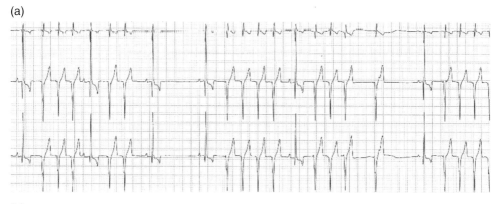

(b)

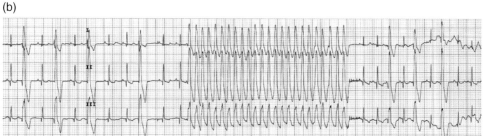

Figure 5.2.8 Ventricular arrhythmias

5.2.8a Couplets and triplets

Leads I, II and III ECG showing couplets, triplets and short runs of ventricular tachycardia with complexes which are wide and bizarre and originating from an ectopic focus in the ventricles (50 mm/s, 5 mm/mV).

5.2.8b Ventricular tachycardia

Leads I, II and III ECG showing intermittent single ventricular premature complexes (VPCs) followed by a run of VPCs at a rate > 180 bpm indicative of ventricular tachycardia (25 mm/s, 5 mm/mV).

- Gastric dilatation-volvulus
- Pancreatitis
- Pheochromocytoma
- Pyometra
- Splenic disease
- Autonomic imbalance
- CNS disease
- Hypoxia
- Systemic inflammation
- Systemic disease is more likely to cause accelerated idioventricular rhythms whereas structural cardiac disease, myocarditis and primary arrhythmias are more likely to cause ventricular tachycardia

Major signs

- May have clinical signs of underlying systemic disease
- May hear the premature beat, but more likely to pick up the pause that follows it
- Pulse deficits associated with ventricular premature complexes
- Weak pulses with sustained ventricular arrhythmias (especially ventricular tachycardia)
- Weakness, lethargy, syncope with ventricular tachycardia
- Usually no clinical signs for single beats, bigeminy, trigeminy, couplets or triplets
- Sustained arrhythmias can cause myocardial failure and result in CHF (right-sided more common than left-sided)
- May have sudden death with ventricular tachycardia often deteriorating to ventricular fibrillation

ORGAN SYSTEMS

Further investigations

- Depends on severity of arrhythmia
  - Ventricular tachycardia will need to be stabilised before further investigations can be performed
  - Less concerning rhythms (e.g. frequent single ventricular premature complexes, runs of accelerated idioventricular rhythm) should be investigated further prior to deciding on treatment plan
- Echocardiography to assess for structural cardiac disease, neoplasia
- Haematology/biochemistry/thoracic imaging/abdominal imaging to assess for systemic disease guided by any reported clinical signs
- Troponin I to assess for myocarditis, *q.v.* section 3.8.2
- 24-hour ECG Holter monitoring to assess for frequency and complexity of rhythm

Treatment

- Depends on the severity of the rhythm disturbance

Single ventricular premature complexes

- Do not require any treatment

Accelerated idioventricular rhythm

- Generally doesn't require anti-arrhythmic treatment; treatment of underlying systemic disease often results in resolution of arrhythmias

Couplets/triplets

- Depends on their instantaneous heart rates and frequency of these arrhythmias and is based on overall assessment of how clinically relevant the rhythm is

Ventricular fibrillation

- Start cardiopulmonary resuscitation immediately

Ventricular tachycardia

- Will need urgent treatment, especially if at high heart rates with pleomorphic or polymorphic complexes

- Lidocaine
  - First-line therapy
  - 2 mg/kg IV, repeat up to total dose of 8 mg/kg if no adverse events (vomiting, seizures); can follow up with continuous infusion
  - Check potassium concentrations and supplement if low; hypokalaemia can be one reason for lidocaine therapy to fail
  - Check magnesium concentrations and supplement if low; hypomagnesaemia can be one reason for lidocaine therapy to fail and as it's often difficult to measure magnesium concentrations in the emergency situation, some cardiologists empirically supplement magnesium in the face of ventricular tachycardia that is not responding to lidocaine therapy
- Procainamide
  - More expensive and less commonly available than lidocaine
  - 2 mg/kg IV over 3–5 minutes, repeat up to total dose of 20 mg/kg – can follow up with continuous infusion
- Either after IV stabilisation or if detected on 24-hour ECG Holter monitoring
  - Sotalol
    - 1–3 mg/kg PO BID
    - Negative inotrope and negative chronotrope; caution if echocardiography shows poor systolic function or left atrial enlargement
    - Often start with low dose and wean up over a week or two
  - Mexiletine
    - 4–8 mg/kg PO BID-TID
    - Give with food to reduce the chances of gastrointestinal side effects
  - Amiodarone
    - Requires loading protocol
      - 10–15 mg/kg BID for 2 days
      - 5–7.5 mg/kg BID for 5 days
      - 5–7.5 mg/kg SID ongoing
    - Significant adverse reactions including hepatic failure, thyroid dysfunction, neutropenia, anaemia, positive Coombs'

test – requires monitoring of hepatic values, thyroid function and haematology
- Stored within fat, resulting in very long half-life (months), therefore usually drug of last resort
- With any anti-arrhythmic, a repeat 24-hour ECG Holter monitor should be performed 7–14 days after treatment of maintenance dose of anti-arrhythmic to make sure good control of arrhythmias and no pro-arrhythmic effect

5.2.5 PERICARDIAL DISEASES

5.2.5A PERICARDIAL EFFUSION

Aetiology
- Accumulation of fluid in the pericardial space between the visceral pericardium (normally adhered to the epicardium of the heart) and the outer parietal pericardium (Figure 5.2.9). A small amount of lubricating fluid in the pericardial space is normal, but a larger volume of fluid is abnormal.

- The parietal pericardium contains a fibrous layer of tissue, making it relatively indistensible. A slowly accumulating pericardial effusion can cause the pericardium to gradually stretch, resulting in limited haemodynamic consequence.
- The pericardium cannot stretch to accommodate a rapidly accumulating pericardial effusion and this leads to a rapid rise in intra-pericardial pressure. When intra-pericardial pressure exceeds right atrial pressure (the lowest pressure cardiac chamber) there is compression of the right atrium, also known as cardiac tamponade.
- Several conditions can lead to pericardial effusion.

Common causes
- Idiopathic pericardial effusion is most common
- Neoplasia: chemodectoma, haemangiosarcoma, mesothelioma

Uncommon causes
- Coagulopathies: anticoagulant poisoning
- Congenital pericardial cyst – very uncommon

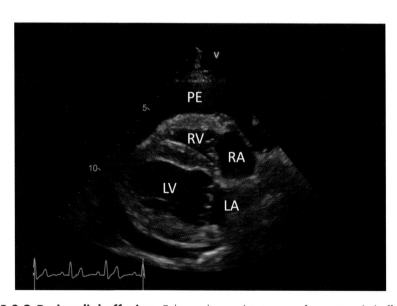

Figure 5.2.9 Pericardial effusion. Echocardiographic image of a pericardial effusion. The effusion is hypoechoic, similar to the echogenicity of the heart chambers.
PE, pericardial effusion; RA, right atrium; RV, right ventricle; LA, left atrium; LV, left ventricle.

ORGAN SYSTEMS

- Effusive constrictive pericardial disease
  - Unknown aetiology: thought to be subsequent to previous inflammation of the pericardium, including recurrent pericardial effusions
- Left atrial rupture
- Metabolic causes are very uncommon
  - Hypothyroidism
  - Renal failure
- Neoplasia: ectopic thyroid carcinoma, lymphoma, sarcoma
- Purulent pericardial effusion/pericarditis is very uncommon
  - Penetrating injury, foreign body (grass awn) or haematogenous spread
- Right-sided CHF: rare manifestation in dogs compared to cats

Major signs
- Ascites
- Dyspnoea (pleural effusion)
- Exercise intolerance/lethargy
- Inappetence
- Syncope
- Weight loss

Minor signs
- Polydipsia without polyuria
- Cough

Potential sequelae
- Right-sided CHF
- Collapse due to reduced cardiac output
- Death

Predisposition
Idiopathic pericardial effusion
- Golden retriever, Saint Bernard
- No age or sex predisposition

Left atrial rupture
- Small-breed dogs with advanced myxomatous mitral valve disease

Neoplasia
- Haemangiosarcoma
  - Right atrium predilection site
  - GSD and Golden retriever
  - Older dogs more likely to be affected
- Chemodectoma, heart base tumours

- Tend to occur in older, brachycephalic dogs but can occur in any dog

Historical clues
- Sudden onset of clinical signs
- Recurrent effusions can be seen with both neoplastic and idiopathic causes

Physical examination
- Apex beat less pronounced than normal
- Heart sounds muffled
- *Pulsus paradoxus* (strength of pulse decreases with inspiration)
- Tachycardia
- Signs of right-sided CHF
  - Ascites
  - Jugular venous distension
  - Hepatomegaly
  - Pleural effusion – reduced heart sounds, dullness on percussion
  - Subcutaneous oedema (uncommon)

Laboratory findings
- Clotting profile to ensure pericardial fluid is not secondary to a coagulopathy
- Pericardial fluid analysis
  - Cytology can be difficult to interpret as reactive mesothelial cells behave in similar manner to neoplastic cells. However, it is useful to rule out lymphoma.
  - Comparison of pericardial fluid haematocrit with peripheral blood haematocrit can be used to assess for the presence of recent acute haemorrhage.
  - Culture to rule out infectious causes.
- Pericardial tissue for histopathology
  - Only way to diagnose mesothelioma
  - Tissue collected during surgical management of pericardial effusion

Imaging
Plain radiographs
- Large, round cardiac silhouette – depends on volume of effusion
- Cardiac outline is sharper than normal- not seen if pleural effusion is present

Echocardiography
- Collapse of right atrium due to cardiac tamponade can be imaged

- Evidence of advanced myxomatous mitral valve disease can be seen in cases of left atrial rupture; a hyperechoic thrombus, often attached to the left atrium, may also be seen within the pericardial space
- Hypoechoic space between pericardium and myocardium

Hyperechoic 'speckles' within the hypoechoic space can suggest a highly cellular fluid

- Masses on the right atrium or at the heart base can see seen; these are best visualised before drainage of the pericardial fluid, as the hypoechoic fluid highlights the soft tissue structures

Special investigations
Electrocardiography
- Electrical alternans: QRS complex voltages alter from beat to beat (reflects swinging heart within pericardial sac with a large effusion)
- QRS voltages may be small due to electrical dampening by fluid

Treatment
- Treatment protocol for left atrial rupture is very different from treatment of all other causes of pericardial effusion and should be ruled out before pericardiocentesis
- Pericardiocentesis for diagnostic and therapeutic purposes
- Diuretics are contra-indicated prior to pericardiocentesis as they reduce circulating volume and therefore reduce right atrial pressures, worsening cardiac tamponade
- Diuretics may be used after pericardiocentesis to reduce ascites but are often not required as the ascites normally resolves without intervention within 24–48 hours
- Prednisolone has been suggested at anti-inflammatory doses for cases of idiopathic pericardial haemorrhage; evidence is lacking
- Pericardial surgery
  - Performed if recurrent effusion: usually ≥3 separate episodes or if effusion recurs within a relatively short time after pericardiocentesis
  - Diagnostic and therapeutic
  - Various options:
    - Balloon pericardiostomy; does not allow for collection of tissue for histology

- Pericardectomy by thoracoscopy
- Pericardial strip at exploratory thoracotomy
- If left atrial rupture suspected
  - Do not perform pericardiocentesis
  - Treatment aimed at keeping patient quiet and lowering systemic BP (to 90–100 mmHg) until tear has begun to heal (usually 24–48 hours)
    - Decreasing systemic BP encourages more blood flow along the aorta and discourages mitral regurgitation, dropping left atrial pressures slightly
    - Sodium nitroprusside continuous rate infusion allows tight control over BP but requires frequent monitoring and can only be used for approximately 24 hours due to the development of cyanide toxicity
    - Sedation with acepromazine and an opioid requires less intense monitoring but may be less effective in reducing BP

Monitoring
- Clinical signs
- Echocardiography

Prognosis
- Idiopathic pericardial effusion may require surgical pericardectomy if recurrent disease, but generally fair to good prognosis
- Neoplasia:
  - Haemangiosarcoma carries a poor prognosis but could consider aggressive surgical resection of right auricle along with pericardectomy if possible
  - Chemodectoma carries a relatively good prognosis; pericardectomy may be required to control clinical signs
  - Mesothelioma carries a fair prognosis but is ultimately fatal
- Left atrial rupture: very poor prognosis, often rapidly fatal; if not fatal, the patient can recover but may have further tears in the future
- Pericarditis: prognosis depends on underlying cause; often require surgical pericardiectomy for effective treatment

ORGAN SYSTEMS

ORGAN SYSTEMS

5.2.5B PERITONEAL PERICARDIAL DIAPHRAGMATIC HERNIA (PPDH)

Aetiology
- May be congenital or acquired
- Congenital is usually due to incomplete development of the septum diaphragm leading to a persistent connection between the peritoneal cavity and the pericardium
- Acquired is usually secondary to trauma, and is, strictly, a rupture not a hernia
- In true PPDH, abdominal contents end up in the pericardium, surrounding the heart. The most common organ to herniate into the pericardium is the liver, followed by the gall bladder, SI, spleen, stomach, and omentum.
- Clinical signs depend on the organs herniated into the pericardium

Major signs
- May have no clinical signs
- Anorexia
- Coughing
- Diarrhoea
- Dyspnoea
- Lethargy
- Vomiting

Minor signs
- Right-sided CHF

Potential sequelae
- Many animals may never show signs
- Gastrointestinal obstruction, strangulation or torsion is possible

Predisposition
- Congenital PPDH: Weimaraner

Historical clues
- Clinical signs developing after a major trauma may suggest an acquired defect
- Intermittent clinical signs in a young patient can be explained by organs moving in and out of the pericardium

Physical examination
- Displaced apical beat
- 'Empty' abdominal palpation
- Muffled heart sounds

Laboratory findings
- Haematology and biochemistry generally unremarkable
- May see increased ALT activity in some patients

Imaging
Plain radiographs
- Enlarged cardiac silhouette
- Loss of distinction between heart and diaphragm
- May see gas-filled bowel within cardiac silhouette
- Small hepatic silhouette
- Other abdominal organs (spleen, intestine) may not be present on abdominal radiography

Echocardiography
- Abdominal organs adjacent to heart; the liver is most commonly seen and must be distinguished from a consolidated lung lobe
- Small volume of pericardial effusion may be present

Special investigations
Barium swallow
- Demonstrates the presence of GI tract within the pericardium
- Generally not needed for diagnosis as thoracic radiographs and echocardiography usually sufficient

Treatment
- Surgical repair is indicated if the patient is showing clinical signs.
- In older animals without clinical signs, surgical repair may not be the best option due to likely adhesions that will have formed between the organs in the pericardium. In these cases, monitoring for clinical signs is generally optimal.

Monitoring
- Clinical signs

Prognosis
- Good prognosis with surgical repair

5.3   ENDOCRINE SYSTEM

Problems

Endocrine disorders may be the result of:
- A lack of a specific hormone, often due to the immune-mediated destruction of the gland

or

- Inappropriate secretion of a specific hormone which may be the result of a functional tumour, although the clinical signs are mostly an effect of the hormone excess

Presenting complaints

q.v. section 1
1.2 Alopecia
1.5 Anorexia
1.22 Exercise intolerance
1.36 Polyphagia
1.37 Polyuria/polydipsia (PU/PD)
1.42 Seizures
1.45 Stunting
1.51 Weakness, collapse and syncope
1.52 Weight gain
1.53 Weight loss

Physical abnormalities

q.v. section 2
2.1 Abdominal enlargement
2.4 Arrhythmias: bradycardia
2.7 Eye lesions
2.8 Hepatomegaly
2.10 Hypertension
2.27 Skin pigmentation changes

Laboratory abnormalities

q.v. section 3
3.7 Calcium
3.9 Chloride
3.11 Cortisol (basal)
3.17 Glucose
3.19 Lipids
3.20 Liver enzymes
3.23 Potassium
3.24 Sodium
3.26 Thyroid hormone

Diagnostic Approach

- Suspect endocrinopathy from problem list
- Screening by routine laboratory testing
- Perform specific endocrine tests

Diagnostic Methods

History, Physical examination, Laboratory findings
q.v. individual diseases sections 5.3.1 to 5.3.7.

Imaging

Plain radiographs
- Altered fat distribution
- Calcification
  - Adrenals
  - Aortic wall
  - Calcinosis cutis
  - Pulmonary
  - Soft tissues
- Hepatomegaly in diabetes mellitus (DM) and hyperadrenocorticism (HAC)
- Osteopenia in hyperparathyroidism and HAC

Ultrasound
- Endocrine organ enlargement
- Hepatomegaly in DM and HAC

Special investigative techniques

- Specific hormone assays and dynamic function tests are used as indicated to confirm the diagnosis
q.v. individual diseases in sections 5.3.1 to 5.3.7

5.3.1   DIABETES INSIPIDUS (DI)

- Antidiuretic hormone (ADH) is produced by the pituitary in response to increases in plasma osmolality
- ADH increases water reabsorption by the renal collecting ducts

ORGAN SYSTEMS

Notes on Canine Internal Medicine, Fourth Edition. Victoria L. Black, Kathryn F. Murphy, Jessie Rose Payne, and Edward J. Hall.
© 2022 John Wiley & Sons Ltd. Published 2022 by John Wiley & Sons Ltd.

Aetiology
- A lack of ADH or failure of renal collecting ducts to respond to ADH
- Can be partial or complete
- True DI is rare but is sometimes mistakenly diagnosed and treated with desmopressin (DDAVP, i.e. synthetic ADH) without having ruled out HAC or psychogenic polydipsia

Central DI (CDI)
- Absolute or relative deficiency of ADH (rare)

Causes
- Congenital
- Hypophysectomy for pituitary-dependent HAC (PDH), but usually transient as hypothalamus-neurohypophysis can still secrete ADH
- Idiopathic
- Secondary to head trauma or expanding pituitary or hypothalamic tumour

Nephrogenic DI (NDI)
- Results from a defect in renal tubular receptor that leads to an insensitivity to ADH

Causes
- Congenital (rare)
- Secondary to renal, metabolic and electrolyte disorders
  - Chronic kidney disease (CKD)
  - Fanconi syndrome
  - Hepatic failure
  - HAC
  - Hypercalcaemia
  - Hypokalaemia
  - Pyelonephritis
  - Pyometra

Major signs
- PU/PD

Minor signs
- Dehydration
- NDI: signs referable to inciting disease may be present
- Nocturia
- Restlessness and weight changes secondary to severe polydipsia
- Urinary incontinence if urine volume overwhelms urethral sphincter mechanism

Potential sequelae
- CNS signs
  - Expanding tumour of pituitary or hypothalamus
  - CNS signs due to gradual water restriction causing chronic hypernatraemia, *q.v.* section 3.24.1
    - Aimless wandering
    - Incoordination
    - Seizures
    - Visual deficits

Predisposition
- Congenital CDI recognised
- No age, sex or breed predisposition for idiopathic CDI

Historical clues
- Onset of profound PU/PD
- Other major signs absent in CDI unless hypernatraemic

Physical examination
- Often unremarkable unless hypernatraemic
- With secondary NDI there may be clinical findings referable to the underlying disease

Laboratory findings
Haematology and serum biochemistry
- To rule out other causes of PU/PD
- Slight increases in PCV, total proteins and plasma osmolality may be seen secondary to mild dehydration with DI
- If total water is depleted, urea, creatinine, sodium and chloride may be increased
- Further assessment of hepatic function or the pituitary-adrenal axis may be indicated

Urinalysis
- Hyposthenuria: urine specific gravity (USG) 1.001–1.007
- Urine osmolality 40–200 mOsm/kg

Imaging
Thoracic and abdominal radiographs
- Performed to assess for other diseases causing PU/PD
- In many cases a large bladder will be observed due to overstretching from severe PU

Special investigations
Water deprivation test
- Should *never* be performed in azotaemic or hypercalcaemic animals
- Aims to establish if ADH is released in response to dehydration and therefore distinguish psychogenic polydipsia from DI
- Before performing a water deprivation test it is essential, in the authors' view, to rule out HAC conclusively by means of ACTH stimulation *and* low-dose dexamethasone suppression (LDDS) tests, *q.v.* section 5.3.4A
- Dogs with HAC will not fully concentrate urine in response to water deprivation and this may lead to a misdiagnosis of partial DI
- The ADH response test is commonly performed after the water deprivation test to classify whether the dog with DI has CDI or NDI

Absolute water deprivation test
- This test acutely restricts water intake and assesses any increase in USG
- Failure to concentrate the urine may indicate:
  - CDI
  - NDI
  - Medullary washout causing a false positive: prolonged polyuria depletes the renal medulla of sodium, so that urine-concentrating ability is disabled
- Rarely performed, as potentially dangerous and medullary washout may give a false positive result

Modified water deprivation test
- Medullary washout is a controversial concept, but the modified test is preferred to avoid false positives.
- The modified test gradually restricts water intake for several days before complete water restriction to rule out medullary washout as an explanation for failure to concentrate urine

  Day 1: Weigh dog and allow 120 ml water/ kg body weight (BW) given as small amounts during 24 hour period

  Day 2: Weigh dog and allow 90 ml water/ kg BW as above

  Day 3: Weigh dog and allow 60 ml water/ kg BW as above

  Day 4: Remove all water and perform water deprivation test as below

Hydration and USG are monitored on a daily basis
- Dogs with psychogenic polydipsia often stop drinking excessively and concentrate their urine > 1.030 within 24–48 hours of hospitalization, obviating the need to perform a full water deprivation test
- The full test is rarely performed as DI is largely a diagnosis by exclusion, and is only indicated if psychogenic polydipsia can't be distinguished from DI

Protocol for water deprivation test (absolute or end of modified)
- The dog is hospitalised and receives no food or water for the duration of the test
- An indwelling urinary catheter is preferred over repeated catheterisations
- It is preferable to measure urine osmolality and plasma osmolality during this protocol if the equipment is available
1 The bladder is emptied, then the USG is measured and the dog weighed every hour; results are recorded
2 All water and food are withheld
3 The test is stopped when:
   - 5% of the initial body weight has been lost, usually within 3–8 hours for true DI cases

     or
   - USG increases to > 1.030, indicating normal concentrating ability
   - The dog shows CNS signs, i.e. depression, stupor, seizures
4 ADH response test is commonly performed immediately after the water deprivation test

Interpretation
- USG at the end of water deprivation
  - < 1.010 is highly suggestive of CDI or NDI
  - 1.020–1.030 is equivocal, but may be seen with partial ADH deficiency, medullary washout, or HAC
  - > 1.030 is normal and indicates psychogenic polydipsia

ORGAN SYSTEMS

ADH response test
- Indicated for dogs failing to concentrate urine adequately in response to dehydration at the end of the water deprivation test, i.e. psychogenic polydipsia has been ruled out
  1. Catheterise and empty bladder
  2. Check USG and, preferably, osmolality as above
  3. Desmopressin (DDAVP) administered: 1–4 µg IV or IM
  4. Empty bladder every 15–30 minutes for 2 hours
  5. Collect urine for SG and osmolality every 15–30 minutes
  6. Collect plasma samples for osmolality concurrently
  7. Check hydration and CNS status
- Interpretation
  - Failure to increase USG above 1.030 after DDAVP is highly suggestive of NDI
  - Increase of USG > 1.030 is indicative of CDI
- At end of test
  - Introduce small amounts of water every 30 minutes for 2 hours
  - Monitor for vomiting and CNS signs
  - Return to *ad lib* water after 2 hours if dog is well

Therapeutic trial with desmopressin
- Because of the difficulty and risks of the water deprivation test, trial treatment with desmopressin for 5–7 days is reasonable once all other causes of PU/PD have been excluded, although water intoxication is a hypothetical risk with psychogenic polydipsia

Treatment
CDI or partial NDI
- DDAVP
  - subcutaneously 0.5–2 µg once or twice daily, or
  - intranasal drops (via conjunctival sac): 1–4 drops once or twice daily, or
  - tablets @ 10 µg/kg given before food twice daily
- Duration of action is variable (8–24 hours); maximal effect usually between 6 and 10 hours
- Side effects uncommon

- Thiazide diuretics (see below) may decrease water intake by 50% but are often unavailable

NDI
- Treat underlying disease
- Reduce water intake by 30–50% in some cases
- Salt intake should be restricted
- Thiazide diuretics, but are often unavailable
  - Hydrochlorothiazide @ 2.5–5 mg/kg twice daily
  - Chlorothiazide @ 10–20 mg/kg twice daily
  - Mechanism
    - Thiazides reduce total body sodium by inhibiting reabsorption in the ascending loop of Henle
    - Decreased sodium and plasma osmolality inhibit the thirst centre and reduce water consumption
    - This results in decreased glomerular filtration rate, increased proximal tubular reabsorption of sodium and water, and decreased delivery of sodium to distal tubule with net reduction in urine volume

Monitoring
- Urine specific gravity (USG)
- Water intake

Prognosis
- Water intake can be reduced by more than 50% in some cases
- CNS signs may develop in some cases of CDI secondary to tumour growth

5.3.2 DIABETES MELLITUS (DM)

- Insulin is secreted by the pancreas in response to hyperglycaemia
- It acts to lower blood glucose, promoting uptake of glucose by peripheral tissues

Aetiology
- Hyperglycaemia due to:
  - Absolute lack of insulin [equivalent to Type I, insulin-dependent DM (IDDM)]
  - Insulin resistance [equivalent to Type II, non-insulin-dependent DM (NIDDM)]
- IDDM is the more common form in dogs

- NIDDM is secondary, but prolonged hyperglycaemia ultimately and irreversibly exhausts insulin production
- Signs relate to:
  - Diabetic ketoacidosis (DKA) if untreated
  - Disturbance of intermediary metabolism
  - Osmotic diuresis

Causes of IDDM
- Idiopathic
- End-stage chronic pancreatitis

Causes of NIDDM
- Acromegaly
- Glucagonoma
- HAC
- Growth hormone (GH) secretion
  - Neoplastic mammary tissue may secrete GH
  - Progesterone can induce mammary tissue to secrete GH
    - During metoestrus and pregnancy
    - Iatrogenic
- Obesity

Major signs
Early
- Polyphagia
- PU/PD
- Weight loss

Late
- Cataracts
- Ketoacidosis
  - Anorexia
  - Collapse
  - Dehydration
  - Depression
  - Ketotic breath
  - Vomiting

Minor signs
- Exercise intolerance/decreased activity
- Inappropriate urination
- Peripheral neuropathies
- Recurrent infections, e.g. urinary tract, conjunctivitis

Potential sequelae
- Acute kidney injury in DKA
- Cataracts

- Gall bladder mucocoele
- Hepatic disease can occasionally complicate DM therapy
  - Hepatocutaneous syndrome can be associated with DM due to glucagonoma
- Hyperosmolar DM: rare condition causing severe hyperglycaemia without ketosis and with a very poor prognosis
- Hypoglycaemia is a potential complication with insulin therapy
- Predisposition to infection
  - Conjunctivitis
  - Cystitis
  - Pyoderma
  - Stomatitis
  - Urinary tract infection

Predisposition
- Breeds over-represented: cross-bred terriers, Boxers, Poodles, Schipperke, but geographical variations
- Breeds under-represented: GSD, Golden retriever
- Females may be at greater risk of developing DM than males, but this is age-related, i.e. < 7 years equal risk for both sexes
- Entire females at 8–10 years are 3 times more likely to develop DM than neutered females of the same age
- Peak incidence of idiopathic DM is > 7 years

Historical clues
- Initially well and polyphagic
- Owner notices extreme PU/PD, polyphagia and weight loss
- Sometimes cataracts are the first sign noted
- Later, DKA causes anorexia, depression and vomiting
- Long history of chronic GI signs suggests end-stage chronic pancreatitis

Physical examination
- Cataracts
- Emphysematous cystitis: bladder 'crackles' on palpation
- Hepatocutaneous syndrome, *q.v.* sections 2.26, 5.6
  - Hyperkeratotic foot pads
  - Lameness because of foot pain from cracked pads

- Hepatomegaly
- Hyperosmolar
  - Extreme lethargy to comatose state
- Ketoacidosis
  - Depression
  - Deydration
  - Ketotic breath
  - Tachypnoea
  - Vomiting
  - Weakness
- Obesity or weight loss depending on severity/chronicity of disease

Laboratory findings
Haematology
- Dehydration may lead to increased haematocrit
- Infection may cause leukocytosis ± left shift
- Non-regenerative anaemia associated with chronic disease
- If severe hypophosphataemia (during treatment of DKA), haemolysis can occur

Serum biochemistry
- Hyperglycaemia
- Hypercholesterolaemia
- Hypertriglyceridaemia
- Ketonaemia
  - Increased acetoacetate, β-hydroxybutyrate and acetone
- Increased liver enzyme activities (ALP and ALT) due to hepatic lipid storage ('hepatic lipidosis')
- Lipaemic blood samples
- DKA causes marked abnormalities of serum electrolytes and azotaemia
  - Initial hyperkalaemia changing to hypokalaemia after insulin therapy
  - Initial hyperphosphataemia changing to hypophosphataemia after insulin therapy

Urinalysis
- Glucosuria when blood glucose is greater than renal threshold of 10–12 mmol/l
- Ketonuria, but increases during initial treatment of DKA, reflecting conversion of acetone and β-hydroxybutyrate back to acetoacetate, which urine strips are more sensitive at detecting
- Sediment suggestive of urinary tract infection: bacteriuria, haematuria, proteinuria, pyuria

Imaging
Plain radiographs
- Generally unremarkable except diffuse hepatomegaly
- Emphysematous cystitis seen occasionally
- Emphysematous cholecystitis seen very occasionally

Ultrasound
- Adrenals for suspected HAC
- Pancreas to try to identify pancreatitis as underlying disease

Special investigations
Arterial blood gas analysis
- Acid/base information in the ketoacidotic diabetic

Glycosylated serum proteins
- Fructosamine: marker of average glycaemic control over 2–3 weeks, q.v. section 3.16
- Glycated haemoglobin marker of average glycaemic control over several months

Serum insulin concentrations
- Not helpful as most cases are IDDM

cPL
- May be increased with pancreatitis

cTLI
- Decreased with end-stage chronic pancreatitis causing concurrent DM and EPI

Other investigations
- Should aim to identify concurrent diseases, e.g. HAC, infections, if insulin resistance occurs

Treatment
Diabetic ketoacidosis (DKA)
It is beyond the scope of this book to detail management of DKA; the reader is advised to refer to other texts.
1 Correct fluid/electrolyte losses
  - 0.9% sodium chloride with potassium/phosphate supplementation as indicated
  - Rate depends on degree of dehydration.
  - IV fluid requirements normally 1.5–2× maintenance

ORGAN SYSTEMS

2 Insulin
- Aim to normalise intermediary metabolism with regular/soluble insulin
  - Intermittent IM regime
  - CRI of low-dose regular/soluble insulin
  - Intermittent high-dose IM/SC protocol with regular insulin
  - Insulin Lispro may be an alternative when regular insulin is unavailable
3 Longer-acting insulin started once the dog is stable and eating voluntarily: initial dose in the range of 0.25 to 0.5 units per kg
4 Correct acidosis: IVFT ± cautious use of bicarbonate
5 Identify any precipitating factors for the DM
6 Provide carbohydrate substrate when dictated by insulin therapy
7 Aim to return parameters to normal SLOWLY: too-rapid correction can be harmful and can create osmotic and biochemical problems

Non-ketotic diabetic
Stabilisation period
1 Diet
- Daily regime constant in dietary composition, volume and timing of meals
- Greater content of complex carbohydrates including fibre to slow digestion and absorption, giving smoother glycaemic curve
2 Exercise
- Avoid exercise at times of expected low blood glucose, e.g. 6–8 hours after lente insulin
- Constant in duration and intensity once stabilised
3 Insulin
- Preparation
  - Intermediate acting, e.g. lente
  - Longer acting, e.g. protamine zinc, if lente's duration of action is too short
- Frequency
  - Twice-daily injections recommended over once daily
- Plan
  - Twice-daily lente insulin with 50% food each time
- Monitoring
  - Flash glucose monitor, e.g. Freestyle Libre
  - Glucose curve

- Spot blood glucose checks at time of suspected nadir
- Adjustment doses
  - Usually takes some time to obtain a consistent response to a specific dose of insulin; therefore, wait 2–3 days before considering changing the dose unless marked hypoglycaemia occurs
  - Most dogs stabilise at 1–1.5 units/kg of lente insulin twice daily
  - 24-hour blood glucose curve after the initial stabilisation period to assess duration of action of insulin and stability and help to determine ideal meal times
1 Maintenance therapy: insulin
- Adjust dose as above, based on:
  - occasional or serial nadir blood glucose concentrations initially weekly, then every 2 weeks, then once a month
  - glucose curve
  - Freestyle Libre monitor
  - serum fructosamine
- Maintenance dose > 2.0 units/kg indicates insulin resistance or incorrect administration
2 Neutering
- Unspayed bitches should be neutered before their next season to avoid rapid and unpredictable changes in insulin requirement at the beginning and end of metoestrus

Monitoring
- Routine clinical examination
- Occasional minimum database including urinalysis to identify problems early
- Occasional or serial nadir blood glucose concentrations

Fructosamine
- Measure of plasma proteins which have undergone non-enzymatic glycation
- It reflects the mean blood glucose in the lifetime of those proteins, i.e. usually 1–3 weeks
- Can be assessed at any time of day
- > 400 µmol/l suggests poor control

Glycated haemoglobin
- Reflects control over the preceding 1–3 months

- Useful for animals that are not rechecked frequently
- Lack of availability of validated assays

Prognosis
- Survival times are likely to be decreased compared to the unaffected dog population
- DM can be very difficult to control after oestrus in unspayed bitches
- Cataracts frequently develop and phacoemulsification may be needed to restore sight, although rare cases will also develop retinal blindness
- Hepatocutaneous syndrome is difficult to manage
- Underlying diseases, e.g. HAC, pancreatitis, infections, can make DM difficult to manage

5.3.3 GROWTH HORMONE DISORDERS

- Lack of or excessive secretion of growth hormone (GH) are rare disorders but can cause significant skeletal, soft tissue and metabolic abnormalities
- A commercial assay for GH is not readily available and serum IGF-1 concentration is used as a surrogate marker

5.3.3A ACROMEGALY (HYPERSOMATOTROPISM)

Aetiology
- A rare condition due to the chronic secretion of excess GH causing slow overgrowth of bony and soft tissues, and insulin resistance leading to DM
- The dog is unusual in that GH is secreted by the pituitary and also by mammary tissue during the progesterone phase of metoestrus

Common causes
- Iatrogenic chronic progestagen administration
- Metoestrus (luteal/progesterone phase)

Uncommon causes
- Functional pituitary mass: rare compared to diabetic cats

- GH-secreting mammary tumour
- Secondary to hypothyroidism: increases GH and IGF-1

Major signs
- Diabetes mellitus: initially transient during metoestrus, but if dog is not spayed DM will become permanent after the next season
- Prognathism and increased interdental spaces
- Soft tissue swelling
  - Abdominal swelling
  - Changes in facial features
  - Increased soft tissue in pharyngeal area
  - Thickened skin folds
- PU/PD with or without DM
- Respiratory stridor
  - Dyspnoea
  - Snoring

Minor signs
- Cardiac hypertrophy but rarely signs of heart disease
- Gigantism, as seen in human acromegalics, is very rare as increased GH in dogs typically occurs after bone growth has ceased
- Stiffness, difficulty rising, neck rigidity
  - Articular cartilage proliferation
  - Periarticular periosteal reaction
  - Spondylosis deformans

Potential sequelae
- CNS signs rarely if pituitary mass
- DM
- Upper airway obstruction

Predisposition
- Entire female dogs
- Middle-aged and older dogs

Historical clues
- Chronic progestagen administration, e.g. megestrol
- Onset of snoring in older age
- Recent oestrus

Physical examination
- Prognathism and increased interdental spaces
- Soft tissue swelling, especially in throat
- Thickened skin folds

Laboratory findings
- Unremarkable unless DM has developed, *q.v.* section 5.3.2

Imaging
Plain radiographs
- Prognathism and widened interdental spaces
- Excess soft tissue in neck

Ultrasound
- Cardiac hypertrophy

Special investigations
- IGF-1 assay

Treatment
- Stop any exogenous progestagen treatment
- Manage DM
- Ovariectomy: ideally performed either before DM develops or after the first metoestrus when the dog shows signs of DM, as it can be prevented or reversed; after the second season the DM will become permanent because of insulin exhaustion
- Progesterone receptor blocker, e.g. aglepristone
- Pituitary mass
  - Hypophysectomy for pituitary mass
  - Octreotide (somatostatin analogue)
  - Radiation
- Treat hypothyroidism causing secondary acromegaly

Monitoring
- Check for the development of DM

Prognosis
- Good if due to progesterone

5.3.3B PITUITARY DWARFISM

A rare condition due to an absence of growth hormone (GH) secretion.

Aetiology
- Congenital pituitary cyst (Rathke's pouch) causing pressure atrophy
- Genetic: mutation in LHX3 gene

- Usually a concurrent lack of thyroid-stimulating hormone (TSH) and prolactin, and impaired release of gonadotropins; ACTH secretion is unaffected

Major signs
- Proportional stunting, *q.v.* section 1.45

Minor signs
- Ataxia due to cervical cord compression from atlanto-axial instability
- Decreased appetite and activity at 2–3 years due to concurrent hypothyroidism
- Poor hair coat
  - Gradual development of truncal alopecia
    - Lack of primary or guard hairs
    - Retention of lanugo or secondary hairs that are easily epilated by wear and tear
- Poor behavioural training
- Progressive skin hyperpigmentation and scale
- Secondary pyoderma

Potential sequelae
- CNS signs rarely if pituitary mass
- DM
- Upper airway obstruction

Predisposition
- GSD, Karelian Bear Dog, Miniature Pinscher, Spitz and Wolfdog (Czechoslovakian, Saarloos),

Historical clues
- Retarded growth: retains puppy size but in normal proportion

Physical examination
- Proportional stunting

Laboratory findings
- Usually unremarkable, but increased creatinine due to renal abnormal glomerular development

Imaging
- Proportionally small bones on radiographs
- CT is better than MR for imaging the pituitary

ORGAN SYSTEMS

Special investigations
- DNA test for LHX3 gene mutation
- Decreased IGF-1 concentration as a marker of GH deficiency is not definitive
- GH assay but not commercially available
  - Decreased GH concentration is not definitive
  - GH stimulation test using GHRH, clonidine or xylazine is definitive
- Decreased cTSH and T4

Treatment
- Canine GH is not available, but porcine GH injections can be trialled
- Progestins, but bitches should be spayed first
  - Medroxyprogesterone acetate may increase GH and body size, and improve coat
  - Proligestone can cause development of an adult hair coat, increased body weight, and increased IGF-1 concentrations
- Treat
  - Hypothyroidism
  - Pyoderma

Monitoring
- During treatment, monitor IGF-1, blood glucose and GH if assay available

Prognosis
- Untreated: poor with euthanasia often at 3–5 years
  - Bald, dull and thin
    - Progressive hair loss
    - Progressive loss of pituitary functions, continuing expansion of pituitary cysts
    - Progressive renal failure
- Treated: guarded

5.3.4 ADRENAL GLAND DISORDERS

The adrenal gland produces:
- Glucocorticoid
  - Cortisol is the major hormone
  - Controlled by ACTH secretion from pituitary
- Mineralocorticoid
  - Aldosterone

- Part of renin-angiotensin-aldosterone system (RAAS) stimulated in response to sodium delivery to the renal juxtaglomerular apparatus
- Sex hormones

5.3.4A HYPERADRENOCORTICISM (HAC)

- The main glucocorticoid, cortisol, is produced by the adrenal cortex
  - Its secretion is controlled by ACTH from the pituitary
  - It exerts negative feedback on ACTH release

Aetiology
- Excessive production of endogenous glucocorticoids
  - Adrenal-dependent HAC; tumour is usually unilateral but can be bilateral
  - Pituitary-dependent HAC (PDH), i.e. excess ACTH secretion overstimulating both adrenals to secrete cortisol
- Iatrogenic: administration of exogenous glucocorticoids both orally and topically

Major signs
- Abdominal enlargement ('pot-belly') due to muscle weakness and hepatomegaly
- Alopecia
- Hepatomegaly
- Lethargy/exercise intolerance
- Muscle atrophy and weakness
- Panting
- PU/PD causing nocturia/incontinence/inappropriate urination
- Polyphagia

Minor signs
- Blindness
  - Cataracts
  - Sudden acquired retinal degeneration syndrome (SARDS)
- Calcinosis cutis: white/cream skin plaques, surrounded by erythema, developing cracks and secondary infection
- Comedones

- Myotonia: rare
- Neurological signs due to expansion of pituitary macroadenoma
- Reproductive failure
- Slow wound healing or wound breakdown
- Thin skin

Potential sequelae
- Progression of major signs
- DM from insulin resistance
- Gall bladder mucocoele
- Immunosuppression with secondary infections
  - Pyoderma
  - Urinary tract infection
- Neurological signs due to expansile pituitary macroadenoma (Nelson's syndrome)
  - Decreasing levels of consciousness
  - Decreasing appetite
  - Seizures
- Pancreatitis
- Pulmonary thromboembolism (PTE)
- Sudden death due to PTE

Predisposition
- < 20% of cases develop adrenal-dependent HAC
- > 80 % of cases develop PDH
- Adrenal-dependent HAC
  - Females > males
  - More frequently in large-breed dogs: 50% weigh > 20 kg
  - Tend to be older than PDH: median 11–12 years
- PDH
  - Dachshund, Poodle, Samoyed and small terriers at increased risk
  - No sex predisposition
  - Usually mid- or old-aged dogs (median 7–9 years)

Historical clues
Owner often feels dog is generally well
- Eating
- Gaining weight
but is concerned by
- Exercise intolerance/lethargy
- Hair loss
- Panting

- Polyphagia
- PU/PD
- Poor wound healing

Dogs that are anorexic, unwell, or losing weight do not normally have HAC as the primary cause of their problem but could have a pituitary macroadenoma.

Physical examination
- Alopecia: usually bilaterally symmetrical, affecting flank, ventral abdomen and thorax, perineum and neck
- Bruising after blood sampling
- Calcinosis cutis occasionally
  - Predilection sites: axilla, neck, inguinal, ventrum
- Comedones
- Decreased muscle mass, especially on limbs, spine and temporal region
- Excessive surface scale
- Hepatomegaly
- Myotonia: stiff, stilted hindlimb gait (rare)
- Pot-bellied appearance
- Thin skin over ventrum

Laboratory findings
Haematology
- Stress leukogram
  - Eosinopenia
  - Lymphopenia
  - Neutrophilia
  - Mild monocytosis
- Red blood cells (RBCs): normal or increased numbers
- Platelets: mild increases

Serum biochemistry
- Alkaline phosphatase (ALP) activity increased in > 90% of cases
  - 5–40× upper end of reference range
  - Induction of hepatic isoenzyme of ALP (steroid-induced)
- Alanine aminotransferase (ALT) activity
  - Mild increase, possibly secondary to glycogen accumulation in hepatocytes
- Bile acids
  - Mild/moderate increases; rarely > 50 µmol/l
- Cholesterol and triglycerides increased

- Glucose
  - Blood concentration usually slightly increased but below renal threshold
  - DM develops in ~10% of cases due to insulin antagonism by cortisol
- Urea and creatinine
  - Low-normal due to increased urinary loss with PU

Urinalysis
- USG usually < 1.015 and often hyposthenuric (< 1.008)
- Glucosuria only in cases with DM
- Urinary tract infection
  - Asymptomatic bacteriuria present in ~50% of cases
  - Sediment may appear inactive due to immunosuppression

Imaging
Thoracic radiographs
- Pulmonary metastasis from adrenocortical carcinoma
- Tracheal/bronchial wall/pulmonary mineralisation
- PTE: rarely identified on plain films; CT more sensitive
- Congestive heart failure (rare)

Abdominal radiographs
- Hepatomegaly
- Good contrast: excess fat in abdomen
- Large, distended bladder secondary to PU/PD
- Pot-bellied appearance
- General poor bone density = osteoporosis (lumbar vertebral bodies good place to assess)
- Soft tissue mineralisation
  - Adrenal tumour
  - Aorta
  - Calcinosis cutis
  - Kidneys

Ultrasonography
Adrenals
- Bilateral enlargement = hyperplasia in PDH
- Unilateral enlargement = likely tumour causing adrenal-dependent HAC, as bilateral tumours are rare
- Invasion of caudal vena cava and/or phrenicoabdominal vein with advanced neoplasia

Liver
To assess hepatomegaly and, if an adrenal tumour, to check for visible metastasis

Special investigations
Assess the hypothalamo-pituitary-adrenal axis by measuring changes in plasma cortisol caused by stimulation and suppression tests, and interpreting the results in conjunction with clinical signs and imaging findings

Hypothalamo-pituitary-adrenal test protocols
Basal cortisol
Cannot be used to diagnose HAC as marked variation, *q.v.* section 3.11

ACTH stimulation test
1 Collect plasma or serum for basal cortisol concentration.
2 Inject synthetic ACTH (tetracosactide, Cosacthen® Synacthen®) slowly intravenously.
3 Collect a second sample for cortisol concentration @ 30–90 minutes after ACTH, depending on lab protocol.
   - Interpretation
     - Stimulation of the cortisol concentration above the upper reference interval is highly suggestive of HAC, but can be caused by severe illness; values post-ACTH cortisol > 700 nmol/l are highly consistent with HAC
   - Identifies ~50% of cases with adrenal-dependent HAC as tumour may be autonomous
   - Identifies ~85% of cases with PDH
   - Recent administration of glucocorticoids will affect results

Low dose dexamethasone suppression test (LDDS)
- Dexamethasone exerts negative feedback on the hypothalamus and pituitary, decreasing the secretion of ACTH and thus cortisol. It does not cross-react in the cortisol assay.
1 Collect plasma or serum for basal cortisol concentration.
2 Inject 0.01 mg/kg dexamethasone intravenously; it can be a very small volume, so

may need diluting 1 in 10 for a measurable volume, and place IV catheter to ensure IV administration.

3 Collect further samples for cortisol determination @ 3 or 4 hours and @ 8 hours after dexamethasone administration.

4 The dog should be kept quiet and unstressed during the test period.

5 This test can be modified to be performed at home, with the owner administering oral dexamaethasone and collecting urine samples for urine cortisol:creatinine ratio (UCCR) measurements, but is not routinely performed in the UK.

- Interpretation
  - The critical finding is lack of suppression below 40 nmol/l at 8 hours indicative of either PDH or adrenal-dependent HAC, i.e. confirms HAC. NB: Cutoff may vary with laboratory.
  - Further information:
    - < 50% suppression at 3–4 hours consistent with normality, PDH or adrenal-dependent HAC
    - > 50% suppression at 3–4 hours is consistent with PDH or normality
  - Diagnostic in ~100% of adrenal-dependent HAC cases and ~90% of PDH cases

High-dose dexamethasone suppression test (HDDS)

- As for LDDS but 0.1 mg/kg dexamethasone is injected intravenously
- Interpretation
  - Discriminatory test for adrenal-dependent HAC versus PDH
  - Suppression @ 8 hours with PDH
  - 20–30% of PDH cases will still not suppress even at 0.1 mg/kg dexamethasone, although a much higher percentage of PDH cases will suppress than with LDDS test
  - No suppression with adrenal-dependent HAC

High-high dose dexamethasone suppression test (HHDDS)

- As for LDDS but 1.0 mg/kg dexamethasone is injected IV
- Interpretation
  - Discriminatory test for adrenal-dependent HAC versus PDH if HDDS test does not give an answer

- Almost 100% of PDH cases will suppress at this dose of dexamethasone but very rarely performed

Plasma endogenous ACTH concentration

1 Collect blood into cooled plastic EDTA tube and centrifuge immediately @ 4° C.

2 Separate plasma and freeze $< -20^\circ$ C in plastic tube.

3 Transport frozen to the laboratory

- Interpretation
  - Increased in PDH
  - Decreased in adrenal-dependent HAC

Urine cortisol:creatinine ratio (UCCR)

- Screening test
  - A morning urine sample is collected, urine cortisol and creatinine are measured and their ratio calculated. False positives are cause by non-adrenal disease and stress, and the test should be performed at home and not within approximately a week following a stressful event, e.g. veterinary consultation, surgery.
  - Only useful if negative as this rules out HAC
  - A positive result could be HAC, non-adrenal illness or simply stress

Imaging
CT/MRI

- Head to identify pituitary tumour
- CT abdomen to identify
  - Adrenal tumour: usually unilateral but occasionally bilateral
  - Bilateral adrenomegaly in PDH
  - Invasion of draining veins with adrenal-dependent HAC

Treatment
Medical
Trilostane

- Competitive enzyme inhibitor in the steroid synthesis pathway
- Only licensed product in UK (Vetoryl®)
- Licensed for once-daily usage, but some dogs respond better to twice-daily split dosing
- If overdosed, withdrawal of the drug and administration of IV fluids and prednisolone should reverse signs within 24–48 hours

- Permanent adrenal necrosis and hypoadrenocorticism can occur

Mitotane (o,p'-DDD)
- Selective destruction of zona fasciculata and reticularis of adrenal cortex
- Complete chemical adrenalectomy with high daily doses of mitotane until dog has hypoadrenocorticism; reduces chance of relapse but is potentially fatal
- Standard therapy
  - Induction: orally @ 50 mg/kg/daily with food as fatty meal aids absorption
  - Then dose @ 50 mg/kg/week with food as maintenance when one or more of the following develop:
    - ACTH stimulation suppressed
    - Lethargy/depression
    - Reduced appetite (taking longer to eat food)
    - Water intake reduced to < 60/ml/kg/day
    - Vomiting/diarrhoea
- Average 6–14 days for dogs to respond to induction
- Adjust dosage based on results of ACTH stimulation testing; some dogs require ~75 mg/kg weekly for maintenance
- If relapse give a short re-induction course or increase maintenance dose
- Higher doses required for adrenal tumours
- Overdose can lead to hypoadrenocorticism (5–17% of cases)

Pituitary irradiation
- If showing neurological signs

Surgical
Hypophysectomy
- Significant morbidity and mortality, especially with macroadenoma, but can be curative

Bilateral adrenalectomy for PDH
- Treat as hypoadrenocorticism for rest of life
- Glucocorticoid and mineralocorticoid supplementation peri- and post-operatively

Unilateral adrenalectomy for adrenal-dependent HAC
- Glucocorticoid supplementation peri- and immediately post-operatively

- If successful excision, all steroid replacement therapy can be gradually withdrawn

Monitoring
- ACTH stimulation
- Alkaline phosphatase
- Clinical signs
- Pre-pill cortisol now recommended for monitoring trilostane therapy

Prognosis
- Improvement in appetite and drinking seen soon after effective treatment commences
- Median survival time of 30 months (range: days to 7 years)
- Minimum of 6–8 weeks on treatment before marked improvement in dermatological signs and hepatomegaly/pot belly
- Highest mortality in first 16 weeks of treatment with mitotane
- Possible sudden death after initiation of trilostane due to adrenal necrosis
- Successful treatment may unmask steroid-responsive disease, e.g. flea bite hypersensitivity, osteoarthritis
- Prognosis with adrenal-dependent HAC depends on the ability to remove tumour surgically and the absence of metastases

5.3.4B HYPOADRENOCORTICISM (ADDISON'S DISEASE)

Aetiology
- Adrenocortical insufficiency: lack of cortisol and aldosterone
- Clinical signs are only evident when 90% of the adrenal cortex is non-functional

Primary
- Destruction of the adrenal cortices
  - Idiopathic/(auto)immune-mediated
    - Typical = lack of glucocorticoid and mineralocorticoid production
    - Atypical Addison's = hypocortisolaemia without mineralocorticoid deficiency and electrolyte changes (rare); may progress to typical
  - Infectious/infiltrative/bleeding diseases: rare cause of disease

Secondary (rare)

- Deficient ACTH secretion by the pituitary
  - Destructive lesion in pituitary or hypothalamus, e.g. neoplasia/inflammation/trauma
  - Iatrogenic secondary to long-term glucocorticoid therapy causing suppression of the normal adrenal axis – effect can last for weeks after cessation of therapy
- Only glucocorticoid production affected, as RAAS intact

Major signs

- Initially signs may wax and wane, but if untreated a crisis will occur

Initial signs

- Anorexia
- Diarrhoea
- Lethargy
- PU/PD
- Vomiting
- Weight loss

Crisis

- Bradycardia
- Collapse
- Hypovolaemic shock

Minor signs

- Melaena/haematochezia
- Shaking/shivering

Potential sequelae

- AKI
- Hypovolaemic shock
- Death

Predisposition

- Average age 2–7 years
- Females > males
- Castrated males more than intact males
- Genetic predisposition suggested in some breeds by a familial occurrence: Leonberger, Nova Scotia Duck Tolling retriever, Standard Poodle
- Increased risk suggested in other breeds: Great Dane, Saint Bernard, Springer spaniel, WHWT and others

Historical clues

1. Vague/non-specific signs
2. Clinical signs compatible with many other diseases
   e.g. primary gastrointestinal/renal or neuromuscular disease
3. Waxing-waning course of disease probably due to progressive destruction of the adrenal cortex, which ultimately cannot cope with "stress"
4. Temporary improvement with intravenous fluid therapy and/or glucocorticoids may mask diagnosis
5. Eventual crisis with profound collapse

Physical examination

- Abdominal pain
- Bradycardia in up to 30% of cases
- Collapse
- Depression
- Hypothermia
- Weak peripheral pulse
- Weakness

Minimum database

Haematology

- Mild to severe normochromic, normocytic anaemia in 20–30% of cases
  - Non-regenerative anaemia of chronic disease
  - GI blood loss, which can be severe
- Hypovolaemia may mask anaemia due to haemoconcentration; recheck after rehydration
- Reverse stress leukogram (lymphocytosis) would be expected but only seen in < 20% of cases
- However, in a dog with severe illness the presence of normal or increased lymphocyte and eosinophil counts (instead of decreased) should alert the clinician to the possibility of hypoadrenocorticism

Serum biochemistry

- Hyperkalaemia: 90% of cases
- Hyponatraemia: 83% of cases
  - Concurrent hypochloraemia: 46% of cases

- Decreased sodium/potassium ratio: 92% of cases
  - normal > 27:1, hypoadrenocorticism < 23:1
- Pre-renal azotaemia: 60–80% of cases, but progressing to AKI if hypovolaemia untreated
- Inorganic phosphate increased: 66% of cases
- Hypoglycaemia: 20% of cases but rarely of clinical significance
- Hypercalcaemia: 30% of cases, correlating with hyperkalaemia and severity of disease
- Hypoalbuminaemia: < 40% of cases – various mechanisms
- Mild to moderate increases in ALT and ALP activities: 30–50% of cases; could be secondary to poor tissue perfusion or may reflect primary hepatic disease

Urinalysis
- USG should be > 1.030 as azotaemia is prerenal in origin
- Often < 1.030 due to impaired concentrating ability as a result of chronic sodium loss reducing the renal medullary concentrating gradient
- Ultimately AKI may occur due to renal ischaemia, and urine may be isosthenuric

Imaging
Thoracic radiography
- Changes reflect hypovolaemia and decreased tissue perfusion, or muscle weakness, i.e. not specific for hypoadrenocorticism
  - Hypoperfusion of the lung fields
  - Megaoesophagus is present in < 1% of cases
  - Microcardia
  - Narrowed caudal vena cava and descending aorta

Abdominal radiography
- Liver and kidneys may appear slightly small due to hypovolaemia

Ultrasonography
- Significant decrease in the length and width of the adrenal glands

Special investigations
Blood pressure
- Hypotension common

Arterial blood gas analysis
- Mild to moderate acidosis common
- Total CO_2 and serum bicarbonate values reduced

ECG
- Classical ECG changes due to hyperkalaemia, but influenced by acid–base status and other electrolyte changes
- The ECG changes occur as listed below: the higher the potassium the more changes are evident
  1. Peaking of T wave
  2. Shortening of QT interval
  3. Increased QRS duration
  4. Decreased P wave amplitude
  5. Prolonged PR interval
  6. Absence of the P wave (sinoatrial standstill)
  7. Severe bradycardia

Hormone assays
ACTH stimulation test
- Follow the protocol of the laboratory analysing the samples
- Perform after intravenous fluid replacement, ideally before glucocorticoids are administered but cross-reactivity of dexamethasone with cortisol in the assay is negligible compared with other glucocorticoid preparations so can be used for emergency treatment before ACTH stimulation test
- Diagnosis of hypoadrenocorticism
  - Low basal cortisol and lack of response/ stimulation to exogenous ACTH
  - Does not differentiate between primary and secondary disease

Aldosterone assay
- Concentration should be normal after ACTH stimulation with secondary hypoadrenocorticism and decreased in cases of primary hypoadrenocorticism

- Can be used in cases with an ACTH stimulation suggestive of hypoadrenocorticism but with normal serum electrolytes

Endogenous ACTH

- Useful in dogs with abnormal ACTH stimulation and normal electrolytes. Cases of primary hypoadrenocorticism should have markedly increased concentrations of plasma ACTH (> 90% of cases) and low or unmeasurable concentrations of plasma ACTH in secondary hypoadrenocorticism. Follow laboratory directions for handling of the sample; blood must be spun and frozen quickly and shipped to the lab on ice.

Treatment

Acute crisis

- Hypovolaemia and shock is life-threatening

Fluid therapy

- 0.9% normal saline is fluid of choice
- Initial rate repeated boluses of 20 ml/kg depending on severity
- 1.5–2.0× maintenance once hypovolaemia is corrected
  - Monitor urine output
- Fluid therapy is gradually reduced and stopped when hydration, urine output, serum electrolytes and serum creatinine concentrations are normal

Glucocorticoid therapy

- One of the following drugs:
  - Hydrocortisone @ 5–10 mg/kg IV repeated every 6 hours or 0.5 mg/kg/hour is preferred, as it has glucocorticoid and mineralocorticoid effects
  - Methyl prednisolone sodium succinate @ 1–2 mg/kg IV
  - Dexamethasone @ 0.5–2 mg/kg IV single dose
- Methyl prednisolone and dexamethasone can be repeated 2–6 hours later according to response

Mineralocorticoid therapy

- One of the following drugs:
  - Hydrocortisone IV is preferred as it provides some mineralocorticoid action

- Oral administration of fludrocortisone, but it must be swallowed and is slower acting
- Desoxycorticosterone acetate (DOCA) a short-acting injectable mineralocorticoid is ideal, but the preparation is unavailable in UK

Management of hyperkalaemia

- Usually resolves with repeated fluid boluses (10–20 mg/kg per bolus)
- If the hyperkalaemia does not respond to fluid therapy or there are severe bradydysrhythmias, specific therapy may be indicated, e.g. insulin/dextrose, bicarbonate
- The ability to measure potassium concentrations and acid–base is important for safe correction of the hyperkalaemia
- The reader is advised to refer to critical care textbooks for management of hyperkalaemia

Maintenance therapy

Mineralocorticoids

- Desoxycorticosterone pivalate (DOCP)
  - Longer-acting depot mineralocorticoid preparation
  - Licensed @ 2.2 mg/kg every 25–28 days SC, although maintenance dose is generally less
  - Adjust dose and/or frequency based on serum electrolyte concentrations
- Fludrocortisone acetate
  - @ 0.015–0.02 mg/kg daily (once daily or divided twice daily)
  - Adjust dose by 0.05–0.1 mg/day
  - Recheck electrolytes 1–2 weeks after discharge and at this frequency until electrolytes are stable
- Once stable, electrolytes should be checked at least 2–3 times yearly
- Required dose usually increases during first 6–18 months of therapy
- Side effects PU/PD, polyphagia and hair loss

Glucocorticoids

- Use in all cases in the early stages of stabilisation and with maintenance DOCP
- Only ~50% of cases on maintenance fludrocortisone therapy require glucocorticoid supplementation long-term
- Prednisolone
  - @ 0.2 mg/kg/day

- Hydrocortisone
  - @ 500 μg/kg twice daily: benefit of mineralocorticoid action which may help to reduce the requirements for DOC pivalate or fludrocortisone
- All owners should have a small supply for 'at home' use during stressful episodes e.g. exertion, trauma, surgery, illness
- Increase dose 2- to 10-fold during stressful periods (illness, hospitalization, etc.)

Salt (NaCl)
- Mild and persistent hyponatraemia can be corrected by adding salt to the diet @ 0.1 mg/kg/day

Secondary hypoadrenocorticism
- Only glucocorticoid supplementation required

Monitoring
- Clinical signs
- Creatinine and urea initially
- Sodium/potassium

Prognosis
- Excellent after stabilisation once maintenance therapy has been started
- Owner education is important with regard to the necessity for lifelong treatment and the risk factors and signs of destabilisation
- Acute addisonian crisis can result in intrinsic renal damage if hypovolaemia is not rapidly addressed: this alters the prognosis for full recovery
- It is important to consider hypoadrenocorticism in animals that appear to have an AKI, as the prognoses for these two conditions are very different

5.3.5 HYPOTHYROIDISM

- Thyroid hormone secretion is regulated by the circulating concentration of thyroid-stimulating hormone (TSH) produced by the pituitary gland.
- T4 and triiodothyronine (T3) are highly protein-bound and only the free hormone is active.

- Thyroid hormones have an effect in most metabolic reactions.
- NB: Hyperthyroidism is a rare condition in dogs and is caused by:
  - Iatrogenic overdosing of hypothyroid dog
  - Thyroid carcinoma, although most tumours are non-functional
  - Inadvertent ingestion of exogenous thyroid tissue in raw-fed dogs

Aetiology
- Decreased production of (T4) and (T3) by the thyroid gland.
- Primary hypothyroidism (95% of cases)
  - Congenital
  - Idiopathic thyroid atrophy
  - Lymphocytic thyroiditis (at least 50% of cases)
    - Believed to have an immune-mediated basis: anti-thyroglobulin antibody present
- Secondary hypothyroidism due to inadequate pituitary TSH secretion is rare
- Tertiary hypothyroidism due to decreased hypothalamic secretion of thyroid releasing hormone (TRH) is very rare
- Total thyroid hormone concentrations are also decreased in non-thyroidal illnesses, so-called euthyroid sick syndrome

Major signs
- Alopecia
- Cold intolerance
- Exercise intolerance
- Lethargy
- Pyoderma
- Seborrhoea
- Weight gain/obesity

Minor signs
- Disproportionate dwarfism in congenital hypothyroidism
- Female infertility
- Myxoedema: thickened, oedematous dermis
- Neuromuscular dysfunction: possible association, but cause-and-effect rarely shown
  - Peripheral neuropathy
    - Facial paralysis
    - Megaoesophagus
    - Vestibular disease

- Ocular disorders
  - Corneal lipodystrophy

Potential sequelae
- Myxoedema coma is rare but is associated with a poor prognosis

Predisposition
- Castrated males and neutered females may be at greater risk
- Decreased risk in greyhounds
- High incidence in Dobermann, Golden retriever
- Lymphocytic thyroiditis inherited in laboratory Beagles and a family of Borzois
- Middle-aged (mean 7 years), purebred dogs over-represented

Historical clues
- Weight gain
- Lethargy
- Bilaterally symmetrical alopecia
- 'Heat-seeking'
- Response to empirical therapy is an unreliable diagnostic criterion

Physical examination
Dermatological
- Alopecia
- Change in haircoat colour/quality
- Comedones
- Dry/scaly, thickened skin
- Hyperkeratosis
- Hyperpigmentation
- Myxoedema: classically facial, i.e. 'tragic face'
- Otitis externa
- Poor wound healing/increased bruising
- Seborrhoea
- Superficial pyoderma

Cardiovascular
- Bradycardia
- Pallor and slow CRT
- Poor peripheral pulse volume

Neurological
- Central nervous disease
- Peripheral neuropathy: local (e.g. facial paralysis) or generalised

Ocular
- Corneal lipid dystrophy
- Other lesions secondary to hyperlipidaemia, e.g. retinopathy

Laboratory findings
Haematology
- Mild, non-regenerative, normocytic, normochromic anaemia
- Mild increase in platelet count and decrease in platelet size

Serum biochemistry
- Hypercholesterolaemia: in 75% of cases, it is often > 10 mmol/l
- Hypertriglyceridaemia is also common
- Mild increases in creatine kinase activity can be seen due to myopathy or reduced clearance
- Serum ALP activity is often mildly increased

Imaging
- Likely to be unremarkable apart from increased subcutaneous and intracavitary fat

Special investigations
Hormone assays
Basal thyroid hormone concentrations
- Total T3
  - Less informative than TT4
- Total T4 (TT4)
  - If well within normal range, likely to be euthyroid (unless rare cases of cross-reaction of antithyroid antibodies)
  - Decreased TT4 does not give a diagnosis of hypothyroidism as nonthyroidal disease/drugs can cause this, i.e euthyroid sick syndrome
  - Greyhounds and Scottish deerhounds have lower TT4 compared with other breeds
  - Small breeds have higher TT4 than medium/large breeds
- Free (unbound) T4 (fT4)
  - Active hormone, therefore more representative of true thyroid function
  - Only reliable if equilibrium dialysis method is used
  - Other methods underestimate fT4 level and so have no benefit over TT4

ORGAN SYSTEMS

- Problems of test interpretation
  - Drugs, e.g. prednisolone, phenobarbitone, trimethoprim sulphonamides, etc., can alter thyroid hormone concentration
  - Any drug that may decrease thyroid hormone levels should be stopped (if possible) before testing for hypothyroidism
  - Dogs with non-thyroidal illness may have decreased TT4 levels; investigation of thyroid disease should be postponed to allow recovery from the illness or, if that is not possible, stabilisation of the pre-existing disease

Endogenous canine thyroid-stimulating hormone (cTSH)

- Increased cTSH with decreased TT4 or fT4 is specific for hypothyroidism
- Increased cTSH with normal TT4 may be early hypothyroidism with TT4 maintained in normal range by increased cTSH or could reflect drug therapy or recovery from non-thyroidal illness
- Up to one third of hypothyroid dogs have normal cTSH concentration

TSH response/stimulation test

- Was considered the 'gold standard' but is rarely performed now
  - TSH is expensive, difficult to obtain
  - Using a non-medical grade TSH can cause anaphylaxis
- Minimum response expected is two-fold increase and TT4 > 30 nmol/l post-TSH
- If dog is receiving L-thyroxine supplementation, it must be stopped for 6–8 weeks before TSH stimulation is performed

TRH response test

- TRH stimulates release of TSH and thus TT4 but the increases are much smaller than with TSH stimulation
- cTSH also increases after TRH administration; again, this is a small response
- Follow laboratories' protocol
- Interpretation of TRH response test is more difficult than the TSH stimulation test due to smaller magnitudes of change

Other tests
Antibodies

- Anti-thyroglobulin and anti-thyroid hormone antibodies can be measured
- Detect immune-mediated thyroid damage, but do not predict hypothyroidism
- Clinical value is limited, but may help direct breeding choices

Thyroid biopsy
- Rarely indicated clinically

Treatment
L-thyroxine

- Treatment of choice because it results in normalisation of T4 and T3
- Bioavailability can vary with products – use a licensed product
- Consider twice-daily administration because half-life of T4 is 9–15 hours
- If concurrent disease, e.g. CHF, DM, hypoadrenocorticism:
  - Start at 25% dose and increase by 25% every 2 weeks until full dose is achieved at 6 weeks

Response to treatment

- Increased activity/improved attitude within 1 week
- Weight loss within 2–4 weeks
- Dermatological improvement will take months
- Improved cardiovascular function by 8 weeks
- Peripheral neuropathies should improve in 8–12 weeks

Monitoring

- Collect blood samples for therapeutic monitoring 4–6 weeks after starting therapy, either pre-pill, 4–6 hours post-pill, or both
- TT4 should be within reference range immediately before pill and at high end/above reference range for 4–6 hours after administration
- Check TT4 every 6–8 weeks for first 6–8 months, as metabolism of T4 will alter as the metabolic rate stabilises
- Once stable, check TT4 levels 1–2 times yearly

Prognosis
- Oral therapy is effective in most cases
- Resolution of clinical signs in puppies with congenital disease depends on early recognition and treatment

5.3.6 INSULINOMA

Aetiology
- Most common functional neuroendocrine tumour in dogs, primarily arising in the pancreatic beta cells
  - Other neuroendocrine tumours arising in the pancreas (e.g. gastrinoma, glucagonoma) are very rare.
- Approximately 80% are solitary, arising in one limb of the pancreas, but almost all are malignant, with a metastatic rate of between 45 and 70% at the time of diagnosis.
- Signs relate to recurrent episodes of hypoglycaemia caused by episodic, inappropriate release of insulin

Major signs
Neuroglycopenia
- Disorientation, mental dullness, and visual disturbances
- Seizures
- Weakness–ataxia–collapse

Minor signs
- Hunger
- Nervousness
- Tremors
- Weight gain

Potential sequelae
- Peripheral neuropathy (rare)
- Death

Predisposition
- Middle-aged to older, female
- No breed predisposition

Historical clues
- No history of insulin administration
- Recurrent episodes of weakness, especially if unfed

Physical examination
- Often unremarkable except being overweight

Laboratory findings
- Decreased fructosamine
- Mild hypokalaemia and increased ALP
- Profound hypoglycaemia, *q.v.* section 3.17.2
  - Rule out artefactual decreased blood glucose, and other causes, especially hypoadrenocorticism and xylitol toxicity

Imaging
- Combined radiographs and ultrasound have ~50% sensitivity

Radiographs
- Pancreatic mass often not visible

Ultrasound
- Hepatic and LN metastasis sometimes noted
- Pancreatic mass often not visible

Special investigations
- Serum insulin concentration
  - Increased or high-normal insulin is inappropriate in the face of simultaneous hypoglycaemia and confirms the diagnosis
  - Calculation of amended insulin:glucose ratio not needed
- Contrast-enhanced CT most sensitive for identifying pancreatic mass and metastatic disease

Treatment
Acute crisis
- Constant rate IV infusion of 2.5% or 5% dextrose
- Boluses of 50% dextrose should be avoided if possible as they can cause a rebound insulin secretion

Medical
1. Frequent small meals containing complex carbohydrate
2. Prednisolone starting at low doses (0.2 mg/kg) and escalating as needed
3. Diazoxide: limited availability and variable efficacy

ORGAN SYSTEMS

- 10 to 40 mg/kg/day PO divided q8–12 hours
- ~70% of treated dogs exhibit a response
4 Streptozotocin
  - Specifically destroys pancreatic islet cells
  - Nephrotoxic so must be given with IVFT to promote diuresis
  - Success rate of ~50% but success is the creation of DM
5 Octreotide

Surgical excision
- First-choice treatment
- May still be indicated even if confirmed metastatic disease
  - Reduces the main source of insulin, but hypoglycaemia recurs within a few days of surgery
- Post-operative pancreatitis quite common
- ~10% develop DM postsurgically

Monitoring
- Blood glucose concentration
- Clinical signs

Prognosis
- Good if surgery successful
- Ultimately fatal, but survival of many months up to 5 years is possible with medical management after partial pancreatectomy

5.3.7   PARATHYROID DISEASES

- Parathormone (PTH) is secreted by the parathyroid glands in response to hypocalcaemia
- PTH increases serum calcium by stimulating its release from bone and the conversion of 25-hydroxy vitamin D into 1,25-dihydroxy vitamin D (calcitriol), thereby enhancing intestinal calcium absorption, whilst inhibiting the reabsorption of phosphate by renal tubules
- Assay of PTH requires special handling requirements: blood must be spun and frozen quickly and shipped to the lab on ice

5.3.7A   PRIMARY HYPERPARATHYROIDISM (PHPT)

Aetiology
- PHPT is caused by autonomous secretion of excess PTH by one or more of the four parathyroid glands
  - Carcinoma
  - Hyperplasia
  - Solitary adenoma most common
- Secondary HPT is caused by inappropriate nutrition or CKD, and is not discussed here

Major signs
- PU/PD, but often not profound
- Urinary infection or urolithiasis
  - Pollakuria
  - Stranguria

Minor signs
- Gastrointestinal signs
  - Constipation
  - Inappetence
  - Vomiting
- Neuromuscular signs
  - Depression
  - Muscle twitching
  - Shivering
  - Stiff gait
- Other signs
  - Dental pain
  - Dysphagia
  - Exercise intolerance

Potential sequelae
- Nephrocalcinosis and CKD
- Urinary obstruction

Predisposition
- Familial PHPT in Keeshonden

Historical clues
- Hypercalcaemia found during health check
- Urinary signs

Physical examination
Parathyroid masses are rarely palpable
- Dull mentation
- Stiffness and gait abnormalities
- Muscle wastage
- Weakness

Laboratory findings
Haematology
- Unremarkable

Serum biochemistry
- Hypophosphataemia
- Total and ionised hypercalcaemia

Imaging
- Ultrasound of ventral neck to identify parathyroid nodule/mass

Special investigations
- PTH assay
  - Increased or high-normal PTH is inappropriate in the face of hypercalcaemia
  - PTHrp, a marker for malignant hypercalcaemia, will be low
  - Follow laboratory directions for handling of the sample
- DNA test for familial PHPT in Keeshonden

Treatment
- Pre-surgical lowering of calcium with IVFT and bisphosphonates
- Surgical parathyroidectomy of one or more glands
- Transient hypoparathyroidism may need to be managed, with calcium and vitamin D supplementation, especially if surgical trauma or ischaemia impair the remaining glands, *q.v.* section 5.3.7B

Monitoring
- Ionised calcium
- PTH

Prognosis
- Good if affected gland can be identified and removed
- Metastasis of carcinoma is exceptionally rare

5.3.7B HYPOPARATHYROIDISM

Aetiology
- Decreased production of PTH

Causes
- Congenital agenesis very rare
- Idiopathic: lymphocytic infiltration suggests (auto)immune process and is most common
- Metastatic disease
- Trauma, especially during neck surgery; may be transient

Major signs
- Neuromuscular excitability
  - Intermittent fasciculations and tremors of individual muscle groups
  - Progression to generalised tetany
  - Weakness

Minor signs
- Ataxia
- Facial rubbing and biting at paws
- Nervous and restless
- Panting
- Stiff gait
- Vomiting and diarrhoea

Potential sequelae
- Convulsions
- Death

Predisposition
- Females
- Small terriers, Miniature Schnauzers, and Poodles over-represented but there are geographic differences in breed predisposition, and large and giant breeds, including Saint Bernard, can be affected

Historical clues
- Episodic signs
- Nervousness and may growl or snap
- Tetany triggered by exercise or excitement

Physical examination
- Hyperthermia
- Jaw champing
- Muscle fasciculations and tremors

- Punctate cataracts
- Tetanic seizure

Laboratory findings
Haematology
- Unremarkable

Serum biochemistry
- Decreased total and ionised calcium
- Increased phosphate

Imaging
- Unremarkable

Special investigations
PTH assay
- Subnormal or low-normal, which is inappropriate in the face of hypocalcaemia
- Follow laboratory directions for handling of the sample; incorrect handling will result in an artefactually low PTH concentration and a false positive result for HPT

Treatment
During tetany
- IV calcium gluconate to effect

Maintenance
- Oral calcium salts (carbonate most commonly or gluconate or lactate)
- Vitamin D: Calcitriol (D_3) is preferred, but formulation size may necessitate using vitamin D_2

Monitoring
- Clinical signs
- Ionised calcium

Prognosis
- Good once stabilised
- Life-long treatment

5.4   HAEMOPOIETIC SYSTEM

Problems

Presenting complaints
q.v. section 1
1.4 Altered consciousness
1.5 Anorexia/hyporexia/inappetence
1.9 Bleeding
1.18 Dyspnoea/tachypnoea
1.21 Epistaxis
1.22 Exercise intolerance
1.25 Haematemesis
1.26 Haematochezia
1.27 Haematuria and discoloured urine
1.28 Haemoptysis
1.31 Melaena
1.32 Nasal discharge
1.44 Stiffness, joint swelling and generalised lameness
1.51 Weakness, collapse and syncope
1.53 Weight loss

Physical abnormalities
q.v. section 2
2.1 Abdominal enlargement
2.4 Arrhythmias
2.7 Eye lesions
2.8 Hepatomegaly
2.13 Icterus/jaundice
2.14 Lymphadenopathy
2.15 Murmur
2.17.1 Abdominal pain
2.18 Pallor
2.25 Pyrexia and hyperthermia
2.28 Splenomegaly

Laboratory abnormalities
q.v. section 3
3A Biochemical tests
3.5 Bile acids
3.6 Bilirubin
3.11 Cortisol (basal)
3.18 Iron profile
3.20 Liver enzymes
3.26 Thyroid hormone
3.27 Total protein (albumin and globulin)

3.B Haematology
3.30 Red blood cells (RBCs)
3.31 Platelets
3.32 White blood cells (WBCs)
3.33 Pancytopenia

Diagnostic Approach
- For anaemia, *q.v.* section 3.30
- For bleeding disorders, *q.v.* section 5.5
- For leukocytosis, *q.v.* section 3.32.1
- For leukopenia, *q.v.* section 3.32.2
- For WBC neoplasia, *q.v.* section 5.7
- For pancytopenia, *q.v.* section 3.33

Diagnostic Methods
q.v. individual diseases in sections 5.4.1 to 5.4.7

Special investigative techniques
- Bone marrow aspirate and core biopsy
- Erythropocitin
- Serum ferritin (not readily available)
- Immunological tests, e.g. Coombs' test
- Serum iron and total iron-binding capacity

5.4.1   ANAEMIA OF CHRONIC KIDNEY DISEASE (CKD)

Aetiology
- The hormonal stimulus for RBC production, erythropoietin (EPO), is normally synthesised by the kidney. In CKD, the production of EPO declines, leading to a non-regenerative anaemia.
- Secondary hyperparathyroidism associated with renal disease can lead to myelofibrosis and may have a direct inhibitory effect on erythropoiesis.
- Gastric ulceration secondary to CKD can result in blood-loss anaemia.
- Anaemia of chronic inflammation (iron trapping in enterocytes).

Major signs

- Anorexia
- Lethargy
- Pallor
- PU/PD
- Tachycardia
- Tachypnoea
- Weakness
- Weight loss

Predisposition/signalment

- GI bleeding in uraemic dogs can contribute to development of anaemia
- Middle- to older-aged dogs with CKD
- Younger dogs with familial/congenital nephropathies

Potential sequelae

- Anaemia develops gradually and can be profound
- Death/euthanasia from uraemia is the usual end result

Physical examination

- Typical signs of anaemia as above
- May be signs of uraemia, *q.v.* section 5.12.1B
- Systolic heart murmur if severe anaemia

Laboratory findings

Haematology

- Assess degree of anaemia and type (usually normocytic-normochromic) and non-regenerative (check reticulocyte count)
  NB: Often the dog is dehydrated and this may mask the anaemia, therefore re-evaluate after rehydration.

Serum biochemistry,
q.v. section 5.12.1

- Azotaemia expected if renal disease advanced enough to cause anaemia
- If urea is disproportionately increased compared to creatinine, this suggests GI blood loss
- Hypoalbuminaemia may suggest blood loss

Urinalysis

- Urine specific gravity (USG) is likely to show submaximal concentration in an azotaemic animal, suggesting loss of concentrating ability
- USG in advanced CKD is usually isosthenuric

Imaging

Radiography

- Small kidneys associated with chronic kidney disease
- Osteopenia occasionally
- Renal calcification sometimes
- Ultrasonography of the kidneys and urinary tract is indicated

Special investigations

Blood pressure assessment

- Arterial hypertension is reported in up to 69% of dogs with chronic kidney disease
- Retinal examination for evidence of hypertension, *q.v.* section 2.10

ACTH stimulation test

- Rule out hypoadrenocorticism, which can also present with azotaemia, isosthenuria and anaemia

PTH concentration

- May be helpful for identifying secondary hyperparathyroidism
  NB special collection and transport for this sample to the laboratory

Serum erythropoietin (EPO) concentration

- If EPO level is increased, further investigation for a cause of the anaemia other than renal disease should be carried out

Iron profile

- Serum iron, total iron-binding capacity (TIBC)
- Assessment of transferrin saturation (serum iron, TIBC), *q.v.* section 3.18

Treatment

- Treat renal disease, *q.v.* section 5.12.1

Gastrointestinal and other blood loss

- Reduce gastric ulceration with gastric protectants, etc.
- If iron-deficient: supplement with oral iron, e.g. ferrous sulphate 100–300 mg/day/dog

Blood transfusion

- Whole blood or packed RBCs
  - Useful for acute cases requiring rapid improvement

- Difficult to restore PCV to normal in these dogs
- Repeated transfusions are usually required and even with cross-matching, incompatibility can occur
- Availability of donors often limits the number of transfusions that can be given

Recombinant human erythropoietin
- PCV usually increases by 0.5–1% per day with red cell mass restored in 1 month
- Improves appetite, physical activity and general well-being
- Used in patients with moderate to severe anaemia due to EPO deficiency
- Long term, dogs can develop anti-EPO antibodies that reduce the benefit of therapy. Recombinant canine EPO is not yet available commercially so recombinant human EPO is used. Additionally, seizures are described as a side effect.
- Iron supplementation is essential

Monitoring
- PCV
- Progression of renal disease, *q.v.* section 5.12.1

Prognosis
- Poor to guarded, as the renal disease is usually advanced and will progress regardless of the management of the anaemia

5.4.2   IMMUNE-MEDIATED HAEMOLYTIC ANAEMIA (IMHA)

There are numerous causes of haemolytic anaemia (*q.v.* section 3.30.1), but the most common is IMHA. This is typically a regenerative anaemia, with the haemolysis being either intra- or extra-vascular. A non-regenerative form occurs with precursor-targeted immune-mediated anaemia (PIMA), where the immune target is RBC precursors in the bone marrow.

Aetiology
- IMHA can be:
  - Primary/autoimmune/non-associative
  - Secondary/associative: sometimes a precipitating event can be identified
    - Drugs, e.g. cephalosporins, penicillins, trimethoprim-sulfa

- Infectious or parasitic, e.g. *Babesia, Dirofilaria, Ehrlichia, Leishmania,* haemotropic *Mycoplasma*
- Immunological, e.g. transfusion reaction, post-vaccine
- Neoplastic, e.g. lymphoma, leukaemia

Major signs
- Bounding pulse
- Lethargy
- Pale mucous membranes
- Tachycardia
- Tachypnoea
- Weakness

Minor signs
- Collapse: acute onset, severe cases
- Dyspnoea
- Haemic heart murmur
- Lymphadenopathy
- Pyrexia

Potential sequelae
- Failure to respond to therapy with immunosuppressive drugs or recurrence once treatment stops should prompt a thorough search for possible underlying disease and an assessment of the adequacy of immunosuppression
- Pulmonary thromboembolism (PTE)
- Disseminated intravascular coagulation (DIC) and death

Predisposition
- Common in some breeds: Cocker spaniel, Collies, English Springer spaniel, Poodles, Old English sheepdog
  NB: American Cocker spaniels and English Springer spaniels are predisposed to phosphofructokinase (PFK) deficiency, which can also cause recurrent haemolysis and regenerative anaemia.
- Young adult to middle-aged dogs; may be more common in females

Historical clues
- Recent drug or vaccine administration should be considered in dogs diagnosed with IMHA and should be used with caution in future
- Further studies are needed to determine if and when vaccine-associated IMHA occurs
- Travel and infectious disease exposure should be reviewed

Physical examination
- Bounding pulse
- Heart murmur
- Hepatosplenomegaly
- Jaundice and discoloured urine
- Lymphadenopathy
- Pallor
- Pyrexia
- Tachycardia
- Tachypnoea

Imaging
- Radiographs and ultrasound may demonstrate hepatosplenomegaly
- Screening radiographs and abdominal ultrasound are indicated to search for underlying disease
- Identify zinc foreign body as cause of haemolysis

Minimum database
Haematology
- Moderate to severe anaemia which is usually regenerative, *q.v.* section 3.30.1, Figure 3.1
  - Anisocytosis
  - Polychromasia
  - High corrected reticulocyte count
  - Increased numbers nucleated RBCs
    NB: It can take 3–5 days from onset for marrow regeneration to be evident.

- Spherocytosis (round, dense RBCs) and agglutination are consistent with diagnosis of IMHA and indicate immune-mediated destruction, Figure 5.4.1
- Neutrophilic leukocytosis, as haemolysis is 'inflammatory'
- Platelets are usually normal unless concurrent IMTP (Evans syndrome), *q.v.* section 5.5.5

Serum biochemistry
- Haemoglobinaemia with intravascular haemolysis
- Hyperglobulinaemia but usually normal albumin
- Mild to moderate increases in liver enzymes secondary to hepatic hypoxia
- Mild to moderate hyperbilirubinaemia is a sign of haemolysis; it is usually transient but seen with severe and acute anaemia, until liver adjusts to the increased bilirubin turnover

Urinalysis
- Bilirubinuria
- Haemoglobinuria with intravascular haemolysis

Special tests
- Slide agglutination test (SAT) to differentiate agglutination and rouleaux:
  if positive it is highly suggestive of IMHA

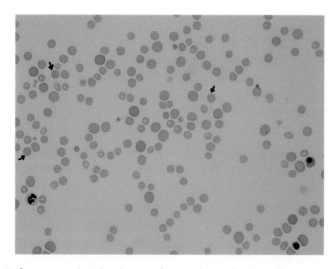

Figure 5.4.1 Spherocytosis. Blood smear from a dog with IMHA demonstrating the presence of spherocytes (arrows).

ORGAN SYSTEMS

- Immunological testing
  - Coombs' test/direct antiglobulin test (DAT): positive result confirms IMHA but not primary autoimmune haemolytic anaemia
  - Negative Coombs' test/DAT are sometimes reported with IMHA
- Lymph node cytology/biopsy to try and identify underlying disease
- Infectious disease testing e.g. *Babesia* spp by PCR
- Bone marrow analysis
  - Bone marrow neoplasia
  - Myelodysplasia
  - Precursor-targeted immune-mediated anaemia (PIMA), also known as non-regenerative IMHA or pure red cell aplasia

Criteria for diagnosis of IMHA

- Signs of haemolysis, i.e. hyperbilirubinaemia, bilirubinuria or icterus without hepatic disease/cholestasis or sepsis, haemoglobinaemia, haemoglobinuria, RBC ghosts
- Signs of immune mediated destruction
  - spherocytes
  - positive SAT without washing or that persists after washing
  - positive Coombs' test/DAT
  - flow cytometry
- Level of confidence
  - ≥ 2 signs of destruction and ≥ 1 sign of haemolysis is considered diagnostic for IMHA
  - ≥ 2 signs of destruction and no sign of haemolysis is supportive of IMHA if other cause cannot be found
  - 1 sign of destruction and ≥ 1 sign of haemolysis is supportive of IMHA if other cause cannot be found
  - 1 sign of destruction and no sign of haemolysis is suspicious of IMHA if other cause cannot be found
  - No signs of destruction: this is not IMHA

Treatment

- Start treatment as soon as diagnostic samples have been collected
- Manage underlying/predisposing disease, e.g. treat infectious disease, lymphoma, etc.

Immunosuppressive therapy

- Glucocorticoids
  - Prednisolone @ 2–3 mg/kg/day or 40–60 mg/m²/day for dogs > 25 kg per os, given once or split twice daily
  - Initially may want to use intravenous preparation if oral not tolerated, e.g. dexamethasone @ 0.2–0.4 mg/kg/day
  - Prednisolone should be reduced to ≤ 2 mg/kg within 1–2 weeks of treatment
  - Should see response with increased PCV by 7–10 days
  - Tailor therapy according to response, gradually decreasing to alternate-day therapy
- Other immunosuppressants are used if inadequate response to prednisolone alone
  - Ongoing clinical signs
  - $\geq 5\%$ decrease in PCV within 24 hours in the initial 7 days of treatment
  - Continued need for blood transfusions > 7 days into treatment
  - Develops adverse effects from glucocorticoids

  NB: Due to lag period before they are effective, some clinicians start them immediately.
  - Administration of three or more immunosuppressants at the same time should be avoided.
    - Azathioprine 2 mg/kg/day or 50 mg/m²/day PO reducing after 2–3 week to every other day until treatment is discontinued
    - Ciclosporin 5 mg/kg q12h PO, therapeutic drug monitoring can be used to adjust dose
    - Leflunomide 2 mg/kg q24h PO, therapeutic drug monitoring can be used to adjust dose
    - Mycophenolate mofetil 8–12 mg/kg q12h PO
    - Cyclophosphamide is not recommended

Supportive therapy

- Cage rest to reduce oxygen demand
- Oxygen supplementation for very severe cases, but lack of RBCs needs addressing
- Fluid therapy to maintain urine output

  NB: These patients are normovolaemic so cautious intravenous fluid therapy is recommended.

ORGAN SYSTEMS

- Thromboprophylaxis should be provided for all dogs with IMHA unless severe thrombocytopenia ($< 30 \times 10^9/l$) is present and continued for at least 2 weeks or until the dog is no longer receiving prednisolone
  - Unfractionated heparin with monitoring with Anti Xa Assay or direct Xa inhibitors e.g. rivaroxaban is advised.
- Anti-platelet drugs can be used, e.g. clopidogrel 1.1–4.0 mg/kg PO q24h

Blood transfusion

- Indicated in patients with severe, acute onset anaemia showing clinical signs of compromise/impaired tissue oxygen delivery or with PCV < 10–12%
- Transfused cells have a short life in dogs with IMHA and potentially can increase the rate of haemolysis but can be lifesaving in critical situations
- Packed RBCs are preferable to whole blood or bovine haemoglobin solutions, as patients are normovolaemic
- Plasma is not indicated unless haemorrhagic DIC is present
- Blood typing and cross-matching should be performed, particularly if multiple transfusions are anticipated, but consider the impact of agglutination on blood-typing kits and refer to guidance from kit manufacturers

Alternatives for refractory cases

- Intravenous immunoglobulin (IVIG) at 0.5–1 g/kg as single infusion can be considered for salvage in dogs not responding to two immunosuppressive medications
- Splenectomy: spleen is the major site of red cell destruction and an important site of antibody production; there is weak evidence that this is a beneficial treatment
- Plasmapheresis, liposomal clodronate, hyperbaric oxygen and melatonin are sometimes suggested but current evidence is weak

Monitoring

- When the PCV/HCT has remained stable and > 30% for 2 weeks after starting treatment with improvement in indicators of disease activity then prednisolone can be reduced by 25% every 3 weeks

- Side effects are common and periodic urinalysis is recommended
- If a second drug is being used, it should not be changed at the same time and there is weak evidence for tapering the dose of these medications other than the reduction of azathioprine to every-other-day treatment after the first few weeks.
- Typically, treatment will be continued for 3–6 months with prednisolone and 4–8 months for all immunosuppressive treatment
- If using azathioprine, monitor for development of myelosuppression and hepatoxicity, i.e. increased ALT enzyme activity
- If using ciclosporin, monitor for GI adverse effects and gingival hyperplasia
- If using mycophenolate, monitor for GI adverse effects and haematology every 2–3 weeks then every 2–3 months
- If using leflunomide, monitor haematology and biochemistry (particularly ALT/ALP activity) every 2 weeks for 2 months then every 1–2 months
- PCV should be monitored after stopping therapy
- Some dogs remain Coombs' positive for a very long period of time, possibly indefinitely
- Dogs with bone marrow immune-mediated disease, i.e. PIMA, may require transfusion and up to 3 months before improvement is seen in the PCV

Prognosis

- Can develop DIC: grave prognosis
- Negative prognostic indicators include profound jaundice, haemoglobinaemia, haemoglobinuria, poor regenerative response and positive slide agglutination
- Mortality rates are high: 33–50% of all presented cases die or are euthanased because of severe anaemia or PTE during the acute crisis, or recurrent/persistent disease, or unacceptable drug side effects
  - High-risk for developing PTE: if an anaemic patient develops severe and persistent dyspnoea consider a PTE. Prognosis is grave.
- Relapse should prompt investigation for underlying trigger factors and repeat treatment

5.4.3 IRON-DEFICIENCY ANAEMIA

Aetiology

- Insufficient intake of iron, e.g. newborn puppies
- Chronic blood loss
  - External parasites, e.g. severe flea infestation
  - Internal parasites, e.g. *Ancylostoma* hookworm
  - Chronic GI bleeding, e.g. neoplasia, ulcer
  - Excessive bleeding of blood donors
- Rapid erythropoiesis
  - EPO therapy in anaemia (increased demand for iron)

Gastrointestinal tract blood loss is the most common reason for iron-deficiency anaemia

Major signs

- Evidence of bleeding, e.g. melaena, haematemesis, etc.
- Lethargy
- Pallor
- Weakness

Predisposition

- Chronic NSAID therapy
- EPO supplementation without iron supplementation
- Parasitism

Potential sequelae

- Severe anaemia

Historical clues

- Melaena
- NSAID administration

Physical examination

- Depends on underlying cause: may be normal
- Abdominal mass may be palpable with bleeding intestinal neoplasms
- Evidence of external parasitism, e.g. parasite, flea dirt
- Pallor
- Tachycardia/tachypnoea/weakness/lethargy

Laboratory findings

- Decreased reticulocyte haemoglobin is an early indicator
- Early normocytic, normochronic and increased reticulocytes
- Later microcytic, hypochromic, non-regenerative anaemia
- Morphological changes may affect RBCs, e.g. microcytes, schistocytes, target cells and keratocytes
- Reactive thrombocytosis may be present
- Biochemical abnormalities may be present relating to the underlying disease, e.g. GI blood loss is often associated with hypoalbuminaemia
- Faecal parasitology to assess for hookworm ova or perform ELISA testing

Imaging

- Radiographs may demonstrate the cause
  - Intestinal mass
  - GI ulcer
- Ultrasonography is indicated for a thorough abdominal evaluation for evidence of GI disease, particularly focal tumours

Special investigations

q.v. section 3.18

- Serum iron concentration is low, but also seen with acute/chronic inflammatory reactions
- Total iron-binding capacity (TIBC) indicates the amount of iron bound to transferrin plus the amount of iron needed to saturate the bindings sites on transferrin; it does not reflect tissue iron levels
- % saturation (serum iron bound to transferrin) is low: less than 20% (normal ~30%)
- Serum ferritin concentrations are decreased and correlate well with iron stores in the body
- Bone marrow iron stores are depleted/absent
- Endoscopy/surgery to look for source of GI bleeding and to obtain biopsies

Treatment

- Treat underlying cause
  - Gastroprotectants, etc. if gastric ulceration
  - Resection of localised neoplasm
  - Treat for internal and external parasites

- Iron supplementation @ 100–600 mg/dog q24h PO or 10–20 mg/kg IM once only and then continue with oral therapy
  - Food reduces iron absorption, therefore give on an empty stomach
- If dog has malabsorption or does not tolerate oral medication, inject with iron dextran initially as above

Monitoring

- Reticulocytosis normally develops within 3–4 days
- If inadequate response, reassess diagnosis
- Supplementation is recommended for 1–3 months to allow replacement of body stores and not just correction of PCV or until signs have resolved

Prognosis

- If underlying disease is appropriately managed and iron is supplemented, the prognosis can be good

5.4.4 LYMPHOID LEUKAEMIA

Aetiology

- Lymphoid neoplasm arising in the bone marrow, manifested in blood, and spreading to the liver, spleen and lymph nodes

Acute lymphoblastic leukaemia (ALL)

- Acute malignant disease characterised by immature lymphoid cells (lymphoblasts) present in large quantities in circulating blood, lymphoid tissue and bone marrow
- Can present similarly to Stage V lymphoma, *q.v.* section 5.7.2A
  - ALL
    - WBC count normally > 50×10⁹/l
    - Other cytopenias are more common with ALL
    - Most ALL cases are unwell
  - Lymphoma
    - B cell is more common
    - Can affect GI tract, CNS and bone as well as intramedullary sites
    - Lower numbers of circulating atypical cells

Chronic lymphocytic leukaemia (CLL)

- Neoplastic proliferation of small lymphocytes, usually of T-cell origin, in the peripheral blood and haemopoietic tissues

Intermediate-grade leukaemia

- Circulating cells are less mature than in CLL but marrow infiltration and haematological changes are less marked than in ALL. Probably should be treated as ALL.

Major signs

Clinical signs with ALL are acute/severe, but with CLL are often vague

- Anorexia
- Dyspnoea
- Lameness
- Lethargy
- PU/PD
- Vomiting and diarrhoea
- Weight loss

Predisposition

- ALL has wide age range: mean age at presentation of 6 years, and more commonly reported in large-breed dogs
- CLL more common in middle-aged to older dogs

Historical clues

- CLL can often be an incidental finding on a blood screen

Physical examination

May be normal

- Hepatosplenomegaly
- Mild lymphadenopathy
- Neurological abnormalities
- Pallor
- Pyrexia

Laboratory findings

ALL

- Leukocytosis due to circulating blasts
  - 10% of cases are aleukaemic, i.e. no circulating neoplastic cells
- Usually there is accompanying thrombocytopenia and neutropenia due to myelophthisis

(marrow "crowding") and variable degrees of anaemia

- Increased liver enzyme activity, mild azotaemia and hypercalcaemia can be found
- ALL is differentiated from lymphoma on the basis of severe marrow infiltration, lack of markedly enlarged lymph nodes and acute clinical progression
- Differentiation of lymphoblast and myeloblasts can be difficult and (immuno)cytochemistry may be necessary to differentiate the cells

CLL

- Moderate to marked peripheral lymphocytosis with small, mature lymphocytes
  - Counts can be $10-300 \times 10^9/l$
- Marrow infiltration and splenic, hepatic and lymph node enlargement
- If high tumour burden in marrow, thrombocytopenia and anaemia (usually normocytic, normochromic) ± neutropenia can also be present
- Occasionally there is hyperglobulinaemia, which can be due to a monoclonal spike and increased calcium and liver enzymes
- Bence-Jones proteinuria also reported with CLL

Imaging

- Hepatosplenomegaly and lymphadenopathy sometimes present

Special investigations

- Bone marrow aspirate and core biopsy: > 30% lymphoblasts is diagnostic
- Immunophenotyping to distinguish between B cell and T cell
- ALL is normally CD34 positive, most lymphomas are CD34 negative
- Clonality testing, i.e. flow cytometry or PARR, to confirm neoplastic and not inflammatory/reactive; flow cytometry can provide additional classifying information

Treatment

- ALL is treated with various chemotherapy protocols: the reader is advised to refer to current texts for the current treatment recommendations.

- Treatment of CLL is controversial. Chemotherapy is used but it is suggested that only symptomatic or cytopenic dogs should be treated or if lymphocyte count is $> 60 \times 10^9/l$

Monitoring

- Haematology
- Regular physical examination

Prognosis

- Poor for ALL: median survival times of 16 days, range 3–128 days
- CL: much better than ALL, usually 1–3 years regardless of treatment with good quality of life, can transform to ALL which then progresses rapidly

5.4.5 OTHER HAEMOPOIETIC NEOPLASMS

Aetiology

Acute myeloid leukaemia (AML)

- Accumulation of blast cells (myeloblasts, monoblasts, megakaryoblasts) in the circulation and extramedullary tissues

Chronic myeloid/granulocytic leukaemia (CML/CGL)

- Rare neoplasm of granulocytes

Chronic eosinophilic leukaemia

- Malignant cells of eosinophilic origin in bone marrow and peripheral blood distinguished from hypereosinophilic syndrome where the infiltrating cells are mature
- May be organ infiltration, e.g. liver, spleen, intestines, mesenteric lymph nodes with mature and immature eosinophils

Myelodysplastic syndrome (MDS)

- Characterised by abnormal maturation of cells and production resulting in anaemia, thrombocytopenia, neutropenia or pancytopenia

Major signs

- Anorexia
- Lameness
- Lethargy
- PU/PD

ORGAN SYSTEMS

- Vomiting and diarrhoea
- Weight loss

Potential sequelae
- Clinical course in MDS can be prolonged for months
- Death

Predisposition
- No specific predisposition noted

Historical clues
- None

Physical examination
- May be normal
- Hepatosplenomegaly
- Mild lymphadenopathy
- Pallor
- Pyrexia

Laboratory findings
- AML: peripheral leukocytosis, anaemia and thrombocytopenia
- CML/CGL: marked neutrophilia with left shift
- Chronic eosinophilic leukaemia: marked peripheral eosinophilia with immature forms in peripheral blood and cytopenia of other cell lines

Imaging
- Hepatosplenomegaly in some cases

Special investigations
- Biopsy of infiltrated organs: liver, spleen, LN
- Bone marrow examination
  - Classes of AML are based on the percentage of each type of blast cell in the marrow
    - Blast cells are identified with cytochemical stains for a specific diagnosis
  - Bone marrow shows granulocytic hyperplasia and erythroid hypoplasia ± disordered maturation in CML/CGL

Treatment
- Chemotherapy; consult specialist text for latest advice

Prognosis
- Guarded to poor

5.4.6   LEUKOPENIA

- For causes of leukopenia and approach to investigation, *q.v.* section 3.32.2

Treatment of neutropenia
- Consider antibiotic therapy: prophylactic antibiotics against intestinal flora if neutrophil count $< 1 \times 10^9/l$
- Isolation/high hygiene if high risk of acquiring infection from other animals
  - Generally dogs are better at home if no concerns of sepsis as in hospital situation they risk nosocomial infections with potentially resistant organisms
- Manage underlying disease
  - Stop potentially responsible drugs
    - Chemotherapy
    - Phenobarbitone; transition to another antiepileptic
- Recombinant haemopoietic factors to stimulate neutrophil production
  - Recombinant G-CSF @ 2.5–10 µg/kg/day subcutaneously for 3–5 days
- Treatment of immune-mediated neutropenia is similar to that of IMHA or IMTP

5.4.7   THROMBOSIS

Aetiology
- Thrombi (fibrin-platelet masses) tend to form when Virchow's triad, three broad categories of factors, are met:
  - Endothelial injury/dysfunction
  - Hypercoagulability
    - Hyperadrenocorticism (HAC)
    - Hypoproteinaemia
    - Systemic inflammatory conditions
  - Haemodynamic changes, i.e. stasis, turbulence
    - Dilated cardiomyopathy (DCM)
    - Cardiac valvular disease
- Thrombosis is the ischaemic condition caused by intravascular deposition of a thrombus

- Thromboembolism is fragmentation of a thrombus producing emboli that may cause ischaemia at remote sites

Major signs
- Depend upon site, i.e. which organs involved and to what extent vessels are occluded
- Common sites
  - Aortic thrombus
    - Painful, cool, paretic, pulseless, pale hindlegs
  - PTE
    - Acute respiratory distress
    - Dyspnoea, haemoptysis, tachycardia, tachypnoea, pyrexia
  - Renal thrombosis
    - Haematuria, flank pain
- Uncommon sites
  - Neural thrombosis
    - Neurological deficits dependent upon site of thrombosis
      NB: Transient vascular events in the brain are more often related to bleeding.
  - Visceral arterial thrombosis
    - Abdominal pain, vomiting

Potential sequelae
- Thrombosis of other organ systems
  - Pulmonary hypertension ± tricuspid regurgitation
- Worsening signs and death

Predisposition
- Chronic inflammatory enteropathy/inflammatory bowel disease
- Dislodged catheter tips
- Diabetes mellitus
- HAC
- IMHA ± corticosteroids
- Neoplasia
- Nephrotic syndrome causing antithrombin deficiency
  - Amyloidosis, glomerulonephritis
- Vascular endothelial damage
  - Bacterial endocarditis, *Dirofilaria*, immune complex vascular disease

Physical examination
- *q.v.* Major signs as above

Laboratory findings
- Assessment for proteinuria
- Haematology and biochemistry to assess for co-existent disease, e.g. hypoalbuminaemia, thrombocytopenia
- Screening coagulation tests are usually normal but may be slightly shortened and fibrin degradation products (FDPs) and D-dimer increased

Imaging
- Thoracic radiographs/contrast CT in case of PTE may be normal or may show acute truncation of the pulmonary vessels or increased lung density
- Ultrasonography of affected areas and other predilection sites

Special investigations
- Angiography or Doppler of the affected area
  - High-velocity pulmonic and/or tricuspid regurgitation
- Arterial blood gas analysis
- Antithrombin measurement. reduced in 50–70% of cases of nephrotic syndrome
- Nuclear imaging (scintigraphic) perfusion scan
- Platelet aggregation

Treatment
- Correct underlying predisposing factors/diseases
- Limit further thrombus formation
  - Heparin, warfarin, aspirin, clopidogrel
- Direct thrombolytic therapy
  - Urokinase, streptokinase and tissue plasminogen activator
- Supportive therapy
  - Oxygen, analgesia, fluids, etc.

Monitoring
  - Perfusion and function of affected organ

Prognosis
- Prognosis is guarded but depends upon location, severity and underlying cause
- Unless the underlying cause can be managed, the prognosis is poor

5.5 HAEMOSTATIC SYSTEM

- Haemostasis is the maintenance of vascular integrity and blood fluidity that is necessary for the normal functions of blood.
- There are three stages of repairing a vascular injury causing bleeding:
  - Primary haemostasis = the formation of a platelet plug at the injury site; platelet number and function are important.
  - Secondary haemostasis = stabilisation of the plug with a mesh of fibrin formed via the coagulation cascade.
  - Fibrinolysis = the balance between clot formation and clot dissolution.
- Dysfunction of one or more of these stages may lead to prolonged bleeding.

Problems

Presenting complaints

q.v. section 1
1.4 Altered consciousness
1.5 Anorexia/hyporexia/inappetence
1.9 Bleeding
1.10 Blindness
1.13 Coughing
1.15 Diarrhoea
1.18 Dyspnoea/tachypoea
1.21 Epistaxis
1.22 Exercise intolerance
1.25 Haematemesis
1.26 Haematochezia
1.27 Haematuria and discoloured urine
1.28 Haemoptysis
1.31 Melaena
1.32 Nasal discharge
1.34 Paresis/paralysis
1.40 Red eye (and pink eye)
1.42 Seizures
1.44 Stiffness, joint swelling and generalised lameness
1.49 Vomiting
1.50 Vulval discharge
1.51 Weakness, collapse and syncope

Physical abnormalities

q.v. section 2
2.1 Abdominal enlargement
2.2 Abdominal masses
2.4 Arrhythmias
2.7 Eye lesions
2.8 Hepatomegaly
2.14 Lymphadenopathy
2.16 Oral masses
2.17 Pain
2.18 Pallor
2.26 Skin lesions
2.28 Splenomegaly

Laboratory abnormalities

q.v. section 3
3.27.2 Hypoproteinaemia
3.30.1 Anaemia
3.31.1 Thrombocytopenia
3.33 Pancytopenia

Diagnostic Approach

q.v. section 1.9
1 Determine whether bleeding is localised or generalised
2 Detemine if bleeding is due to a local or systemic problem
  - Local
    - Foreign body
    - Infection
    - Neoplasia/ruptured mass
    - Post-surgery
    - Trauma
    - Ulcer
  - Generalised
    - Hypertension
    - Hyperviscosity
      - Hyperproteinaemia: macroglobulinaemia, multiple myeloma
      - Infectious disease: *Angiostrongylus*, *Ehrlichia*, *Leishmania*
    - Toxicity

ORGAN SYSTEMS

Notes on Canine Internal Medicine, Fourth Edition. Victoria L. Black, Kathryn F. Murphy, Jessie Rose Payne, and Edward J. Hall.
© 2022 John Wiley & Sons Ltd. Published 2022 by John Wiley & Sons Ltd.

3 Differentiate platelet problems (primary haemostasis) from coagulopathy (secondary haemostastis) by nature of the bleeding
  • Primary haemostasis: pinpoint bleeds, i.e. petechiae, ecchymoses, surface/mucosal bleeds, multiple small bleeds, prolonged bleeding
  • Secondary haemostasis: single large bleeds which can appear localised, e.g. deep/cavity bleeds, haematomas, re-bleeding, widespread subcutaneous bleeds
4 Assess platelet function and numbers and clotting times as appropriate

Diagnostic Methods
For history, physical examination, laboratory findings, *q.v.* section 1.9

Special investigative techniques
Tests of primary haemostasis
Buccal mucosal bleeding time (BMBT)
• Time taken for bleeding to stop from a standardised superficial incision
  • Reflect upper lip and hold in place with a gauze bandage
  • Make an incision in non-vascular part of mucosa with spring-loaded cutting device (template) or no. 11 scalpel blade
  • Use filter paper to absorb blood (do not touch incision, dab below)
  • Time for bleeding to stop is recorded
• 1.7–4.2 minutes is normal, but it is an insensitive test
• Prolonged times with qualitative platelet defects, thrombocytopenia, von Willebrand disease (vWD)

Platelet number and morphology
• Automated platelet counts
  • Use veterinary laboratories or validated in-house machines
    NB: CKCSs have macrothrombocytes that are not included in automated counts which thus gives an appearance of a lower count.
• Manual platelet count
  • Lyse RBCs and then manual count using haemocytometer chamber
• Smear evaluation
  • One platelet in oil immersion field (1000× total magnification) approximates to 15 × 10^9/l platelets

• Normal: 11–25 platelets per oil immersion field ($\cong 165 \times 10^9$/l platelets)
• Platelet morphology should be assessed by an experienced haematologist from smear

Platelet function
• Clot retraction is a crude method of assessing platelet function when numbers are normal
• Platelet function analysers can be used but are rarely available in the clinic

Platelet aggregation tests
• Specialist assay to assess ability to aggregate and release granule contents by adding reagents to induce these responses rarely available in the clinic

von Willebrand factor (vWF) antigen
• Assayed by electroimmunoassay or ELISA
• vWF antigen concentrations are low in patients with bleeding disorders caused by vWF deficiency
• Clinical signs are not usually seen until vWF antigens concentrations are < 20%
• Genetic tests have been developed for certain breeds
• vWF concentrations can be increased by exercise, liver disease, etc., so do not sample within 2 weeks of any systemic illness/stress or from females during oestrus or pregnancy as they can have increased vWF concentrations

Tests of secondary haemostasis
Activated clotting time (ACT)
• Time taken for whole blood to clot in the presence of a substance (diatomaceous earth) that initiates contact activation of coagulation
  • Pre-warm ACT tube to 37°C in water bath
  • Minimise tissue factor collection when taking blood sample, i.e., discard first 0.5 ml of blood
  • Add 2 ml blood to ACT tube; start timing as soon as blood enters tube
  • Mix sample by inversion and place in 37°C water bath
  • Tilt sample every 10 seconds till first clot is observed
  • Normal = 60–110 seconds

- Prolongation suggests abnormalities of intrinsic and common clotting pathways
- Prolonged by severe thrombocytopenia and hypofibrinogenaemia also

Coagulation profile

- Tested by measuring the activated partial thromboplastin time (aPTT) and one-stage prothrombin time (OSPT/PT)
  - Collect sample into sodium citrate anticoagulant and follow manufacturers or reference laboratory guidance for sample handling
  - Use appropriate reference intervals for the methodology used

Activated partial thromboplastin time (aPTT)

- Identifies coagulation disorders of intrinsic (VIII, IX, XI, XII) and common pathways (II, V, X)
- Prolongation relative to laboratory reference indicates a significant deficiency of factors (< 30% normal concentrations)
- Prolonged time
  - DIC
  - Dilutional coagulopathy
  - Dogs receiving unfractionated heparin
  - Haemophilia
  - Liver disease
  - Rodenticide toxicity: OSPT/PT prolongs first
- Can be artefactually prolonged =s
  - Difficult venepuncture
  - Hand-held analyzer
  - Inappropriate anticoagulant:blood ratio
  - Sample from heparinised catheter
  - Storage of sample
- Will not detect carriers of haemophilia with 40–60% or higher of normal concentrations of Factor VIII or IX activity

One-stage prothrombin time (OSPT/PT)

- Identifies coagulation disorders of extrinsic (VII) and common pathways (II, V, X)
- Prolongation relative to laboratory reference indicates a significant deficiency of factors if < 30% of normal concentrations
- Prolonged
  - Acquired vitamin K deficiency
  - DIC

- Dilution
- Liver disease
- Specific factor deficiencies

Whole blood clotting time

- Glass tube, not ACT or plastic tubes: add 1 ml blood to each of two tubes and tilt every 30 seconds till blood has coagulated.
- Normal = 6–7 minutes
- Prolonged for same reasons as ACT

Specific factor assays

- Contact specialist laboratory

Tests of fibrinolysis
Antithrombin (AT) (formerly known as antithrombin III)

- Circulating natural anticoagulant, main inhibitor of thrombin
- Decreased in hypercoagulable diseases compared to normal pooled plasma
  - DIC
  - Hepatic disease: reduced synthesis
  - Protein-losing conditions (PLE, PLN) due to similarity in size to albumin, and being lost with albumin

D-dimer

- Assay for cross-linked fibrin degradation products (FDPs), indicating clot formation and dissolution is occurring
- Negative D-dimer suggests no evidence of thromboembolism
- Increased/positive D-dimer indicates increased fibrinolysis
  - DIC is an important cause
  - Pulmonary thromboembolism (PTE) possible

Fibrin degradation products (FDPs)

- Includes product of fibrin and fibrinogen breakdown so not as indicative as D-dimers
- Healthy dogs FDP concentrations < 10 µg/ml
- FDP > 40 µg/ml indicates increased fibrinolysis
- Increased FDPs
  - Coagulopathy secondary to vitamin K antagonism hepatic disease
  - DIC: main cause of increased fibrinolysis
  - Thrombotic disease

ORGAN SYSTEMS

Fibrinogen
- Fibrinogen is synthesised in the liver and is an acute-phase protein
- Fibrinogen concentration ranges from 1.5 to 3.0 g/l in healthy dogs
- Congenital hypofibrinogenaemia
- Acquired hypofibrinogenaemia with increased consumption
  - Advanced liver disease
  - Blood loss
  - DIC
  - Dilution
  - Sepsis
  - Trauma

Thrombin clot time (TCT)
- Time taken for citrated plasma to clot when exogenous thrombin and calcium are added
- Only assesses ability of thrombin to convert fibrinogen to fibrin
- Insensitive: requires > 70% factor loss to be prolonged
- Prolonged TCT
  - Hypofibrinogenaemia
  - Dysfibrinogenaemia
  - Inhibition of thrombin, e.g. by abnormal serum proteins, fibrin degradation products (FDPs), heparin
- PIVKAs (protein induced by vitamin K absence or antagonism)
  - Non-functional factors which cannot be activated due to lack of vitamin K and accumulate in the blood
  - Can be detected via the TCT test

Global assessment of coagulation
Viscoelastic testing
with thromboelastography (TEG) or
rotational thromboelastometry (ROTEM)
- Dynamic assessment of haemostasis providing information on speed and strength of clot formation including cellular and plasma components and assesses fibrinolysis
- Can indicate bleeding and thrombotic tendencies
- Considered a patient-side test but not widely available in practice

5.5.1 ANTICOAGULANT RODENTICIDE POISONING

Aetiology
- Vitamin K is a fat-soluble vitamin absorbed in the gut and stored in the liver. Vitamin K is regenerated to ensure sufficient amount is available for haemostasis.
- Factors II, VII, IX and X are produced in the liver in an inactive form; they become activated in the presence of vitamin K.
- Functional deficiency of any of the coagulation factors leads to severe impairment of secondary haemostasis.
- Anticoagulant rodenticides inhibit the enzymatic process that regenerates vitamin K.
- Fat maldigestion/malabsorption can also cause vitamin K deficiency,
  e.g. lymphangiectasia, exocrine pancreatic insufficiency, extrahepatic bile duct obstruction

Anticoagulant rodenticides
- First generation
  - Coumarins: coumatetralyl, warfarin
    - Single ingestion of massive dose or, more commonly, repeated ingestion of small doses
    - Clinical signs usually develop after 4–5 days unless massive exposure
    - Warfarin half-life ≈ 12 hours, once exposure is discontinued, toxicity unlikely to persist > 1 week
- Second generation
  - Coumarins: brodifacoum, bromadiolone, difenacoum, flocoumafen
  - Indanediones: chlorophacinone, diphacinone, pindone
  - Thiochromenones: difethialone
    - All highly potent compared with warfarin
    - Clinical signs within 24 hours of ingestion
    - Toxicity can persist > 1 month
    - Secondary poisoning from ingestion of poisoned rodents is possible

Major signs
- Spontaneous bleeding
  - Major episodes of acute haemorrhage into body cavities, e.g. joints, pericardium, pleural space, peritoneal cavity
    - Acute severe dyspnoea: pleural or sub-mucosal tracheal bleeds
    - Coughing: pulmonary/mediastinal/tracheal/laryngeal bleeding
    - Development of large subcutaneous/intramuscular haematomas at injection sites
  - Superficial or external manifestations of bleeding
    - Cutaneous ecchymoses
    - Ocular haemorrhage: conjunctival/scleral bruising, hyphaema
    - Oral bleeding, epistaxis, haemoptysis, haematemesis, haematuria, melaena, vaginal/preputial bleeding
- Hypovolaemic shock, i.e. pallor, collapse, poor pulse volume, tachycardia

Minor signs
- Lameness: muscular or joint bleeds
- Neurological signs: bleeds into CNS
- Weakness, exercise intolerance

Potential sequelae
- Death

Predisposition
- Farm/rural environment

Historical clues
- Access to rodenticide
- Some baits contain blue/green dyes that colour the faeces if ingested

Physical examination
- Usually, no petechial haemorrhages as primary haemostasis should be intact
- Dyspnoea, cough
- Hypovolaemia
- Ocular haemorrhage
- Pallor
- Subcutaneous bleeds or swellings
- Swollen joints

Laboratory findings
Haematology
- Anaemia
  - May take 12 to 24 hours for PCV to decrease significantly with acute blood loss
  - Anaemia becomes regenerative within 5 days
- Consumptive thrombocytopenia can be seen with rodenticide toxicity

Serum biochemistry
- Bilirubin and bile acids to ensure no biliary obstruction causing secondary vitamin K deficiency or severe hepatic failure with failure to produce coagulation factors
- Folate and cobalamin for SI malabsorption
- Hypoproteinaemia

Coagulation profile
- All these tests will become prolonged
  - ACT
  - aPTT
  - PT
- Factor VII has the shortest half-life and as a component of the extrinsic clotting pathway, PT will be prolonged before the aPTT and ACT

Imaging
Abdominal radiographs
- Abdominal distension and loss of detail: haemoperitoneum

Thoracic radiographs
- Pleural effusion due to haemothorax ± pericardial effusion
- Increased mediastinal density due to haemomediastinum
- Generalised mixed alveolar/interstitial opacities due to pulmonary haemorrhage and intra-airway bleeding
- Tracheal narrowing due to sub-mucosal haematoma

Ultrasonography
- Thorax, heart, abdomen to identify or locate internal bleeding or assess for concurrent disease, e.g. rule out large bleed from tumour

ORGAN SYSTEMS

Special investigations
- Joint tap/thoracocentesis/abdominocentesis/ pericardiocentesis or aspiration of haemato- mas to identify the nature of the fluid/ swelling
  NB: Caution – there is a risk of further bleed- ing: avoid jugular venepuncture and thoraco- centesis is only performed to relieve signs of extreme respiratory distress.
- PIVKAs
- Toxicology to detect presence of anticoagu- lants in liver, kidney, stomach contents, unclotted blood, urine

Treatment
Vitamin K
- Use vitamin K_1 as K_3 is very much less effective
- Follow dosing and administration guidance of the product being used, starting by injec- tion and transitioning to oral therapy
- IM administration is possible but is associated with increased risk of haematoma formation
- IV administration may trigger anaphylaxis depending on the specific product used
- Treat for the duration the toxin will remain in body
  - First generation (warfarin): 1–2 weeks
  - Second generation: at least 1 month
- Vitamin K orally is absorbed better if given with a fatty meal
  - Dose
    - 3–5 mg/kg q24h can be given as divided doses
    - Administer with food to improve absorp- tion
    - Refer to formulary and dosing regime for the product being used
    - Higher doses and longer duration recom- mended with second-generation products

Transfusion therapy
- Even with prompt vitamin K therapy it may take 12–24 hours for the generation of func- tional clotting factors
- If the dog is severely dyspnoeic, etc., provi- sion of functional clotting factors must be provided by transfusion
- Fresh or fresh-frozen plasma is most suitable but whole blood can be used if needed or if oxygen-carrying support is needed

Management of toxic incident
- Gastric emesis/lavage/activated charcoal with recent suspected or confirmed ingestion < 4 hours after event
  - If recognised early after ingestion and effec- tively decontaminated, 90% of dogs do not need vitamin K
    - Monitor clotting times and, if prolonged, vitamin K is indicated
  - If dogs present with bleeding it is likely > 12 hours post-ingestion and emesis is not indicated

Symptomatic therapy
- Dyspnoeic animals are likely to benefit from oxygen
- Minimise injections/blood sampling/external haemorrhage, surgery until haemostatic defect is corrected
- Strict cage rest
- Therapeutic centesis, e.g. of pleural or peri- cardial cavity, is only indicated if situation is life threatening
- Treat shock with appropriate fluid therapy

Monitoring
- Coagulation parameters return to normal within 1–2 days of starting appropriate therapy
- Monitor haematology
- Monitor PT 2 days after stopping vitamin K therapy and, if it is prolonged, continue main- tenance therapy for a further 2 weeks and repeat the process

Sequelae
- If recognised and an adequate course treat- ment is administered, the prognosis is good
- Mortality is estimated at 10–20% due to fail- ure of prompt diagnosis or inadequate dura- tion and/or dosage of vitamin K

5.5.2 DISSEMINATED INTRAVASCULAR COAGULATION (DIC)

Aetiology
- DIC occurs when there is:
  - Procoagulant activation

- Fibrinolytic activation
- Inhibitor consumption
- Microvascular thrombosis
- End-organ failure
- Numerous factors produce an overwhelming thrombotic process, depleting clotting factors and hence promoting bleeding elsewhere and organ failure
  - Endotoxin
  - Exogenous toxins
  - Hypoxia
  - Pyrexia
  - Sepsis
  - Tissue necrosis
  - Vascular stasis

Major signs
- Relate to haemorrhage or thrombosis

Acute
- Acute organ failure due to microcirculatory obstruction with thrombi, e.g. acute oliguric renal failure, coma, dyspnoea, haemorrhagic vomiting and diarrhoea
- Often bleeding is late in the course of disease
  - Severe fulminant DIC: generalised bleeding from body orifices, mucosal petechiation or ecchymoses, haematuria

Chronic
- Minimal clinical signs
- Low-grade consumption of platelets and clotting factors can lead to unexpected bleeding after surgery

Potential sequelae
- End-organ failure
- Uncontrollable haemorrhage
- Death

Predisposition
- Associated with many diseases of varying severity:
  - Immune-mediated disease, e.g. immune-mediated haemolytic anaemia (IMHA)
  - Infectious disease, e.g. heartworm, bacterial sepsis, rickettsial diseases
  - Inflammatory disease, e.g. pancreatitis
  - Neoplasia, e.g. haemangiosarcoma, acute leukaemias

- Miscellaneous, e.g. heatstroke, severe trauma, snake envenomation
- Tissue trauma, ischaemia and necrosis, e.g. GDV, intestinal infarction or volvulus

Physical examination
- Dyspnoea/tachypnoea
- Ecchymoses/petechiae
- External bleeding, e.g. epistaxis, haematuria, melaena
- Abdominal pain/abdominal distension
- Pallor

Laboratory findings
Haematology
- Moderate to severe thrombocytopenia < 100 × 10^9/l
- ± Anaemia
- Fragmented red cells: schistocytes
- ± Leukocytosis

Serum biochemistry
- Indicate underlying disease process or organ damage, e.g. liver, kidneys

Coagulation screen
- aPTT, PT prolonged
- Antithrombin decreased
- Increased FDPs
- Increased D-dimer
- Hypofibrinogenaemia
- Thromboelastography (TEG or ROTEM) can detect hyper- and hypo-coagulable states

Imaging
- Thoracic and abdominal radiographs to identify evidence of underlying disease

Special investigations
- Histological evidence of microthrombi

Treatment
- Remove/treat underlying cause/disease
- Control hypovolaemia, hypoxia, endotoxaemia, acidosis
- Oxygen administration
- Factor replacement
  - Transfusion whole blood or plasma

ORGAN SYSTEMS

- No general consensus, e.g.,
  - Heparin – to reduce the process of intravascular coagulation
    - Low-molecular-weight heparin @ 50–200 IU/kg SC TID
    - Requires adequate antithrombin (AT) concentrations to be effective

Monitoring
- Clinical signs
- Coagulation screen, especially D-dimer, FDPs, platelets, PT and aPTT

Prognosis
- Often high mortality which is likely associated with poor control of underlying disease or insufficiently prompt therapy

5.5.3 FACTOR VIII DEFICIENCY (HAEMOPHILIA A)

Aetiology
- Haemophilia is an inherited, sex-linked deficiency of a specific coagulation protein
  - Haemophilia A is a deficiency of Factor VIII
  - Haemophilia B is a deficiency of Factor IX
    - Rarer than haemophilia A, but clinical signs are similar
  - Deficiencies of factors X, XI and XII are extremely rare
- Severity of signs in any haemophiliac depends on which factor and degree of deficiency
  - Factor VIII deficiency can cause fatal haemorrhage

Major signs
Severe disease
- Perinatal death: bleeding from umbilicus
- Gingival haemorrhage when teeth are shed
- Haematoma formation in puppies once they interact with littermates
- Mediastinal haemorrhage, haemothorax and retroperitoneal bleeds are common causes of death
- Persistent navel bleeding at birth
- Shifting/recurrent lameness due to haemarthrosis, intramuscular haematoma
- Subcutaneous bleeds/ecchymoses

Moderate disease
- Bleeding tendency after trauma/surgery
- Prolonged bleeding during oestrus in carrier females
- Recurrent lameness

Potential sequelae
- Recurrent bleeding episodes in less severely affected patients
- Degenerative osteoarthroses following haemarthroses
- Death before adulthood in severe cases

Predisposition
- Commonest inherited coagulopathy
- Sex linked: affects males; female carriers
- Self-limiting: affected males rarely survive to adulthood and reproductive capacity
- GSD: moderately severe form occurs and affected males may survive until adulthood and be used for breeding

Historical clues
- Recurrent episodes of bleeding with no history of access to anticoagulants

Physical examination
- Ecchymoses
- Haematomas
- Heart murmur
- Joint effusions
- Pallor
- Pleural effusion, etc.
- Prolonged bleeding from wounds/surgery sites
- Tachycardia, tachypnoea, weak pulses, collapse

Laboratory findings
Haematology
- Normal platelet numbers
- Normal red cell parameters unless recent haemorrhage

Coagulation profile
- Prolonged clotting times that assess the intrinsic system, e.g. aPTT
- PT normal
- BMBT normal

Imaging
Thoracic and abdominal radiographs and ultrasound
- To investigate intracavitary bleeds
- Joints to assess for effusion ± degenerative changes

Special investigations
- Measure Factor VIII activity levels: less than normal plasma pool in affected animals
  - < 20% in affected animals; 40–60% in carrier females
- Factor VIII-related antigen (vWF antigen) is normal or increased in affected animals
- DNA test for affected and carrier dogs
- Pedigree analysis to try and identify female carriers

Treatment
- Gene therapy has been used successfully, but only short-term expression (1–2 weeks) of the gene occurred due to development of antibodies
- Tranexamic acid (TXA [unlicensed]): inhibitor of fibrinolysis has been used to control bleeding episodes in haemophiliac patients @ 15–20 mg/kg orally 2–4 times daily

Transfusion
- Packed red cells or fresh whole blood if severe anaemia
- Fresh or fresh-frozen plasma @ 6–15 ml/kg over 30–120 minutes and repeated q12–24h or until bleeding stops
- Cryoprecipitate (if available)
  - Higher levels of factor VIII; less incidence of side effects
  - 1–5ml/kg IV over 1 hour

Monitoring
- Clinical signs
- At risk for spontaneous haemorrhage or bleeding with trauma/surgery and should be pre-treated with cryoprecipitate before elective surgery
- Avoid intramuscular injections
- Screen for carriers/affected dogs in susceptible dogs before breeding

Prognosis
- Guarded to grave, depending on severity of deficiency

5.5.4   HYPERFIBRINOLYSIS

Aetiology
- Accelerated breakdown of clots, which can result in bleeding syndrome and potentially significant blood loss
- Associated with:
  - Acute coagulopathy of trauma and shock (ACOTS)
  - Delayed post-operative bleeding in Greyhounds, presumed to be due to increased fibrinolytic activity
  - DIC

Major signs
- Spontaneous bleeding associated with trauma/shock
- Widespread post-operative subcutaneous bleeding

Potential sequelae
- Severe bleeding requiring transfusion
- Can be fatal

Predisposition
- Greyhounds and probably other sight hounds

Physical examination
- Widespread ecchymotic haemorrhage in delayed post-operative bleeding from wound and extending peripherally
- Intracavitary bleeds in trauma/shock causing signs of poor oxygenation, impaired ventilation

Laboratory findings
- Coagulation times usually normal
- D-dimers and FDPs often increased
- TEG or ROTEM can demonstrate excessive fibrinolysis
- Other changes reflecting primary disease or secondary to acute blood loss

ORGAN SYSTEMS

Imaging
- May be normal

Treatment
- Antifibrinolytic drugs (aminocaproic acid [ACA] and TXA) can slow fibrinolysis
- In at-risk dogs, e.g. greyhounds, perioperative administration of TXA can decrease incidence of post-operative bleeding
  - TXA is dosed at 15–20 mg/kg q8h for 5 days starting on the day of surgery

Monitoring
- Clinical signs and extent of haemorrhage
- Viscoelastic coagulation testing, i.e. TEG or ROTEM

Prognosis
- Prophylaxis reduces severity of post-operative bleeding.

5.5.5 IMMUNE-MEDIATED THROMBOCYTOPENIA (IMTP)

Aetiology
- Auto-immune/primary
- Secondary *q.v.* section 3.31.1

Major signs
- Ecchymotic and petechial haemorrhages on oral, penile or vulval mucous membranes and the skin
- Epistaxis
- Haematemesis
- Haematochezia
- Haematoma
- Haematuria
- Melaena

Minor signs
- Anorexia
- Concurrent anaemia
  - Blood loss
  - Concurrent IMHA (Evans syndrome)
- Hepatosplenomegaly
- Lethargy and weakness
- Lymphadenopathy
- Ocular bleeds: hyphaema, blindness
- Seizures

Potential sequelae
- Recovery
- Recurrence
- Persistent haemorrhage
- Death
  - Blood loss
  - CNS haemorrhage

Predisposition
- Commonly middle-aged dogs for primary IMTP
- Female predisposition for immune-mediated disease
- Breed association: Cocker spaniel, Miniature and Toy poodles, Old English sheepdog

Historical clues
- Recent drug therapy or vaccination
- Infectious disease exposure
- Presence of petechiation is cardinal sign of thrombocytopenia

Physical examination
- Ecchymoses
- External blood loss, e.g. epistaxis, etc.
- Hyphaema
- Mucous membrane pallor
- Petechiae
- Pyrexia
- Retinal haemorrhages

Laboratory findings
Haematology
- Low platelet count; commonly $< 10 \times 10^9/l$
  - Confirm with evaluation of a blood smear, *q.v.* section 3B
  - $< 3–4$ platelets per high-power field = increased risk of bleeding
  - Spontaneous bleeding is not usually seen until platelets $< 50 \times 10^9/l$
- If significant blood loss, regenerative anaemia may be seen
  - Part of immune-mediated process: IMTP plus IMHA = Evans syndrome
  - Response to bleeding due to thrombocytopenia
- Microplatelets possibly suggest primary IMTP
- Macroplatelets indicate marrow regeneration
- Pancytopenia may be seen with bone marrow hypoplasia/aplasia

- Schistocytes and thrombocytopenia may suggest DIC

Serum biochemistry
- Evidence of concurrent disease

Urinalysis
- Evidence of haematuria

Imaging
- Blood loss into body cavities
- Assess for evidence of neoplasia
- Splenomegaly often seen with immune-mediated disorders

Special investigations
- APTT normal to slightly increased
- BMBT increased
- FDPs normal unless DIC
- PT normal
- Platelet count decreased
- Blood cultures, infectious disease screening
- Bone marrow biopsy
  - If immune-mediated/infectious cause cannot be identified as the cause of the thrombocytopenia
  - If other cytopenias without evidence of immune/infection causes
- Coombs' and ANA tests to evaluate for immune-mediated disease
- Platelet antibody tests
  - Anti-platelet antibodies can be detected using flow cytometry but the test is not very specific
- Platelet factor 3 (PF3) release test
  - Detects anti-platelet antibody but is not reliable

Treatment
- Identify underlying/concurrent disease and manage that specifically
- Withdraw any drug therapy which may have induced thrombocytopenia
- Severe bleeding may require transfusion of fresh frozen plasma or platelet-rich plasma where available, fresh whole blood or packed red cells if severe anaemia
- Immunosuppressive therapy to suppress phagocytic activity of reticulo-endothelial system

- Prednisolone @ 40–60 mg/m^2 if < 25 kg or 2 mg/kg q24h or split into q12h, tapering once platelet count returns to normal
- Equivalent dose of dexamethasone can be used initially
- Vincristine, single-dose 0.02 mg/kg IV dogs < 15 kg and 0.5 mg/m^2 if > 15 kg to increase platelet numbers
- Other immunosuppressive therapy
  - Azathioprine @ 2 mg/kg daily per os, reduce to 1 mg/kg daily or to every-other-day treatment when in remission
    - Regular haematology as myelosuppressive
  - Ciclosporin 5 mg/kg q12h PO
  - Mycophenolate mofetil 8–12 mg/kg q12h PO
- Human intravenous immunoglobulin infusion (IVIG) can be used to block antibody mediated platelet phagocytosis when available
- Minimise venepuncture or invasive diagnostics due to risk of significant haemorrhage
- Cage rest

Monitoring
- Clinical signs
- Haematology including platelet count: daily platelet count until > 50 × 10^9/l usually achieved within 7–10 days, and then before every dose reduction
- Taper medications once platelet count is normalised gradually over 4–6 months

Prognosis
- Up to 30% of cases with IMTP die or are euthanased during the initial episode or during recurrence
- > 70% of dogs with primary IMTP will have a platelet count > 100 × 10^9/l after initial therapy with immunosuppressive agents
- ~40% of cases have recurrent disease
- Prognosis when concurrent IMHA

5.5.6 VON WILLEBRAND DISEASE

Aetiology
- von Willebrand factor (vWF, Factor VIII-related antigen) is an endothelial factor required for the binding/adhesion of platelets

ORGAN SYSTEMS

- von Willebrand disease is an inherited, autosomal trait
- vWF deficiency can cause generalised bleeding
- Range of severity is dependent upon the vWF concentration and the type of multimer deficient, i.e. more severe if lacking high-molecular-weight multimer
  - Type I vWD is partial quantitative deficiency of all vWF multimers: bleeding severity is variable and is most common; seen in Dobermann
  - Type II vWD has a low concentration of high-molecular-weight vWF multimers and has severe bleeding problems; seen in German short-haired and wire-haired pointers
- Type III vWD is most severe with severe deficiency of all vWF multimers; seen in Chesapeake Bay retriever, Dutch Kookier, Scottish terrier and Shetland sheepdogConcurrent disease can accentuate signs, e.g. hepatic disease, renal disease, possibly hypothyroidism

Major signs
Excessive bleeding from mucosal surfaces
- Haematuria
- Epistaxis
- Melaena
- Uterine or gingival haemorrhage

Excessive bleeding after surgery or trauma
Minor signs
- Lameness
- Intracranial haemorrhage – neurological signs
- Poor wound healing

Potential sequelae
- Depends on severity
  - Asymptomatic
  - Bleeds after trauma/surgery
  - Spontaneous bleeding
  - Fatal bleeding

Predisposition
- No sex predisposition
- Prevalent in Dobermann, Irish Wolfhound and GSD in the UK

Historical clues
- Episodes of bleeding following previous traumatic events

Physical examination
- Signs as for bleeding, e.g. haematomas, haemarthroses

Laboratory findings
- Platelet count normal

Coagulation screen
- Coagulation times normal
- BMBT
  - Useful as a presurgical assessment in dogs from susceptible breeds with unknown vWD status
  - Mild decreases in vWF:Ag concentration may have normal BMBT
  - Moderate/severe decreases in vWF:Ag concentration prolong BMBT

Imaging
- Normal unless intracavitary bleed, etc.

Special tests
- vWF:Ag testing quantifies plasma vWF levels but not its function
  - Levels range from 70 to 180% in normal dogs
  - Levels 50–60% are borderline normal
  - Levels < 50% are abnormal
  - Levels < 35% increased risk of bleeding
  - Levels can be increased in late pregnancy and sepsis
- Genetic testing
  - Gene defects identified in certain breeds, e.g. Dobermann, Dutch Kooiker, Manchester terrier, Pembroke Welsh Corgi, Poodle, Shetland sheepdog, Scottish terrier
  - No evidence for a link between genetic defect and severity of clinical disease, therefore check vWF:Ag levels also

Treatment
- Increase vWF:Ag concentration to a level to stop or prevent haemorrhage
  - Infusion of cryoprecipitate or fresh frozen plasma

- Cryoprecipitate is preferred at 1 U/10 kg IV q6–12h
- Plasma at 10–12 ml/kg IV q8–12h
  - Avoid whole blood as risk of sensitising to further transfusions; use only if severe anaemia
- Desmopressin (DDAVP)
  - Increases plasma vWF:Ag and Factor VIII levels by inducing release of vWF from endothelial cells
  - Only effective in dogs with Type I vWD who have endothelial stores
  - Repeat injections have reducing benefit due to depletion of stores
  - Can be used for pre-surgical treatment of 'at-risk' Dobermanns or for donor dogs before transfusion is collected
  - 1 µg/kg diluted to 1 ml with sterile saline injected subcutaneously 30 minutes before surgery (intranasal preparation) – may shorten BMBT for up to 4 hours
  - Response is unpredictable
- Local haemostatic control

Monitoring
- Clinical signs

Prognosis
- Good to grave, depending on severity

5.5.7 VASCULITIS

Aetiology
Vasculitis is inflammation of vessel walls which can occur as an immune/hypersensitivity response. It is typically Type III hypersensitivity with antigen-antibody complex deposition, and can affect skin and other organs or be systemic only with no skin signs.

NB: A vasculopathy is ischaemic damage to vessel walls without inflammation present.
- Vasculitis can have a variety of triggers:
  - Infections: bacterial, viral, fungal, mycobacterial, rickettsial, parasitic
  - Drugs, vaccine, food/additives
  - Neoplasia
  - Immune-mediated disease
  - Burns/trauma
  - Idiopathic

Major signs
- Erythema
- Haemorrhagic bullae
- Petechiae/ecchymoses
- Plaques
- Swelling
- Urticaria

Minor signs
- Alopecia
- Anorexia
- Fever
- Lameness
- Lethargy
- Nail changes, e.g. onychodystrophy
- Pain
- Pigment changes
- Scaling

Potential sequelae
- Necrosis and ulceration
- Death (euthanasia)

Predisposition
- Cutaneous and renal glomerular vasculopathy (CRGV)
- Cutaneous vasculitis of Jack Russell terrier
- Dermal arteritis or nasal philtrum in Saint Bernard and related breeds
- Familial cutaneous vasculopathy of GSD
- Nasal vasculitis of Scottish terrier
- Ischaemic dermatopathies are specific syndromes
  - Familial dermatomyositis in Collie, Shetland sheepdog and other breeds
  - Generalised idiopathic ischaemic dermatopathy
  - Generalised vaccine-induced ischaemic dermatopathy
  - Juvenile onset non-familial dermatomyositis
  - Post-injection panniculitis
- Pinnal thrombovascular necrosis

Historical clues
- Infectious disease risks based on local and travel history
- Investigate any triggers, e.g. anti-parasitics, drugs, recent vaccination, supplements

ORGAN SYSTEMS

Physical examination
Dermatological examination
- Lesions do not blanch with pressure
- Localised or generalised lesions
- Variable size and distribution of lesions
  - Erythema
  - Haemorrhagic bullae
  - Plaques
  - Petechiae and ecchymoses
  - Swelling
  - Ulceration and necrosis
  - Urticarial lesions

Ophthalmic examination
- Retinal haemorrhages

Laboratory findings
Haematology
- Anaemia
- Leukocytosis
- Thrombocytosis or thrombocytopenia

Biochemistry
- Evidence of organ involvement, e.g. azotaemia, increased liver enzymes, hypoalbuminaemia

Urinalysis
- Proteinuria
- Haematuria

Imaging
- To evaluate for organ damage, neoplasia

Specialised tests
- Skin biopsy/histopathology: early lesions without significant ulceration/necrosis are preferred; if sampling ulcerated lesion, sample margin
- Infectious disease screening
- Test antinuclear antibody (ANA) if suspicious of systemic lupus erythematosus (SLE)

Treatment
- Avoid drugs, etc., that were implicated in causing vasculitis
- Manage underlying disease
- Systemic treatment:
  - Pentoxyfilline: 1–30 mg/kg q8–12h; can take 4–6 weeks for response; taper to once daily before stopping
  - Niacinamide (give with doxycycline): ≤ 10 kg 25 0mg PO q8h, or > 10 kg 500 mg PO q8h
  - Doxycycline (give with niacinamide): 5 mg/kg q8–12h; can take up to 12–16 weeks to respond; taper to once daily before stopping
  - For more severe cases immune suppression, e.g., glucocorticoids are used as for treating IMHA/IMTP
  - Other treatments exist for more complex cases; readers are advised to seek specialist advice
- Topical treatment for skin lesions alone or with systemic treatment, e.g. tacrolimus, glucocorticoids
- Supportive treatment
  - Essential fatty acids (180 mg EPA/5 kg PO once daily) and Vitamin E 400–800 IU PO q12h may help
  - Topical keratolytic/plastic shampoo can be used for scale and crust
  - Treatment of secondary infections may be required

Monitoring
- Clinical improvement
- Medication side effects

Prognosis
Guarded, depending on underlying trigger

5.6 HEPATOBILIARY SYSTEM

Problems

Presenting complaints

q.v. section 1
1.4 Altered consciousness
1.5 Anorexia/hyporexia/inappetence
1.9 Bleeding
1.10 Blindness
1.15 Diarrhoea
1.25 Haematemesis
1.27 Haematuria and discoloured urine
1.31 Melaena
1.35 Perinatal death
1.37 Polyuria/polydipsia (PU/PD)
1.42 Seizures
1.44 Stunting
1.49 Vomiting
1.51 Weakness, collapse and syncope
1.53 Weight loss

Physical abnormalities

q.v. section 2
2.1 Abdominal enlargement
2.5 Ascites
2.7 Eye lesions
2.8 Hepatomegaly
2.13 Icterus/jaundice
2.17.1 Abdominal pain

Laboratory abnormalities

q.v. section 3
3A Biochemical tests
3.2 Ammonia
3.5 Bile acids
3.6 Bilirubin
3.17.2 Hypoglycaemia
3.19.2 Hypocholesterolaemia
3.20 Liver enzymes
3.27.1B Hyperglobulinaemia
3.27.2A Hypoalbuminaemia
3.29 Urea
3B Haematology
3.30.1 Anaemia
3.32.1 Leukocytosis

Diagnostic Approach

1 Identify potential hepatic disease from clinical signs and increased liver enzymes
2 Check for primary hepatopathy by liver function test, e.g. bile acids
3 Evaluate by imaging and rule in/out portosystemic shunt (PSS)
4 Liver biopsy for chronic cases

Diagnostic Methods

History
Clinical signs
- Often acute in onset, which may reflect either acute disease or tipping point in chronic process
- A detailed history usually reveals subtle signs of ill-thrift preceding presentation for chronic disease
- Drug administration, e.g. barbiturates
- Environment, e.g. access to toxins
- Vaccination status: canine adenovirus (CAV), leptospirosis

Age
- Young
  - Congenital PSS
  - Infections
    - Canine viral hepatitis: CAV-1 (infectious canine hepatitis)
    - Canine herpes virus (neonates)
  - Ductal plate abnormalities
  - Gall bladder (GB) agenesis
  - Lobular-dissecting hepatitis
  - Portal vein hypoplasia
    - Microvascular dysplasia
    - Non-cirrhotic portal hypertension/juvenile hepatic fibrosis
    - Portal vein atresia: fatal at very young age
- Older
  - Chronic hepatitis
  - Cirrhosis
  - Neoplasia
- Breed-associations
  - See specific conditions below

ORGAN SYSTEMS

Notes on Canine Internal Medicine, Fourth Edition. Victoria L. Black, Kathryn F. Murphy, Jessie Rose Payne, and Edward J. Hall.

Specific clinical signs
- Jaundice, *q.v.* section 2.13
  - Prehepatic cause in haemolytic jaundice
  - Not invariably present in severe liver disease
- Acholic faeces indicate biliary obstruction or rupture
- Ascites if portal hypertension ± hypoalbuminaemia
- Poor growth/stunting, especially with congenital PSS
- Hepatocutaneous syndrome, *q.v.* section 2.26
- Hepatoencephalopathy (HE)
  - Bizarre neurological signs
    - Pacing, restlessness, intermittent blindness, head pressing, stupor, seizures, coma
    - Exacerbation by dehydration, azotaemia, hypokalaemia, GI bleeding, constipation and dietary protein intake

Non-specific clinical signs
- Bleeding diatheses, especially GI bleeding (haematemesis, melaena), disseminated intravascular coagulation (DIC)
- Fever
- Loss of appetite
- PU/PD
- Weight loss

Clinical examination
Visual inspection
- General body condition
- Icterus
- Neurological/behavioural signs suggestive of hepatoencephalopathy

Physical examination
- Abdominal palpation
  - Abdominal enlargement
  - Ascites
  - Hepatomegaly
  - Cranial abdominal pain in acute disease
- Ecchymoses
- Icteric mucous membrane
- Murmur over cranial abdomen with AV fistula
- Renomegaly in PSS
- Weight loss/stunting

Laboratory findings
All dogs suspected of having hepatic disease should undergo laboratory investigation

Haematology
- Anaemia of chronic disease
  - Microcytosis, especially in PSS
  - Target cells and poikilocytosis
- Leukocytosis if infectious/inflammatory disease

Serum biochemistry
- Crude markers of liver function
  - Hypoalbuminaemia
  - Hyperglobulinaemia
  - Hypoglycaemia
  - Low urea
  - Hypo- or hyper-cholesterolaemia
- Liver function tests, *q.v.* sections 3.2, 3.5 and 3.6
  - Ammonia
  - Bile acids
  - Bilirubin
- Markers of cholestasis: ALP and GGT
- Markers of hepatocellular damage: ALT and AST

Urinalysis
- Absence of urobilinogen in biliary obstruction: unreliable
- Bilirubinuria but small amount is normal in male dogs
- Urate crystalluria

Imaging
Radiographs
Plain
- Liver size related to gastric axis: normally parallel to ribs, *q.v.* section 4.1.1A
  - Microhepatica tilts axis cranially
  - Hepatomegaly tilts axis caudally
- Gallstones
- Emphysematous cholecystitis

Portovenography or CT angiography
- AV fistula
- Single congenital PSS
- Multiple secondary (acquired) shunts

Ultrasound
- Bile ducts
  - Choleliths or sludge
  - Dilated and tortuous if obstructed
  - Mineralisation: incidental or suggestive of cholangitis

- Hepatic parenchymal architecture
  - Diffuse changes in echogenicity, compared to kidneys and spleen
  - Heterogeneous changes in echogenicity
  - Masses and nodules
- GB wall and contents
  - Choleliths
  - Limy bile
  - Mucocoele
  - Sludge
- Liver size
- Portal and hepatic veins and flow
- Portosystemic shunts

Special investigative techniques
- Abdominocentesis
  - Bile from biliary rupture
  - Protein-rich 'modified' transudate if hepatic or post-hepatic portal hypertension
  - Transudate if pre-hepatic portal hypertension
- Coagulation times are mandatory before liver biopsy
- GB aspirates for cytology and culture
- Liver biopsy for histology with staining for copper, fluorescent *in situ* hybridisation (FISH) analysis and culture
  - Fine needle aspirate (FNA)
  - Tru-cut
  - Laparoscopic
  - Surgical

Treatments
- Antibacterials
  - Bacterial cholangiohepatitis
  - Leptospirosis
- Anti-fibrotic
  - Prednisolone
  - Colchicine (no evidence)
- Anti-inflammatory
  - Prednisolone
- Antioxidants
  - S-Adenosyl methionine (SAME)
  - Sylibin
  - Vitamin E
- Choleretic
  - Ursodeoxycholic acid (UDCA)
- Control hepatoencephalopathy; start with all three and de-escalate, stopping antibacterials first

1 Dietary protein modification and restriction
2 Lactulose
3 Neomycin, ampicillin or metronidazole
- Decoppering
  - D-penicillamine
  - Trientine
  - Zinc
- Immunosuppressant
  - Azathioprine
  - Ciclosporin
  - Prednisolone

5.6.1 CHRONIC HEPATITIS (CH)/CIRRHOSIS

Aetiology
- Chronic inflammatory disease of the liver, characterised by a lymphoplasmacytic infiltrate, with progression to bridging fibrosis and ultimately cirrhosis
- Cirrhosis is characterised by bands of fibrosis and regeneration nodules
- Many cases of CH are idiopathic, but a variety of potential causes have been identified
  - Autoimmune
    - Suspected in Dobermann due to presence of anti-histone antibodies
  - Bacterial cholangitis/cholangiohepatitis
  - Copper accumulation
  - Drugs
    - Halothane
    - Mebendazole
    - Phenobarbitone and, historically, primidone
  - ICH
  - Metabolic defects
  - Toxins
    - Aflatoxin

Major signs
Signs may wax and wane
- Ascites
- Bleeding diatheses
- HE
- Icterus
- PU/PD

Minor signs
- Hepatocutaneous syndrome: cracked hyper-keratotic footpads secondary to liver disease
- Variable appetite or anorexia
- Weight loss

Sequelae
- Cirrhosis
- End-stage liver failure and death

Predisposition
- Idiopathic: Cocker spaniel, English Springer spaniel, female Dobermann
- Copper accumulation: Bedlington terrier, Dobermann, Labradors and WHWT
- Lobular dissecting hepatitis in young dogs: GSD, Standard poodle

Historical clues
- May be asymptomatic and liver enzyme increases detected on routine blood testing
- Episodes of vague illness before presentation in acute crisis

Physical examination
Changes consistent with chronic liver disease – see above

Laboratory findings
- Anaemia of chronic disease
- Abnormal liver function tests
- Hyperbilirubinaemia
- Hypoalbuminaemia
- Persistently increased liver enzymes, but can be mild at end-stage
- Terminal hypoglycaemia

Imaging
Ultrasound
- Acquired porto-caval shunts
- Ascites
- Heterogeneous echogenicity
- Small liver with irregular borders

Special investigations
- Abdominocentesis
  - Modified transudate
- Liver biopsy
  - Culture
  - Special stains for collagen, copper, etc.

Treatment
The most effective treatment is unknown due to lack of controlled studies.

Control HE
1 Dietary modification
2 Lactulose
3 Antibacterials

Immunosuppression
- Azathioprine
- Ciclosporin
- Prednisolone: avoid high doses as it causes steroid hepatopathy

Manage ascites
- Ensure adequate protein intake
- Diuretics: spironolactone preferred over fru-semide, which can precipitate HE by causing dehydration and hypokalaemia
- Paracentesis only recommended if massive ascites causing dyspnoea

Non-specific
- Anti-oxidants
- UDCA

Monitoring
- Clinical signs
- Serum albumin concentration
- Serum liver enzyme activities
    NB: Changes in bile acids cannot be used to quantify changes in hepatic function.

Prognosis
- Ultimately grave, but treatment may prolong life

5.6.2 CHOLANGITIS/ CHOLANGIOHEPATITIS

Aetiology
- Infection of bile ducts primarily, but inflammation may extend into the hepatic parenchyma
- Often associated with cholecystitis, and perhaps predisposed by cholelithiasis and bile sludge

- Presumed ascending bacterial infection from SI as enteric organisms usually found, but haematogenous spread via portal vein is possible

Major signs
Signs may wax and wane
- Icterus
- Pyrexia
- Variable appetite – anorexia

Minor signs
- HE uncommon
- Weight loss

Sequelae
- Persistent or recurrent infection causing hepatic fibrosis

Predisposition
- May be more prevalent in small-breed dogs

Historical clues
- Episodes of vague illness with pyrexia

Physical examination
- Icterus
- Pyrexia

Laboratory findings
- Anaemia of chronic disease
- Abnormal liver function tests
- Hyperbilirubinaemia
- Persistently increased cholestatic liver enzymes > hepatocellular enzyme increases

Imaging
- Bile ducts
  - Dilated and containing cholelith or sludge
  - Mineralisation, but can also be an incidental finding
- Thickened GB wall if concurrent cholecystitis

Special investigations
- FNA of bile from GB for culture-sensitivity and cytology
- Liver biopsy
  - Culture
  - Histopathology

Treatment
- Antibacterials, ideally based on bile culture/sensitivity (C/S) results
- Anti-oxidants
- UDCA
- Surgical removal of GB if suspected source of recurrent infection

Monitoring
- Clinical signs
- Liver enzymes

Prognosis
- Guarded because antibiotic resistance and recurrent infections likely

5.6.3   CHOLECYSTITIS

Aetiology
- Inflammation of the GB due to cholelithiasis and/or bacterial infection
- Cystic mucosal hyperplasia may be trigger or consequence
- May predispose to GB mucocoele

Major signs
- Abdominal discomfort
- Icterus if GB ruptures or cholelith obstructs common bile duct
- Pyrexia

Minor signs
- Variable appetite – anorexia
- Weight loss

Sequelae
- Extrahepatic bile duct obstruction (EHBDO)
- GB mucocoele
- GB rupture

Predisposition
No known predispositions

Historical clues
Episodes of vague illness with pyrexia

Physical examination
- Icterus
- Pyrexia

Laboratory findings
- Anaemia of chronic disease
- Hyperbilirubinaemia and hypercholesterolaemia if EHBDO
- Persistently increased cholestatic liver enzyme activities > hepatocellular enzymes

Imaging
- Cholelithiasis
- Empty GB if ruptured
- Thickened, irregular GB mucosa

Special investigations
- GB FNA for culture-sensitivity and cytology
- Liver biopsy
  - Culture
  - Histopathology

Treatment
- Antibacterials, ideally based on bile C/S results
- Anti-oxidants
- UDCA
- Ultimately, cholecystectomy if cholelithiasis, ruptured GB or recurrent episodes

Monitor
- Clinical signs
- Liver enzymes

Prognosis
- Good unless GB ruptures

5.6.4 CONGENITAL PORTO-SYSTEMIC SHUNT (PSS)

Aetiology
- Congenital abnormalities of the portal circulation (porto-systemic shunts) leading to bypass of the liver
- Delivery of ammonia and other toxins from the GI tract to the systemic circulation causes HE
- The liver fails to develop because of lack of nutrients and trophic factors
- Signs of PSS are related largely to HE and, eventually, to hepatic failure
- Congenital anomalies comprise:

- Intrahepatic microvascular dysplasia
  - Vascular changes are found on liver biopsy in dogs with a single PSS, reflecting a common pathological response to reduced portal blood flow
- Single porto-systemic shunts, which may be:
  - Extra-hepatic (EHPSS)
    There are a number of variations but the basic patterns are:
    - Porto-azygos
    - Porto-caval, including porto-gastric and porto-splenic
    - Porto-phrenic
  - Intra-hepatic (IHPSS), inserting into hepatic vein or, more uncommonly, the phrenic vein
    - Left divisional: persistent ductus venosus
    - Central divisional
    - Right divisional: most common

Major signs
- HE
- PU/PD
- Stunting

Minor signs
- Haematuria from renal and/or cystic urate calculi
- Intermittent pyrexia from repeated bacteraemia
  NB: Ascites is rare and related to hypoalbuminaemia.
  - Icterus is *not* a feature
- Vomiting and diarrhoea

Potential sequelae
- Ascites
- Rarely, discospondylitis following bacteraemia
- Seizures and hepatic coma
- Death

Predisposition
- Young dogs, usually less than one year
- Extra-hepatic shunts in small-breed dogs
  - Lhasa Apso and Shih Tzu
  - Miniature schnauzer
  - Pug
  - Terrier breeds

- Extra- or intra-hepatic shunts in medium- and large-breed dogs
  - Australian cattle dogs
  - Retrievers
  - Irish setter
  - Old English sheepdog
- Intrahepatic shunts in giant breeds
  - Irish Wolfhound; heritability proven
  - Golden retriever

Historical clues
- Recurrent illnesses since early life
- Failure to thrive
- Intermittent neurological signs

Physical examination
- Often unremarkable except for reduced body size, unless showing HE as microhepatica not palpable
- Association with cryptorchidism
- Flow murmur due to volume overload
- Renomegaly reflecting increased GFR

Laboratory findings
Haematology
- Microcytic anaemia

Serum biochemistry
- Abnormal liver function
  - Post-prandial bile acids are as sensitive as ammonia and less prone to laboratory artefact
- Hypocholesterolaemia
- Liver enzyme activities generally only mildly increased, but age-related increase in ALP activity anyway
- Decreased urea
- Urate crystalluria

Imaging
Radiography
- Microhepatica
- Nephroliths and/or cystoliths (ammonium biurate)
- Renomegaly

Contrast radiography
- Identification of a single shunt by portovenography or CT angiography

Ultrasound
- PSS may be demonstrated but less sensitive than CT angiography
- Renomegaly
- Urolithiasis

Special investigations
- Liver biopsy if no macroscopic shunt identified

Treatment
- Control hepatoencephalopathy medically if ligation not possible or unaffordable
  1 Dietary protein modification
     - Vegetable protein
     - Hydrolysed diet if formulated for growth
     - Mild restriction
  2 Lactulose
  3 Antibacterials
- Interventional radiology to occlude IHPSS with coils
- Surgical ligation (complete/partial/staged)
  - Ameroid constrictor
  - Cellophane banding
  - Silk ligature

Sequelae
- Gradual improvement after immediate post-operative recovery
- Irreversible neurological signs post-surgery or after prolonged hepatic coma
- Secondary acquired shunts if portal hypertension after surgical ligation
- Ultimately, liver failure if not corrected surgically

Prognosis
- Medical management may prolong life for years but requires daily treatment
- Surgical correction offers the best prognosis if the dog survives the peri-operative period as there are significant risks
  - Ascites due to portal hypertension or kinking of portal vein by Ameroid constrictor
  - Bleeding
    - Gastric ulceration
    - Intra-operative

- Intestinal infarction following portovenogram
- Post-op seizures

5.6.5 COPPER-ASSOCIATED CHRONIC HEPATITIS

Aetiology
- Accumulation of copper in the liver is potentially hepatotoxic
- In some breeds the failure to excrete copper is the primary event
- In other breeds copper accumulation is believed to follow chronic cholestasis, and to help perpetuate chronic hepatitis
- Mutation of MURR/COMMD1 gene in Bedlington terrier and suspected mutations in ATP7A and ATP7B in Labrador retriever

Major signs
- Anorexia
- Icterus
- PU/PD
- Weight loss

Minor signs
- Acute haemolytic crisis is rare

Predisposition
- Increasing incidence with age due to progressive copper accumulation
- Primary copper accumulation in Bedlington terrier and Labrador retriever
- Probably secondary to cholestasis in Dobermann and WHWT

Potential sequelae
- CH/cirrhosis
- Death

Historical clues
- Episodes of vague illness before presentation in acute crisis
- May be asymptomatic and be detected on routine blood testing

Physical examination
- Asymptomatic or signs of CH

Laboratory findings
- As for chronic hepatitis
- There are no characteristic changes in blood copper or caeruloplasmin concentrations

Imaging
- As for chronic hepatitis

Special investigations
- DNA test for MURR/COMMD1 mutation
- Liver biopsy
  - Histopathology
  - Quantitative copper analysis
  - Staining for copper with rhodanine or rubeanic acid

Treatment
- As for chronic hepatitis
- Decoppering
  - Low-copper/high-zinc diet
  - Oral zinc acetate or gluconate
  - D-penicillamine or 2,2,2-tetramine (Trientine)

5.6.6 EXTRA-HEPATIC BILE DUCT OBSTRUCTION (EHBDO)

Aetiology
- Obstruction of the extra-hepatic biliary tree results in post-hepatic jaundice
- Rupture of GB or cystic or common bile ducts also causes post-hepatic jaundice with bile peritonitis developing gradually over 1–2 weeks

Common causes
- Acute pancreatitis
- Cholelithiasis
- GB mucocoele, *q.v.* section 5.6.7
- Traumatic rupture of gall bladder or cystic or common bile duct by road traffic accident

Uncommon causes
- Aberrant *Toxocara* migration
- Bile duct carcinoma
- Chronic fibrosing pancreatitis
- Liver fluke (not in UK)
- Pancreatic carcinoma

- Perforation of duodenum near major papilla, e.g. NSAIDs or foreign body
- Obstruction of duodenal papilla by foreign body

Major signs
- Jaundice
- Vomiting
- Ascites develops gradually if ruptured biliary tree

Minor signs
- Anorexia
- Weight loss

Sequelae
- Death if untreated

Predisposition
- Pancreatitis: obese, sedentary, middle-aged bitches
- Pancreatic carcinoma in old dogs

Historical clues
- History of trauma for ruptured biliary tree

Physical examination
- Ascites
- Hepatomegaly
- Icterus
- Palpable pancreatic mass

Laboratory findings
- Hyperbilirubinaemia
- Increased ALP and GGT activities >> ALT and AST activity increases
- Hypercholesterolaemia

Imaging
Radiograph
- Cranial abdominal mass
- Loss of peritoneal detail
- Radiodense choleliths

Ultrasound
- Dilated GB and common bile duct
- Choleliths
- Free fluid if bile peritonitis
- Free abdominal fluid

Special investigations
- Abdominocentesis: bile-stained fluid if bile peritonitis
- Exploratory laparotomy

Treatment
- Surgery: repair, cholecystectomy, cholecystoduodenostomy
- Euthanasia

Monitor
- Clinical signs
- Bilirubin

Prognosis
- Guarded

5.6.7   GALL BLADDER MUCOCOELE

Aetiology
- Progressive accumulation of tenacious mucin-laden bile in the GB
- May be secondary to underlying condition
  - Endocrinopathy
  - GB dysmotility and/or and cystic hyperplasia
- May extend into the cystic, hepatic, and common bile ducts, resulting in variable degrees of bile duct obstruction
- May lead to cholecystitis and GB rupture

Major signs
Initially, vague episodic signs for months, but can be asymptomatic and an incidental finding
- Anorexia
- Vague abdominal discomfort
- Vomiting
Later as cholecystitis develops
- Abdominal pain
- Jaundice
Dogs progressing to GB rupture
- Jaundice
- Pyrexia
- Tachycardia
- Tachypnoea

Minor signs
- Abdominal distension
- Diarrhoea
- PU/PD

ORGAN SYSTEMS

Predisposition
- Breed associations
  - Border terrier in UK
    - Gluten sensitivity and reduced cholecystokinin release may lead to GB dysmotility
  - Cocker spaniels
  - Miniature schnauzer
  - Shetland sheepdogs in United States
    - Mutation in the ABCB4 (MDR3) phospholipase flippase transporter gene
- Cholecystitis
- Endocrinopathy
  - Diabetes mellitus (DM)
  - Hyperadrenocorticism (HAC)
  - Hyperlipidaemia
  - Hypothyroidism

Historical clues
- Vague history of poor appetite and abdominal discomfort

Physical examination
- Abdominal pain
- Jaundice

Laboratory findings
Haematology
Leukocytosis with a mature neutrophilia and monocytosis and sometimes a left shift

Serum biochemistry
- Hyperbilirubinemia
- Hypercholesterolemia inconsistent
- Increased liver enzyme activities

Imaging
Radiographs
- Hepatomegaly

Ultrasound
- Either a heterogeneous or hyperechoic hepatic parenchyma
- Non-mobile GB contents often with characteristic stellate ('kiwi fruit') appearance (Figure 5.6.1)
- Not always possible to identify GB rupture

Special investigations
- Cholecystocentesis is contra-indicated
- Culture of GB contents after cholecystectomy
- Tissue transglutaminase antibody to test for gluten sensitivity

Treatment
- Conservative management (analgesia, antibacterials, UDCA) if asymptomatic
  - Controversial as the mucocoele can resolve but risk of GB rupture

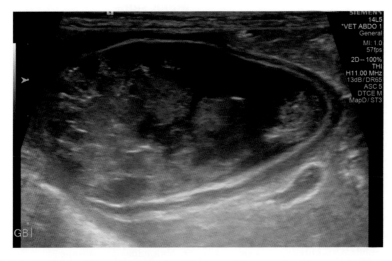

Figure 5.6.1 Gall bladder mucocoele. Ultrasound image of a GB mucocoele with the characteristic stellate ('kiwi fruit') appearance.

ORGAN SYSTEMS

- Cholecystectomy with antibacterial cover modified as needed after culture and sensitivity
  - Significant morbidity and mortality if GB already ruptured

Prevention of recurrence
- Mucoid bile could still cause an EHBDO after cholecystectomy
- Avoid high-fat diets
- Continue UDCA life-long
- Gluten-free diet in Border terriers
- Treat any underlying endocrinopathy

Monitoring
- Abdominal discomfort
- Temperature
- Ultrasound of liver and evidence of free fluid

Prognosis
- Guarded, as GB can be adherent to the liver, causing bleeding when resected
- Poor if GB already ruptured

5.6.8 HEPATIC NEOPLASIA

Aetiology
- Primary neoplasia of the liver is uncommon, but because of its highly vascular nature, it is a common site of metastatic disease and the third most common site of origin for haemangiosarcoma.
- Hepatic tumours may be:
  - Primary
    - Hepatoma
    - Hepatocellular carcinoma
    - Biliary carcinoma
  - Infiltrative
    - Histiocytic
    - Lymphoma
    - Mast cell
  - Secondary
    - Vascular
      - Haemangiosarcoma
    - Metastatic
      - Carcinoma of pancreas, ovary, prostate, intestine, and insulinoma, seminoma, or osteosarcoma

Major signs
- Non-specific signs of liver dysfunction
- Hepatomegaly
- Intra-abdominal haemorrhage in haemangiosarcoma
- Signs of primary organ if metastatic disease

Minor signs
- Anorexia
- Weight loss

Predisposition
- Older dogs

Historical clues
- Often asymptomatic until advanced disease

Physical examination
- Hepatomegaly
- Primary tumour may be palpable

Clinicopathological findings
Haematology
- Anaemia of chronic disease or haemorrhage

Serum biochemistry
- Increased liver enzyme activities
  - Hepatocellular carcinoma: ALT
  - Biliary carcinoma: ALP
- Liver function tests often normal as not all liver affected

Imaging
Radiography
- Hepatomegaly
- Irregular outline/masses
- Chest radiographs for metastatic disease

Ultrasound
- Nodules/masses of altered echogenicity

Special investigations
- FNA
- Liver biopsy

Treatment
- Combination chemotherapy for lymphoma
- Surgical lobectomy if tumour localised
- Euthanasia

Monitoring
- Liver size and function

Prognosis
- Usually poor unless complete resection possible

5.6.9   INFECTIOUS CANINE HEPATITIS

Aetiology
- Infectious canine hepatitis (ICH) caused by canine adenovirus 1 (CAV1) infection
- Rare in the UK because of vaccination

Differential diagnoses
- Bacterial cholangitis, *q.v.* section 5.6.2
- Canine herpes virus infection: only causes hepatitis as a perinatal infection, *q.v.* section 1.35
- Leptospirosis, *q.v.* section 5.11.9

Major signs
- Anorexia
- Cranial abdominal discomfort
- Lethargy
- Pyrexia

Minor signs
- Anorexia
- Conjunctivitis
- Jaundice not common
- Vomiting and diarrhoea

Potential sequelae
- Recovery
- Corneal oedema ('blue eye') due to immune complex deposition
- Chronic hepatitis
- Death

Predisposition
- Young unvaccinated dogs

Historical clues
- Failure to vaccinate

Physical examination
- Cranial abdominal discomfort
- Enlarged tonsils
- Icterus

- Petechiation
- Pyrexia
- Tachycardia

Laboratory findings
Haematology
- Inflammatory leukogram
- Leukopenia

Serum biochemistry
- Increased liver enzyme activities
- Thrombocytopenia

Imaging
- Swollen liver, but may be unhelpful

Special investigations
- Serology or PCR
- Liver FNA or biopsy to show intranuclear inclusions not necessary, but proof on post mortem examination

Treatment
- Supportive care for viral hepatitis
- Prevention with modified live CAV-2 vaccine

Monitoring
- Clinical signs
- Bilirubin
- Liver enzymes

Prognosis
- Guarded, but full recovery possible

5.6.10   NODULAR HYPERPLASIA

Aetiology
- A benign, age-related change in the liver
- Its only significance is that it may misleadingly suggest HAC

Major signs
- Asymptomatic

Minor signs
- Hepatomegaly

Predisposition
- Older dogs > 8 years

Historical clues
• Asymptomatic

Physical examination
• Hepatomegaly if multiple nodules

Clinicopathological findings
• Increased ALP activity
• Other liver enzymes and function tests unremarkable

Imaging
Radiographs
• Hepatomegaly may be noted

Ultrasound
• Nodules may or may not be apparent

Special investigations
• Liver biopsy generally not indicated

Treatment
• None

Monitor
• Not required

Prognosis
• Excellent

5.6.11 PORTAL VEIN HYPOPLASIA (PVH)

Aetiology
• Decreased blood flow to the liver via the portal vein is associated with microvascular dysplasia (MVD)
  • MVD is present in the liver of dogs with a single congenital PSS
  • PVH causing MVD can also occur in the absence of a congenital PSS
• A spectrum of disease, depending on the degree of PVH, is postulated
  • MVD causes no or minimal clinical signs
  • Non-cirrhotic portal hypertension (juvenile hepatic fibrosis) causing hepatic fibrosis and portal hypertension
  • Portal vein atresia is a lethal condition, with death occurring in the perinatal period

5.6.11A MICROVASCULAR DYSPLASIA (MVD)

A congenital vascular anomaly, with intrahepatic, microscopic shunting due to abnormal development of the fine (tertiary) branches of the intrahepatic portal veins. Its main significance is that unexpected bile acid increases necessitate investigation even if the dog is asymptomatic.

Major signs
• Asymptomatic: most often an incidental finding on blood testing
• HE: usually mild or absent
• PU/PD

Minor signs
• Picky appetite

Predisposition
• Bichon Frise, Chihuahua, small terrier breeds especially Yorkshire and Maltese

Historical clues
• None or signs of HE

Physical examination
• Unremarkable unless encephalopathic

Laboratory findings
• Bile acids increased but rarely > 80 µmol/l
• All other parameters unremarkable

Imaging
Radiographs
• Unremarkable

Portovenogram or CT angiography
• No single congenital PSS

Ultrasound
• Unremarkable

Special investigations
• Liver biopsy shows vascular anomaly, but a congenital PSS has to be ruled out by CT angiography before MVD can be diagnosed

Treatment
• May not need treatment
• Management of HE

Monitoring
- Not required

Prognosis
- Excellent

5.6.11B NON-CIRRHOTIC PORTAL HYPERTENSION/JUVENILE HEPATIC FIBROSIS

Aetiology
- Development of hepatic fibrosis in the absence of an inflammatory response seen in young dogs
- Hypothesised to be a severe variant of PVH
- Signs are related to hepatic function impairment and portal hypertension

Major signs
- Abdominal enlargement
- Hepatoencephalopathy
- Late-onset icterus
- Stunting
- Weight loss

Minor signs
- Loss of appetite
- Diarrhoea

Potential sequelae
- Ascites and secondary acquired shunts from portal hypertension
- Death

Predisposition
- Young pure-bred dogs under 1 year of age
- GSD, Rottweiler

Historical clues
- Signs consistent with congenital PSS

Physical examination
- Ascites
- Icterus
- Neurological signs of HE
- Undersized/underweight

Clinicopathological findings
- Abnormal function tests: ammonia, bile acids
- Ascitic fluid is modified transudate
- Hypoalbuminaemia, but insufficient to cause ascites alone suggesting portal hypertension
- Increased liver enzymes
- Microcytic anaemia
- Prolonged PT and PTT

Imaging
- Ascites
- Microhepatica
- Increased echogenicity
- Multiple secondary, acquired PSSs

Special investigations
- Liver biopsy
- Special stain for collagen

Treatment
- Antioxidants
- Diuretics
- Manage HE
- Prednisolone

Monitor
- Clinical signs
- Serum albumin

Prognosis
- Guarded/poor, depending on response to treatment

5.6.12 STEROID HEPATOPATHY

Aetiology
- The canine liver can be exquisitely sensitive to the effects of glucocorticoids, which cause accumulation of glycogen
- However, individual dogs vary in their response to specific dosages, and there is a suggestion that repeated exposure is more likely to cause changes

Causes
- HAC
- Exogenous glucocorticoids: parenteral, oral or topical

Major and minor signs
- The same as for HAC, *q.v.* section 5.3.4A

- The enlargement of the liver and signs of PU/PD may misleadingly suggest a primary hepatopathy

Predisposition
- Same as for HAC
- Dog on chronic steroid therapy, e.g. atopic

Potential sequelae
- Progressive enlargement of liver

Historical clues
- Known administration of steroids

Physical examination
- Hepatomegaly
- Signs of HAC

Clinicopathological findings
- Marked increase in ALP activity >> ALT activity increase
- Mild increase in bile acids (usually < 50 μmol/l)

Imaging
- Hepatomegaly
- Variable, diffuse alteration in echogenicity

Special investigations
- ACTH stimulation test: no stimulation as pituitary-adrenal axis suppressed
- Steroid-induced ALP isoenzyme measurement unreliable

Treatment
- Withdrawal of exogenous steroids, but can take 6–8 weeks to normalise

Monitoring
- ALP activity
- Liver size

Prognosis
- Excellent, completely reversible

5.6.13 VACUOLAR/REACTIVE HEPATOPATHY

Aetiology
- A common histopathological change, reactive to metabolic and systemic diseases

- DM
- Drugs, e.g. phenobarbitone
- Hypothyroidism
- Hypoxia
- Inflammatory disease elsewhere
- Malnutrition
- Over-nutrition

Major and minor signs
- The signs reflect the primary disease

Potential sequelae
- Vacuolar hepatopathy leading to hepatocellular carcinoma in Scottish terriers

Predisposition
- As related to primary disease

Historical clues
- Depends on primary disease

Physical examination
- Depends on primary disease

Laboratory findings
- Changes related to primary disease, e.g. hyperglycaemia and glucosuria in DM
- Secondary increase in liver enzymes
- No or mild changes in liver function tests

Imaging
- Normal or increased liver size
- Diffuse or patchy changes in echogenicity

Special investigations
- Look for underlying disease

Treatment
- Treat primary disease

Monitoring
- Signs of underlying disease

Prognosis
- Good if underlying disease can be treated

ORGAN SYSTEMS

5.7 IMMUNE SYSTEM

The immune system is not confined to a specific organ; immune cells are an integral part of all organs and the circulation. Disorders of the immune system fall into two major categories:
- Immune-mediated
  - Autoimmune
  - Immune-mediated (secondary to a trigger)
- Neoplasia of specific cell lines

Thus the impact of an immune system disorder is far-reaching and the following is not an exhaustive list of conditions. Some disorders are covered in detail elsewhere in this book, e.g. eosinophilic bronchopneumopathy, IMHA, IMTP, immune-mediated neutropenia, leukaemia, glomerulonephritis, meningoencephalitis of unknown origin (MUO) and steroid-responsive meningitis-arteritis (SRMA) (*q.v.* sections 5.4, 5.8, 5.10 and 5.12). Immunological processes may also be involved in a number of chronic diseases, e.g. chronic hepatitis, chronic inflammatory enteropathy (inflammatory bowel disease), hypoadrenocorticism and hypothyroidism.

The following immune-mediated skin disorders are listed as differentials (*q.v.* section 2.26) but are not covered in detail as they fall outside the scope of internal medicine, and the reader is advised to consult dermatological textbooks.
- Dermatomyositis
- Erythema multiforme
- Exfoliative cutaneous lupus erythematosus
- Juvenile cellulitis
- Lupoid onychodystrophy
- Pemphigus complex
- Sebaceous adenitis

Problems
Presenting complaints
q.v. section 1
1.8 Ataxia
1.9 Bleeding
1.10 Blindness
1.11 Constipation
1.13 Coughing
1.15 Diarrhoea
1.17 Dysphagia
1.31 Melaena
1.37 Polyuria/polydipsia (PU/PD)
1.44 Stiffness, joint swelling and generalised lameness
1.49 Vomiting
1.53 Weight loss

Physical abnormalities
q.v. section 2
2.1 Abdominal enlargement
2.2 Abdominal masses
2.3 Abnormal lung sounds
2.5 Ascites
2.9 Horner's syndrome
2.13 Icterus/jaundice
2.14 Lymphadenopathy
2.17 Pain
2.20 Peripheral oedema
2.25 Pyrexia and hyperthermia

Laboratory abnormalities
q.v. section 3
3.7.1 Hypercalcaemia
3.14 C-reactive protein
3.27.1B Hyperglobulinaemia
3.30.1 Anaemia
3.31.1 Thrombocytopenia
3.32.1 Leukocytosis
3.32.2 Leukopenia
3.33 Pancytopenia

Diagnostic approach
- Suspect immune system disorder from problem list
- Screening by routine laboratory testing
- Perform specific tests, in particular biopsy for cytology, histopathology and immunohistochemistry

Diagnostic methods
History
- Onset of clinical signs and progression
  - Gradual-onset progressive signs may increase suspicion of neoplastic disorder

ORGAN SYSTEMS

- Presence of previous episodes may increase suspicion of immune-mediated disorder (often waxing and waning) or recurrent opportunistic infections due to immunodeficiency
- Response to previous treatment, in particular antimicrobial therapy or corticosteroids

Physical examination
- Thorough clinical examination with particular attention to lymphoid organs: lymph nodes, spleen, and liver

Laboratory findings
Haematology
- RBCs
  - Anaemia of chronic disease
  - Non-regenerative anaemia due to bone marrow involvement
- Platelets
  - Thrombocytopenia
- WBCs
  - Leukocytosis
  - Leukopenia
  - Mastocytosis

Biochemistry
- Changes dependent on organ systems affected, e.g. infiltrative disorders affecting liver
- Hypercalcaemia in lymphoma and multiple myeloma

Urinalysis
- For urine protein:creatinine (UPC) ratio and specific disorders
- Bence-Jones proteins in cases of suspected multiple myeloma

Imaging
Plain radiographs
- Intra-thoracic or intra-abdominal lymphadenomegaly or organ enlargement
- Bone lucency or destructive lesions: multiple myeloma, hypertrophic osteopathy
- Soft tissue swelling and periarticular erosive lesions: IMPA

Ultrasound
- Intra-thoracic or intra-abdominal lymphadenomegaly, lymphadenopathy or organ enlargement

Special investigative techniques
- Biopsy for cytology and histopathology
- Infectious disease screening: serology, PCR, culture, FISH
- Serum protein electrophoresis
- Immunocytochemistry and immunohistochemistry
- Flow cytometry
- PCR for antigen receptor gene rearrangements (PARR)

5.7.1 (AUTO)IMMUNE-MEDIATED DISORDERS

Either true autoimmune conditions, or immune-mediated disorders triggered by drugs, infection, neoplasia, or perhaps vaccination.

5.7.1.1 IMMUNE-MEDIATED POLYARTHRITIS (IMPA)

Aetiology
IMPA is thought to be caused by a Type III hypersensitivity reaction. The deposition of these immune complexes in the joint space results in recruitment of leukocytes and cytokines. The presence of this inflammatory response results in the clinical signs observed.

IMPA may occur secondary to a trigger (vaccination, drug, infectious disease, GI disease, or neoplasia), or, in some cases, may be primary, i.e. no trigger detected on screening.

Major signs
- Shifting lameness
- Pain: generalised, joint, back
- Joint effusions
- Pyrexia

Minor signs
- Lethargy
- Inappetence
- Spontaneous vocalisation

Potential sequelae
- Erosive joint disease
- Ligament laxity

Predisposition
- Young to middle-aged dogs appear to be predisposed to idiopathic IMPA

Historical clues
- In some cases clinical signs of joint pain may be subtle. Questions to detect changes in ambulation can be useful, e.g. willingness to walk up and down stairs or to jump up or down from furniture or car
- In some cases systemic signs, e.g. lethargy, inappetence, may not be reported

Physical examination
- Careful examination may be required to detect joint effusions and pain
- IMPA tends to have a predilection for distal joints; therefore, manipulation of digits can be useful
- May detect lymphadenopathy
- In some cases systemic signs, e.g. pyrexia, may not be detected

Laboratory findings
Haematology
- Neutrophilia

Serum biochemistry
- Acute phase protein response
  - Hypoalbuminaemia/hyperglobulinaemia
  - Increased C-reactive protein (CRP) is evidence of systemic inflammation

Urinalysis
- Proteinuria may be present; increased UPC ratio

Imaging
Plain radiographs
- Erosive changes in affected joints (rare)
- Periarticular soft tissue swelling and periosteal new bone
- May detect a trigger for IMPA in secondary disease (i.e. infection, neoplasia) on thoracic and abdominal imaging

Ultrasound
- May detect a trigger for IMPA in secondary disease, i.e. infection, neoplasia, changes in GI wall layering for enteropathy

Special investigations
- Arthrocentesis for joint fluid cytology, proteins ± culture
- Troponin and/or echocardiogram to screen for vegetative valve lesions in cases with a suspicion of endocarditis (novel heart murmur, arrhythmia)
- Infectious disease screening depending on tick exposure and travel history (*Anaplasma*, *Borrelia*, *Ehrlichia*, *Leishmania*)
- Blood cultures in dogs with a suspicion of haematogenous infection, e.g. endocarditis
- Rheumatoid factor may be performed in dogs with erosive joint disease as one criterion for diagnosis of rheumatoid arthritis

Treatment
- Where a trigger is detected, treatment initially aimed at resolution of this, e.g. antimicrobial therapy for endocarditis
- In cases where no trigger is found, immunosuppressive therapy is advised; drugs typically used include:
  1 Prednisolone
  2 Ciclosporin
  3 Leflunomide, azathioprine, and mycophenolate mofetil

Monitoring
- Remission assessed by:
  - Clinical response
  - CRP
  - Repeated arthrocentesis for joint cytology

Prognosis
Prognosis in primary IMPA is mixed
- 50–60% achieve remission following immunosuppression which persists following tapering
- ~25% require long-term immunosuppression or experience relapse either during tapering of immunosuppression or later
- ~ 15% appear refractory to therapy

5.7.1.2 IMMUNODEFICIENCY

Aetiology
Immunodeficiencies are rare and are most frequently breed-related disorders. Clinical signs

are most often apparent in young animals presenting with opportunistic infection; this typically occurs after maternally derived antibodies wane (8–16 weeks), although in some cases clinical signs may present later in life.

Primary immunodeficiencies are poorly documented in dogs; immunoglobulin deficiencies are rare, and defects in cell-mediated immunity are poorly characterised. Defects in neutrophil and macrophage killing activities are also poorly documented but are thought to be predisposing factors in, for example, granulomatous colitis of Boxers.

5.7.1.2A CANINE LEUKOCYTE ADHESION DEFICIENCY (CLAD)

Canine leukocyte adhesion deficiency (CLAD) is a fatal immunodeficiency disease found in Irish setters and Irish Red and White setters. The condition is caused by a mutation in a gene encoding a leukocyte surface molecule, leading to a dysfunction of the granulocytes.

- Affected dogs show severe infections including omphalophlebitis, skin infections, osteomyelitis and gingivitis from an early age, and die early in life from multiple severe infections, even if treated with antibiotics.
- There is a DNA test for the condition. In the UK, all Kennel Club registered setters are tested 'clear' or are 'hereditarily clear' of the CLAD gene. However, CLAD carriers are found in other countries and should be tested before breeding.

5.7.1.2B CYCLIC HAEMATOPOIESIS (CYCLIC NEUTROPENIA)

Aetiology
- Inherited disease that cyclically affects bone marrow cell production. As neutrophils have the shortest half-life, the 14- to 21-day cycle affects this cell line preferentially.

Major signs
- Failure to thrive
- Opportunistic infections due to neutropenia with pyrexia
- Shifting lameness with joint swelling

Minor signs
- Acute pyrexia following vaccination
- Intermittent gastrointestinal signs

Predisposition
- Grey or merle border collies

Historical clues
- Recurrent opportunistic infections

Physical examination
- Bilateral keratitis
- Gingival ulceration
- Poor body condition score, small stature

Laboratory findings
- Neutropenia: occurs on a 10- to 14- (up to 21-) day cycle with 4–5 days of neutropenia and resultant illness
- Increased ALP enzyme activity: may be related to age of dog diagnosed, or increased bone turnover
- Neutrophilic joint inflammation on arthrocentesis
- Proteinuria due to amyloidosis

Imaging
- May detect evidence of opportunistic infection
- Osteomyelitis especially at the metaphysis

Special investigations
- Genetic test

Treatment
- Most dogs respond temporarily to antibiotic therapy
- G-CSF and gene therapy has been described

Prognosis
- Long-term prognosis is guarded, with most dogs succumbing to recurrent infections

5.7.1.2C HEREDITARY SELECTIVE COBALAMIN MALABSORPTION (IMERSLUND-GRÄSBECK SYNDROME)

q.v section 3.10

Major signs
- Inappetence
- Intermittent diarrhoea
- Failure to thrive

Minor signs
- Impaired swallowing
- Mucosal ulceration
- Opportunistic infections, e.g. hepatic or pulmonary fungal infection, due to neutropenia

Predisposition
- Known mutations in Australian shepherd, Beagle, Border collie, Giant schnauzer and Komondor but also reported in a Yorkshire terrier and mixed breeds
- Cobalamin deficiency in Shar pei associated with GI disease

Historical clues
- Intermittent GI signs in a small-stature dog of relevant breed
- Recurrent opportunistic infection, in particular fungal

Physical examination
- Bradyarrhythmia
- Forebrain signs on neurological examination
- Poor body condition score
- Small stature

Laboratory findings
Haematology
- Neutropenia

Biochemistry
- Undetectable serum cobalamin
- Increased ammonia
- Hypoglycaemia
- Mild increase in AST activity
- Metabolic acidosis
- Mild proteinuria

Imaging
Evidence of opportunistic infection

Special investigations
- Breed-specific genetic tests
- Increased urine or blood methylmalonic acid and homocysteine

Treatment
Oral or injectable cobalamin supplementation

Monitoring
- Serum cobalamin
- ± Repeat methylmalonic acid

Prognosis
- Poor in untreated dogs
- Good in those identified prior to severe infection where cobalamin supplementation is provided

5.7.1.2D IMMUNOGLOBULIN DEFICIENCY

The absence of one or more immunoglobulin classes.

Major signs
- Opportunistic infection, in particular dermatological and respiratory infections (cough, exercise intolerance, dyspnoea, cyanosis)

Minor signs
- Pyrexia is uncommon

Predisposition
- Mucosal IgA deficiency has been suspected in GSDs with CIE but not proven
- CKCS and Dachshunds are thought to be predisposed to *Pneumocystis carinii* respiratory infections due to an immunoglobulin deficiency
- Beagle, Shar pei and Weimaraner have been documented to have immunoglobulin deficiencies and recurrent skin infections

Historical clues
- Affected littermates

Physical examination

- Abnormal thoracic auscultation
- Concurrent skin disease, e.g. demodecosis

Laboratory findings

- Neutrophilia, monocytosis

Imaging

- In CKCS with *Pneumocystis carinii* infection there may be a hazy interstitial lung pattern ± pneumothorax or pneumomediastinum

Special investigations

- Serum immunoglobulin quantitation, but there are no established reference intervals in dogs younger than 12 months of age
- Bronchoalveolar lavage and lung fine needle aspiration (FNA) for *Pneumocystis carinii*: lung FNA appears to be superior
- Special stains for *Pneumocystis carinii* (e.g. Grocott-Gomori methanemine silver, PAS) and PCR

Treatment

- Antimicrobial
  - Trimethoprim sulphonamides for *Pneumocystis carinii*
- ± Corticosteroids

Prognosis

Reasonable with early treatment, may need repeated courses of antimicrobial therapy

5.7.1.2E   TRAPPED NEUTROPHIL SYNDROME

Aetiology

Functional impairment of release of neutrophils from the bone marrow.

Major signs

- Failure to thrive
- Opportunistic infections due to neutropenia with pyrexia
- Shifting lameness with joint swelling

Minor signs

- Acute pyrexia following vaccination
- Intermittent GI signs

Predisposition

- Border collies

Historical clues

- Recurrent opportunistic infections
  - Physical examination
- Abnormal craniofacial development ('ferret face')
- Poor body condition score, small stature

Laboratory findings

- Neutropenia
- Increased ALP activity: may be related to age of dogs diagnosed, or increased bone turnover
- Hypercholesterolaemia
- Neutrophilic joint inflammation on arthrocentesis

Imaging

- May detect evidence of opportunistic infection
- Osteomyelitis especially at the metaphysis

Special investigations

- Bone marrow aspiration compatible with myeloid hyperplasia
- Genetic test

Treatment

- Most dogs respond temporarily to antibiotic and glucocorticoid therapy

Prognosis

- Long-term prognosis is guarded, with most dogs succumbing to recurrent infections

5.7.1.3   LYMPHADENITIS

Aetiology

Lymphadenitis is defined as the infiltration of lymph nodes by one or more non-lymphoid inflammatory cells.

- The following cut-offs are described based on proportion of the cellular population of the lymph node:
  - Neutrophilic lymphadenitis: > 5% neutrophils

- Granulomatous lymphadenitis: > 2% macrophages
- Pyogranulomatous: mixed neutrophilic and macrophagic infiltration

Major signs
- Lymphadenopathy
- Pyrexia

Minor signs
- Lethargy and inappetence
- Signs of concurrent systemic disease may be detected
  - Cough
  - Dermatopathy (skin or facial swelling, ulceration)
  - Epistaxis, sneezing, nasal discharge
  - Ophthalmologic disease
  - Shifting lameness
  - Vomiting and/or diarrhea

Potential sequelae
- Dogs may develop hypercalcaemia due to activated macrophages and increased serum vitamin D, and resultant polyuria and polydipsia

Predisposition
- English Springer spaniels are thought to be predisposed to sterile steroid-responsive lymphadenitis
- Juvenile cellulitis occurs in young dogs

Historical clues
- A diagnosis of sterile steroid-responsive lymphadenitis is achieved through exclusion of infectious causes
  - History should focus on establishing risk of infectious disease, e.g. travel history, tick exposure

Physical examination
- Evidence of concurrent systemic involvement, e.g. dermatological changes
- Lymphadenopathy
  - Lymphadenopathy in some cases is restricted to intrathoracic or intrabdominal lymph nodes and may not be appreciable on clinical examination
- Pyrexia

Laboratory findings
Haematology
- Inflammatory leukogram may be present: neutrophilia and monocytosis, lymphopenia and eosinopenia
- Mild non-regenerative anaemia of chronic disease

Biochemistry
- Acute-phase response: hypoalbuminaemia and hyperglobulinaemia
- Increased ALP activity
- Increased CRP
- Hypercalcaemia (uncommon)

Imaging
Plain radiographs
- Evidence of intrathoracic lymphadenopathy
- Screening for triggers (infectious, neoplastic)

Ultrasound
- Evidence of intrabdominal lymphadenopathy
- Screening for triggers (infectious, neoplastic)

Special investigations
- Infectious disease screening depending on risk factors
  - *Anaplasma*
  - *Bartonella*
  - *Borrelia*
  - *Ehrlichia*
  - Fungal disease, e.g. *Aspergillus*
  - *Leishmania*
  - *Mycobacterium*
  - *Toxoplasma*

Treatment
- Where a trigger is identified, treatment should be directed at this
- Prednisolone (0.5–2 mg/kg per day), with tapering typically performed over 3–6 months

Monitoring
- Reassess lymphadenopathy, repeat sampling if concerned over relapse

ORGAN SYSTEMS

Prognosis
- Where no trigger identified
  - Typically respond positively to immuno-suppressive therapy
  - Some may require adjunctive therapy
  - Relapse is not uncommon

5.7.1.4 SYSTEMIC LUPUS ERYTHEMATOSUS (SLE)

Aetiology

Production of excessive immune complexes overwhelms the monocytic clearance system, resulting in deposition of these complexes in the joints, glomerulus, skin, and blood vessels resulting in a Type III hypersensitivity reaction and resultant tissue inflammation affecting multiple organ systems.
- SLE is diagnosed when there are two major signs with positive ANA or one major sign and two minor signs with positive ANA
- SLE is suspected when there is one major sign with positive ANA or two major signs with negative ANA

Major signs
- Skin lesions with biopsy findings consistent with SLE
- Non-erosive immune-mediated polyarthritis
- Glomerulonephritis
- Polymyositis
- Leukopenia
- Thrombocytopenia

Minor signs
- Neurologic disorders, in the absence of a known cause
- Oral ulceration
- Immune-mediated haemolytic anaemia
- Serositis (i.e. inflammation of any serous membrane – e.g. pericarditis, pleuritis)

SLE is rarely diagnosed in dogs; treatment is based on immunosuppressive therapy.

5.7.2 NEOPLASIA OF IMMUNE CELLS

5.7.2.1 LYMPHOMA

Aetiology
- Spontaneous neoplasm of a single lympho-cyte clone (B or T cells), resulting in abnormal lymphoid cells
- Typically intermediate- or large-cell
- Small-cell lymphoma is also recognised, with a more indolent clinical course and improved prognosis, but is rare in dogs
- Lymphoma may be confined to:
  - Lymph nodes
  - Solid organs
    - CNS
    - GI tract
    - Kidneys
    - Liver
    - Lungs
    - Skin (epitheliotropic)
    - Spleen
- Multicentric lymphoma involves more than one site, and is staged:
  - Stage 1 – limited to single lymph node or lymphoid tissue of single organ
  - Stage 2 – two or more lymph nodes in same region
  - Stage 3 – multiple lymph nodes (generalised)
  - Stage 4 – involvement of liver and/or spleen
  - Stage 5 – any of the above and including bone marrow and blood or non-lymphoid solid organ
  - Subclassify each stage as (a) without systemic signs or (b) with systemic signs
- For lymphoid and myeloid leukaemias, *q.v.* sections 5.4.4, 5.4.5

Major signs
- Lymphadenomegaly may result in functional changes, e.g. dyspnoea
  - Pleural effusion
  - Respiratory obstruction
  - Caval syndrome, causing facial swelling in mediastinal lymphadenomegaly and vena cava compression

- May present with no clinical signs aside from lymphadenomegaly
- In solid organ disease, signs may reflect organ involved, e.g. neurological signs
- PU/PD may be present due to paraneoplastic hypercalcaemia
- Secondary immune-mediated disease may be triggered on rare occasions
  - IMHA and/or IMTP
  - IMPA
  - Myasthenia gravis
  - Polyneuropathy
- Signs related to pancytopenia in cases with bone marrow involvement
  - Bleeding diathesis due to thrombocytopenia
  - Lethargy and exercise intolerance due to anaemia
  - Opportunistic infection due to neutropenia

Minor signs
- Anorexia/inappetence
- Lethargy
- Weight loss

Potential sequelae
- Acute kidney injury due to hypercalcaemia
- Haemorrhage due to thrombocytopenia
- Respiratory obstruction
- Death

Predisposition
Boxer, Bernese Mountain dog, Bullmastiff, Dobermann, Golden retriever and Rottweiler

Historical clues
- May be gradual- or acute-onset lymphadenomegaly
- Clinical signs pertaining to the organ involved
- Transient response to prednisolone

Physical examination
- Lymphadenopathy
- Hepatosplenomegaly
- Pallor if anaemic

Laboratory findings
Haematology
- Anaemia
- Neutropenia ± thrombocytopenia

- Leukocytosis
- Circulating atypical cells may be detected (rare)

Serum biochemistry
- Acute-phase protein response (hypoalbuminaemia, hyperglobulinaemia)
- Azotaemia
- Changes may reflect organ involvement (e.g. hypoproteinaemia in gastrointestinal lymphoma, increased liver enzyme activities in hepatic lymphoma, etc.)
- Hypercalcaemia (T-cell lymphoma)

Imaging
Plain radiographs
- Enlargement of lymph nodes
  - Mediastinal mass
  - Bronchial, sternal, mesenteric, sublumbar
- Hepatosplenomegaly
- Lung infiltrate (most commonly interstitial or alveolar, although can be any)

Ultrasound
- Enlargement or abnormal echotexture of lymph nodes
- Hepatosplenomegaly
- Loss of GI wall layering, or thickened mucosal layer
- Renomegaly

Special investigations
- Lymph node FNA for cytology
- Less commonly, lymph node biopsy required for diagnosis most often required in small-cell lymphoma where cells have normal gross morphology
- Bone marrow aspirate
- Immunophenotyping
  - Immunohistochemistry
  - Flow cytometry
  - PCR for antigen receptor rearrangements (PARR)
- Serum PTHrp in cases investigating hypercalcaemia

ORGAN SYSTEMS

Treatment

- Chemotherapy protocol dependent on lymphoma location, phenotype, and response to previous therapy
  - Examples of protocols:
    - Cyclophosphamide, vincristine, prednisolone (COP)
    - Cyclophosphamide, doxorubicin, vincristine, prednisolone (CHOP)
    - Lomustine, vincristine, procarbazine, prednisolone (LOPP)
  - Normally administered as an intensive induction phase with discontinuation or less intense maintenance phase, with rescue therapy on relapse
- Prednisolone will result in a transient improvement in some dogs; sole therapy may increase likelihood of resistance to chemotherapy if selected in the future
- Readers are advised to consult oncology texts for further guidance on safe administration of combination chemotherapy protocols

Monitoring

- Haematology
- Lymph node size
- Canine lymphoma blood test: scoring system including CRP and haptoglobin
- Thymidine kinase activity

Prognosis

- Grave with no treatment (weeks)
- Improved with small-cell (indolent) lymphoma
- Chemotherapy will achieve remission for a period in 80–90% of dogs, with prognosis depending on stage and solid organ involvement (median 6–14 months)
- Prognosis poorer with:
  - Anaemia
  - Hypercalcaemia
  - Increasing stage, especially stage V
  - Substage b
  - T-cell phenotype
  - Young dogs

5.7.2.2 MAST CELL TUMOUR (MCT)

Aetiology

- Neoplastic proliferation of mast cells
- Mast cells arise as progenitors from the bone marrow, and under the influence of cytokines within the tissues differentiate to mast cells; they are uncommonly detected in the circulation
- Mast cells contain cytoplasmic granules containing heparin, histamine and proteases which, when released, may have local or systemic effects

Major signs

- Mass lesion
  - Most commonly dermal, less commonly subcutaneous when it can be mistaken for a lipoma
  - Well differentiated: slow-growing solitary hairless lesions
    or
  - Poorly differentiated: rapidly growing, ulcerated
  - Multiple primary or satellite lesions in some cases
- Less commonly can have splenic, hepatic, intestinal, or mediastinal MCT with associated signs pertinent to the organ involved

Minor signs

- Local bleeding
- Erythema
- Pruritus
- Scaling

Potential sequelae

- Acute anaphylaxis (especially in dogs with high tumour burden)
- Gastric ulcer: abdominal pain, anorexia, haematochezia and melaena
- Iron deficiency anaemia
- GI perforation
- Tumour recurrence after surgical removal
- Lymph node ± systemic metastasis

Predisposition
- Usually older dogs
- Typically low- or intermediate-grade: Boxer and Pug
- Typically high-grade and/or multiple: Boston terrier, Pit bull terriers and Shar pei:
  - Shar pei typically younger with a poor prognosis due to aggressive disease

Historical clues
- Skin mass, may be pruritic
- Paraneoplastic signs

Physical examination
- Dermal or subcutaneous skin mass ± ulceration ± hairless skin
- Local lymphadenomegaly
- Rarely, manipulation may produce mast cell degranulation, resulting in erythema and wheal (Darier's sign)

Laboratory findings
- Usually unremarkable

Haematology
- Regenerative anaemia if severe GI bleeding
- Occasionally eosinophilia
- Rarely circulating mast cells

Serum biochemistry
- Hypoproteinaemia and increased urea if GI bleeding

Imaging
Plain radiographs
- In dogs with nodal metastasis, full staging includes thoracic and abdominal imaging, although thoracic metastasis is rare

Ultrasound
- In dogs with nodal metastasis, full staging includes abdominal imaging and splenic and liver fine needle aspirates (FNAs) regardless of appearance

Special investigations
- FNA for cytology of mass
- FNA for cytology of local lymph nodes ± liver and spleen
- Incisional if cytology non-diagnostic
- Excisional biopsy if cytology non-diagnostic, or therapeutic
- Additional markers may be helpful in exploring the clinical behaviour of the MCT, but must be interpreted in combination with the overall clinical picture
  - Argyrophilic nucleolar organiser regions (AgNORs)
  - c-KIT mutation
  - Mitotic index
  - Proliferating cell nuclear antigen (PCNA)

Treatment
- Surgical excision with adequate margins where possible
- Radiotherapy of mass on distal limb may be considered where complete surgical excision is not possible
- Chemotherapy
  - May be used in three settings:
    - Prior to surgery to aid achievement of margins
    - To treat residual microscopic disease where further surgery is not possible
    - To address systemic disease in metastatic mast cell tumour, in particular high-grade
  - Most commonly prednisolone and vinblastine or lomustine
- Tyrosine kinase inhibitors (masitinib, toceranib) are not considered first-line treatment but appear to be beneficial in scenarios where surgical excision is not possible with the aim of achieving stable disease
- Tigilanol tiglate to be administered by injection directly into the mass can be considered in non-resectable, non-metastatic, subcutaneous MCTs located at or distal to the elbow or hock and non-resectable, non-metastatic, cutaneous MCTs less than 8 cm^3

Monitoring
- Haematology and biochemistry for dogs on chemotherapy and tyrosine kinase inhibitors
- Urinalysis also in dogs on tyrosine kinase inhibitors to monitor for proteinuria

Prognosis
- Clinical progression and behaviour of MCTs is highly variable

- High-grade disease prognosis is guarded, with median survival times of 4 months
- Surgical excision may be curative, especially with low-/intermediate-grade

5.7.2.3 MULTIPLE MYELOMA

Aetiology
- Spontaneous neoplasm of plasma cells within the bone marrow
- Isolated extramedullary plasmacytomas occur rarely, most commonly in the skin, stomach and large intestine

Major signs
- Bleeding diatheses, e.g. hyphaema, haematuria
- Shifting lameness

Minor signs
- Anorexia
- Lethargy
- Pain
- Pyrexia

Potential sequelae
- Immunoparesis may result in opportunistic infection
- Pathological fractures due to osteolysis

Predisposition
- Older dogs

Historical clues
- History should focus on establishing risk of infectious disease (e.g. travel history, tick exposure) as it is an important differential diagnosis for hyperglobulinaemia

Physical examination
- Splenomegaly may be present
- Bone pain, e.g. back pain
- Pyrexia
- Ophthalmic examination for evidence of hyperviscosity: retinal haemorrhage, tortuous retinal vessels

Laboratory findings
Haematology
- Non-regenerative anaemia

- Leukopenia
- Thrombocytopenia
- Pancytopenia

Biochemistry
- Hyperglobulinaemia
- Hypercalcaemia

Imaging
Plain radiographs
Osteolytic bone lesions

Ultrasound
Hepatosplenomegaly may be present

Special investigations
- Infectious disease screening depending on risk factors
  - *Ehrlichia*
  - *Leishmania*
- Diagnosis is achieved when three of the four following criteria are met:
  - Bence-Jones proteinuria
  - Hyperglobulinaemia with monoclonal gammopathy on serum protein electrophoresis
  - Multiple osteolytic bone lesions
  - Bone marrow biopsy with increased plasma cells, i.e. > 5%

Treatment
Melphalan and prednisolone

Monitoring
- Clinical signs
- Hyperglobulinaemia

Prognosis
Treatment can control signs, although cure is rare; median survival is 220–930 days with treatment

5.7.2.4 THYMOMA

Aetiology
- Spontaneous neoplasm of thymic epithelial cells that is usually slow-growing and does not spread.
- Aggressive and metastatic thymic carcinomas are exceptionally rare.

Major signs
- Tachypnoea, cough, dyspnoea due to mass effect
- Myasthenia gravis
  - Focal: regurgitation due to megaoesophagus
  - Generalised: regurgitation and exercise-induced collapse due to fatigue of muscles after stimulation

Minor signs
- Anorexia
- Facial oedema due to caval syndrome
- Laryngeal paralysis
- Lethargy

Potential sequelae
- Aspiration pneumonia due to megaoesophagus
- Fulminant respiratory failure due to generalised myasthenia gravis
- Paraneoplastic conditions, e.g. hypercalcaemia, myasthenia gravis

Predisposition
- Older dogs

Historical clues
- Generalised myasthenia gravis can sometimes present as a short choppy gait rather than exercise-induced fatigue of muscles

Physical examination
- Assessment for evidence of aspiration pneumonia
- Neurological examination to assess for evidence of myasthenia gravis
  - Fatiguability of blink reflex can be useful

Laboratory findings
Haematology
- Thymoma-associated lymphocytosis (rare)

Biochemistry
- Hypercalcaemia (rare)

Imaging
Plain radiographs
- Cranial mediastinal mass
- Megaoesophagus in conscious dog
- Metastasis rare

Ultrasound
- Thoracic ultrasound may detect a mediastinal mass
- Metastasis rare

Special investigations
- Nicotinic acetylcholine receptor (AChR) antibody test for acquired myasthenia gravis
  - Can have false negative results, especially with focal disease or early in the clinical course
- CT scan for surgical planning and metastasis screen
- Cytology: differentiation between lymphoma and thymoma from cytology alone may be challenging
- Incisional biopsy or surgical resection and histopathology

Treatment
- Anticholinesterase treatment for myasthenia gravis
- Surgical resection where appropriate
- Radiation therapy is described in non-surgical cases

Monitoring
Repeat AChR antibody test post-operatively to assess for remission of myasthenia gravis

Prognosis
- Surgical resection in dogs without evidence of metastasis is associated with a favourable outcome
- Remission of myasthenia gravis is not guaranteed with surgical resection
- Dogs with megaoesophagus are more likely to suffer post-operative complications

5.8 NEUROLOGICAL SYSTEM

Problems

Presenting complaints

q.v. section 1

1.3 Altered behaviour

1.4 Altered consciousness

1.8 Ataxia

1.10 Blindness

1.14 Deafness

1.17 Dysphagia

1.30 Head tilt

1.33 Nystagmus

1.34 Paresis/paralysis

1.41 Regurgitation

1.42 Seizures

1.47 Tremors

1.48 Urinary incontinence

Physical abnormalities

q.v. section 2

2.4 Arrhythmias

2.9 Horner's syndrome

2.10 Hypertension

2.17 Pain

2.25 Pyrexia and hyperthermia

2.30 Stridor and stertor

Laboratory abnormalities

q.v. section 3

3.20.1B Aspartate aminotransferase (AST)

3.12 Creatine kinase

3.14 C-reactive protein

Diagnostic Approach

After standard history and physical examination a neurological examination should be performed to:

- Distinguish neurological disease from non-neurological causes of signs
- Localise any lesion

1 Assess mentation, gait and posture (e.g. presence of head tilt) during walk and whilst interacting with the environment

2 Postural reactions
  - Hemi-walking or wheelbarrowing

- Hopping
- Paw positioning

3 Spinal reflexes
  - Cutaneous trunci (panniculus), triceps, patella and withdrawal reflexes

4 Pain perception
  - Spinal reflexes and pain perception must be considered separately, and both be assessed
  - Assess the dog's conscious perception of a painful stimulus, e.g. does the dog dislike its toe being pinched? This should not be confused with the spinal reflexes
  - A paraplegic dog may have lost the ability to withdraw its leg but still feel pain as demonstrated by visible changes in demeanour
  - It may be able to withdraw its leg but not have consciously perceived the pinching

5 Cranial nerves
  - Facial movement: blink, muzzle and ear movement
  - Gag reflex
  - Jaw tone
  - Oculocephalic reflex
  - Resting and positional strabismus
  - Spontaneous and positional nystagmus
    - Positional nystagmus can be assessed by placing the dog on its back and looking closely for nystagmus to unmask more subtle vestibular dysfunction
  - Voice

6 Response to nasal stimulation
  - Conscious perception of this, i.e. resentment response involves the forebrain

7 Eye
  - Eye position: enophthalmos, exophthalmos, strabismus
  - Third eyelid position
  - Pupil size: appropriateness, symmetry
  - Pupillary light responses: direct and consensual

8 Menace response
  - Only present from ~12 weeks of age
  - Will be abnormal in

Notes on Canine Internal Medicine, Fourth Edition. Victoria L. Black, Kathryn F. Murphy, Jessie Rose Payne, and Edward J. Hall.
© 2022 John Wiley & Sons Ltd. Published 2022 by John Wiley & Sons Ltd.

- Cerebellar lesions
- Facial movement disorders
- Forebrain lesions
- Ocular issues affecting vision

9 Visual fixation

10 Spinal pain
- Neck or back pain

Diagnostic Methods

History

Signalment in conjunction with the clinical course of any neurological disorder is highly informative when prioritising differential diagnoses; key areas to focus on are:

- Duration
- Onset: gradual, acute
- Progression: deteriorating, improving, waxing and waning

Physical examination

- Evidence of systemic disease, e.g. pyrexia, lymphadenopathy
- Rectal examination especially useful in dogs with hindlimb signs: may identify intrapelvic mass lesions
- Ophthalmic examination may be useful, especially in dogs with forebrain or multifocal localisation

Modified Glasgow Coma Scale

- Useful in providing prognostic information and assessing for trends in neurological status. Has been employed in the context of traumatic brain injury (suggested prognosis following brain injury: < 8 grave, 9–14 guarded, 15–18 good)

Modified Glasgow Coma Scale	Score
Motor activity	
Normal gait, normal spinal reflexes	6
Hemiparesis, tetraparesis, or decerebrate activity	5
Recumbent, intermittent extensor rigidity	4
Recumbent, constant extensor rigidity	3
Recumbent, constant extensor rigidity with opisthotonus	2
Recumbent, hypotonia of muscles, depressed or absent spinal reflexes	1
Brainstem reflexes	
Normal pupillary light reflexes and oculocephalic reflex	6
Slow pupillary light reflexes and normal to reduced oculocephalic reflex	5
Bilateral unresponsive miosis with normal to reduced oculocephalic reflex	4
Pinpoint pupils with reduced to absent oculocephalic reflex	3
Unilateral, unresponsive mydriasis with reduced to absent oculocephalic reflex	2
Bilateral, unresponsive mydriasis with reduced to absent oculocephalic reflex	1
Level of consciousness	
Occasional periods of alertness and responsive to environment	6
Depression or delirium, capable of responding but response may be inappropriate	5
Semicomatose, responsive to visual stimuli	4
Semicomatose, responsive to auditory stimuli	3
Semicomatose, responsive only to repeated noxious stimuli	2
Comatose, unresponsive to repeated noxious stimuli	1

ORGAN SYSTEMS

Laboratory findings
Haematology and biochemistry
- Changes uncommon in primary neurological disease; more likely systemic disease if abnormal
- May demonstrate a suspicion of an inflammatory focus in inflammatory disorders, e.g. steroid-responsive meningitis (SRMA)

Imaging
Plain radiographs
- Multiorgan involvement in metastatic disease or infection
- Spinal cord disease (e.g. neoplastic, discospondylitis, disc extrusion) but poor sensitivity

Ultrasound
Multiorgan involvement in disseminated neoplasia or infection

Special investigative techniques
- Cerebrospinal fluid (CSF) sampling for cytology and protein analysis
- CT scan
- Electrodiagnostics
  - Electroencephalogram (EEG)
  - Electromyography (EMG)
  - Nerve conduction
  - Brainstem auditory evoked response (BAER)
  - Electroretinogram (ERG)
- Infectious disease screening (serology, PCR, CSF analysis)
- MRI
- Myelogram

5.8.1 CEREBROVASCULAR DISEASE

Aetiology
Cerebrovascular disease encompasses ischaemic and haemorrhagic events resulting in reduced brain perfusion.
- Ischaemic cerebrovascular disease occurs due to obstruction of blood supply; loss of perfusion results in injury and necrosis
- Haemorrhagic cerebrovascular disease occurs due to rupture of blood vessels, with compression of the surrounding tissue with blood, resulting in ischaemia

Major signs
Depend on the location of the cerebrovascular event:
- Brainstem signs: vestibular disease, postural deficits
- Cerebellar signs: vestibular disease, loss of menace response, proprioceptive deficits
- Forebrain signs: mentation change, postural deficits, circling, ataxia

Potential sequelae
- Cushing reflex (hypertension and bradycardia) due to increased intracranial pressure
- Status epilepticus

Predisposition
- *Angiostrongylus* infection
- Greyhounds are predisposed to cerebrovascular events

Historical clues
- May progress during the initial 48-hour period but typically onset of signs is acute and can then improve
- Suspicion of underlying disorder that may have predisposed to a cerebrovascular event
  - Endocrine disease: hyperadrenocorticism (HAC), hypothyroidism
  - Liver disease
  - Neoplasia
  - Protein-losing enteropathy (PLE)
  - Protein-losing nephropathy (PLN)

Physical examination
- Assess for suspicion of underlying disorder as above
- Blood pressure measurement

Neurological examination
Abnormal asymmetrical signs localising to the site of the vascular event

Laboratory findings
Haematology and serum biochemistry
- Bile acid stimulation test
- Folate and cobalamin: PLE
- Thrombocytopenia: IMTP, etc.
- Hypoalbuminaemia: PLE, PLN

Urinalysis
UPC ratio: PLN

Imaging
Plain radiographs and ultrasound
Screen for underlying disorders as above

Special investigations
- *Angiostrongylus vasorum* ± *Dirofilaria immitis*
- Coagulation testing: PT and aPTT
- Echocardiogram: cardiac disease rare cause for cerebrovascular disease
- Endocrine testing where clinical suspicion, e.g. signs of HAC
- MRI and CSF to assess for other disorders

Treatment
- Supportive care with treatment for increased intracranial pressure as needed
- Treat underlying cause

Monitoring
Repeat neurological examination

Prognosis
- Prognosis is fair to guarded and depends on lesion location and severity of signs
- Dogs with hypertension appear to experience a poorer prognosis

5.8.2 CORTICOSTEROID-RESPONSIVE TREMOR SYNDROME

Aetiology
Acquired disorder characterised by acute-onset whole body tremors, and vestibular dysfunction. Formerly referred to as idiopathic cerebellitis and 'little white shaker syndrome'. Based on the findings of mild inflammatory pleocytosis on CSF analysis in some dogs and response to glucocorticoids, an autoimmune condition is suspected.

Major signs
- Whole-body tremors, may be exacerbated by stress and excitement
- Vestibular signs

Potential sequelae
Severe tremors may result in hyperthermia

Predisposition
- Young dogs (1–5 years) appear to present most commonly
- Small-breed, white-haired dogs appear to be predisposed (e.g. Maltese terrier, Poodle, WHWT), although any breed or coat colour can be affected

Historical clues
- Typically, acute-onset tremors with exacerbation during excitement and stress, discriminated from MUO as neurological signs all localise to cerebellum, i.e. abnormal mentation, seizures or spinal cord localisation are *not* expected

Physical examination
- Clinical examination expected to be normal; may detect hyperthermia

Neurological examination
- Whole-body tremors, exacerbated by excitement or stress
- Loss of menace response bilaterally
- ± Nystagmus, head tilt and strabismus

Laboratory findings
Haematology and biochemistry
- Within reference ranges
- Useful to exclude other causes of seizure or tremor

Imaging
Plain radiographs and ultrasound
No abnormalities

Special investigations
- CSF sampling for cytology and proteins: may detect mononuclear pleocytosis or increased protein
- MRI may reveal hyperintensity or mild contrast enhancement of the cerebellum
- Useful to exclude other causes, i.e. causes of seizure or tremor
  - Exclusion of neoplastic and infectious disease
  - EEG (electroencephalogram) may discriminate seizure disorders from differential diagnoses, e.g. post-anaesthesia involuntary movements in dogs recovering from general anaesthesia

Treatment

Prednisolone is the mainstay of treatment, with short tapering courses (over 2–3 months) described to result in favourable responses

Monitoring

- Repeat assessment and neurological examination
- Repeat CSF analysis rarely performed

Prognosis

- Generally good with favourable response typically observed within 3 days of starting treatment, although some dogs will relapse

5.8.3 HYDROCEPHALUS

Aetiology

Hydrocephalus is characterised by accumulation of CSF; this may be congenital due to excessive production or reduced absorption of CSF or related to obstruction of outflow due to a space-occupying lesion or abnormal anatomy.

Major signs

- Circling
- Dull mentation
- Head pressing
- Restlessness
- Seizures
- Visual deficits
- Vomiting

Potential sequelae

- May have acute deterioration in signs in some dogs as vulnerable to subdural haematoma
- Status epilepticus

Predisposition

- Toy breeds, e.g. Chihuahua, Pomeranian, Yorkshire terrier
- Boston terrier, English bulldog

Historical clues

Difficulty training the puppy, in particular house training

Physical examination

- Abnormal dome-shaped head and strabismus (bilateral, ventrolateral) may be appreciated
- Open fontanelle may be present, but is also seen without hydrocephalus, e.g. Pomeranian

Neurological examination

- Abnormal forebrain signs
- Strabismus

Laboratory findings

- Unremarkable
- Important to rule out PSS and hypoglycaemia in affected dogs

Imaging

Radiographs and ultrasound

- Radiographs may be suspicious with domed calvarium and thinned cortical bone
- May be able to scan through persistent open fontanelle

Special investigations

- CT or MRI to assess ventricle size
- Caution must be employed when discerning significance of hydrocephalus, in particular in toy breeds; it may be an incidental finding, as ventricle size has not been found to correlate with clinical signs

Treatment

- Medical management: glucocorticoids, omeprazole, and diuretics may achieve temporary palliation in obstructive hydrocephalus with masses or in some cases with congenital hydrocephalus where surgery is not an option
- Surgical management with a ventriculoperitoneal shunt achieves a fair to good outcome in dogs

5.8.4 IDIOPATHIC EPILEPSY

Aetiology

Idiopathic epilepsy is a seizure condition where an underlying trigger is not detected.

- Age of onset of the first seizure is typically 6 months to 6 years of age

- Channelopathy resulting in an abnormal excitatory neuronal activity is hypothesised to contribute
- Genetic predisposition suspected in some breeds
- In between seizures the dog is considered normal

Major signs
- Seizures, *q.v.* section 1.42
  - Dogs are expected to be normal between post-ictal phase and next seizure
  - May be generalised or focal
  - Prodrome-ictal-post ictal stages
- Status epilepticus: seizure lasting more than 5 minutes, or two or more discrete seizures with incomplete recovery of consciousness in between

Minor signs
Anxiety-related behaviour is reported more commonly in dogs diagnosed with idiopathic epilepsy

Potential sequelae
- Some dogs may be refractory to anti-epileptic therapy; in these cases the disorder may result in euthanasia
- Prolonged status epilepticus can result in severe systemic (heat stroke, non-cardiogenic pulmonary oedema, hypoglycaemia) and neurological (hypoxic and post-excitatory brain injury) consequences
- Cognitive dysfunction has been described in dogs with idiopathic epilepsy

Predisposition
- Border collie, GSD
- Some breeds appear to be predisposed to juvenile-onset epilepsy: Lagotto Romagnolo

Historical clues
- Age of onset of the first seizure is typically 6 months to 6 years of age
- Dogs diagnosed with idiopathic epilepsy are expected to have normal neurological signs between seizures following recovery from the post-ictal period
- Dogs with status epilepticus refractory to diazepam are less likely to have idiopathic epilepsy, i.e. are more likely to have reactive or symptomatic seizure disorder

Physical examination
- Clinical examination expected to be normal

Neurological examination
- Normal following the post-ictal period
- During the post-ictal period neurological abnormalities may be detected (e.g. vision changes, proprioceptive deficits); however, these are expected to be symmetrical

Laboratory findings
Haematology and biochemistry
- Most frequently within normal reference interval, with prolonged status epilepticus may detect hypoglycaemia
- Muscle enzyme activities (AST and CK) and UPC (urine protein:creatinine) ratio may increase transiently post seizures
- Bile acid stimulation to exclude hepatic dysfunction

Imaging
Plain radiographs and ultrasound
Abnormalities not detected; however, may be rewarding if multisystemic disease is suspected to be a differential diagnosis (e.g. disseminated neoplasia or infection)

Special investigations
- CSF sampling for cytology and proteins
- EEG may be useful in discriminating seizure disorders from differential diagnoses (e.g. post-anaesthesia involuntary movements in dogs recovering from general anaesthesia)
- Exclusion of neoplastic and infectious disease
- MRI

Treatment
- Antiepileptic therapy is suggested if:
  - Acute repetitive seizures or status epilepticus
  - Two or more seizures in 6 months
  - Prolonged, severe, or unusual aggressive or distressing post-ictal signs
- Drug therapy
  - Phenobarbital (first-line drug)

ORGAN SYSTEMS

- Monitoring of serum concentrations recommended at 2 and 6 weeks after dose changes and every 6 months
- Side effects include hepatotoxicity and bone marrow suppression, PU/PD, sedation, ataxia and polyphagia
- Potassium bromide (first-line drug)
  - Monitoring recommended at 1 and 3 months after every dose change and every 12 months to keep within the therapeutic range
  - Side effects include pancreatitis, sedation and ataxia
  - Affects plasma chloride measurement in laboratory testing
- Imepitoin (first-line drug)
  - Incremental dose increases may be required for seizure control, monitoring not required
  - Side effects include ataxia, vomiting, sedation and polyphagia
- Levetiracetam
  - Not licensed for veterinary medicine but is used in short-term management of seizure disorders in dogs, with minimal side effects reported
  - However, the dose interval (q8h) and suspected loss of efficacy over time means that it is not recommended for sole long-term therapy in idiopathic epilepsy
- Non-pharmacological treatment
  - Dietary alteration, e.g. ketogenic diet
  - Omega-3 fatty acid supplementation
  - Vagal nerve stimulation (surgical device)

Monitoring

- Drug monitoring recommended as above
- Seizure diary may be useful

Prognosis

Prognosis depends on degree of seizure control
- Dogs with poor seizure control appear to have survival times ~2 years shorter
- Border collies have been found to be the least likely to achieve remission
- Median lifespan of 5.2 years
- Median survival 2.1 years after seizure onset

5.8.5 IDIOPATHIC HEAD TREMOR

Aetiology

Idiopathic head tremor is a paroxysmal movement disorder with no known underlying cause, with some similarity to essential tremor and dystonia disorders in people. There are breed predispositions, implying some genetic basis to this presentation.

Episodes are characterised by:
- Sudden-onset vertical ('yes'; may also be called head bobbing) or horizontal ('no') head movements, without loss of consciousness
- Events may be precipitated by stress
- Typically, can be distracted to curtail the movement, e.g. with a ball or food

Major signs

Involuntary head movements (vertical or horizontal) with no loss of consciousness and ability to distract the dog

Potential sequelae

Clinical remission occurs spontaneously in some dogs, whereas in others quality of life may be of concern due to the frequency of events

Predisposition

Any breed may present with idiopathic head bobbing, but especially Boxer, Bulldog, Dobermann, Labrador retriever

Historical clues

- Dogs should be normal between events unless the stress of systemic illness has precipitated an increased frequency
- Maintenance of consciousness during the tremors and ability of owner to distract most dogs

Physical examination

- Clinical examination expected to be normal

Neurological examination
- Normal

ORGAN SYSTEMS

Laboratory findings
Haematology and biochemistry
- Typically within normal reference interval
- May detect abnormalities if systemic illness has resulted in increased frequency of tremors
- Useful to exclude other causes (e.g. causes of seizure or tremor)

Imaging
Plain radiographs and ultrasound
- Abnormalities not detected

Special investigations
- Owner video may be typical of disorder
- Useful to exclude other causes (e.g. causes of seizure or tremor)
  - CSF sampling for cytology and proteins
  - EEG (electroencephalogram) may be useful in discriminating seizure disorders from differential diagnoses (e.g. post-anaesthesia involuntary movements in dogs recovering from general anaesthesia)
- Exclusion of neoplastic and infectious disease
- MRI

Treatment
- No treatment needed in most cases
- Imepitoin may be helpful in reducing frequency in a small number of dogs

Prognosis
- Generally good, non-progressive condition, although dogs may be severely affected in rare cases

5.8.6 IDIOPATHIC VESTIBULAR DISEASE

Aetiology
Idiopathic vestibular disease is a disorder characterised by peripheral vestibular dysfunction where no underlying cause it detected. The aetiology is unknown, although it appears to affect older dogs more commonly and is sometimes termed 'old dog vestibular disease'.

Major signs
- Vestibular disease
  - Head tilt
  - Ataxia
  - Nystagmus
  - Falling
- Vomiting and nausea

Minor signs
- Dogs may have concurrent facial nerve dysfunction

Predisposition
- Affects dogs of any age but typically older

Historical clues
- Typical onset is acute, non-progressive, improving
- Occasionally dogs may display transient abnormal vestibular function in the 48 hours preceding presentation
- Any history of metronidazole therapy as it can cause vestibular dysfunction

Physical examination
- Unremarkable
- Otoscopy helpful to rule in/out for otitis media

Neurological examination
- Localisation is peripheral, therefore mentation and proprioception (paw positioning) is unaffected

Laboratory findings
- Unremarkable

Imaging
Plain radiographs and ultrasound
- Unremarkable

Special investigations
- MRI and CSF as diagnosis of idiopathic vestibular disease is a diagnosis of exclusion;

however, age, neurolocalisation and clinical course is highly suggestive

Treatment
- Anti-emetics
- Nursing if recumbent

Prognosis
Prognosis is expected to be good
- Most dogs begin to improve within 2–3 days, with recovery over a few weeks
- Some dogs may display a permanent head tilt

5.8.7 INFECTIOUS DISEASES AFFECTING THE NERVOUS SYSTEM

Aetiology
Infectious diseases may affect the nervous system through multiple mechanisms:
1 As part of a multisystemic infection
   - *Brucella*
   - Distemper
   - *Neospora*
   - Rabies
   - *Toxoplasma*
2 Extension of local infection due to iatrogenic causes (e.g. injection, etc.), migrating foreign body or bite wounds
   - Bacterial otitis media
   - Cryptococcosis
   - Discospondylitis
   - Empyema
3 Infections through haematogenous spread
   - Abscess due to endocarditis
   - Discospondylitis
4 Infections with consequences on the nervous system due to coagulable states or viscosity
   - *Angiostrongylus*; may also have aberrant larvae migration
   - *Leishmania*

Major signs
- Altered behaviour
- Altered consciousness
- Ataxia
- Blindness
- Circling
- Deafness
- Head tilt
- Nystagmus
- Pain
- Paresis/paralysis
- Seizures
- Tremors
- Weakness, collapse

Minor signs
- Anorexia
- Depression
- Lethargy
- Weight loss
- Pyrexia
- Concurrent systemic disease depending on cause

Potential sequelae
Status epilepticus

Predisposition
- Lifestyle and exposure to vectors increases risk of infection
- A litter of puppies may be affected by *Neospora*, typically at 3–9 weeks of age

Historical clues
Typically acute-onset progressive signs

Physical examination
- May detect evidence of multisystemic disease
- Pyrexia may be present

Neurological examination
Abnormal asymmetrical examination findings anticipated in space-occupying lesions affecting the brain (abscess, empyema)

Ophthalmic examination
- May detect evidence of inflammation or concurrent ocular involvement (e.g. chorioretinitis in toxoplasmosis) or systemic consequences of infection (e.g. vessel tortuosity in leishmaniasis and hyperviscosity)

ORGAN SYSTEMS

Laboratory findings
Haematology and biochemistry
- May detect evidence of multisystemic disease (e.g. inflammatory leukogram), or specific organ involvement (e.g. increased muscle enzyme activities in neosporosis, hyperglobulinaemia in leishmaniosis)

Imaging
Plain radiographs and ultrasound
- May detect evidence of multisystemic disease or specific organ involvement
- Discospondylitis may be apparent on plain spinal radiographs (sensitivity early in disease poor, can take more than 8 weeks to detect changes)

Special investigations, treatment, monitoring and prognosis
- Depends on specific infectious agent, *q.v.* section 5.11
- Bacterial infection treatment is ideally tailored by tissue sampling and culture for targeted antimicrobial therapy
- Surgery may be useful to provide drainage of infection and stabilisation

5.8.8   MOVEMENT DISORDERS

Aetiology
Movement disorders are characterised by involuntary abnormal movement (dyskinesia), lasting minutes to hours, with no loss of consciousness and no post-ictal period. In people, the underlying cause is thought to either reflect a transient dysfunction of the basal nuclei or a channelopathy similar to an epileptic disorder.
- Genetic causes for movement disorders have been identified in
  - Episodic falling syndrome in CKCS
  - Paroxysmal dyskinesia in Soft-coated Wheaten terriers
- Gluten sensitivity appears to play a role in paroxysmal gluten-sensitive dyskinesia in Border terriers
- Drug-induced movement disorders have been reported related to phenobarbital and propofol

Major signs
- Abnormal involuntary movements with preservation of consciousness
- Breed-related disorders are described with some specific characteristics
  - Border terriers may present with borborygmi, vomiting, or diarrhoea during or immediately after a period of abnormal movement

Potential sequelae
- Spontaneous clinical remission occurs in some dogs
- In others, quality of life may be of concern due to the frequency of events

Predisposition
- Border terrier, Boxer, CKCS, Dalmatian, Golden retriever, German short-haired pointer, Jack Russell terrier, Soft-coated Wheaten terrier

Historical clues
- Dogs should be normal between events
- Maintenance of consciousness during the tremors, although ability to distract a dog out of the event is not often reported

Physical examination
- Clinical examination expected to be normal

Neurological examination
- Normal

Laboratory findings
Haematology and biochemistry
- Within reference intervals
- Useful to exclude other causes of seizure or tremor

Imaging
Plain radiographs and ultrasound
- Abnormalities not detected

Special investigations
- Owner video may be typical of movement disorder
- Useful to exclude other causes (e.g. causes of seizure or tremor)
  - CSF sampling for cytology and proteins

- EEG may be useful in discriminating seizure disorders from differential diagnoses (e.g. post-anaesthesia involuntary movements in dogs recovering from general anaesthesia)
- Exclusion of neoplastic and infectious disease
- MRI

Treatment
- Acetazolamide described to be effective in episodic falling syndrome in CKCS
- Clonazepam, acetazolamide and fluoxetine described variably as treatment trials in dogs
- Gluten-free diet in Border terriers

Prognosis
- Generally good, non-progressive condition, although dogs may be severely affected in rare cases

5.8.9 MENINGOENCEPHALITIS OF UNKNOWN ORIGIN (MUO)

Aetiology
Meningoencephalitis of unknown origin (MUO) is a term assigned to non-infectious inflammatory disorders of the central nervous system (CNS) where the diagnosis is presumed in the absence of histopathology as this is rarely performed pre-mortem. The disorder is thought to be due to an aberrant immune response against CNS tissues.

Post-mortem histopathology in dogs has classified MUO as:
- Granulomatous meningoencephalitis (GME): characterised by perivascular accumulation of macrophages and lymphocytes
- Necrotizing encephalitis (NE): characterised by perivascular and meningeal necrotic lesions with mononuclear infiltration

Major signs
- Altered behaviour
- Altered consciousness
- Ataxia
- Blindness
- Deafness
- Head tilt

- Nystagmus
- Pain
- Paresis/paralysis
- Seizures
- Tremors
- Weakness, collapse

Minor signs
- Anorexia
- Depression
- Lethargy
- Pyrexia; uncommon in MUO

Potential sequelae
- Aspiration pneumonia due to loss of protective gag reflex
- Cushing reflex due to increased intracranial pressure: hypertension and bradycardia
- Respiratory arrest due to brain herniation

Predisposition
- GME may occur in any breed of dog, although a predisposition for toy and terrier dogs is suspected. Middle-aged dogs (4–8 years) appear to be most commonly affected.
- NE occurs most commonly in Pugs, Yorkshire terriers and Maltese terriers but has been described in other toy-breed dogs. Young dogs (< 4 years) appear to be most commonly affected.

Historical clues
- Typical clinical course is waxing and waning or progressive neurological signs
- May be acute or gradual onset

Physical examination
- May detect signs suspicious for Cushing reflex, concerning for brain herniation, causing hypertension and bradycardia
- Pyrexia is uncommon
- Systemic signs uncommon

Neurological examination
- Typically asymmetrical neurological examination findings; can be forebrain, brainstem or multifocal
- Minority of affected dogs may present with signs of spinal cord involvement

ORGAN SYSTEMS

Ophthalmic examination
- May detect papilloedema, raising concerns of increased intracranial pressure

Laboratory findings
Haematology and biochemistry
  - Most frequently within reference interval

Imaging
Plain radiographs and ultrasound
- Abnormalities not detected
- May be rewarding if multisystemic disease is suspected to be a differential diagnosis (e.g. disseminated neoplasia or infection)

Special investigations
- CSF sampling for cytology and proteins
- Exclusion of neoplastic and infectious disease
- MRI
- Stereotactic CT-guided or free hand brain biopsy is described but rarely performed

Treatment
- Immunosuppression is the mainstay of treatment
  - Protocols describe prednisolone alone or in combination with adjuvant therapy, most commonly cytosine arabinoside (cytarabine) or ciclosporin
- Radiation therapy has been described in one case series

Monitoring
- Clinical response and resolution of neurological deficits
- MRI and CSF rarely repeat due to risks and financial costs

Prognosis
Highly variable although likely overall guarded prognosis
  - Some dogs do very poorly and others experience extended survival
  - Around 25–33% of dogs are reported to die within 1 week of diagnosis

5.8.10 MYASTHENIA GRAVIS (MG)

Aetiology
Congenital myasthenic syndromes:
- Defective synthesis of acetylcholine
- Acetylcholinesterase deficiency
- Inherited lack of nicotinic acetylcholine receptors
Acquired myasthenia gravis (MG)
- Autoimmune destruction of nicotinic acetylcholine receptors: no trigger detected
  - Generalised
  - Focal affecting the oesophagusor pharynx or both, *q.v.* section 5.1.3B
- Paraneoplastic disorder, in particular due to thymoma, *q.v.* section 5.7.2D

Major signs
- Exercise-induced fatigue
- Regurgitation due to megaoesophagus
- Cough, dyspnoea, pyrexia due to aspiration pneumonia

Minor signs
- Stiffness rather than classic major signs
- Focal MG: megeoesophagus without evidence of exercise induced fatigue
- Rarely, facial, pharyngeal or laryngeal dysfunction alone

Potential sequelae
Dogs may present with acute crisis with rapidly progressive muscle weakness, and vulnerable to acute death
  - Severe aspiration pneumonia
  - Respiratory muscle weakness

Predisposition
- Breed-related congenital myasthenic syndromes (rare)
- Fulminant acquired MG in Golden retriever

Historical clues
- May present with range of signs from regurgitation alone (focal myasthenia gravis), a stiff gait with exercise-induced fatigue, or rapid fulminant myasthenic crisis

ORGAN SYSTEMS

Physical examination
- Assess for evidence of aspiration pneumonia

Neurological examination
- Fatiguability of palpebral reflex: repeated stimulation in dogs with MG results in fatigue
- Observe effect of exercise: weakness, 'bunny-hopping' gait
- Reduced gag reflex

Laboratory findings
Haematology and biochemistry
- May be evidence of inflammatory disease in dogs with aspiration pneumonia: inflammatory leukogram, acute-phase response

Imaging
Plain radiographs and ultrasound
- Assess for presence of megaoesophagus; must be taken conscious as sedation or GA can result in false positives
- Assess for cranial mediastinal mass: 3–5% of cases have thymoma-related acquired MG

Special investigations
- Acetylcholine receptor antibody serology
- Acetylcholinesterase inhibitor response test (edrophonium/Tensilon test)
  - Not suitable for congenital and focal acquired MG
- Electrophysiology; fatigue on repetitive nerve stimulation

Treatment,
q.v. section 5.1.3B
- Acetylcholinesterase inhibitor
  - May cause cholinergic crisis
  - Titrating dose can be challenging as drug side effects can be difficult to discriminate from the disease
- Value of immunosuppression is unclear as spontaneous remission is reported
- Surgical removal recommended in dogs with thymoma, although remission is not guaranteed and there is increased risk with general anaesthesia

Monitoring
- Serial acetylcholine receptor antibody titres may be useful at assessing remission

- Re-assessment for megaoesophagus and aspiration pneumonia may be useful

Prognosis
- Dogs with non-thymoma-related MG may experience remission; the prognosis for dogs with thymoma is uncertain
- Regardless of the type of acquired MG (focal or generalised), the prognosis is guarded
  - 1-year mortality approximately 50%
  - Cause of death most commonly aspiration pneumonia

5.8.11 NEOPLASIA OF THE NEUROLOGICAL SYSTEM

Aetiology
- Primary brain tumours
  - Abnormal unregulated proliferation of cells normally found in the brain
    - Glioma
    - Lymphoma
    - Meningioma
- Secondary brain tumours
  - Direct extension from adjacent tissue
    - Pituitary adenoma or adenocarcinoma
    - Nasal tumours
  - Metastatic disease
    - Any carcinoma, but especially mammary
    - Haemangiosarcoma
    - Histiocytic sarcoma
- Spinal cord
  - Haemangiosarcoma
  - Lymphoma
  - Nephroblastoma
  - Osteosarcoma
- Peripheral nerves
  - Nerve sheath tumour
    - Benign
      - Haemangiopericytoma, but locally invasive and likely to recur
      - Neurofibroma
      - Schwannoma
    - Malignant
      - soft-tissue sarcoma

Major signs
- Altered behaviour
- Altered consciousness
- Ataxia

- Blindness
- Circling
- Deafness
- Head tilt
- Lameness
- Nystagmus
- Pain
- Paresis/paralysis
- Seizures
- Tremors
- Weakness, collapse

Minor signs
- Anorexia
- Depression
- Lethargy
- Weight loss

Potential sequelae
- Cushing reflex due to increased intracranial pressure, resulting in hypertension and bradycardia
- Respiratory arrest
- Status epilepticus

Predisposition
- Older dogs
- Primary brain tumours: Boxer, Dobermann, Golden retriever, Old English sheepdogs, Scottish terriers
- Secondary brain tumours: Golden retrievers

Historical clues
- Typically, gradual-onset progressive signs
- Seizures most common presenting sign in dogs with primary forebrain tumours, also abnormal consciousness
- Dogs may be neurologically abnormal between seizures
- Dogs with secondary brain tumours may present with signs related to the nature of the tumour:
  - Functional pituitary tumours: PU/PD, polyphagia and panting
  - Invading nasal tumours: epistaxis, stertor, sneezing
- Dogs with peripheral nerve sheath tumours typically present with progressive severe lameness

Physical examination
- Clinical examination expected to be normal in primary brain tumours; may detect cachexia, or evidence of HAC in dogs with pituitary tumours
- Clinical examination in dogs with secondary brain tumours may detect multi-organ involvement (e.g. lymphoma, histiocytic sarcoma, haemangiosarcoma)
- Dogs with peripheral nerve sheath tumours often display marked, localised muscle wastage
- Suspicion of Cushing reflex: hypertension and bradycardia

Neurological examination
- Abnormal asymmetrical examination findings anticipated localising to the site of the brain tumour: forebrain, cerebellum, brainstem
- Spinal cord tumours can be intramedullary or extramedullary and may present with paresis or paralysis as well as ataxia and spinal pain. Intramedullary lesions may also present with signs such as Horner's syndrome, depending on lesion location.
- Abnormal Modified Glasgow Coma Scale score may raise suspicion of herniation

Ophthalmic examination
- May detect papilloedema, raising concerns of increased intracranial pressure

Laboratory findings
Haematology and biochemistry
- Within reference interval for primary brain tumours
- Changes with secondary brain tumours due to multi-organ involvement
- Paraneoplastic disease: hyperadrenocorticism, hypercalcaemia, hypoglycaemia

Imaging
Plain radiographs and ultrasound
Abnormalities may detect metastatic disease or multi-organ involvement

Special investigations
- CSF sampling for cytology and proteins
  - May occasionally detect neoplastic cells
  - May detect lymphoma

- Excisional biopsy, in particular for extra-axial or extradural masses or peripheral nerve sheath tumours
- Exclusion of infectious disease
- Lymph node or mass-lesion sampling distant to the brain
- MRI most sensitive for intracranial neoplasia, CT poorer sensitivity
- Stereotactic CT-guided or free-hand brain biopsy is described but rarely performed

Treatment
- Symptomatic treatment with anti-inflammatory glucocorticoids and anti-epileptic drugs
- Surgery may be an effective treatment modality, in particular in pituitary masses and extradural or extra-axial masses
- Radiation therapy has been described as effective modality, in particular in extra-axial masses or pituitary tumours but also in some intra-axial tumours
- Chemotherapy has been described, in particular use of hydroxyurea in meningiomas and lomustine in gliomas
- Dogs with HAC due to large functional pituitary masses (macroadenomas) may neurologically deteriorate following introduction of trilostane due to loss of negative feedback effect of cortisol and resultant expansion of tumour (similar to Nelson's syndrome in humans)

Monitoring
- Repeat assessment and neurological examination
- Dogs undergoing radiation may undergo repeated advanced imaging (CT scan)

Prognosis
- Surgically resectable tumours or those amenable to radiation therapy may enjoy extended survival (years) in some cases, in particular extra-axial and pituitary tumours
- Most other brain tumours are associated with a guarded prognosis: weeks-to-months survival with treatment

5.8.12 POLYRADICULONEURITIS

Aetiology
Polyradiculoneuritis is a diffuse disorder of the myelin of the ventral nerve roots. A similar disorder in humans is Guillain-Barré syndrome.
- In dogs *Campylobacter* and *Toxoplasma* have been explored as potential triggers
- In North America there is a link with a recent raccoon bite ('Coonhound paralysis')
- Tick paralysis is a differential diagnosis in many countries

Major signs
q.v. section 1.34
- Tetraparesis or tetraplegia with loss of peripheral reflexes

Potential sequelae
- Respiratory arrest may occur due to progressive hypoventilation

Predisposition
- Jack Russell terriers, WHWT

Historical clues
- Acute-onset progressive, ascending (hindlegs affected first) tetraparesis or tetraplegia with loss of peripheral reflexes and flaccid tone in all four limbs
- Autonomic function (urination and defaecation) and tail tone is typically preserved
- Hunting dogs in North America bitten by raccoons

Physical examination
- Unremarkable aside from neurological changes, may detect hypoventilation

Neurological examination
- Autonomic function (urination and defaecation) and tail tone are typically preserved
- Tetraparesis or tetraplegia with loss of peripheral reflexes
  - Flaccid tone in all four limbs
  - Sensation is preserved, e.g. toe pinching will elicit behavioural response but limb withdrawal not present

ORGAN SYSTEMS

Laboratory findings
• Unremarkable

Imaging
Plain radiographs and ultrasound
• Unremarkable

Special investigations
• Blood gas (monitor pCO_2 as marker of hypoventilation)
• CSF sampling (albumin/cytological dissociation)
• Electrodiagnostics

Treatment
Treatment is primarily aimed at supportive care, in particular nursing the recumbent patient; rare cases may need mechanical ventilation due to respiratory failure

Prognosis
• Guarded; some dogs will die of respiratory failure unless ventilated
• Incomplete recovery and failure to improve has been reported
• Most dogs will begin to improve within 3 weeks of onset of signs, with full recovery within 6 months

5.8.13 STEROID-RESPONSIVE MENINGITIS-ARTERITIS (SRMA)

Aetiology
• SRMA is a presumed autoimmune disorder occurring due to infiltration of the meninges with inflammatory cells
• No environmental trigger has been detected
• The disorder almost exclusively affects dogs under 2.5 years of age

Major signs
• Cervical hyperaesthesia
• Pyrexia

Minor signs
• Tail pain (less common)
• Lethargy

• Inappetence
• Obtundation

Potential sequelae
• Spinal cord haemorrhage has been described (very rare)

Predisposition
• Beagle, Border collie, Boxer, Jack Russell terrier, Springer spaniel, Nova Scotia Duck Tolling retriever, Weimaraner and Whippet
• Disorder highly age-associated, with most cases identified in dogs under 2.5 years of age

Historical clues
• Previous similar episodes may be reported by the owner given the waxing and waning course of the disorder
• Partial response to NSAIDs or steroids in previous events may be reported

Physical examination
• Neck pain ± back pain or, in rare cases, tail pain
• Pyrexia
• Neurological deficits are not expected in SRMA
• A chronic form has been described, in particular in Boxers, but is not typical

Laboratory findings
Haematology and biochemistry
• Evidence of systemic inflammation
  • Acute phase protein response: hypoalbuminaemia and hyperglobulinaemia
  • Increased C-reactive protein
  • Leukocytosis with neutrophilia and monocytosis

Imaging
Plain radiographs and ultrasound
• Typically unremarkable

Special investigations
• Arthrocentesis for joint cytology in cases with concurrent joint effusions or pain due to concurrent IMPA
• CSF for cytology and protein analysis:

- Increased protein
- Neutrophilic pleocytosis; often high numbers with > 80% non-degenerate neutrophils
- Infectious disease screening (e.g. *Toxoplasma*, *Neospora*)
- MRI scan if concurrent neurological deficits, but not expected with SRMA

Treatment

- Immunosuppressive therapy
  - Typically prednisolone; adjuncts including azathioprine, mycophenolate, ciclosporin and cytarabine, although unlicensed, are described
  - Duration of treatment described is currently 6 months of gradual tapering; however, considerably shorter courses (approximately 6 weeks) appear to be effective in some dogs

Monitoring

- Assessment for relapse can be supported by clinical examination
  - Especially neck pain and pyrexia
  - CRP but not increased in all relapses
- Gradual tapering of immunosuppression: literature suggests reducing dosages to complete a course over 6 months, more rapid tapering over weeks is likely to be adequate in most cases

Prognosis

- Generally excellent with immunosuppressive therapy, although relapse occurs in ~30%

ORGAN SYSTEMS

5.9 REPRODUCTIVE SYSTEM

Problems

Presenting complaints

q.v. section 1
1.1 Abortion
1.3 Altered behaviour
1.5 Anorexia/hyporexia/inappetence
1.7 Anuria/oliguria
1.9 Bleeding
1.11 Constipation
1.19 Dysuria
1.20 Dystocia
1.27 Haematuria and discoloured urine
1.35 Perinatal death
1.37 Polyuria/polydipsia (PU/PD)
1.46 Tenesmus and dyschezia
1.48 Urinary incontinence
1.50 Vulval discharge
1.51 Weakness, collapse and syncope

Physical abnormalities

q.v. section 2
2.1 Abdominal enlargement
2.5 Ascites
2.17 Pain: Abdominal and generalised
2.18 Pallor
2.19 Perineal lesions
2.20 Peripheral oedema
2.25 Pyrexia and hyperthermia
2.23 Prostatomegaly

Laboratory abnormalities

q.v. section 3
3.1 Acid–base
3.4 Azotaemia
3.14 C-reactive protein
3.17 Glucose
3.22 Phosphate
3.25 Symmetric dimethylarginine (SDMA)
3.27 Total protein (albumin and globulin)
3.29 Urea
3B Haematology
3C Urinalysis

Diagnostic Approach

- Identify potential reproductive disease from knowledge of reproductive status of male and female dogs
  - Entire vs neutered
    - If neutered nature of procedure performed, e.g., is stump pyometra possible?
    - Could an ovarian remnant remain?

Diagnostic Methods

History

- Evaluate neuter status
- Associate any cyclical nature with any signs or attractiveness to males
- Evidence of systemic disease: consider infection, e.g. pyometra, prostatitis
- Evidence of dermatological disease: consider syndromes of hormone excess

Physical examination

- Examine reproductive tract for:
  - Any secondary signs, i.e. secondary to hormone excess
  - Any swelling/masses
  - Discharge – nature

Laboratory findings

- See specific disease

Imaging

- See specific disease
- Ultrasound generally more informative than plain radiographs

Special investigative techniques

- Culture of discharge
- Cytology/histopathology
- Hormonal evaluation

5.9.1 MAMMARY GLAND DISEASE

The mammary glands are susceptible to infectious/inflammatory disease (mastitis) and neoplasia.

ORGAN SYSTEMS

Notes on Canine Internal Medicine, Fourth Edition. Victoria L. Black, Kathryn F. Murphy, Jessie Rose Payne, and Edward J. Hall.
© 2022 John Wiley & Sons Ltd. Published 2022 by John Wiley & Sons Ltd.

5.9.1A MASTITIS

Aetiology
- Can affect one or more glands
- Tends to occur *post-partum* or during pseudopregnancy
- Typically caused by an ascending infection, e.g. *E. coli*, staphylococci, streptococci and enterococci

Major signs
Single or multiple abnormal glands
- Discoloured, swollen, firm and painful
- Gangrenous/ulcerated
- Haemorrhagic or purulent discharge

Minor signs
- Failing pups
- If severe: systemic signs, e.g. fever, anorexia, lethargy, vomiting

Potential sequelae
- Necrosis and loss of mammary gland
- Sepsis with severe mastitis

Predisposition
- After death or weaning of puppies
- Dirty environment
- Galactostasis
- Pseudopregnancy
- Trauma to glands

Historical clues
Caudal glands more often affected

Physical examination
See major/minor signs

Laboratory findings
- Neutrophilic inflammation
- Thrombocytopenia with gangrenous mastitis/sepsis

Imaging
Radiography
Rarely performed

Ultrasound
- Abscessation
- Loss of layering of normal tissue and hypoechogenic

Special investigations
- Milk cytology and culture

Treatment
- Analgesia
- Broad-spectrum antibiotics with good penetration into milk, ideally based on culture and sensitivity of milk sample
  - Avoid antibiotics that can harm neonates
- Cabergoline
  - If puppies are weaned, use cabergoline to reduce milk production
  - Do not use if not weaned; simply let the puppies feed
  - If associated with pseudopregnancy
- Local management
  - Expressing milk
  - Warm compresses, gentle massage, cabbage leaf compress
- Surgical debridement for severe necrotic lesions
- Supportive treatment: IVFT, etc.

Monitoring
- Clinical signs

Prognosis
- Good, most resolve within 2–3 weeks
- Guarded if sepsis

5.9.1B MAMMARY NEOPLASIA

Aetiology
Hormone exposure plays a role
- Exposure to exogenous oestrogens and/or progestagens may increase risk of neoplasia
- Neutering before first oestrus believed to reduce risk

Major signs
- Palpable mass in mammary gland ± Local lymphadenopathy
- ± Other affected glands; can be same or different tumour type

Minor signs
- If inflammatory carcinoma, gland can be red, swollen, and painful
- Lymphoedema of limbs
- Metastatic disease: anorexia, dyspnoea, lethargy, weight loss

Potential sequelae
- Metastatic disease: ~50% are malignant

Predisposition
- Females >>> males
- Middle-aged to older
- Sexually intact or neutered after first oestrus
- Boston Terrier, Brittany spaniel, Chihuahua, Cocker spaniel, Dachshund, Dobermann, English setter, GSD, Maltese terrier, Springer spaniel, Pointer, Poodle, Yorkshire terrier

Physical examination
- See major/minor signs

Laboratory findings
- Often unremarkable
- May have coagulation changes

Imaging
Radiography
- Thoracic radiographs to evaluate for metastatic disease: pulmonary nodules, lymphadenopathy
- Both laterals with chest inflation under general anaesthesia improve sensitivity, but CT is preferable

Ultrasound
- To evaluate for intrabdominal metastasis:
  - Liver and kidney
  - Bladder and reproductive tract in inflammatory carcinoma
  - Intra-abdominal lymph nodes

Special investigations
- Cytology: can be challenging to differentiate benign vs malignant mammary masses; more useful for looking for lymph node metastasis
- Histopathology:
  - Essential for identifying tumour type, vascular or lymphatic invasion or local invasion

Treatment
- Surgery to remove the tumour with margins is ideal alongside aspiration/removal of draining lymph nodes
- Consult with an oncologist about adjunctive treatment, e.g. radiotherapy or chemotherapy, or use of NSAIDS or anti-hormone treatment
- Analgesia

Monitoring
- Thoracic imaging, lymph node aspiration ± bloods if having chemotherapy

Prognosis
- Survival improved for:
  - Tumour < 3 cm
  - Well-differentiated (low-grade)
- Poorer prognosis if:
  - Advanced disease stage, i.e. widepread metastasis
  - High AgNOR index
  - Poorly differentiated (high-grade)
  - Tumour > 3 cm
  - Vascular or stromal invasion
- Tumour types: carcinoma survive longer than sarcoma or inflammatory carcinoma

5.9.2 OVARIAN REMNANT SYNDROME

Aetiology
- Failure to remove some or all of an ovary; typically the right ovary
- Small amount of ovarian tissue dropped and remaining in abdomen
- Rarely, ectopic/extra-ovarian tissue

Major signs
- Attractive to males
- Bloody discharge
- Vulval swelling

Minor signs
- Behavioural changes
- Excessive licking of vulva
- Mating posture

Potential sequelae
- Can be challenging to find the remnant

Predisposition
- None

Historical clues
- Repeated/cyclical episodes of oestrus-like behaviour in neutered female dog

Physical examination
- If in pro-oestrus/oestrus:
  - Behavioural changes
  - Bloody vaginal discharge
  - Receptive to male
  - Vulval swelling

Laboratory findings
- No specific changes

Imaging
Plain radiographs
- Usually normal

Ultrasound
- Can identify remnant tissue if experienced ultrasonographer, moderate size of residual tissue and oestrus activity
- Also helpful to identify ovarian neoplasia

Special investigations
- Vaginal cytology during signs of oestrus
- Progesterone measurement: increases on basal or stimulated (by HCG or GNRH) consistent with oestrogen exposure
- Anti-mullerian hormone (AMH) levels if increased indicate presence of gonadal tissue
- Histology of removed tissue to confirm ovarian in nature

Treatment
- Long-term use of medical oestrus-suppressing drugs is *not* recommended
- Removal of remnant is advised
- Laparoscopy makes finding the remnant easier
- Performing during oestrus/luteal phase increases chances of locating abnormal tissue

Prognosis
- Excellent with removal of all remnant tissue
- May develop pseudopregnancy after removal; should resolve within 4–8 weeks

5.9.3 PROSTATIC DISEASE

Aetiology
Benign and malignant causes of prostatic enlargement cause clinical signs through interference with normal urinary and faecal flow.

Conditions
q.v. section 2.23
- Benign prostatic hypertrophy (BPH)
- Cyst ± paraprostatic cyst
- Neoplasia
- Prostatitis/prostatic abscess
- Squamous metaplasia: Sertoli cell tumour, exogenous ocstrogen

Major signs
- Dysuria
- Tenesmus: urinary and/or faecal
- Haematuria
- Intermittent haemorrhage from penis, not associated with urination
- Deformed ('ribbon') stool

Minor signs
- Fever
- Hindlimb lameness
- Hindlimb oedema

Predisposition
- Uncastrated male dog
- Increased incidence with age

Potential sequelae
- Recurrent infection if squamous metaplasia or cysts
- Neoplasia may still occur in neutered dogs

Historical clues
- Disease more likely if older intact male (BPH)
- Dripping blood from penis without urination is characteristic of prostatitis or neoplasia

Physical examination
- Rectal examination
  - Abnormal prostate may be enlarged (may be intra-abdominal), asymmetric, firm, and have areas of fluctuance and pain
  - Sublumbar lymphadenopathy suggestive of neoplasia

Laboratory findings
- Rarely any abnormalities

Haematology
- Inflammatory leukogram in prostatitis

Biochemistry
- Azotaemia and hyperkalaemia if urinary obstruction

Urinalysis
- Abnormal cells in prostatic carcinoma
- Haematuria sometimes in BPH, prostatic cyst
- Pyuria in prostatitis

Imaging
Plain radiographs
- Prostatic enlargement
- Sub-lumbar lymph node enlargement with periosteal reaction on lumbar vertebral bodies
- Thoracic radiographs for metastatic disease

Contrast radiographs
- Asymmetric position of urethra if neoplasia or cyst
- Extravasation of contrast on retrograde urethrogram
- Irregular urethral outline

Ultrasound
- Prostate size and changes in echo architecture
- Cysts, abscess, neoplasia

Special tests
- Prostatic wash for culture and cytology
- Suction biopsy using side-hole of urinary catheter
- (Ultrasound-guided) FNA and Tru-cut biopsy

Treatment
BPH
- Anti-androgens: delmadinone or osaterone
- Castration
- Other hormonal treatments, e.g. deslorelin

Squamous metaplasia
- Castration
- Remove Sertoli cell tumour or discontinue oestrogen therapy

Prostatitis
- Analgesia, e.g. NSAIDs
- Antibacterials
- ± Castration if entire
- Surgical drainage ± omentalisation for abscess or large cyst

Prostatic cyst
None unless infected or causing obstruction

Neoplasia
- Chemotherapy: limited efficacy
- Surgical resection or transurethral resection: limited efficacy
- NSAIDs
- Palliative radiotherapy
- Palliative urethral stenting or cystotomy tube

Monitoring
- Clinical signs
- Rectal digital palpation of prostatic size, shape and pain

Prognosis
- Good for BPH
- Fair to guarded for prostatitis, depending on severity
- Poor for neoplasia (carcinoma)

5.9.4 PSEUDOCYESIS (FALSE PREGNANCY)

Aetiology
- False pregnancy typically occurs at end of dioestrus (6–8 weeks after oestrus) when there is abrupt decrease in progesterone and increased prolactin

Major signs
- Licking abdomen/mammary glands
- Mammary development ± milk production
- Mothering inanimate objects
- Nesting behaviour

Minor signs
- Aggression
- Anxiety
- Polyphagia or inappetence
- PU/PD
- Weight gain

Predisposition

- After exogenous progesterone or after recent neutering
- Intact, sexually mature female dogs
- Increased risk with age
  Potential sequela
  - Possible increased risk of mammary neoplasia

Historical clues

- Entire
- Recent season

Laboratory findings

- No significant findings

Imaging

- Can be used to exclude pregnancy from day 24 (ultrasound) or day 44 (radiography) if there is chance dog was mated

Special tests

- Relaxin assay to detect early pregnancy (from day 20–21 post-mating) and differentiate from pseudocyesis

Treatment

- Most self-resolve in 2–3 weeks
- Anti-prolactin drugs, e.g. cabergoline, can be used to speed up resolution of signs, typically within 4–5 days
- Restriction of food can speed resolution
- Supportive treatment: stop dog from licking mammary glands, no hand-milking or compresses as these stimulate lactation
- Use tight-fitting jacket to reduce licking/stimulation of mammary glands

Monitoring

- Clinical signs

Prognosis

- Good prognosis
- Recurrence is common unless neutered

5.9.5 PYOMETRA

Aetiology

- Cystic endometrial hyperplasia is the accumulation of uterine fluid following hormone-related hypertrophy and hyperplasia of endometrial glands
- Pyometra is bacterial infection of the uterus predisposed to by cystic endometrial hyperplasia

Major signs

- Polyuria/polydipsia
- Vomiting
- Vulval discharge

Minor signs

- Abdominal distension
- Anorexia
- Lethargy

Predisposition

- Entire, nulliparous female dogs
- Recent oestrus (within past 2 months, i.e. metoestrus)
- After administration of progestagens ± oestrogens

Potential sequelae

- Septicaemia, renal failure, shock, and death
- Septic peritonitis if ruptures

Historical clues

- Recent season followed by increased thirst

Physical examination

- Dehydration
- Tubular mass in caudo-ventral abdomen, extending cranially

Laboratory findings

Haematology
- Inflammatory leukogram
- Mild non-regenerative anaemia

Biochemistry
- Azotaemia
- Increased ALP activity
- Rule out diabetes mellitus developing in metoestrus

Urinalysis
- Isosthenuria
- Pyuria

Imaging
Plain radiography
- Fluid-dense tubular structure in caudal abdomen, unless open pyometra

Ultrasound
- Distinguish pyometra from pregnancy
- Fluid-filled uterus lying between bladder and colon

Special tests
- FNA not recommended due to risk of uterine rupture
- Vaginal cytology

Treatment
- Correct dehydration
- Ovariohysterectomy (OHE)
- Medical therapy with prostaglandins or the progesterone receptor blocker, aglepristone and antibiosis only relatively safe for open pyometra, carries risk of recurrence if not bred from, and is generally not preferred

Monitoring
- Renal function post-operatively

Prognosis
- Good if OHE performed successfully

5.9.6 TESTICULAR NEOPLASIA

Aetiology
- Seminomas: arise from seminiferous tubules
  - Semi-firm, bulbous, sometimes lobulated masses
- Interstitial (Leydig) cell tumours: originate from cells between the seminiferous tubules
  - Small, soft, bulbous masses which can be cystic
  - Often an incidental finding
- Sertoli cell tumours: sex-cord stromal tumours
  - Bilateral or unilateral
  - Large, firm, lobulated masses
  - Metastasis can occur but is uncommon

Major signs
- Often incidental/asymptomatic
- One enlarged testicle, the other atrophied

- Signs of oestrogen toxicity with Sertoli cell tumour
  - Attractive to other males
  - Hyperpigmentation
  - Mammary development and discharge
  - Pendulous prepuce
  - Truncal alopecia

Minor signs
- Behavioural changes
- Bone marrow suppression (oestrogen): pyrexia, pallor, bruising/bleeding
- Perineal swelling

Potential sequelae
- Testicular tumours can be functional, producing oestrogen, progesterone, or testosterone
- Oestrogen production by Sertoli cell tumours is more common and can lead to:
  - Bone marrow suppression
  - Feminisation
  - Prostatic changes, e.g. metaplasia, cysts
- Excess testosterone production can be associated with Leydig cell tumours with increased risk of:
  - Prostatic disease
  - Perineal hernia
  - Tail gland/perianal gland hyperplasia/adenoma

Predisposition
- Afghan hound, Boxer, GSD, Maltese terrier, Miniature schnauzer, Shetland sheepdog, Weimaraner
- Cryptorchid testes associated with increased risk
- Older (> 10 years), intact males

Historical clues
- Presence of these findings should prompt assessment of testes for tumours:
  - Perineal hernia
  - Perianal hepatoid adenoma
  - Infertility
  - Testicular torsion: neoplasia is predisposing factor

Physical examination
- Testicular palpation
  - Asymmetric testicular shape or firmness
  - Enlarged testicle
  - Palpable mass
  - Other testicle may be atrophied: small and soft

- Firm mass on abdominal palpation or inguinal palpation if retained testicle
- Perineal hernia or perianal mass
- If hyperoestrogenism
  - Bone marrow suppression (pancytopenia), *q.v.* section 3.33
    - Pallor
    - Petechiae/ecchymoses
    - Pyrexia
  - Signs of feminization
    - Attractive to other males
    - Gynaecomastia, mammary hyperplasia, galactorrhoea
    - Pendulous prepuce, prepuce atrophy
    - Symmetrical alopecia, epidermal thinning

Laboratory findings
Haematology:
- Non-regenerative anaemia, leukopenia, and thrombocytopenia with oestrogen toxicity

Imaging
Plain radiographs
- Mass due to secondary prostatomegaly, retained testicle or metastasis to lymph nodes
- Thoracic imaging for metastasis; CT preferable

Ultrasound
- Evaluate for presence and structure of cryptorchid testes and metastases
- Evaluate testes for presence and size/structure of mass

Special investigations
- Cytology can be performed before castration
- Histopathology performed at time of removal of testes/castration
- Oestradiol, testosterone ± progesterone levels may be measured

Treatment
- Castration is treatment of choice; bilateral is recommended even with unilateral tumours
- Chemotherapy may be considered: consult oncologist
- Granulocyte colony stimulating factor (G-CSF) and lithium have been used for pancytopenia
- Radiation therapy: consult oncologist

- Supportive treatment if bone marrow suppression

Monitoring
- Bone marrow suppression: haematology to assess for improvement
- Imaging every 3–6 months for evidence of metastasis
- None indicated if uncomplicated with no systemic effect and benign histopathology

Prognosis
- Excellent if no distant metastasis or bone marrow suppression
- Feminisation syndrome usually improves in 2–6 weeks post-castration unless metastasis is present
- If oestrogen-induced bone marrow suppression, prognosis is guarded

5.9.7 VAGINITIS

Aetiology
- Juvenile vaginitis is common in puppies pre-puberty and typically resolves after first oestrus
- Neutered bitches at any age; tends to be chronic
- Multifactorial and can be made worse by other treatments
  - Chronic urinary tract infection with urethritis/vestibulitis/vulvitis
  - Cystic, urethral, vaginal, or vestibular neoplasia
  - Extensive perivulvar dermatitis
  - Granulomatous uterine stump (stump pyometra)
  - Vaginal foreign body

Major signs
- Excessive licking of vulva
- Pollakiuria
- Scooting/rubbing perineum
- Stranguria
- Vulval discharge, *q.v.* section 1.50

Minor signs
- Attractive to males
- Perivulval dermatitis
- Reluctance to mate

Potential sequelae
- Recurrent infection/irritation if underlying cause not managed
- Self-trauma

Predisposition
- *Brucella canis* infection in endemic areas
- Hooded vulva
- Juvenile before first oestrus
- Neutered status
- Recurrent use of antibiotics
- Self-trauma
- Topical washing

Historical clues
- See above

Physical examination
- Pain/irritation
- Perivulval dermatitis
- Vaginal examination
  - Examine *per vaginum* for foreign body, discharge, structural lesion, e.g. redundant dorsal vulvar folds/stricture/mass/ectopic ureters or for urine pooling/scalding
  - Palpate per rectum for masses
- Vulval discharge: mucoid/haemorrhagic/purulent

Laboratory findings
- Haematology for evidence of inflammation
- Biochemistry for evidence of organ involvement or acute-phase protein pattern
- Urinalysis (cystocentesis preferred) and culture performed

Imaging
- Contrast radiography using retrograde technique can be useful, or CT

- Ultrasound allows evaluation of other organs and elimination of other causes

Special investigations
- Infectious disease testing, e.g. *Brucella canis*
- Vaginal culture may show overgrowth of an atypical bacteria, e.g. pure growth of gram-negative or resistant organisms, e.g. *Pseudomonas* spp. or *Mycoplasma* spp. or yeast overgrowth
- Vaginal cytology shows neutrophils, some lymphocytes and macrophages, and increased numbers of bacteria
- Vaginal histopathology of pinch biopsies may show non-specific lymphoplasmacytic inflammation, occasionally neutrophilic or eosinophilic

Treatment
- Stop any topical flushes
- Prevent self-trauma with collar or similar
- Antibiotics only to be used based on culture and sensitivity and not for mixed growth
- Oestrogen supplementation may help, e.g. estriol at same doses as for urinary sphincter mechanism incompetence
- Probiotics may be useful
- Consider vulvoplasty if severe
- Weight loss can benefit

Monitoring
- Assess for clinical improvement
- If on estriol, monitor for bone marrow suppression

Prognosis
- Juvenile vaginitis usually resolves after first season
- May be a recurrent issue if underlying cause cannot be addressed

5.10 RESPIRATORY SYSTEM

Problems

Presenting complaints

q.v. section 1

1.13 Coughing

1.18 Dyspnoea/tachypnoea

1.28 Haemoptysis

1.29 Halitosis

1.32 Nasal discharge

1.43 Sneezing

1.53 Weight loss

Physical abnormalities

q.v. section 2

2.3 Abnormal lung sounds

2.6 Cyanosis

2.30 Stridor and stertor

Laboratory abnormalities

q.v. section 3

3.30.1 Anaemia

3.30.2 Erythrocytosis

3.32.1 Leukocytosis

Diagnostic Approach

Identify upper- or lower-airway problem by history and physical examination.

- Upper-airway disease
  - Inspiratory respiratory effort/dyspnoea
  - Non-productive cough
  - Positive tracheal pinch
  - Investigations include radiographs, upper-airway examination under light plane of anaesthesia
- Lower-airway disease
  - Expiratory respiratory effort/dyspnoea
  - Productive cough
  - Cough in response to thoracic percussion
  - Investigations include thoracic radiographs or CT, bronchoscopy and broncho-alveolar lavage (BAL)
    - Culture
    - Cytology
    - PCR for *Bordetella*, *Mycoplasma* and viruses involved in canine infectious respiratory disease (CIRD)

Diagnostic Methods

History

Age

- Young: congenital or infectious disease likely
- Older: bronchitis, neoplasia more likely

Breed-associated disease

- See individual diseases

Environment

- Toxin access, e.g. paraquat, warfarin
- Infectious disease risk factors, e.g. vector-borne disease, parasite access

General details

- Exercise tolerance, weight loss, regurgitation, anorexia, etc.
- Respiratory signs: note previous signs, current signs: nature, timing, duration, etc.
- Vaccination status

Onset of signs

- Acute onset increases suspicion of trauma, foreign body, respiratory infection
- Chronic onset increases suspicion of chronic bronchitis, neoplasia

Clinical signs

- Coughing (noting frequency and nature can be useful)
- Dysphonia
- Dyspnoea
- Exercise intolerance (weakness or collapse uncommon)
- Oculo-nasal discharge
- Orthopnoea
- Respiratory noise
- Sneezing
- Tachypnoea
- Weight loss

Clinical examination

Visual inspection

- Observe general body condition, symmetry of nose, neck, chest

Notes on Canine Internal Medicine, Fourth Edition. Victoria L. Black, Kathryn F. Murphy, Jessie Rose Payne, and Edward J. Hall.
© 2022 John Wiley & Sons Ltd. Published 2022 by John Wiley & Sons Ltd.

ORGAN SYSTEMS

- Evidence of haemoptysis: neoplasia/trauma/ foreign body/coagulopathy
- Examine mucous membranes for cyanosis
- Examine fundus for evidence of retinal lesions, e.g. systemic fungal infections
- Examine oral cavity: note halitosis, tonsils, etc.
- Examine nasal region: facial bone symmetry, pain, bilateral air flow through nares, nasal discharge
- Observe respiratory pattern: depth, effort, rhythm, rate (normal 10–30 per minute)
- Listen (without stethoscope) for respiratory noise (inspiratory or expiratory) and observe breathing pattern
  - Inspiratory dyspnoea suggests upper-airway obstruction, restrictive disease, pulmonary fibrosis or pleural effusion
  - Expiratory dyspnoea suggests lower-airway disease
  - Mixed inspiratory/expiratory pattern (restrictive) suggests pleural space disease or parenchymal lung disease, e.g. pulmonary oedema or pulmonary fibrosis
- Dog's posture
  - Barrel chest: severe dyspnoea
  - Standing, neck extended, lips drawn back: severe dyspnoea
  - Sternal recumbency/elbows abducted: orthopnoea
- Lameness or limb swelling: consider hypertrophic osteopathy (HO)
- Horner's syndrome: consider cervical/thoracic lesion

Physical examination
- Abdomen
  - Assess for abdominal enlargement which may be compromising respiration
- Limbs
  - Assess for thickened distal limbs, if present consider HO
- Lymph nodes
  - Assess for local or generalised enlargement

Respiratory examination
- Airway
  - Larynx: deformity/obstruction/vibration
  - Trachea: collapse/foreign body/deviation/ mass

- Cervical thoracic inlet and thorax
  - Assess for evidence of a dilated oesophagus or displacement of trachea by intrathoracic mass
  - Assess for evidence of swellings/pain/rib fractures/subcutaneous emphysema
- Thoracic auscultation
  - Cardiac abnormalities
    - Murmur, tachycardia, gallop sounds, dysrhythmia
  - Respiratory sounds
    - Normal
      - Airway: harsh/coarse/blowing to-and-fro sounds
      - Airway sounds audible at shoulder level, behind triceps
      - Pulmonary/alveolar/small bronchi: vesicular sounds: quiet, soft to-and-fro rustling sounds
      - Vesicular sounds are difficult to hear
    - Abnormal
      - Crackles (bubbling) suggest small-airway disease: obstruction with exudative material, e.g. bronchitis, pulmonary fibrosis or oedema
      - Wheezes (dry, squeaky and continuous) suggest small-airway obstruction, e.g. bronchitis, secretions, neoplasia
      - Referred obstructive sounds: try to localise to upper respiratory tract with the timing of noise in the respiratory cycle and careful auscultation over the larynx and trachea
- Percussion
  - Detect dull areas, e.g. pleural effusion, mass lesions, atelectasis, pneumonia, ruptured diaphragm
  - Horizontal line with dullness ventrally = fluid line = effusion
  - Hyper-resonance with pneumothorax or emphysema

Laboratory findings
Haematology
- Assess for evidence of leukocytosis, e.g. with inflammation/infection
- Eosinophilia may be present in parasitic or immune-mediated disease, e.g. eosinophilic. bronchopneumopathy, heartworm, lungworm
- May detect thrombocytopenia in *Angiostrongylus* infection

Serum biochemistry
- Assess for organ system involvement
- Hypercalcaemia occasionally in *Angiostrongylus* infection

Imaging
Plain radiographs
- Nasal radiographs under GA if nasopharyngeal disease is suspected, *q.v* section 1.32
- Thoracic radiographs (with care in dyspnoeic patients): minimal two views ideally well-inflated inspiratory views
  - Conscious radiographs to assess tracheal collapse may be challenging and fluoroscopy may be required
  - Consolidation, i.e. localised, homogenous increase in radiodensity
    - Abscess
    - Haemorrhage
    - Lobar collapse
    - Lung lobe torsion
    - Primary lung tumour
  - Imaging patterns, *q.v.* section 4.3
    - Alveolar disease
    - Bronchial disease
    - Interstitial disease
  - Vascularity
    - Hypervascularity may be detected in left-sided congestive heart failure, left-to-right shunts, and heartworm
    - Hypovascularity may be detected in right-to-left shunts or hypovolaemia
    - Pulmonary thromboembolism is typically not detected on radiographs

Ultrasound
- Laryngeal to assess for the presence of laryngeal disease, e.g. cysts, masses, paralysis
- Ultrasound of mass/consolidated tissue ± ultrasound-guided fine needle aspirate/Tru-cut biopsy (particularly useful to assess for mediastinal masses)
- May see B-lines in pulmonary infiltrates, e.g. oedema, or fibrosis

Special investigative techniques
- AngioDetect® blood test
- Arterial blood gas analysis
- Baermann technique

- BAL for cytology and culture
- Bronchoscopy
- CT angiography
- Examine laryngeal function under light plane of general anaesthesia (GA)
- Faecal smear to identify lungworm: not very sensitive
- Fluoroscopy to assess for bronchial collapse, barium swallow for swallowing disorders or gastroesophageal reflux in cases with recurrent aspiration pneumonia
- Rhinoscopy/nasopharyngoscopy, *q.v.* section 1.32
- Serology for specific diseases, e.g. *Aspergillus*
- Thoracocentesis for cytology ± culture in cases with pleural effusion
- Ultrasound guided fine needle aspirate (or lung sampling for histopathology)

5.10.1   NASAL DISORDERS

Diseases of the nose may be infectious, inflammatory or neoplastic in origin and result in nasal discharge and/or epistaxis and/or sneezing. Apart from a nasal FB, most start gradually and progress, and if unilateral initially often become bilateral, *q.v.* sections 1.21, 1.32, 1.43.

5.10.1A   CHRONIC IDIOPATHIC RHINITIS

Aetiology
- Chronic idiopathic rhinitis is characterised by a non-specific infiltration of inflammatory cells (predominantly lymphocytes) within the nasal mucosa but is a diagnosis of exclusion. The underlying cause is uncertain but is considered likely to be the interaction between the environment and immune system and is proposed to be caused by a hypersensitivity reaction to allergens and organisms. Aerodigestive disease (i.e. occult gastro-oesophageal reflux of acidic microdroplets causing airway irritation) may contribute to the condition.

Major signs
- Epistaxis (rare)
- Nasal discharge
- Reverse sneezing
- Sneezing
- Stertor

Minor signs
- Inappetence
- Ocular discharge

Potential sequelae
- Post-nasal drip may result in chronic cough or episodes of aspiration pneumonia

Predisposition
- Dolichocephalic dogs including medium- to large-breed dogs and Dachshunds may be predisposed

Historical clues
- May present with unilateral or bilateral signs from onset
- Environmental change (e.g. moving house, boarding elsewhere) may exacerbate or improve signs

Physical examination
- May detect reduced nasal airflow

Laboratory findings
Haematology and serum biochemistry
- Typically unremarkable
- May detect an inflammatory leukogram in dogs with postnasal drip

Imaging
Plain radiographs
- Soft-tissue opacity
- Turbinate destruction

Special investigations
- CT scan or MRI
- Rhinoscopy for visual assessment and biopsy for histopathology

Treatment
- May be very challenging to treat; multiple treatments are described, including:
  - Allergen desensitization

- Anti-fungal treatment and antibiotics used in line with antimicrobial stewardship practices
- Ciclosporin
- NSAIDs
- Prednisolone (inhaled or oral)
- Topical nose drops
  - Maropitant: no clear evidence
  - Glucocorticoids
- Occult aerodigestive disease may be a cause in some dogs, and treatment guided at this may be helpful, *q.v.* section 5.1.3

Prognosis
Although chronic idiopathic rhinitis is unlikely to result in fatal sequelae, treatment can be very challenging and owners may need to be counselled that remission may not be achieved

5.10.1B SINONASAL ASPERGILLOSIS (FUNGAL RHINITIS)

Aetiology
Aspergillus spp. are ubiquitous soil saprophytes. The reason that some dogs develop fungal rhinitis is unclear. However, high fungal spore load, local immune dysfunction, and an altered nasal environment (e.g. after a nasal foreign body, or presence of neoplasia) are thought to play a role. The presence of fungal plaques and local immune response results in significant turbinate destruction.

Major signs
- Epistaxis
- Nasal discharge
- Sneezing
- Stertor

Minor signs
- Inappetence
- Nasal depigmentation

Potential sequelae
- Cribriform plate erosion resulting in neurological signs (rare)
- Disseminated aspergillosis (rare)

ORGAN SYSTEMS

Predisposition
- Mesocephalic and dolichocephalic dogs most likely to be affected, i.e. longer-nosed dogs
- Golden retrievers may be over-represented
- Typically young to middle-aged dogs

Historical clues
- Gradual onset but progressive
- May be unilateral initially and progress to bilateral
- May demonstrate partial improvement to antibiotic therapy, i.e. nasal discharge may become less mucopurulent

Physical examination
- Loss of nasal airflow
- Nasal depigmentation
- Pain on nasal palpation

Laboratory findings
Haematology and serum biochemistry
- Typically unremarkable
- May detect and inflammatory leukogram

Imaging
Plain radiographs
- Hyperostosis and punctate lucencies within the frontal bones
- Soft tissue density in nasal cavities ± frontal sinuses
- Turbinate destruction

Special investigations
- Aspergillus serology is moderately sensitive but has good specificity, i.e. a negative test does not exclude sinonasal aspergillosis but a positive result is likely to be accurate in the presence of clinical signs
- CT scan or MRI is more sensitive than nasal radiographs
- Fungal culture may result in false positive and negative results
  - Culture of swabs or nasal discharge may give false negatives and positives
  - Culture of tissue obtained during rhinoscopy is more likely to be relevant
- Rhinoscopy for visual assessment and biopsy for histopathology

Treatment
- Topical therapy (e.g. clotrimazole) appears to be associated with the best outcome, although the exact optimal method is not certain
  - Combination of topical therapy after trephination of sinuses and extensive debridement of fungal plaques is considered optimal
- Oral therapy (e.g. itraconazole) typically requires extended treatment, is expensive, can have side effects and has variable success (50–70%)

Monitoring
- Repeat examination ± rhinoscopy
- Serological changes not useful
- Some dogs may require multiple treatments

Prognosis
- Generally good for dogs that achieve cure with initial treatment, although relapse may be observed months to years later and some dogs may experience ongoing nasal discharge despite eradication of infection

5.10.2   UPPER-AIRWAY DISORDERS

Diseases of the upper airways (larynx, trachea, mainstem bronchi) may be conformational, degenerative, infectious or, uncommonly, neoplastic. They typically cause coughing and/or inspiratory effort and noise.

q.v. sections 1.13, 1.18

5.10.2A   BRACHYCEPHALIC OBSTRUCTIVE AIRWAY SYNDROME (BOAS)

Aetiology
Brachycephalic dogs have altered facial conformation as a direct result of deliberate breed selection. As a result dogs are at risk of BOAS:
- Stenotic nares
- Elongated soft palate
- Nasopharyngeal turbinates
- Secondary eversion of laryngeal saccules
- Laryngeal collapse

Although a hypoplastic trachea is not strictly part of BOAS, it may be concurrently observed and will exacerbate signs. Similarly oesophageal redundancy and hiatal hernia may be concurrent congenital abnormalities, although dyspnoea can also provoke a hiatal hernia.

Major signs
- Collapse
- Cyanosis
- Dyspnoea
- Exercise intolerance
- Regurgitation
- Stertor
- Stridor

Minor signs
- Concurrent GI signs (aerodigestive disease), including regurgitation and vomiting
- Heat intolerance
- Sleep deprivation

Potential sequelae
- Aspiration pneumonia due to regurgitation
- Low tolerance threshold for future respiratory disease

Predisposition
- Extreme brachycephalic dogs, in particular English bulldog, French bulldog and Pug
- Obesity

Historical clues
- Often apparent on presentation, may be exacerbated by exercise or heat
- Owners may consider signs to be normal for the dog

Physical examination
- Auscultation over the upper respiratory tract (larynx, trachea, etc.) can help localise site of airflow obstruction

Laboratory findings
Haematology and serum biochemistry
- Typically unremarkable, may detect an inflammatory leukogram in dogs with aspiration

Imaging
Plain radiographs
- Assess tracheal dimensions

- Detect aspiration pneumonia: alveolar lung pattern typically affecting the cranial, ventral, right middle lung fields

Special investigations
- Exercise tolerance test
- Fluoroscopy for barium swallow study may be useful to assess for hiatal hernia and other disorders (e.g. redundant oesophagus) in dogs with regurgitation
- Kennel Club respiratory grading function test
- Upper-airway assessment under a light plane of anaesthesia
- Whole-body barometric plethysmography is used mostly in research studies

Treatment
- Surgery may be indicated in some cases:
  - Alar fold resection
  - Laryngeal sacculectomy
  - Staphylectomy: resection of caudal part of soft palate
- In the presence of severe laryngeal collapse, salvage procedures (e.g. permanent tracheostomy) may be needed
- Management of regurgitation may be advised: acid blockers, prokinetics, diet change, postural feeding
- Weight management is a critical step in some dogs

Prognosis
- Cases with long-standing BOAS may develop irreversible secondary changes (e.g. severe laryngeal collapse) and experience a poor prognosis, even after surgery
- Post-operative complications are not uncommon and careful management in the perioperative period is critical

5.10.2B INFECTIOUS TRACHEOBRONCHITIS

Aetiology
Acute infectious respiratory infection, often called 'kennel cough', but more correctly termed canine infectious respiratory disease (CIRD), as it is caused by a mixture of major and minor pathogens and modulated by environmental and immune factors.

- *Bacteria*
  - *Bordetella bronchiseptica*
  - *Mycoplasma* spp.
  - *Streptococcus equi zooepidemicus*
- Viruses
  - Canine adenovirus 2 (CAV2)
  - Canine respiratory coronavirus
  - Canine herpesvirus
  - Canine influenza
  - Canine pneumovirus
  - Parainfluenza virus
- Opportunistic invaders

Major signs
- Acute onset cough

Minor signs
- Inappetence
- Lethargy

Potential sequelae
- Self-limiting, usually within 10 days to 3 weeks
- Occasionally disease is prolonged
- Can develop bronchopneumonia

Predisposition
- Younger dogs more susceptible
- Lack of vaccination

Historical clues
- Recent kennelling, dog training classes, etc. increase risk due to exposure to other dogs

Physical examination
- Coughing easily stimulated by tracheal palpation
- Mild/transient pyrexia

Laboratory findings
Haematology and serum biochemistry
- Typically unremarkable

Imaging
Plain radiographs
- Typically unremarkable

Special investigations
- Tracheal wash cytology, culture and sensitivity and PCR

- Virus isolation may allow identification of the specific cause in a major outbreak

Treatment
- Antibacterials not indicated unless systemically ill or pneumonia
- Antitussives if cough is persistent
- NSAIDs
- Restrict exercise

Monitoring
- Clinical signs, although cough may persist for weeks

Prognosis
- Excellent for recovery in the long term

5.10.2C LARYNGEAL PARALYSIS

Aetiology
Failure of the arytenoid cartilages of the larynx to abduct during inspiration as part of the normal respiratory cycle, which occurs typically due to dysfunction of the recurrent laryngeal nerve. There is also failure of adduction of the arytenoids during swallowing, which increases risk of aspiration of liquids and solids.

Laryngeal nerve dysfunction may occur as part of a polyneuropathy/neuromuscular junction disorder
- Degenerative
  - The most common cause is a gradual-onset progressive polyneuropathy detected in older dogs, also termed geriatric onset laryngeal paralysis and polyneuropathy (GOLPP)
- Autoimmune, e.g. myasthenia gravis
- Infectious causes
- Impingement of the recurrent laryngeal nerve during its course
  - Disorders within the neck including surgery, trauma, or congenital disorder
  - Intrathoracic disease such as neoplasia
- Toxicity
  - Lead poisoning
  - Unidentified toxins in food, *q.v.* section 5.1.3B

Major signs
- Dysphonia: high-pitched bark

- Dyspnoea
- Exercise intolerance
- Stridor

Minor signs
- May develop cough due to aspiration of liquids or solids, in particular immediately after drinking or eating

Potential sequelae
- Heat stroke
- Acute respiratory distress

Predisposition
- Congenital laryngeal paralysis: Bull terrier, Dalmatian, Siberian husky
- Large-breed dogs appear to be predisposed to GOLPP: Labrador retrievers

Historical clues
- Gradual onset, progressive
- Signs tend to be exacerbated by excitement, stress, and humid or hot environments as dogs struggle to pant to dissipate heat

Physical examination
- Auscultation over the larynx may be useful at identifying increased noise
- Neurological examination to assess for concurrent abnormalities in polyneuropathy
- May present with mild signs only apparent during exercise, to severely dyspnoeic and cyanotic

Laboratory findings
Haematology and serum biochemistry
- Typically unremarkable, may detect an inflammatory leukogram in dogs with aspiration

Imaging
Plain radiographs
- Thoracic radiographs to exclude intrathoracic disease as cause of laryngeal paralysis

Ultrasound
- Conscious laryngeal ultrasound is described although technically challenging

Special investigations
- Laryngeal examination under a light plane of anaesthesia; use of doxapram to stimulate

breathing has been advocated but is not recommended
- Thyroid screening for hypothyroidism may be useful, although link with laryngeal paralysis is controversial
- Electrodiagnostics, i.e. EMG and nerve conduction studies, to assess for polyneuropathy

Treatment
- Conservative treatment may be appropriate in some dogs, including:
  - Avoidance of:
    - Dusty environments
    - Exercising during hot weather
  - Harness instead of neck lead
- Emergency treatment may be required in some cases:
  - Cooling where appropriate
  - Oxygen therapy
  - Sedation
  - Short-term glucocorticoid use where laryngeal inflammation is suspected
- Rarely, intubation ± tracheostomy may be required
- Surgery
  - Arytenoid lateralisation laryngoplasty ('tie back') most commonly performed

Prognosis
- Owners must be counselled of the progressive nature of GOLPP in most dogs although in some dogs this is slow and may not impair quality of life further;
- Laryngeal surgery is a palliative treatment
  - Commitment to aftercare, e.g. avoid swimming
  - Risks of aspiration pneumonia following surgery or if concurrent oesophageal dysfunction

5.10.2D TRACHEAL COLLAPSE

Aetiology
Tracheal collapse occurs due to degeneration of the matrix of the tracheal cartilage rings which, in turn, affects the position of the dorsal tracheal membrane and flattens the tracheal lumen. Narrowing of the tracheal lumen increases the velocity of airflow, especially during coughing, and the consequent fall in intraluminal air pressure (Bernoulli's principle) causes

further collapse and, ultimately, airway obstruction. The disease may extend to affect the cartilages of the bronchi and, in this case, is better referred to as tracheobronchomalacia.

Major signs
- Classic 'goose honk' cough
- Collapse
- Cyanosis
- Dyspnoea
- Exercise intolerance
- Stridor

Minor signs
- Dysphonia due to secondary laryngeal collapse
- Retching

Potential sequelae
- Respiratory distress
- Severe exacerbation may occur after GA due to effect of intubation

Predisposition
- Toy-breed dogs: Lhasa Apso, Pomeranian, Shih Tzu, Toy poodles, and especially Yorkshire terrier
- Typically middle-aged onwards at age of presentation

Historical clues
- Careful questioning should assess for risk factors for deterioration:
  - Dust
  - Infectious tracheobronchitis
  - Recent GA
  - Smoke
  - Stress or excitement
  - Weight gain

Physical examination
- Assess for response to tracheal pinch
- Auscultation over the trachea may localise obstruction

Laboratory findings
Haematology and serum biochemistry
- Typically unremarkable

- Increased liver enzymes and bile acids are reported: may reflect concurrent disease such as portal vein hypoplasia

Imaging
Plain radiographs
- Assess tracheal diameter: conscious (i.e. without intubation) radiographs on inspiration (for extrathoracic trachea) and inspiration (intrathoracic trachea)
- Assess for bronchiectasis

Special investigations
- Fluoroscopy during respiratory cycle, and ideally during cough
- Bronchoscopy ± BAL to assess for airway infection or concurrent inflammation; to be carried out with caution, given risk of exacerbation with GA and endoscopic intubation

Treatment
- Emergency treatment
  - Oxygen therapy
  - Reduce stress
  - Sedation
  - Short-acting glucocorticoids may be beneficial if acute inflammation suspected
  - Cooling where appropriate
- Medical management
  - Address concurrent airway infection or inflammation (antibacterials, inhaled or oral glucocorticoids)
  - Antitussives, e.g. butorphanol, codeine, diphenoxylate
  - Harness rather than neck lead
  - Weight loss
- Surgical management
  - Reserved for dogs that have failed medical management, or display collapse
  - Intraluminal stents: first-choice intervention
  - Prosthetic tracheal rings

Prognosis
- Cure is not achieved with medical or surgical management and the emphasis is long-term management, in particular avoiding risk factors causing coughing and exacerbating further tracheal collapse

ORGAN SYSTEMS

5.10.2E TRACHEOBRONCHIAL FOREIGN BODY

Aetiology
Inhalation of foreign material.
- Radiolucent: grass awns
- Radiodense: stones, toys, teeth, etc.

Major signs
- Cough
- Dyspnoea
- Haemoptysis

Minor signs
- Halitosis
- Inappetence

Potential sequelae
- Migration of grass awn
  - Infection elsewhere, e.g. pyothorax, retroperitoneal abscess
  - Lung abscess
  - Pneumothorax

Predisposition
- Common in working dogs and gun dogs
- Dogs exercising in overgrown fields, cereal fields at harvest time, etc.

Historical clues
- Sudden onset of coughing after being in a field, especially near time of cereal harvest

Physical examination
- Abnormally dull percussion if local consolidation/abscess at foreign body (FB) site
- Halitosis, especially if longer history, where FB may have started to decompose
- If focal consolidation: lack of normal respiratory sounds

Laboratory findings
Haematology and serum biochemistry
- Typically unremarkable
- May detect an inflammatory leukogram in dogs

Imaging
Plain radiographs
- Radio-opaque FBs will be evident

- Radiolucent foreign bodies
  - Lungs may appear relatively normal
    - Focal bronchopneumonia: usually right caudal/diaphragmatic lobe bronchus as route is direct straight line from trachea
    - Ill-defined pulmonary infiltrate caudodorsal to heart base; right mainstem bronchus area

Special investigations
- Bronchoscopy

Treatment
- Bronchoscopy for removal
  - Plant material is often difficult to remove: friable nature and the effect of grass awn spikes embedding in airway
  - Multiple attempts may be necessary
  - If marked inflammation and unable to remove FB, and the dog is stable, treat with antibiotics ± anti-inflammatory dose prednisolone and attempt removal again after several days
- Surgical lobectomy is a last resort but necessary in cases where:
  - Abscess has formed
  - FB too firmly lodged for removal
  - FB detected by imaging but is beyond the reach of the endoscope

Prognosis
- Prognosis excellent to good if removal of the FB is successful
- Surgery carries higher risks of respiratory obstruction from purulent material during surgery, and usual risks of thoracotomy

5.10.3 LOWER-AIRWAY DISORDERS

Diseases of the lower airways (small bronchi, bronchioles and alveoli) may be infectious, inflammatory/allergic or, less commonly, neoplastic. They typically cause a soft or productive cough and/or expiratory effort and noise. *q.v.* sections 1.13, 1.18.

5.10.3A CHRONIC BRONCHITIS

Aetiology
Chronic inflammatory condition of medium-sized airways, causing chronic (> 2 months) cough.
- The exact cause is unknown, but infection or inhalant allergy may precipitate it
- Signs are significantly worsened by obesity and dusty, smoky rooms

Major signs
- Cough: dry, hacking, non-productive
- Worse with exercise, excitement or at night

Minor signs
- Exercise intolerance
- Lethargy

Potential sequelae
- Acute respiratory distress
- Secondary bronchopneumonia with systemic signs (pyrexia, depression, inappetence)

Predisposition
- Typically older dogs
- Small-breed dogs may be at increased risk

Historical clues
- Careful questioning should assess for risk factors for deterioration
  - Dust
  - Infectious tracheobronchitis/CIRD
  - Smoke
  - Weight gain

Physical examination
- Harsh bronchial sounds: inspiratory and expiratory crackles, wheezes
- Prolonged expiratory phase of respiration
- Sinus arrhythmia is usually present

Laboratory findings
Haematology and serum biochemistry
- Typically unremarkable, may detect and inflammatory leukogram in dogs with bronchopneumonia

Imaging
Plain radiographs
q.v. section 4.3.2
- Diffuse bronchial pattern with increased peri-bronchial markings ('doughnuts')
- May be interstitial pulmonary infiltrate
- Severe cases may have bronchiectasis

Special investigations
- Bronchoscopy
- BAL cytology, culture and PCR
- CT scan

Treatment
- Address obesity
- Address secondary infection as appropriate, based on investigations
- Avoid risk factors: smoke, dust
- Corticosteroids: ideally inhaled but may initially require oral therapy

Prognosis
- Chronic bronchitis is typically a progressive condition that requires long-term management
- Dogs are vulnerable to secondary infection, in particular if bronchiectasis is present

5.10.3B EOSINOPHILIC BRONCHOPNEUMOPATHY

Aetiology
Eosinophilic bronchopneumopathy (EBP) is characterised by eosinophilic infiltration into the bronchial mucosa and lung and is thought to represent a hypersensitivity reaction.

Major signs
- Cough
- Dyspnoea
- Gagging
- Nasal discharge
- Retching

Minor signs
- Inappetence
- Lethargy
- Tachypnoea

Potential sequelae
- Acute respiratory distress
- Secondary bronchopneumonia with systemic signs, i.e. depression, inappetence, pyrexia

Predisposition
- Siberian huskies and Alaskan malamutes
- Young adult dogs most commonly affected

Historical clues
- Careful questioning should assess for risk factors for deterioration:
  - Dust
  - Infectious tracheobronchitis/CIRD
  - Smoke
  - Weight gain

Physical examination
- Harsh bronchial sounds: inspiratory and expiratory crackles, wheezes
- Prolonged expiratory phase of respiration
- Sinus arrhythmia is usually present

Laboratory findings
Haematology and serum biochemistry
- Dogs may have a peripheral eosinophilia, otherwise unremarkable

Imaging
Plain radiographs
q.v. sections 4.3.1, 4.3.2
- Areas of consolidation/infiltration (nodular)
- Air bronchograms and poorly defined increased interstitial patterns
- Bronchiectasis in severe cases
- Hilar lymphadenopathy

Special investigations
- Exclude parasitic disease
- Bronchoscopy
- BAL: culture and PCR
- CT scan

Treatment
- Avoid risk factors (smoke, dust, address obesity)
- Address secondary infection as appropriate based on investigation
- Corticosteroids, ideally inhaled for long-term management, typically initially require oral therapy

Monitoring
- Typically monitoring on the basis of clinical signs, in some cases haematology (in those with a peripheral eosinophilia), and thoracic radiographs may be useful

Prognosis
- Dogs typically respond well to oral glucocorticoids; however, relapse is common (50–70% of cases) and lifelong therapy may be required. Dogs are vulnerable to secondary infection, in particular those with bronchiectasis.

5.10.3C LUNGWORM (*ANGIOSTRONGLYLUS VASORUM*)

Aetiology
Angiostrongylus resides in the pulmonary arteries and damages the lungs through larval migration and thromboembolism, so is probably best termed a lungworm. However, it is sometimes called a heartworm, and initially was called the 'French heartworm', as France was where it was first identified. However, it is now spreading further north in mainland Europe and the UK. It should be distinguished from the heartworm *Dirofilaria* (*q.v.* section 5.2.1C), and other true lungworms, e.g. *Crenosoma vulpis* (fox lungworm), *Eucoleus aerophilus* (formally *Capillaria aerophilus*), *Eucoleus boehmi*, *Filaroides hirthi*, and *Oslerus osleri* (formally *Filaroides osleri*)

A nematode that has intermediate stages in molluscs, canine infection is acquired by ingestion, deliberately or accidentally if eating grass, of slugs and snails infected with L3 larvae. After ingestion, the larvae penetrate the gut wall, eventually arriving at the right ventricle and pulmonary arteries via lymphatics and venous return from the gut. Adults reside within the pulmonary artery, where they reproduce. Larvae are carried to the pulmonary parenchyma via the vasculature, where they penetrate the bronchial and alveolar walls and are coughed up, swallowed and eventually pass in faeces. As well as pulmonary disease, lungworm can also cause bleeding episodes by an undetermined mechanism and neurological signs, which may be due to intracranial bleeds or aberrant larval migration. Rare cases of ocular larval migration are reported.

Major signs
- Cough
- Dyspnoea
- Ecchymoses and petechiation
- Neurological signs: seizures, vestibular disease, spinal cord disease
  - Aberrant larval migration
  - Bleeding diathesis
- Tachypnoea

Minor signs
- Ascites
- Exercise intolerance
- Nasal discharge

Potential sequelae
- Hypercalcaemia may result in PU/PD
- Pulmonary hypertension may occur in some dogs and result in syncope
- Severe dyspnoea may result in acute respiratory distress

Predisposition
- Typically younger dogs which perhaps are more indiscriminate eaters
- Chronic enteropathy causing dog to eat grass

Historical clues
- Known ingestion of molluscs (slugs/snails)
- Lack of anti-parasiticide treatment

Physical examination
- Abnormal respiratory noise, e.g. crackles
- Bleeding secondary to coagulopathy
  - Check for evidence or mucosal bleeds or petechiation/ecchymoses
- Ocular/retinal examination: active chorioretinitis lesions may be detected

Laboratory findings
Haematology
- Peripheral eosinophilia
- Regenerative or pre-regenerative anaemia due to haemorrhage
- Thrombocytopenia

Serum biochemistry
- Hyperglobulinaemia
- Hypercalcaemia

Imaging
Plain radiographs
- Patchy, diffuse, peripheral alveolar-interstitial pattern
- Sometimes nodules can be seen: need to differentiate from metastatic neoplasia
- Large pulmonary vessels
- Right-sided cardiomegaly

Special investigations
- Bronchoscopy and BAL but diagnosis should be achieved prior to this
  - Lungworm PCR on BAL fluid
- AngioDetect® blood test
- Coagulation parameters (PT, aPTT, D-dimers) may be abnormal
- Direct faecal smear is a useful, quick and cheap screening test but has lower sensitivity than AngioDetect®
- Echocardiogram may detect adult worms, or evidence of pulmonary hypertension
- Faecal analysis (Baermann technique) for larvae
- Pulse oximetry ± arterial blood gas

Treatment
- Milbemycin oxime, imidacloprid/moxidectin and fenbendazole are all described
- Corticosteroids at anti-inflammatory doses, in theory, to reduce the inflammatory reaction from dying worms
- Management of coagulopathy may be required, i.e. plasma transfusion, tranexamic acid
- Management of pulmonary hypertension may be required

Monitoring
- Monitoring clinical signs
- Repeat Baermann technique on faeces

Prognosis
- Variable, depending on presenting signs
- Thought to be poorer in dogs with neurological signs and those with pulmonary hypertension

5.10.4 PULMONARY PARENCHYMAL DISEASE

Diseases affecting the lung alveoli and interstitium can be inflammatory, infectious, neoplastic or neurogenic. They cause dyspnoea through prevention of gas exchange between the alveoli and pulmonary vasculature. Coughing may not be a major feature, but a soft or productive cough or haemoptysis may be present, *q.v.* sections 1.13, 1.18, 1.28.

5.10.4A PNEUMONIA

Aetiology
Pneumonia is infection and secondary inflammation of the lungs involving the alveoli.
- The most common cause in dogs is aspiration pneumonia
- Other causes
  - Bacterial bronchopneumonia, e.g. extension of *Bordetella* or *Mycoplasma* infection
  - Even less commonly
    - Extension of infection
    - Haematogenous spread
    - Migrating FB
    - Fungal infection, e.g. *Pneumocystis carinii* infection
    - Tuberculosis
    - Viral infection, e.g. canine influenza

Major signs
- Cyanosis
- Dyspnoea
- Pyrexia
- Soft cough
- Tachypnoea

Minor signs
- Inappetence
- Lethargy
- Nasal discharge

Potential sequelae
- Acute respiratory distress
- Pyothorax (parapneumonic)

Predisposition
- Aspiration pneumonia
  - Brachycephalic dogs due to hiatal hernia and BOAS
  - Laryngeal paralysis
  - Megaoesophagus
- Immune disorders
  - Ciliary dyskinesia increases risk of recurrent pneumonia
  - CKCSs and Miniature Dachshunds may be at increased risk of *Pneumocystis carinii* infection, suspected due to underlying immunodeficiency
  - Irish Wolfhounds suspected to have immunodeficiency
- Kennelled greyhounds are most commonly described in *Streptococcus zooepidemicus* infections

Historical clues
- Recent general anaesthetic, vomiting/regurgitation or force-feeding may increase suspicion of aspiration pneumonia
- Dogs with extension of upper respiratory infection may have gradual-onset progressive signs
- Dogs with viral infection or *Streptococcus zooepidemicus* are likely to present with acute onset fulminant signs

Physical examination
- Restrictive breathing pattern (increased effort on inspiration and expiration)
- Pyrexia
- Tachypnoea
- Thoracic auscultation:
  - Reduced sounds (areas of consolidation)
  - Bronchovesicular sounds (crackles and wheezes)

Laboratory findings

Haematology
- Neutrophilia with left shift
- May be consumptive neutropenia ± degenerate left shift

Serum biochemistry
- Acute-phase protein response: hypoalbuminaemia, hyperglobulinaemia
- Increased CRP

Imaging

Plain radiographs
- Alveolar pattern: fluffy, indistinct, air bronchograms, local/diffuse often ventral lobes
- Bronchial and interstitial patterns may also be seen
- Hilar lymphadenopathy

Ultrasound
- B-lines may be visible on thoracic ultrasound scan

Special investigations
- Bronchoscopy and BAL for cytology, culture and PCR (with caution, in particular in dogs with a suspicion of aspiration pneumonia where GA may increase risk of further aspiration events)
- Pulse oximetry to assess oxygenation ± arterial blood gas
- Lung fine needle aspirate (reserved for cases with consolidated lung, in particular those with a suspicion of *Pneumocystis carinii* infection)

Treatment
- Acute treatment
  - Empirical antimicrobial treatment where there is a high index of suspicion of bacterial infection
    NB: Dogs with aspiration may have non-infectious, chemical pneumonitis rather than bacterial pneumonia.
  - Oxygen supplementation
  - Nebulisation and coupage
  - Gentle exercise may help recruit alveoli if dog can tolerate it
- Anti-pyretic therapy may be considered, although pyrexia is an adaptive response to combat infection
- Mechanical ventilation may be considered in specific scenarios but the prognosis is typically guarded in these cases

Monitoring
- CRP may be useful to track response to treatment and may be a more practical solution when compared to repeat radiographs
- Haematology
- Pulse oximetry (± arterial blood gas)
- Repeat radiographs
- Temperature

Prognosis
- Depends on cause and severity of signs
- Dogs with severe BOAS and concurrent hypoplastic trachea may have a guarded prognosis

5.10.4B NON-CARDIOGENIC PULMONARY OEDEMA

Aetiology
Accumulation of fluid within the lung fluid including alveoli. Occurs due to abnormal pulmonary vasculature hydrostatic pressure or vessel permeability, or both.

Causes
- Acute respiratory distress syndrome (ARDS), which may occur due to severe systemic or pulmonary disease, e.g. pancreatitis, aspiration pneumonia, or envenomation
- Electrocution
- Seizures (neurogenic oedema)
- Upper respiratory tract obstruction

Major signs
- Cyanosis
- Dyspnoea
- Tachypnoea
- Tachycardia

Minor signs
- Anorexia

Potential sequelae
• May be fatal if severe

Predisposition
• Laryngeal paralysis causing airway obstruction, *q.v.* section 5.10.2C
• Young puppies tend to present with non-cardiogenic pulmonary oedema due to misadventure (e.g. electrocution, strangulation by neck lead, playing with other dogs)

Historical clues
• Choking, upper respiratory tract obstruction, electrocution, or strangulation event may have been observed, e.g. chewed electric cord, struggling when restrained on table at dog groomers, during play, laryngeal paralysis

Physical examination
• Oral ulceration in electrocution, but may take up to 72 hours to be visible
• Tachycardia
• Tachypnoea

Laboratory findings
Haematology and serum biochemistry
• Typically unremarkable, changes related to underlying cause may be detected, e.g. pancreatitis

Imaging
Plain radiographs
• Diffuse pulmonary-alveolar interstitial pattern
• More likely to occur in caudo-dorsal lung fields

Ultrasound
• B-lines on thoracic ultrasound

Special investigations
• Investigations for underlying cause (where upper respiratory tract obstruction not observed/suspected)
• Pulse oximetry ± arterial blood gas

Treatment
• Oxygen therapy
• Sedation as needed

• Treatment of underlying cause
• Mechanical ventilation may be required in some cases
  NB: Diuretic therapy is not effective.

Monitoring
• Clinical signs
• Track radiographic changes

Prognosis
• Depends on underlying cause
• ARDS associated with poor prognosis but depends on ability to treat underlying cause
• If due to upper respiratory tract obstruction or neurogenic cause and can be supported for first 72 hours, long-term prognosis good

5.10.4C PULMONARY FIBROSIS

Aetiology
Underlying cause unknown, although thought to be an abnormal inflammatory response to an alveolar insult. The fibrosis extends to the alveolar wall and eventually results in abnormal oxygenation of blood due to compromised gas exchange. Aerodigestive disease may exacerbate the condition.

Paraquat poisoning can cause peracute signs of pulmonary haemorrhage with CNS, GI and renal signs, but more commonly causes progressive dyspnoea due to irreversible pulmonary fibrosis, almost inevitably leading to death or euthanasia.

Major signs
• Cyanosis
• Dyspnoea
• Exercise intolerance
• Tachypnoea

Minor signs
• Collapse
• Lethargy

Potential sequelae
• Acute dyspnoea and sudden deterioration may occur in some dogs
• Euthanasia before death

Predisposition
- Idiopathic pulmonary fibrosis: WHWT

Historical clues
- Access to paraquat
- Typically, gradual onset of progressive signs, although some may present in acute crisis

Physical examination
- Cyanosis
- Restrictive breathing pattern
  - Abdominal breathing
- Tachypnoea
- Thoracic auscultation
  - Crackles on inspiration: sounds like crinkling of cellophane
  - May also detect wheezes

Laboratory findings
Haematology and serum biochemistry
- Typically unremarkable
- Erythrocytosis, due to chronic hypoxia,

Imaging
Plain radiographs
- May be unremarkable as not 100% sensitive
- Moderate to severe bronchointerstitial lung pattern
- Pulmonary hypertension: right-sided cardiomegaly, pulmonary artery enlargement

Ultrasound
- B-lines on thoracic ultrasound

Special investigations
- Echocardiogram to assess for pulmonary hypertension
- Lung biopsy for histopathology (rarely performed but gold standard)
- Pulse oximetry ± arterial blood gas
- Thoracic CT

Treatment
- Oxygen therapy in acute deterioration
- Treatment if pulmonary hypertension detected
- Treatment with corticosteroids is described and might be beneficial in a small number of patients

Monitoring
- 6-minute walk test described in WHWT to assess for severity and progression of disease

Prognosis
- Typically guarded as a progressive disease
- Some dogs experience extended survival (years), whereas others present with acute dyspnoea, which appears to be associated with poor survival

5.10.4D PULMONARY NEOPLASIA

Aetiology
- Primary pulmonary tumours arise *de novo* in bronchus or smaller airways
  - Adenocarcinoma is the most common type
  - Chondrosarcoma arising from a tracheal ring is rare
  - Primary rib tumours (chondrosarcoma, osteosarcoma) can cause pleural effusion
- Lymphoma infiltrating the lungs is unusual, but bronchial lymph nodes may be affected in multicentric lymphoma; mediastinal lymphoma and thymomas can cause pleural effusion
- Lungs are a common site for metastatic tumours
  e.g. any carcinoma but especially mammary, haemangiosarcoma
- Clinical signs are related to airway obstruction by tumour, haemorrhage or fluid

Predisposition
- Association with passive smoking not yet proven
- Middle-aged to old dogs

Major signs
- Dry cough
- Dyspnoea more common with metastasis (cough less frequently)
- Exercise intolerance/lethargy/depression
- Increasing tachypnoea/orthopnoea/dyspnoea
- Weight loss

Minor signs
- Lameness: HO or metastasis to bone
- Haemoptysis: most common with primary lung adenocarcinoma, *q.v.* section 1.28

Potential sequelae
- Progressive signs
- Pleural effusion
- Death

Historical clues
- Presence of a primary tumour elsewhere, or history of previous excision

Physical examination
- Areas of increased/decreased or abnormal lung sounds
- Heart sounds may be muffled or in abnormal position due to displacement by mass
- Mediastinal shift due to mass: trachea no longer in midline at thoracic inlet
- Tachypnoea/dyspnoea/orthopnoea
- Thoracic percussion may identify fluid or areas of dullness

Laboratory findings
Haematology
- Abnormal circulating lymphocytes may be seen in stage V lymphoma
- Anaemia if significant haemorrhage
- Inflammatory leukogram may be seen with necrotic centre of tumour

Serum biochemistry
- Usually unremarkable
- Paraneoplastic hypercalcaemia in mediastinal lymphoma

Imaging
q.v. section 4.3
- Left and right lateral, inflated radiographs highlight masses; CT is more sensitive
- Primary lung tumour
  - Lobar consolidation: no air bronchograms
  - Increased pulmonary interstitial markings
  - One or more discrete soft-tissue masses
  - Right caudal lobe more commonly affected than other lobes
  - Pleural effusion
  - Hilar/sternal lymphadenopathy
- Metastatic neoplasia
  - Multiple, discrete, round soft-tissue masses ('cannonballs') or more miliary nodular pattern in interstitium: best seen over other

soft-tissue structures, e.g. diaphragm and heart (DDx pleural nodules, end-on blood vessels)
- Pleural effusion

Special investigations
- Bronchoscopy: neoplastic cells sometimes seen in the BAL
- Transthoracic fine needle aspiration/Tru-Cut biopsy: with ultrasound guidance for cytology/histopathology
- Thoracocentesis of pleural effusion
- Thoracoscopic biopsy
- Thoracotomy and biopsy/resection

Treatment
- Primary lung adenocarcinoma
  - Surgical lobectomy of the affected lobe(s) and removal of associated LNs
  - Adjuvant chemotherapy for patients with non-resectable masses or evidence of lymph node metastasis, e.g. cisplatin, vinblastine
- Secondary/metastatic
  - One or two metastatic masses: excision rarely appropriate as often micrometastasis is already present elsewhere
  - Attempt excision or pleurodesis if metastas
  - Systemic chemotherapy: generally disappointing outcome

Monitoring
- Check for recurrence of tumour by radiographs

Prognosis
- Primary lung tumours tend to have slow growth so even incomplete resection can provide a prolonged period of good-quality life
- Surgical/anaesthetic complications should be considered
- Survival times after surgery
  - Lobe and LN affected: 4 months
  - Lobe only: 12 months
- For metastatic neoplasia the prognosis is guarded/poor

ORGAN SYSTEMS

5.10.5 PLEURAL SPACE DISEASE

Accumulation of fluid or air in the pleural space, causing respiratory compromise due to lung lobe collapse.

Neoplasia within the chest cavity is likely to cause clinical signs of dyspnoea due to the accumulation of pleural fluid. Mediastinal masses occasionally cause caval syndrome, *q.v* section 5.7.2.

5.10.5A IDIOPATHIC CHYLOTHORAX

Aetiology
Abnormal accumulation of lymphatic fluid within the pleural space where other causes are excluded, i.e. cardiac disease, lung lobe torsion, neoplasia and trauma.

Major signs
- Collapse
- Cyanosis
- Dyspnoea
- Tachycardia
- Tachypnoea

Minor signs
- Anorexia
- Lethargy

Potential sequelae
- Lung lobe torsion may be primary or develop secondary to pleural effusion
- Pyothorax may develop with repeated drainage
- Restrictive pleuritis: failure of lungs to re-expand following drainage, due to development of fibrosis of pleura

Predisposition
- Afghan hound, Mastiff, Shetland sheepdog
- Lung lobe torsion: Pug

Historical clues
- Typically gradual onset and may have large-volume effusion at time of diagnosis

Physical examination
- Dull ventral lung sounds
- Dyspnoea
- Restrictive breathing pattern
- Tachypnoea

Laboratory findings
Haematology
- Lymphopenia

Serum biochemistry
- Typically unremarkable, but hyponatraemia and hyperkalaemia may occur due to third-space effect of a large-volume effusion

Imaging
Plain radiographs
- Pleural effusion

Ultrasound
- Presence of pleural fluid which may be strongly echogenic

Special investigations
- Thoracocentesis for cytology and biochemistry
  - Triglycerides are higher and cholesterol lower when compared to serum
- Echocardiogram to exclude cardiac disease (rare in dogs)
- Lymphangiography may be considered to assess thoracic duct leak
- Test for heartworm

Treatment
- Medical management
  - Intermittent thoracocentesis or pleural port placement for drainage
  - Low-fat diet, octreotide, and rutin described although evidence very limited
- Surgical management
  - Any combination of thoracic duct ligation, subtotal pericardectomy, cisterni chyli ligation, and thoracic omentalisation

Prognosis
- Prognosis is fair but recurrence of pleural effusion following surgery is not uncommon (~30%)

5.10.5B PNEUMOTHORAX

Aetiology

Pneumothorax refers to free air in the pleural space and may occur due to direct communication with the external environment due to trauma, or related to an air leak from the major airways and/or lungs due to intrathoracic pathology.

- Iatrogenic
  - Barotrauma during GA or bronchoscopy
  - Thoracocentesis/chest tube placement
  - Thoracotomy
- Spontaneous
  - Lungworm
  - Pulmonary neoplasia
  - Rupture of bullae or pleural blebs
  - Severe pneumonia
  - Tracheal rupture
- Trauma

  Major airway damage can, alternatively, cause pneumomediastinum and/or subcutaneous emphysema.

Major signs

- Dyspnoea
- Tachypnoea
- Tachycardia
- Cyanosis
- Collapse

Minor signs

- Lethargy
- Anorexia
- Pain

Potential sequelae

- Migrating FB may cause pyothorax or retroperitoneal abscess
- Tension pneumothorax may occur and is rapidly fatal if not addressed

Predisposition

- No known predisposition

Historical clues

- Typically acute-onset cardiorespiratory compromise

Physical examination

- Dyspnoea
- Restrictive breathing pattern
- Tachypnoea
- Thoracic auscultation
  - Dull dorsal lung sounds

Laboratory findings

Haematology and serum biochemistry

- Typically unremarkable
- Changes related to underlying cause, e.g. pneumonia

Imaging

Plain radiographs

- Air in pleural space with cardiac-sternal separation on lateral view

Ultrasound

- Loss of pulmonary glide sign

Special investigations

- CT scan may be more sensitive for detecting bullae and blebs, although not 100% sensitive
- Thoracotomy for exploration and treatment

Treatment

- Iatrogenic and traumatic pneumothorax may respond well to thoracocentesis alone
- Treat underlying cause where identified
- Surgery should be considered when underlying pathology not treated, or bulla or bleb identified on imaging
- Blood pleurodesis is described in dogs where surgery is not an option or has failed

Prognosis

- Depends on underlying cause: those with spontaneous pneumothorax surgically managed appear to experience a low risk of recurrence (around 10%)
- Pleurodesis often unsuccessful

5.10.5C PYOTHORAX

Aetiology
Accumulation of purulent material within the pleural space.
- Haematogenous spread
- Migrating FB
- *Nocardia*, *Actinomyces*; may be associated with migrating grass awn
- Penetrating wound, especially bite wounds
- Spread from pneumonia = parapneumonic pyothorax

Major signs
- Dyspnoea
- Pyrexia
- Tachypnoea

Minor signs
- Cough
- Inappetence
- Lethargy
- Vomiting and diarrhoea

Potential sequelae
- Septic shock which may be fatal

Predisposition
- Dogs at increased risk of inhalation of foreign bodies (e.g. those that run in long grass, cereal fields at harvest time) may be predisposed

Historical clues
- Typically relatively acute-onset presentation, may be preceded with respiratory signs, e.g. cough

Physical examination
- Restrictive breathing pattern
- Dyspnoea
- Tachypnoea
- Pyrexia
- Thoracic auscultation: dull ventral lung sounds

Laboratory findings
Haematology
- Neutrophilia with left shift
- May be consumptive neutropenia ± degenerate left shift

Serum biochemistry
- Acute phase protein response: hypoalbuminaemia and hyperglobulinaemia
- Hypoglycaemia in severe cases

Imaging
Plain radiographs
- Pleural effusion
- Hilar lymphadenomegaly
- May detect pulmonary lesions, e.g. abscessed lung lobe

Ultrasound
- Presence of pleural fluid which may be strongly echogenic

Special investigations
- CT scan: may be more sensitive at detecting FB, although not always identified
- Thoracocentesis, as treatment and for cytology and culture

Treatment
- Thoracocentesis
- Medical management
  - Antimicrobial therapy
  - Chest drain: temporary to fully drain chest or indwelling to allow intermittent drainage
- Surgical management
  - Indicated in cases with pulmonary abscess or where evidence of filamentous bacteria on cytology or culture (*Actinomyces* or *Nocardia*) as more likely to be associated with plant material

Monitoring
- Clinical signs
- Haematology
- Imaging
- Volume and cytology of pleural fluid during intermittent drainage

Prognosis
- Typically good provided appropriate treatment, although recurrence is likely if FB not found

5.11 SYSTEMIC INFECTIONS

Systemic infections are not necessarily confined to specific organs and may affect the whole body:
- As part of a multisystemic disorder, e.g. *Brucella*, distemper, *Leishmania*, *Neospora*, rabies, *Toxoplasma*
  - Acquired directly or indirectly from an infected dog or other mammalian host
  - Ingestion of paratenic hosts carrying infective larvae
  - Injection by arthropod hosts
- By extension of local infection, e.g. cryptococcosis, bacterial otitis media, empyema from bite wounds or migrating foreign body
- Secondary to iatrogenic causes, e.g. injection, surgical wound
- Through haematogenous spread, e.g. abscess, discospondylitis or septic arthritis secondary to endocarditis

Systemic infections may cause secondary effects, e.g. due to hypercoagulable states or hyperviscosity

Problems
Presenting complaints
q.v. section 1
1.1 Abortion
1.5 Anorexia/hyporexia/inappetence
1.7 Anuria/oliguria
1.8 Ataxia
1.9 Bleeding
1.10 Blindness
1.13 Coughing
1.15 Diarrhoea
1.16 Drooling
1.17 Dysphagia
1.18 Dyspnoea/tachypnoea
1.19 Dysuria
1.21 Epistaxis
1.25 Haematemesis
1.26 Haematochezia
1.27 Haematuria and discoloured urine
1.28 Haemopytsis
1.31 Melaena
1.32 Nasal discharge

1.34 Paresis/paralysis
1.35 Perinatal death
1.37 Polyuria/polydipsia (PU/PD)
1.39 Pruritus
1.40 Red eye (and pink eye)
1.42 Seizures
1.43 Sneezing
1.44 Stiffness, joint swelling and generalised lameness
1.47 Tremors
1.49 Vomiting
1.50 Vulval discharge
1.51 Weakness, collapse and syncope
1.53 Weight loss

Physical abnormalities
q.v. section 2
2.1 Abdominal enlargement
2.3 Abnormal lung sounds
2.4 Arrhythmias
2.5 Ascites
2.6 Cyanosis
2.7 Eye lesions
2.8 Hepatomegaly
2.10 Hypertension
2.11 Hypotension
2.12 Hypothermia
2.13 Icterus/jaundice
2.14 Lymphadenopathy
2.15 Murmur
2.17 Pain
2.18 Pallor
2.20 Peripheral oedema
2.23 Prostatomegaly
2.25 Pyrexia and hyperthermia
2.26 Skin lesions
2.27 Skin pigmentation changes
2.28 Splenomegaly
2.29 Stomatitis
2.30 Stridor and stertor

Laboratory abnormalities
q.v. section 3
3.4 Azotaemia

ORGAN SYSTEMS

Notes on Canine Internal Medicine, Fourth Edition. Victoria L. Black, Kathryn F. Murphy, Jessie Rose Payne, and Edward J. Hall.
© 2022 John Wiley & Sons Ltd. Published 2022 by John Wiley & Sons Ltd.

3.6 Bilirubin
3.8 Cardiac biomarkers
3.12 Creatine kinase
3.13 Creatinine
3.14 C-reactive protein
3.17.2 Hypoglycaemia
3.20 Liver enzymes
3.25 Symmetric dimethylarginine (SDMA)
3.27 Total protein (albumin and globulin)
3.29 Urea
3B Haematology
3C Urinalysis

Diagnostic Approach
1 Suspect systemic infection based on:
   - Exposure risk
   - History of travel or import history
   - Problem list
2 Screening routine laboratory tests
3 Perform specific tests: the best test varies according to the infection
   - Culture
   - Cytology/histology
   - PCR
   - Serology

Diagnostic Methods
Diagnostic methods
History
- Onset of clinical signs and progression
  - Acute and can progress rapidly typically
  - Organ systems may be affected sequentially
- History of tick or other vector exposure
- Infectious disease risk evaluation based on current and previous geographical locations
- Lifestyle/environment
  - Rural vs urban, i.e. fields, woodland
  - Swimming in open water
- Any response to previous treatment
- Any in-contact pets or owners affected

Physical examination
- Thorough clinical examination with particular attention to lymphoid organs (lymph nodes, spleen, and liver) and assessment for any foci of pain or possible sites of infection/inflammation
- Pyrexia may be present

Laboratory findings
Haematology
- Evidence of anaemia of chronic disease or regenerative anaemia due to haemolysis or haemorrhage, depending on infectious agent
- Leukocytosis or leukopenia
- Thrombocytopenia in some infections

Serum biochemistry
- Changes dependent on organ systems affected, e.g. acute kidney injury and liver damage with leptospirosis, increased muscle enzymes with *Toxoplasma/Neospora*
- Hyperglobulinaemia with some infections, e.g. leishmaniasis, ehrlichiosis

Urinalysis
- Evidence of infection, e.g. *Leptospira*
- UPC

Imaging
Plain radiographs/CT
- Changes secondary to specific and non-specific infections
- Changes to intervertebral discs with discospondylitis
Can lag behind clinical signs by ~6 weeks for plain radiographs and 3–4 weeks for CT

Ultrasound
- Focus of infection/inflammation including migrating foreign bodies
- Intrathoracic or intra-abdominal lymphadenomegaly, lymphadenopathy or organ enlargement

Special investigative techniques
- Infectious disease screening (serology, PCR, culture, fluorescent *in-situ* hybridisation)
Choice of test is disease-dependent
- Sample for cytology and histopathology
- Serum protein electrophoresis in dogs with hyperglobulinaemia

Specific Conditions
q.v. section 5.1
- Bacterial enteritis
- Endoparasites
- Parvovirus

q.v. section 5.2.1C
- *Dirofilaria*

q.v. section 5.10
- *Angiostrongylus*
- Bacterial bronchopneumonia
- Infectious tracheobronchitis

5.11.1 ANAPLASMOSIS

Aetiology
Anaplasmosis is caused by obligate, intracellular, gram-negative bacteria.
- *Anaplasma platys* (tick vector *Rhipicephalus sanguineus*) infects platelets and can cause canine cyclic thrombocytopenia
- *Anaplasma phagocytophilum* (tick vector *Ixodes ricinus*) mainly infects granulocytes, causing granulocytic anaplasmosis and can infect humans

Major signs
- Inappetence
- Lameness
- Lethargy
- Pyrexia
- Reluctance to move

Minor signs
- Bleeding disorders
- Cough
- Diarrhoea/vomiting
- Lymphadenopathy
- Neurological signs

Potential sequelae
- Self-limiting or asymptomatic infections are common

Predisposition
- Retrievers may be over-represented with *A. phagocytophilum* infection

Historical clues
- History of living in or travel in endemic areas
- History of tick exposure

Physical examination
- Evidence of bleeding disorder e.g. petechiae
- Hepato/splenomegaly
- Lymphadenopathy

- Pyrexia

Laboratory findings
Haematology
- Anaemia and leukopenia/leukocytosis may be present
- Blood smear evaluation may reveal presence of the organism, i.e. up to 60% of cases with *A. phagocytophilum* from 4 days post-infection, 20% for *A. platys*
- Thrombocytopenia is common

Serum biochemistry
- Decreased albumin, urea
- Increased ALP and ALT activities, bilirubin, globulins

Imaging
- Non-specific findings

Special investigations
- Blood smear examination; see above
- Serology
  - Confirms exposure not active infection and can be negative in acute infection
  - Rising titre after further 10–14 days
- PCR most sensitive method of confirming infection
  - *A. platys* PCR of bone marrow or splenic aspirates more sensitive than blood
- Co-infections are common

Treatment
- Doxycycline 10 mg/kg q24h or 5 mg/kg q12h for 14–28 days is the most common treatment
- Supportive treatment, e.g. fluids, analgesia and anti-inflammatory treatment
- Occasionally glucocorticoids needed for secondary immune-mediated disease

Monitoring
- PCR can be used to assess response to treatment
- Serology is not appropriate as can remain positive for many months after eradication of infection

Prognosis
- Good response to treatment and chronic infection does not appear to be an issue

ORGAN SYSTEMS

Prevention
- Prevention with use of tick preventatives; checking daily for ticks is advised

5.11.2 BABESIOSIS

Aetiology
Babesiosis (piroplasmosis) is caused by protozoan, intraerythrocytic parasites that are transmitted by ticks but can also pass transplacentally and via blood transfusions and possibly via dog bites. Co-infections are common.
- Babesia are grouped according to size
  - Microbabesiae: *B. conradae*, *B. microti*, *B. vulpes*
  - Small organisms: *B. gibsoni*
  - Large organisms: *B. canis*, *B. rossi*, *B. vogeli*
- *Babesia* (sub)species have variable virulence
  - Mild: *B. vogeli*
  - Moderate to severe: *B. canis*
  - Highly pathogenic: *B. gibsoni*, *B. rossi*
  - Uncertain: microbabesiae
- Babesia species vary in their tick vector
  - *B. canis*: *Dermacentor reticulatus*
  - *B. gibsoni*: *Haemaphysalis* spp., *Rhipicephalus sanguineus*
  - *B. rossi*: *Rhipicephalus sanguineus*
  - *B. vogeli*: *Rhipicephalus sanguineus*

Major signs
- Jaundice
- Lethargy/depression
- Pallor
- Pigmenturia
- Pyrexia

Minor signs
- Diarrhoea/weight loss (*B. gibsoni*)
- Neurological signs
- Petechiae/ecchymoses
- PLN: *B. gibsoni*, *B. microti*-like
- Reduced urine output
- Tachypnoea

Potential sequelae
- Complicated babesiosis has an acute or peracute presentation and can be associated with severe haematological signs as well as systemic inflammatory response syndrome and organ failure
- Uncomplicated babesiosis has acute/subacute presentation, mild anaemia and thrombocytopenia and a good response to treatment

Predisposition
- *B. canis*: GSD and Komondor in Hungary
- *B. canis rossi*, *vogeli*: younger dogs show more severe signs
- *B. gibsoni*: Pit bulls in United States
- *B. rossi*: entire females at lower risk for
- *B. microti-like* infection: older hunting dogs with higher risk of azotaemia

Historical clues
- History of tick exposure
- History of living/travel in endemic areas

Physical examination
- Hepato/splenomegaly
- Icterus
- Lymphadenopathy in chronic cases
- Pallor ± petechiae/ecchymoses
- Signs associated with neurobabesiosis

Laboratory findings
Haematology
- Mild to severe anaemia – haemolytic and will become regenerative
- May auto agglutinate
- May be Coombs' positive
- Parasite may be seen on blood smear
- Thrombocytopenia
- ± Leukopenia (neutropenia) or leukocytosis

Serum biochemistry
- Increased bilirubin and liver enzymes
- Increased creatinine and urea
- Increased cPL if secondary pancreatitis
- Hypokalaemia, hyponatraemia
- Hypoglycaemia

Urinalysis
- Proteinuria and cylinduria

Imaging
- Non-specific findings, e.g. hepato/splenomegaly

Special investigations
- Blood smear
  - Fresh sample from pinnal vein increases the chances of parasite detection in the RBCs
  - Lower levels of detection in chronic cases or cases with low parasite load
- PCR is test of choice with high sensitivity and specificity and can be used to identify infecting *Babesia* spp.
- Serology confirms exposure but not active infection and might be negative in acute infection; cannot be used to identify infecting *Babesia* spp.

Treatment
- Large Babesia spp., e.g. *B. canis*
  - Imidocarb dipropionate 5–6.5 mg/kg SC or IM on two occasions, 14 days apart
- Small *Babesia* spp., e.g. *B. gibsoni*
  - Atovaquone 13.3 mg/kg three times daily and azithromycin 10 mg/kg once daily for 10 days
  - More difficult to treat and several other protocols exist
- Supportive care includes fluid therapy, oxygen support and in some cases blood transfusion
- Treatment of organ failure
- Use rapid-acting acaricide in infected dogs to treat all life stages of ticks, which may be attached but not visible

Monitoring
- Monitor CBC and biochemistry for worsening anaemia, thrombocytopenia and organ failure (kidney/liver)
- Check PCR before stopping treatment and again 2 months after treatment

Prognosis
- Clinical cure is possible but not parasitological cure
- Clinical improvement usually seen within 1–7 days but can take up to 15 days
- Mortality up to 50% with *B. canis*
- Re-infection is possible
- Small *Babesia* spp., particularly *B. gibsoni*, are difficult to clear and can recur during stress

Prevention
- Check daily for ticks
- Screen blood donors with PCR
- Use of tick preventatives
- Vaccines are available but considered non-core

5.11.3 BORRELIOSIS (LYME DISEASE)

Aetiology
Borreliosis (Lyme disease) is a tick-borne (*Ixodes* tick, *I. ricinus* in Europe) infection caused by spirochaete bacteria from *Borrelia* spp., particularly *Borrelia burgdorferi*

Major signs
- Asymptomatic in most cases
- Fever
- Joint swelling
- Lameness which may be shifting

Minor signs
- Anorexia
- Lethargy
- Lymphadenopathy
- Signs of myocarditis: induced arrhythmia
- Signs of nephritis: anorexia, weight loss, lethargy, vomiting

Potential sequelae
- 5–10% of dogs develop clinical signs
- Asymptomatic/self-limiting infection in most dogs
- Can develop Lyme nephritis, which can cause a protein-losing nephropathy with membranoproliferative glomerulonephritis, tubular necrosis and interstitial nephritis
- Important cause of disease in humans, but not zoonotic

Predisposition
- Higher levels of seroconversion reported in Bernese mountain dogs in Switzerland
- More serious complications reported in Labradors and Golden retrievers

Historical clues
- Travel/movement in tick-infested endemic areas

Physical examination
- Pyrexia
- Lymphadenopathy
- Joint swelling
- Shifting lameness

Laboratory findings
Haematology and biochemistry
- Non-specific changes
- Rarely evidence of organisms on blood smear

Urinalysis
- Proteinuria, casts

Imaging
- Nonspecific: may be evidence of joint effusion or renal changes

Special investigations
- Culture of organisms is exceedingly difficult
- Co-infections are common, screening is advised
- Joint fluid analysis shows inflammatory arthropathy
- PCR is a very specific test but limitations mean it is not recommended for diagnosis
  - Low sensitivity on blood; better in joint fluid
  - Can be used on tick bites in skin, connective tissue or joint capsule biopsies
  - Does not differentiate live and dead organisms
- Serology is advised to confirm exposure
  - Can take 3–4 weeks to become seropositive after infection
  - If vaccinated against Lyme disease, check validity of test in vaccinated dogs
  - Quantitative C6 assays can be used before and 3–6 months after treatment to evaluate treatment success

Treatment
- Doxycycline 5 mg/kg twice daily or 10 mg/kg once daily for 28 days
- Alternatively cefovecin: two injections 14 days apart has also been shown to be effective
- Supportive treatment, e.g. analgesia, treatment PLN/Lyme nephritis
- Prevention with use of tick preventatives, checking daily for ticks is advised

Monitoring
- Although dogs can remain infected, infection is generally sub-clinical and there is limited evidence about treatment of these dogs. Follow-up advised if clinical signs persist.

Prognosis
- Improvement is typically seen within 24–48 hours of starting treatment in acute cases
- Clearance of infection is challenging, therefore relapse may be seen
- Chronic kidney disease may develop
- Overall prognosis fair to good but if Lyme nephritis is present guarded to poor

Prevention
- Vaccination is available but is considered non-core

5.11.4   BRUCELLOSIS

Aetiology
Brucellosis is caused by infection with bacteria from the *Brucella* genus.
- *Brucella canis*, *B. melitensis*, *B. suis* and *B. abortus* can infect dogs, with *B. canis* being the most common.
- Transmission can be venereal or via inhalation or ingestion.
- *B. canis* is shed in reproductive secretions, urine, milk and other body fluids and the highest concentration of organisms is in aborted material. It is a potential zoonosis.

Major signs
- Abortion/stillbirths
- Scrotal changes: oedema, pyogranulomatous dermatitis
- Testicular changes: orchitis, epididymitis causing pain and swelling

Minor signs
- Early embryonic death
- Endocarditis
- Infertility: male and female
- Meningitis
- Ocular lesions, e.g. uveitis
- Osteomyelitis
- Pyogranulomatous dermatitis

- Pyrexia
- Signs associated with discospondylitis: pain, neurological deficits, etc.

Potential sequelae
- Abortion
- Infertility
- Stillbirth

Predisposition
- *B. canis* is endemic in the Americas, parts of Asia, Africa and Eastern and Central Europe
- Spayed/neutered animals can carry *B. canis*

Historical clues
- History of abortion or stillbirths
- History of scrotal/testicular disease
- Lived in or travelled in countries with higher levels of infection

Physical examination
- May be normal
- Can develop scrotal dermatitis, scrotal oedema, testicular enlargement
- Chronic disease can result in testicular atrophy
- Hepatosplenomegaly
- Lymphadenopathy

Laboratory findings
Haematology and biochemistry
Non-specific changes consistent with inflammatory disease

Urinalysis
- Bacteriuria
- Proteinuria

Imaging
- Nonspecific, e.g. appendicular osteomyelitis, discospondylitis
- Testicular changes on ultrasound

Special investigations
NB potential zoonosis, contact laboratory before sending samples
- Bacterial culture of blood, semen, vaginal discharge or aborted foetus/placenta can be useful. Bacteraemia is intermittent so false negatives might be obtained.
- Semen analysis

- Culture for *Brucella*
- Cytology: immature sperm, damaged sperm, inflammatory cells
- PCR
- PCR can be performed on body fluids, blood or aborted material but does not differentiate live or dead organisms
- Serology
  - 2–4 weeks for seroconversion so can be negative in acute infection or if pre-treated with antibiotics
  - Can remain positive up to 3 years after infection
  - Different test methodologies exist: discuss results with your laboratory

Treatment
Euthanasia of infected dogs is considered the only way to completely remove the risk of onward transmission
- Antibiotic treatment
  Probably impossible to clear infection; combination treatment used,
  e.g. doxycycline/minocycline and gentamicin or streptomycin and gentamicin
- Neuter intact dogs after treatment
- Consider enucleation with ocular infection as eye can act as nidus of infection
- Supportive management based on presentation, e.g. discospondylitis

Monitoring
- Bacterial culture or agar-gel immunodiffusion serology test (CPAg-AGID) should be repeated at end of antibiotic treatment and every 3 months until two negative tests are obtained

Prognosis
- Prognosis for clinical improvement is good but for elimination of infection is guarded
- Relapse is common
- Potential zoonosis

Prevention
- Clean environment with standard disinfectants
- Do not use infected dogs for breeding, even after treatment
- If an infected dog is identified, the kennels should be quarantined, and infected dogs

identified and removed from breeding; kennels should be closed until the disease is eliminated
- Potential zoonosis so consider euthanasia

5.11.5 DISTEMPER

Aetiology
Distemper is caused by an RNA virus and affects carnivores. It can occur in combination with other respiratory infections as part of canine infectious respiratory disease complex, *q.v.* section 5.10.2B.
- It is easily spread in respiratory secretions via aerosol and droplets and is shed in all body fluids from infected dogs
- It spreads from the respiratory epithelium to lymphoid organs including liver and spleen and then to the gastrointestinal and urogenital tracts and central nervous system and skin, e.g. footpads

Major signs
- Cough
- Dermatological signs
  - Pustular dermatitis
  - Nasal or footpad hyperkeratosis ('hard pad')
- Diarrhoea
- Dyspnoea
- Hypoplasia of dental enamel
- Nasal discharge
- Neurological signs occurring 1–3 weeks after systemic disease or much later in life
  - Ataxia
  - Cerebellar or vestibular signs
  - Cervical rigidity
  - Hyperaesthesia
  - Myoclonus: repetitive jerky limb movements
  - Paresis
  - Seizures
- Pyrexia
- Serous-mucopurulent conjunctivitis
- Vomiting

Minor signs
- Abortion/stillbirth
- Cardiomyopathy
- Dehydration
- Hypertrophic osteopathy

- Ocular signs
  - Keratoconjunctivitis sicca (KCS), uveitis, chorioretinitis, optic neuritis
- Tenesmus
- Weight loss

Potential sequelae
- Can be fatal if adequate immune response is not generated within 14 days after infection
- If an equivocal immune response occurs, some antibodies will be generated but clinical signs still seen. The infection may then be cleared from tissues other than the uveal tract, CNS and skin, where it can persist long-term
- If adequate immune response is generated, no clinical signs may be evident, and the virus may be cleared from the tissues

Predisposition
- Unvaccinated dogs
- Younger or immunosuppressed dogs

Historical clues
- Unvaccinated dogs
- Outbreaks in area/kennels

Physical examination
- A combination of signs is highly suggestive: starting with oculo-nasal discharge, coughing and GI signs, neurological signs may follow and, in survivors, hard pad and enamel hypoplasia are indicative of past infection

Laboratory findings
Haematology
- Leukopenia ± anaemia, thrombocytopenia, monocytosis and neutrophilia

Serum biochemistry
- Hyperphosphataemia, hypoproteinaemia and hypoalbuminaemia can be present

Imaging
- Interstitial/alveolar pattern may be seen on thoracic radiographs
- Signs consistent with hypertrophic osteodystrophy/metaphyseal osteopathy may be present

Special investigations

- CSF analysis
  - Increased protein, cell counts and antibody titres can be assessed on non-blood-contaminated samples in dogs displaying late-onset neurological signs
- Distemper inclusion bodies may be seen in cells on blood smears and conjunctival cytology
- Immunofluorescent antibody tests and immunochromatographic tests may be available
- PCR can be performed on buffy coat smears, conjunctival swabs, CSF, whole blood and urine sediment. A cut-off discriminates between wild-type infection and vaccine interference
- Serology can indicate protective levels of antibodies after vaccination, or previous or current infection (after seroconversion occurs), so they are non-specific
- Virus isolation/culture is difficult to perform

Treatment

- No specific treatment is available
- Supportive treatment, e.g. fluid therapy, treatment of secondary infections, nebulisation/coupage for bronchopneumonia and other treatment based on clinical signs

Monitoring

Clinical signs

Prognosis

- Variable and depends on strain and severity
  - Mortality up to 50% is reported
  - Neurological signs are associated with guarded to poor prognosis
- More severe in puppies or immunocompromised older dogs

Prevention

- Vaccination has been effective in reducing the incidence of disease

5.11.6   EHRLICHIOSIS

Aetiology

Ehrlichiosis is caused by intracellular, gram-negative *Ehrlichia* spp. bacteria which are tick-transmitted, mainly by *Rhipicephalus sanguineus* in Europe. Canine monocytic ehrlichiosis is most commonly caused by *Ehrlichia canis*.

Major signs

- Anorexia
- Bleeding disorders: petechiae/ecchymoses, epistaxis, ocular bleeds
- Lethargy
- Pyrexia
- Weight loss

Minor signs

- Neurological signs
- Ocular signs: conjunctivitis, uveitis

Potential sequelae

- Subclinical, acute and chronic phases of infection exist
- Incubation period is 1–4 weeks but transmission can start within hours of tick attachment
- Some dogs clear the infection after acute or subclinical phase
- With severe chronic disease, bone marrow aplasia can result in pancytopenia and high mortality

Predisposition

- GSD and Siberian Husky dogs appear predisposed to severe disease

Historical clues

- Living in or travel in endemic areas
- Tick exposure

Physical examination

- Hepato/splenomegaly
- Lymphadenopathy
- Ocular inflammation/haemorrhage
- Pallor
- Peripheral oedema
- Petechiae/ecchymoses
- Pyrexia

Laboratory findings

Haematology
- Leukocytosis/leukopenia
- Granular lymphocytosis
- Intracellular bacteria (morulae) may very rarely be seen in monocytes
- Non-regenerative anaemia: autoagglutination, Coombs' positive
- Pancytopenia (chronic)
- Thrombocytopenia

Biochemistry

- Azotaemia
- Hyperglobulinaemia: polyclonal gammopathy
- Hypoalbuminaemia
- Mild increase in ALT/ALP activities

Urinalysis

- Proteinuria

Imaging

- Non-specific findings, e.g. hepato/splenomegaly

Special investigations

- Lymph node FNA; sensitivity 50% if performed by skilled person
- Organisms in blood smear: low sensitivity, buffy coat may increase chances
- PCR of EDTA blood or tissue aspirates
  - Positive from 4–10 days post-infection
  - Positive result is specific and consistent with active infection
  - Quantitative PCR allows bacterial load to be monitored
- Serology: IFAT or ELISA
  - Antibodies develop by 3–4 weeks post-infection
  - Confirms exposure, not necessarily active infection
    - Four-fold increase in titres over 2 weeks consistent with active infection
  - Cross-reactivity between *Ehrlichia* spp. and *Anaplasma phagocytophilum* possible
  - Quantitative results allow assessment of changes over time
- Testing for co-infections recommended

Treatment

- Doxycycline 10 mg/kg daily for 28 days
  - Antibody titres persist for years post-infection even with treatment and re-infection can occur
  - Recheck haematology
    - Two weeks after starting treatment
    - At end of treatment
    - Four weeks after end of treatment
- Glucocorticoids for immune-mediated components, e.g. uveitis, thrombocytopenia
- Supportive treatment for organs affected
  - Blood transfusion
  - Iron supplements

- Prophylactic antibiotics if severe neutropenia < 1 × 10⁹/l
- Renal support

Monitoring

- Clinically well, seropositive, no haematological changes
  - Monitor clinically, haematology and serology at least every 6 months
- Four-fold increase in titre or PCR evidence in blood/tissue = infection = treat
- Repeat PCR blood and/or other tissues ideally 1–2 months post-treatment
  - Still positive
    - Further 3–4 weeks treatment
    - Then try to prevent re-infection
  - Still positive, try another treatment

Prognosis

- Clinical/haematological cure possible but not parasitological cure
- Prognosis depends on whether infection is acute or chronic
  - Acute infection
    - Good prognosis
    - Normally clinical improvement within 24–48 hours of treatment
    - Haematological changes improve over 1–3 weeks
  - Chronic infection
    - Poor prognosis
    - Antibody titres can persist for months to years
    - Haematological changes are very slow and can take months to improve, if ever
    - Hyperglobulinaemia may take 3–6 months to improve
- Reinfection is possible

Prevention

- Check and remove ticks at least q24h in endemic areas
- Consider screening blood donors
- Tick prevention product, which ideally repels and kills ticks

5.11.7 HEPATOZOONOSIS

Old World hepatozoonosis is a tick-borne disease caused by the protozoal agent *Hepatozoon canis*. It is transmitted by ingestion of the brown dog tick, *Rhipicephalus sanguineus*, and so is geographically restricted to countries harbouring the tick. It typically causes subclinical infection, with signs only occurring in immunosuppressed dogs.

New World hepatozoonosis is an emerging, potentially fatal infection caused by *Hepatozoon americanum*. It is transmitted via the Gulf Coast tick, *Amblyomma maculatum*, and consequently is most common in the Gulf states of North America and is probably also present in Central and South America.

Neither form of hepatozoonosis has been recorded in the UK. Refer to standard textbooks for information on clinical signs, diagnosis and treatment.

5.11.8 LEISHMANIOSIS

Aetiology

Leishmaniosis is a zoonotic infection caused by *Leishmania infantum*, a protozoan parasite. The incubation period is long and dogs can present with disease many years after the initial exposure. The outcome of infection is determined by the hosts own immune response.

It is transmitted:
- Naturally by sandflies
- Possibly via other vectors
- Vertical transmission
- Via infected blood transfusion

Major signs
- Cutaneous lesions
  - Food pad hyperkeratosis
  - Onychodystrophy
  - Papular/pustular dermatitis
  - Periocular alopecia
  - Poor hair coat
  - Scaling/exfoliative dermatosis
  - Ulceration
- Lymphadenopathy
- Pallor
- Splenomegaly

Minor signs
- Epistaxis
- Lameness/polyarthritis

- Ocular changes
  - Blepharitis
  - Conjunctivitis
  - Eyelid nodules
  - Keratitis
  - Uveitis
- PU/PD
- Signs of kidney failure/glomerulonephritis
- Signs of meningitis
- Signs of vasculitis
- Vomiting/diarrhoea
- Weight loss

Potential sequelae
- Infected dogs may:
  - Clear the infection due to a competent immune system
  - Develop subclinical infection if they have an adequate cell-mediated immune response but which can become active at periods of stress/immune suppression
  - Develop progressive disease where they develop a humoral immune response which is associated with development of immune complex disease

Predisposition
- Breeds susceptibility: Boxer, Cocker, GSD, Rottweiler
- Breed resistance: Ibizan hound
- Immunocompromised dogs are more susceptible to developing clinical disease
- Reported in Foxhounds in United States
- More common in dogs under 3 years or over 8 years of age

Historical clues
- History of living in or travel to endemic areas

Physical examination
- Epistaxis
- Lameness
- Lymphadenopathy
- Masticatory muscle wastage
- Neurological signs
- Ocular lesions as above
- Pallor
- Petechiation/ecchymoses
- Pyrexia
- Skin and nail lesions as above

- Splenomegaly
- Stomatitis

Laboratory findings
Haematology
- Non-regenerative anaemia
- Impaired secondary coagulation and fibrinolytic disorders reported
- Leukocytosis/leukopenia
- Thrombocytopenia, thrombocytopathy

Biochemistry
- Azotaemia
- Hyperglobulinaemia with polyclonal gammopathy
- Hypoalbuminaemia
- Increased C-reactive protein
- Increased liver enzymes

Urinalysis
- Low USG
- Proteinuria

Imaging
- Non-specific findings

Special investigations
- PCR
  - More useful in lesional tissue than in blood, e.g. bone marrow, lymph node, nasal/conjunctival, skin
  - Negative PCR does not exclude infection
  - Positive result confirms infection but is not correlated with disease stage
  - Recommended screening in blood donors
- Serology
  - Antibodies against *Leishmania* can take 5–7 months for seroconversion, i.e. false negative early in disease
  - Highly sensitive in clinically affected cases and can be used for long-term follow-up
  - Quantitative serology recommended over qualitative, i.e. positive/negative
- Cytology/histology
  - Lymphoid hyperplasia and granulomatous inflammation can indicate infection but demonstration of organisms in macrophages (intracellular amastigotes) or extracellular from lymph nodes, liver, spleen, bone marrow and skin samples is definitive

Treatment
Refer to Leishvet.org or Canine Leishmaniasis Working Group for up-to-date information on staging and treating *Leishmania* infection.
- Use a leishcidal and leishstatic drug
- Leishcidal drug
  - Miltefosine 2 mg/kg PO q24h for 4 weeks
  or
  - Meglumine antimonate 75–100 mg/kg SC q24h for 4 weeks
- Leishstatic drug
  - Allopurinol
    - 10–15 mg/kg BID for minimum 6–12 months in addition to Leishcidal drug
    or
    - As sole therapy (10–20 mg/kg BID) in mild cases
    or
    - As sole therapy at lower dose of 5 mg/kg q12h in advanced cases with severe CKD
  - Domperidone: improves immune response
  - Nucelotide supplements can be used
- Low-purine diet to reduce risk of xanthine crystals/uroliths when using allopurinol
- Symptomatic treatment, e.g. management of CKD, proteinuria

Monitoring
Refer to Leishvet.org or Canine Leishmaniasis Working Group
- Clinical examination and repeat bloods based on stage of disease and severity of abnormalities at diagnosis, but at least every 3–6 months
- Repeat serology after at least 6 months of treatment and then every 6–12 months; PCR optional
- Serum protein electrophoresis can be used in addition to laboratory monitoring at earlier stage than serology
- Urinalysis ± imaging for xanthine crystals/uroliths

Prognosis
- Prognosis is variable and depends on the severity at diagnosis
  - Parasitological cure is rare and relapse is possible
  - Renal disease is the main cause of death

ORGAN SYSTEMS

Prevention
- Collars or spot-on products with synthetic pyrethroids that repel sandflies
- Domperidone can reduce risk of developing disease
- Keep dogs indoors from sunset till dawn (April to November); use mosquito nets on doors
- Vaccinations available: some interfere with further use of serology for diagnosis and reduce risk of developing disease rather than prevention of infection

5.11.9 LEPTOSPIROSIS

Aetiology
Leptospirosis is caused by infection with spirochaete bacteria from the genus *Leptospira* and can cause peracute, acute, subacute and chronic disease. It is a zoonotic infection.

The dog is the definitive host for *Leptosira interrogans* (serogroup canicola, serovar canicola) but there is a variety of pathogenic serogroups (and their important serovars) infecting dogs in Europe.
- *Leptospira interrogans*
  - Australis (australis, bratislava)
  - Canicola (canicola)
  - Icterohaemorrhagiae (icterohaemorrhagiae)
  - Pomona
  - Sejroe
- *Leptospira kirschneri*
  - Grippotyphosa
- The organisms grow well in warm, moist environments and can be found in stagnant slow-moving water. Flooding and heavy rainfall can be associated with higher levels of contamination and increased incidence of infection
- Endemic infection may persist in wild rats and in other domesticated and wild species
- Organisms penetrate via mucous membranes and wet or damaged skin
  - Direct transmission
    - Bites
    - Eating infected tissue
    - Infected urine; contamination of wounds or mucous membranes
  - Placental transfer
  - Venereal
- Indirect transmission can occur via contaminated bedding, food, soil and water

Major signs
- In peracute, minimal clinical signs before death
- Abdominal pain
- Anorexia
- Anuria
- Bleeding
- Icterus
- Muscle pain
- Pyrexia or hypothermia
- Shivering
- Vomiting/diarrhoea, including acute haemorrhagic diarrhoea syndrome

Minor signs
- Abortion/infertility
- Conjunctivitis/uveitis
- Cough
- Dyspnoea
- Neurological signs
- Ophthalmological signs
- Stiff gait/lameness
- Tachypnoea/dyspnoea
- Weight loss

Potential sequelae
- CKD and chronic hepatitis after recovery from acute illness
- Organ failure, systemic inflammatory response syndrome and DIC
- Pulmonary haemorrhage syndrome rare
- Ultimately, death

Predisposition
- More severe disease in younger dogs
- Mixed-breed, working/hunting dogs at increased risk
- Possibly entire males at higher risk
- Increased risk in unvaccinated dogs

Historical clues
- Exposure to farm animals and wildlife, including rodents
- Recent heavy rainfall or flooding
- Unvaccinated animal

ORGAN SYSTEMS

Physical examination
- Abdominal pain
- Arrhythmia
- Dehydration
- Hepatomegaly/pain
- Hypovolaemia
- Icterus
- Petechiae/ecchymoses/mucosal bleeds
- Pyrexia
- Renomegaly/pain

Laboratory findings
Haematology
- Anaemia and thrombocytopenia
- Initial leukopenia then leukocytosis ± left shift

Serum biochemistry
- Azotaemia common
- Bilirubin may be increased
- Electrolyte abnormalities and hypocalcaemia can be seen
- Hypoglycaemia with severe liver disease/sepsis
- Liver enzymes can increase, often 6–8 days after renal disease
- Myositis can occur with increased CK and AST
- Pancreatitis can occur with increased pancreatic lipase
- Prolonged coagulation times and increased D-dimer, fibrinogen and FDPs

Urinalysis
- Bilirubinuria
- Glucosuria
- Inflammation and casts
- Proteinuria

Imaging
- Interstitial-alveolar pulmonary infiltrates associated with leptospiral pulmonary haemorrhage syndrome, initially in caudodorsal lung fields
- Ultrasonography can show
  - Changes in intestines, liver, gall bladder, spleen and lymph nodes
  - Pancreatic changes: enlargement, variable echogenicity

- Renal changes: renomegaly, pelvic dilation, hyperechoic cortices, reduced corticomedullary definition, perirenal effusion

Special investigations
- Culture is exceedingly difficult and dark-field microscopy of fresh urine is generally not available
- PCR testing
  - Blood: positive up to 10 days after infection
  - Urine: positive after 10 days from infection or
  - Testing both if the chronology is unknown
  - Pre-treatment with antibiotics can result in false negatives and chronic carrier status can be associated with positive urine PCR
- Serology
  - Microscopic agglutination test (MAT) is most commonly used
    - A single serovar titre ≥ 1:800 in a serogroup not included in vaccine or > 4 months since vaccination is consistent with active infection
    - Negative titres can be seen early in disease, so repeating serology after 2 weeks to assess for rising titre is recommended
  - Patient-side serological tests are available and may be more able to detect early infection

Treatment
- Antibiotics
  - Doxycycline 5 mg/kg BID for 2 weeks is the treatment of choice as it can aid clearance of renal carrier status
  - Initial therapy with penicillin-based antibiotic can be used, but must be followed up by 2 weeks of doxycycline
- Supportive treatment
  - Fluid therapy and treatment of AKI when present
  - Symptomatic treatment, e.g. analgesia, anti-emetics, hepatic antioxidants, treatment of bleeding disorders

Monitoring
- Initially bloods are repeated every 24–48 hours with more frequent electrolyte/acid–base evaluation as needed

- Monitor urine output and adjust fluid therapy accordingly
- Urinalysis and bloods should be repeated at 1 week, then at 1, 3 and 6 months after discharge as CKD can develop

Prognosis
- Prognosis is good, with survival of 80–90% with early recognition and treatment
- Dogs with pulmonary signs or severe renal disease have a poorer prognosis

Prevention
- Control of rodent populations and reducing access to stagnant and flood water is advised
- Isolation of infected dogs and use of protective clothing/gloves/eye protection can reduce environmental contamination and spread of infection to other pets and people
- Prevention includes using multi-serogroup vaccinations according to manufacturers' guidance
  - Duration of immunity with vaccination is 6–8 months, with some protection up to 12 months, so annual revaccination is important

5.11.10 NEOSPOROSIS

Aetiology
Neosporosis is caused by a protozoan parasite, *Neospora caninum*. It causes primarily neuromuscular disease and can be fatal. Transmission can occur vertically and horizontally via contaminated water and ingestion of infected tissues. Faecal transmission may also occur.

Major signs
- Neuromuscular signs, *q.v.* section 5.8
  - Hyperaesthesia
  - Muscle wasting/swelling
- Hindlimbs worse than forelimbs
  - Limb paralysis
  - Progressive muscular rigidity/muscle contraction
- Neurological signs: ataxia, cerebellar signs, cranial nerve deficits, meningitis, seizures, vestibular signs, weakness

- Dyspnoea
- Diarrhoea

Minor signs
- Cervical weakness
- Dysphagia
- Megaoesophagus
- Paralysis
- Cardiac disease
- Ulcerative dermatitis, exudative nodules
- Ultimately, death

Potential sequelae
- Myocarditis
- Neurological consequences
- Peritonitis
- Pneumonia
- Severe muscle contracture
- Ultimately, death is possible

Predisposition
- Clinical signs are more common in young dogs < 6 months of age
- Clinical disease is more severe in immuno-compromised dogs

Historical clues
- Living in rural environment, particularly with cattle
- Raw diet

Physical examination
As above

Laboratory findings
Haematology
- Mild non-regenerative anaemia
- Mild eosinophilia
- Monocytosis

Serum biochemistry
- Increased ALT/CK/AST activities from muscle damage
- Hyperglobulinaemia and hypoalbuminaemia less commonly

Imaging
- Radiographs may show evidence of pneumonia or megaoesophagus

- Advanced imaging/MRI should be considered with neurological signs: multifocal lesions may be seen

Special investigations
- Cytology of skin lesions or other lesional tissue may demonstrate intracellular organisms
- Faecal samples for oocysts
- Histology and IHC to demonstrate organisms in tissue samples
- PCR on CSF other body fluids and tissue
- Serology
  - Seroconversion occurs up to 3 weeks after infection
  - Repeat serology may be needed to show rising titre in acute disease

Treatment
- It is difficult to effectively treat: long-term treatment is often needed and relapses are seen
- Treatment is more effective before muscle contracture occurs
  - Clindamycin at 15–22 mg/kg q12h for 4–8 weeks alone or with trimethoprim sulphonamide at 15–20 mg/kg q24h for 4–8 weeks
    or
  - Sulfonamide at 15–30 mg/kg q12h for 4–8 weeks combined with pyrimethamine at 1 mg/kg q24h
- Supportive treatment with analgesia and nutritional/fluid support

Monitoring
- Test littermates of affected neonates in view of vertical transmission

Prognosis
- Prognosis is poor to guarded
  - Cutaneous signs are associated with better prognosis
  - Once muscle contracture has developed, treatment will not reverse this
  - Relapses are common

Prevention
- Avoid immunosuppression in seropositive dogs
- Avoid raw/undercooked offal and meat

- In known positive dams, avoid the pups nursing
- Remove faeces to maintain hygiene in the environment

5.11.11 RABIES

Aetiology
Rabies is a Lyssavirus, a genus of RNA viruses in the family *Rhabdoviridae*, and can infect warm-blooded animals. It is neuroinvasive and invariably fatal.
- It is transmitted via bites from an infected animals, although transmission via wounds/ mucous membranes with infected saliva or neural tissue is possible
- It is a fatal zoonotic infection

Major signs
- Altered behaviour
  - Aggression
  - Anxiousness/nervousness
  - Ataxia
  - Hyperacsthesia
  - Photophobia
- Anorexia
- Inability to swallow
- Paresis/paralysis
- Seizures

Minor signs
- Change in voice
- Cranial nerve deficits
- Disorientation
- Mandibular paralysis

Potential sequelae
- Coma then death

Predisposition
- None

Historical clues
- Dogs are the main infectious source for humans
- Living in an endemic area or recent travel
- Recent bite

ORGAN SYSTEMS

Physical examination
- Prodromal phase
  - Anxious
  - Behavioural changes
  - Fever
- Furious phase
  - Aggressive but unpredictable
    - Attacking enclosure
    - Snapping at imaginary things
  - Incoordination/disorientation
  - Hyperaesthesia
  - Muscle tremors
- Paralytic phase 2–4 days after onset of signs
  - Hypersalivation/dysphagia
  - Paralysis spreading from site of bite and becoming generalised
  - Other neuropathies
    - Cranial nerve deficits
    - Dropped jaw
    - Laryngeal paralysis
    - Altered voice

Laboratory findings
- Non-specific

Imaging
- Non-specific

Special investigations
- Direct fluorescent antibody test (DFA) on brain tissue (chilled after death)
- Direct IHC: similar to DFA but more rapid test
- Histopathology for evidence of rabies inclusion (Negri bodies)
- Mouse inoculation and virus isolation: virus isolation more available

Treatment
- No treatment exists and euthanasia is recommended where a high suspicion exists

Monitoring
- Not applicable

Prognosis
- Prognosis is poor and euthanasia is recommended

Prevention
- Vaccination is an effective method of preventing infection in dogs and for reducing the reservoir of infection as this is an important worldwide cause of human deaths

5.11.12 TOXOPLASMOSIS

Aetiology
Toxoplasmosis is caused by the protozoan parasite *Toxoplasma gondii* and typically causes neuromuscular disease but can affect many organs.
- Transmission is via ingestion of intermediate hosts, raw feeding, or ingestion of cat faeces
- *Toxoplasma* has zoonotic potential

Major signs
- Dyspnoea/tachypnoea/cough
- Neuromuscular signs
  - Hyperaesthesia
  - Muscle stiffness/pain
  - Spinal/neck pain
- Uveitis

Minor signs
- Abortion/stillbirth
- Cutaneous lesions

Potential sequelae
- Can develop more severe disease with pneumonia and CNS disease

Predisposition
- Multiple dog/pet environments
- Poor hygiene

Historical clues
- Raw feeding

Physical examination
- Arrhythmia
- Ataxia
- Cutaneous lesions
  - Nodules
  - Panniculitis
  - Ulcers
- Depression

- Dyspnoea
- Gait abnormalities
- Hindlimb hyperextension
- Lethargy
- Lymphadenopathy
- Muscle pain
- Paresis
- Pyrexia
- Stiffness
- Uveitis

Laboratory findings
Haematology
- Non-specific changes

Biochemistry
- Non-specific changes
- Acute phase protein response
- Changes consistent with pancreatitis
- Increased ALT/ALP activities and bilirubin with hepatic involvement
- Increased ALT/AST/CK activities due to myositis

Imaging
- Non-specific findings on routine imaging: may be evidence of pneumonia
- Consider advanced imaging/MRI when neurological signs are present

Special investigations
- Histology
  - Inflammation and associated tachyzoites in tissues
  - Immunohistochemistry can demonstrate organisms
- PCR can be performed on tissues, CSF, and other fluids (aqueous humor, respiratory secretions as well as cytology
- Serology
  - In acute phase of infection, negative results may be obtained
  - Assess IgM and IgG titres as IgM rises early and then drops as IgG rises

- Assessing for a rise in titre after 2 weeks can be useful
- Positive IgG with low IgM results confirm exposure, not necessarily active infection

Treatment
- Treatment of clinical signs can be effective, but the parasite is not cleared from the body
- First-line treatment is usually clindamycin at 12.5 mg/kg q12h for 4 weeks
- Trimethoprim sulfonamides, pyrimethamine and ponazuril are alternatives

Monitoring
- Reassess physical examination and any laboratory results that were abnormal at diagnosis
- Serology is not useful to monitor response to treatment as IgG titres can remain elevated for a long time
- If re-infection is suspected, evidence of a rising IgM titre can be useful

Prognosis
- Improvement is typically seen within 48 hours of starting treatment, and clinical cure is common
- Prognosis is worse for dogs with systemic infection, CNS or respiratory disease
- Tissue cysts persist even with clinical improvement and so the disease is not fully eliminated, and immunosuppression should be avoided as relapse can be seen

Prevention
- Oocysts can be resistant to many disinfectants
- Tissue cysts persist even with clinical improvement and so the disease is not fully eliminated, and immunosuppression should be avoided as relapse can be seen
- Prognosis is worse for dogs with systemic infection, CNS or respiratory disease

5.12 URINARY SYSTEM

Diseases of the urinary tract can be congenital, degenerative, infectious, inflammatory, mechanical or neoplastic. Disorders typically affect the:
- Kidneys
- Lower urinary tract comprising ureters, bladder, urethra (and prostate, *q.v.* section 2.23)
- Whole urinary tract
  Urinary tract infection (UTI) can affect part or all of the urinary tract. Urolithiasis may be solitary or multiple and can occur anywhere from the renal pelvis to the urethra.

5.12.1 KIDNEY DISEASES

- Azotaemia is the increase in the plasma concentration of nitrogenous substances, *q.v.* section 3.4
- Uraemia is the clinical syndrome associated with azotaemia
- The kidneys have significant reserve capacity, and azotaemia only occurs when glomerular filtration is < 25% of normal

Problems
Presenting complaints
q.v. section 1
1.5 Anorexia/hyperexia/inappetence
1.11 Constipation
1.15 Diarrhoea
1.19 Dysuria
1.25 Haematemesis
1.27 Haematuria and discoloured urine
1.29 Halitosis
1.37 Polyuria/polydipsia (PU/PD)
1.42 Seizures
1.48 Urinary incontinence
1.49 Vomiting
1.51 Weakness, collapse and syncope
1.53 Weight loss

Physical abnormalities
q.v. section 2
2.1 Abdominal enlargement
2.5 Ascites
2.10 Hypertension
2.17.1 Abdominal pain
2.18 Pallor
2.20 Peripheral oedema
2.21 Pleural effusion
2.25 Pyrexia and hyperthermia
2.29 Stomatitis

Laboratory abnormalities
q.v. section 3
3.4 Azotaemia
3.7.1 Hypercalcaemia
3.13 Creatinine
3.19.1 Hyperlipidaemia and hypercholesterolaemia
3.23.1 Hyperkalaemia
3.24.1 Hypernatraemia
3.27.2A Hypoalbuminaemia
3.29 Urea
3.30.1 Anaemia
3.32.1 Leukocytosis
3.36 Urine protein:creatinine (UPC) ratio

Diagnostic Approach
- Identify renal disease from clinical signs, azotaemia and urinalysis
- Identify significant proteinuria caused by protein-losing nephropathy (PLN)
- Distinguish acute kidney injury (AKI) and chronic kidney disease (CKD)

Diagnostic Methods
History
Clinical signs
- Endocrine and metabolic disturbances
  - Muscle atrophy
  - Osteodystrophy
  - Weight loss
- Fluid, electrolyte disturbances
  - Dehydration
  - PU/PD
  - Nocturia
- GI disturbances
  - Anorexia

Notes on Canine Internal Medicine, Fourth Edition. Victoria L. Black, Kathryn F. Murphy, Jessie Rose Payne, and Edward J. Hall.
© 2022 John Wiley & Sons Ltd. Published 2022 by John Wiley & Sons Ltd.

ORGAN SYSTEMS

- GI bleeding
- Halitosis
- Oral ulceration/stomatitis
- Vomiting
- Haematological disturbances
  - Pallor due to anaemia in CKD
- Hypertensive complications
  - Blindness
  - Hyphaema
- Neuromuscular disturbances
  - Depression
  - Lethargy
  - Weakness

Physical examination
- Dehydration: depression/lethargy, skin tent, sunken eyes, tacky mucous membranes
- Halitosis
- Loss of muscle mass
- Oral ulceration in uraemic patients: buccal mucosa around molars and premolars, and tongue ulceration and necrosis
- Osteodystrophy: thickened bones with abnormal flexibility ('rubber jaw'), especially in young, growing puppies with uraemia
- Pallor
- Pyrexia: pyelonephritis, neoplasia

Bladder palpation
- Absent or small bladder in a dog with a history of not producing urine raises concerns of anuria (or urinary tract rupture) in dogs with acute kidney injury (AKI)

Rectal examination
- Anal sac adenocarcinoma associated with paraneoplastic hypercalcaemia and nephrocalcinosis

Renal palpation
- Small
  - Suspect CKD
- Large
  - Haematoma
  - Haemorrhage
  - Hydronephrosis
  - Neoplasia
  - Perirenal cysts
  - Polycystic disease
- Pain on palpation: acute hydronephrosis, large renal calculi, pyelonephritis, ureteral obstruction

Laboratory findings
Haematology
- Moderate non-regenerative normocytic, normochromic anaemia with CKD due to lack of erythropoietin production and failure of RBC production
  - PCV may be normal at presentation due to dehydration (haemoconcentration)
    - Assess PCV and total plasma protein to allow recognition of anaemia in dehydrated patient and after rehydration
  - Post-renal causes of azotaemia and AKI are not associated with anaemia unless secondary GI blood loss or combined anticoagulant and cholecalciferol toxicity
- Moderate to severe neutrophilia may indicate septic process or urinary tract infection

Serum biochemistry
- Calcium may be high, low or normal in uraemic patients
  - Ionised calcium is more appropriate to assess in renal patients as calcium complexed with phosphate, which is part of the total calcium, is altered
- Hyperkalaemia most likely in AKI (oliguric or anuric) or post-renal azotaemia
- Hypokalaemia most likely in CKD and may result in weakness, inappetence and polymyopathy
- Hyperphosphataemia can be seen with all forms of azotaemia
- Increased SDMA, *q.v.* section 3.25

Urinalysis
- Dehydrated patient with azotaemia and concentrated urine should be investigated for causes of pre-renal azotaemia
- Dehydrated patient with azotaemia producing no urine following IV fluid therapy suggests anuric renal failure or post-renal causes
- Dilute isosthenuric urine (SG 1.007–1.016) in dehydrated patient with azotaemia suggests renal dysfunction

Imaging
Radiography
- Abdominal radiography
  - Assess renal size ± shape
  - Presence of radiopaque calculi

- Urinary tract rupture: intrapelvic soft tissue swelling, caudal peritonitis, ascites
  - Perform positive contrast studies to identify the site of leakage
- Thoracic radiography
  - If cardiorespiratory signs or checking for metastasis from urinary tract neoplasia
  - Uraemic pneumonitis is a very rare finding in advanced disease: patchy alveolar and diffuse interstitial pulmonary infiltrates
- Contrast radiography
  - Excretory urogram to identify ureteric obstruction and ectopic ureters
  - Contraindicated in renal azotaemia
  - Lower urinary tract contrast studies to assess presence of bladder pathology, urinary tract obstruction and urethral rupture

Ultrasonography
- Bladder size, mural lesions
- Calculi: renal pelvis, ureters, bladder
- Prostate enlargement and echoarchitecture
- Renal size, shape and echoarchitecture
- Sublumbar lymph node size
- Ureteral emptying into bladder neck (ureteral jets) to assess ectopic ureters

Special investigative techniques
- Systemic blood pressure (BP) indicated in all azotaemic patients
- GFR assessment
  - Creatinine clearance
  - Iohexol clearance
- Blood gas for acid–base status
- Pyelocentesis for cytology ± culture
- Renal FNA for cytology
- Renal biopsy (ultrasound guidance or surgical) for histology including electron microscopy and IHC in non-azotaemic PLN where underlying triggers excluded

5.12.1A   ACUTE KIDNEY INJURY

Aetiology

Acute kidney injury (AKI) was formerly termed acute renal failure, and refers to an abrupt decline in renal function, resulting in increased creatinine and changes in urine volume.

AKI may be:
- Volume-responsive: abnormal renal perfusion, formerly termed pre-renal
  - Alterations in renal blood flow
    - Angiotensin converting enzyme (ACE) inhibitors
    - Congestive heart failure
    - NSAIDs
    - Renal vessel thrombosis
  - Hypotension
    - GA
    - Haemorrhage
    - Hypoadrenocorticism
    - Hypovolaemia
    - Sepsis
- Intrinsic: morphological changes to renal tissue; all causes may result in intrinsic renal injury
  - Amyloidosis
  - Glomerulonephritis
  - Hypercalcaemia
  - Leptospirosis
  - Neoplasia, in particular lymphoma
  - Pyelonephritis
  - Pyometra
  - Toxins, including iodinated radiographic contrast agents
- Post-renal: abnormal handling of filtrate after renal nephrons
  - Urinary tract obstruction or rupture
    - Obstruction is more likely to result in back pressure across the glomerulus and resultant reduced glomerular filtration

Major signs
- Abdominal or lumbar pain
- Haematuria
- PU/PD
- Pyrexia
- Seizures
- Stranguria
- Vomiting
- Weakness

Minor signs
- Anorexia/inappetence
- Lethargy

ORGAN SYSTEMS

Potential sequelae

- Anuria, which may result in:
  - Accumulation of uraemic toxins and hyperkalaemia; may result in fatal cardiac disturbances
  - Volume overload with development of effusions (e.g. peripheral oedema, pleural effusion, ascites)
- Ureteric obstruction: uroliths composed of blood clot, inflammatory cells and bacteria

Predisposition

- No reported breed, age or sex predispositions

Historical clues

- Recent onset signs
- May be a history of an event that exposed the dog to risk of an acute injury, e.g. drugs, general anaesthesia, toxin

Physical examination

- Abdominal or lumbar spinal pain
- Bradycardia
- Dehydration
- Hypothermia
- Pyrexia (pyelonephritis)
- Renal pain or asymmetry (renomegaly) on palpation where conformation allows
- Signs of volume overload: ascites, peripheral oedema, pleural effusion

Laboratory findings

Haematology

- May be mild to moderate poorly regenerative anaemia
- May be haemoconcentration
- May be leukocytosis, neutrophilia ± left shift (band neutrophils and toxic change) in infectious causes of AKI (pyelonephritis, leptospirosis)

Serum biochemistry

- Azotaemia depending on International Renal Interest Society (IRIS) AKI grading:
  - Grade I AKI: non-azotaemic dog (creatinine < 140 µmol/l, < 1.6 mg/dl) with an increase in creatinine within the non-azotaemic range within a 48-hour period (> 26.4 µmol/l, 0.3 mg/dl), or reduced urine production over 6 hours and compatible history and investigation findings
  - Grade II AKI: mildly azotaemic dog (creatinine 141–220 µmol/l, 1.7–2.5 mg/dl) with increase from baseline creatinine (> 26.4 µmol/l, 0.3 mg/dl) or reduced urine production over 6 hours and compatible history and investigation findings
  - Grade III AKI: moderate to severe acute kidney injury (creatinine 221–439 µmol/l, 2.6–5.0 mg/dl)
  - Grade IV AKI: moderate to severe acute kidney injury (creatinine 440–880 µmol/l, 5.1–10 mg/dl)
  - Grade V AKI: moderate to severe acute kidney injury (creatinine > 880 µmol/l, > 10 mg/dl)
  - Each grade of AKI is sub-graded as non-oliguric or oligo-anuric
- Electrolyte disturbances
  - Hypercalcaemia
  - Hyperkalaemia
  - Hyperphosphataemia
- Increased SDMA
- Depending on cause, may detect hepatopathy
  - Leptospirosis, toxin

Urinalysis

- Each grade of AKI is sub-graded as non-oliguric or oligo-anuric
- Glucosuria may be present and suggests proximal tubular injury if euglycaemic
- Isosthenuria or hyposthenuria
- Sediment examination may reveal haematuria, bacteriuria, pyuria
- Renal casts may be present
- Urine culture

Imaging

Plain radiographs

- May detect renomegaly, or small kidneys in dogs with AKI superimposed on CKD

Ultrasound

- Altered renal size: small or large
- Increased renal hyperechogenicity
- Perirenal fluid
- Pyelectasia (renal pelvis dilatation)
- Reduced corticomedullary differentiation
- Ureteral dilatation

Special investigations
- ACTH stimulation test to exclude hypoadrenocorticism
- BP to assess for hypotension or hypertension
- Contrast studies may be useful
  - Intravenous urography should be used with caution due to increased risk of further renal injury
  - Retrograde urography may be useful to assess lower urinary tract for rupture where there is a clinical concern
- Renal biomarkers are described (e.g. neutrophil gelatinase-associated lipocalin) and are used in people
- Renal fine needle aspirate to assess for lymphoma
- Test for leptospirosis including PCR and/or serology, *q.v.* section 5.11.9
- Toxicology screening
- Venous blood gas to assess anion gap

Treatment
- Aimed at supporting renal perfusion and fluid status to allow time for renal recovery
  - This needs to be employed early in the course of renal injury to be successful
- Dialysis (renal replacement therapy or peritoneal dialysis) may be considered but is not widely practised
- Fluid therapy is aimed at correcting dehydration and addressing ongoing losses whilst avoiding volume overload; once euhydration is achieved, fluid therapy should be gradually tapered
- For anuric patients, diuretics (furosemide, mannitol) may be used to attempt to convert the dog to a non-oliguric state once rehydrated
  - May be useful in establishing whether there are functional nephrons; there is no evidence this improves outcome in patients
  - Not used in cases with contrast- or aminoglycoside-induced AKI
- Treatment may be required to address hyperkalaemia: essential when > 8 mmol/l
- Sodium bicarbonate therapy is rarely used but may be useful in a small cohort of patients
- Supportive therapy
  - Anti-emetics
  - Electrolyte supplementation
  - Enteral tube feeding

- Gastroprotectants
- Prokinetics
- Therapy specific to the cause may be used
  - Antimicrobials for leptospirosis or pyelonephritis
  - Fomipazole and/or ethanol for ethylene glycol toxicity

Monitoring
- Close monitoring in the initial phases is required, including BP urine output, electrolytes and body weight
- Once a stable creatinine is documented, frequency of monitoring can be reduced
- Full renal recovery may take months

Prognosis
- Generally fair to guarded prognosis: survival around 40–50%
- Infectious and NSAID-induced AKI appear to have a better prognosis
- Poor for ethylene glycol toxicity once anuria occurs

5.12.1B CHRONIC KIDNEY DISEASE

Aetiology
Chronic kidney disease (formerly chronic renal failure) describes a chronic (> 3 months) state of reduced glomerular filtration due to loss of renal function. This may occur as the downstream effect of a heterogenous group of disorders, including congenital, familial or acquired causes.

Major signs
- PU/PD
- Urinary incontinence
- Vomiting
- Weakness

Minor signs
- Anorexia, inappetence
- Halitosis
- Lethargy
- Weight loss

Potential sequelae
- Blindness due to target organ damage from hypertension
- Cachexia due to poor appetite and muscle wastage
- Osteodystrophy and pathological fractures due to renal secondary hyperparathyroidism
- Tachycardia and pallor due to anaemia

Predisposition
- More common in older dogs (> 12 years)
- Breed-related disorders are described, e.g. juvenile nephropathy in Boxers

Historical clues
- Chronic, progressive signs in most dogs
- Some dogs may present with no apparent history of PU/PD, especially in early stages

Physical examination
- Dehydration
- Halitosis
- Hypothermia
- Oral ulceration

Laboratory findings
Haematology
- May be mild to moderate poorly regenerative anaemia

Serum biochemistry
- Analysis should be carried out on a fasted dog that is stable and euhydrated, ideally on at least two occasions
- Azotaemia, depending on IRIS stage:
  - Stage 1: non-azotaemic dog (creatinine < 125 µmol/l, 1.4 mg/dl) with evidence of abnormal renal architecture (including imaging), increasing creatinine, or persistently increased SDMA
  - Stage 2: normal or mild increase in creatinine, may be within laboratory reference range (creatinine 125–250 µmol/l, 1.4–2.8 mg/dl), may be increased SDMA
  - Stage 3: moderate renal azotaemia, clinical signs likely to be present at this stage (creatinine 251–440µmol/l, 2.9–5.0mg/dl)
  - Stage 4: moderate to marked azotaemia with increasing risk of clinical signs (creatinine > 440 µmol/l, > 5.0 mg/dl)

- Increased electrolyte disturbances
  - Hypercalcaemia or hypocalcaemia
  - Hyperphosphataemia
  - Hypokalaemia
- SDMA

Urinalysis
- Urine protein:creatinine (UPC) ratio to allow sub-staging, *q.v.* section 3.36
  - UPC < 0.2, non-proteinuric
  - UPC 0.2–0.5, borderline proteinuric
  - UPC > 0.5, proteinuric
  - Must be interpreted:
    - In combination with sediment analysis: suspicion of urinary tract infection
    - In light of method of collection, e.g. free catch in male entire dogs with be increased)
    - In light of gross blood contamination
- Isosthenuria or hyposthenuria
- Sediment examination may reveal haematuria, bacteriuria, pyuria
- Urine culture

Imaging
Plain radiographs
- May detect small kidneys

Ultrasound
- Small kidneys and, sometimes, an irregular outline
- Hyperechoic renal cortex
- Loss of corticomedullary differentiation
- Renal calculi
- Pyelectasia (dilated renal pelvis)

Special investigations
- BP to assess for hypertension for substage of CKD
- Retinal examination complements indirect BP measurement to assess for target organ damage
- Parathyroid hormone and vitamin D panel, may be considered in particular in cases with osteodystrophy
- Renal biopsy for histopathology and culture, rarely performed once azotaemic

Treatment
- Discontinue nephrotoxic drugs
- Address hypertension if detected

- Address and investigate proteinuria if detected
- Manage dehydration with plentiful access to water and encourage drinking; subcutaneous fluid therapy is used less commonly in dogs than cats
- Rule out pyelonephritis and ureteric obstruction
- Supportive treatment
  - Anti-emetics
  - Appetite stimulants
  - Gastroprotectants
- Depending on IRIS stage, reduce phosphate intake
  - Restricted-phosphate renal diet
  - Phosphate binders
- Calcitriol may be considered in specific cases
- Recombinant erythropoietin if significantly anaemic

Monitoring
- Monitoring of renal parameters and phosphate should be implemented following adjustment of therapy, in particular dose adjustment of ACE inhibitors and phosphate binders
- BP, haematocrit, renal parameters, urinalysis should be monitored regularly every 3–6 months depending on clinical progression

Prognosis
- Prognosis is associated with IRIS stage and rate of progression of CKD in dogs
- Median survival
  - Fair (11–15 months) for stages 2 and 3 CKD
  - Poor (2 months) for stage 4 CKD
- Underweight body condition score and hypoalbuminaemia associated with a poorer prognosis

5.12.1C GLOMERULAR DISORDERS

Aetiology
Glomerular disorders in dogs encompass pathology of any cause localising to the glomerulus and are characterised by the presence of proteinuria arising from loss of the normal glomerular filtration barrier. Disorders may be categorised based upon electron microscopy findings as immune-complex glomerulonephritis (ICGN), non-immune-complex glomerulonephritis (non-ICGN), glomerulosclerosis and amyloidosis. This discrimination is beneficial as aetiology and, therefore, treatment is likely to be different.

Renal proteinuria is suspected in dogs with persistent (i.e. > two occasions) UPC >2 where the following has been excluded:
- Extra-urinary proteinuria, excluded with cystocentesis sample
- Pre-renal proteinuria: haemoglobuniuria, myoglobinuria, hyperglobulinaemia
- Post-renal proteinuria: lower urinary tract infection, prostatic disease, vaginitis, urolithiasis, haematuria, neoplasia

Major signs
- May be asymptomatic, particularly early in disease
- May present due to thrombotic disease, e.g. cerebrovascular disease or iliac thrombosis due to hypercoagulable state
- Renal insufficiency may be present
  - Halitosis
  - Oral ulceration
  - PU/PD
  - Vomiting

Minor signs
- Lethargy
- Weight loss

Potential sequelae
- Hypercoagulable state may result in catastrophic thrombotic event, e.g. aortic thromboembolism
- May develop nephrotic syndrome
  - Proteinuria
  - Hypoalbuminaemia
  - Hypercholesterolaemia
  - Extravascular fluid accumulation: ascites, pleural effusion or peripheral oedema

Predisposition
- Chinese Shar pei dogs are predisposed to amyloidosis
- Familial nephropathy is described in a number of breeds including Bernese mountain dog, Dalmatians, English Cocker spaniels, Rottweilers

Historical clues

- Amyloidosis is typically associated with higher-magnitude UPC and lower serum albumin compared to other non-ICGN disorders and ICGN
- Chinese Shar pei dogs may have history of pyrexic episodes (potentially with joint, in particular hock, swelling)
- Consider drugs or diets that may predispose to hypertension or glomerular disease
  - Phenylpropanolamine
  - Raw-food diet
  - Steroids
  - Sulfonamides
  - Tyrosine kinase inhibitors, e.g. masitinib, toceranib

Physical examination

May be normal
- Ascites/peripheral oedema
- Dyspnoea (pleural effusion)
- Reduced BCS
- Signs of thromboembolism
  - Neurological signs
  - Hind limb paresis/paralysis with reduced/absent femoral pulses

Laboratory findings

Haematology
- Thrombocytopenia may increase suspicion of vector-borne disease or leptospirosis if low

Biochemistry
- Azotaemia: this is prognostic
- Hyperglobulinaemia may increase suspicion of vector-borne disease
- Changes due to concurrent organ disorders (e.g. hepatopathy), may increase suspicion of infectious disease (e.g. leptospirosis) or trigger (infection or neoplasia)

Urinalysis
- Urine culture and sediment examination critical in diagnosing renal proteinuria

Imaging

Plain radiographs
- Thoracic radiographs to screen for trigger, in particular neoplasia

Ultrasound
- Abdominal ultrasound to screen for trigger
- Adrenal gland size in cases with a suspicion of hyperadrenocorticism (HAC)
- Assess renal and lower urinary tract

Special investigations

- Assess for immune-mediated disease causing ICGN when an index of suspicion exists, e.g. IMPA in dogs with shifting lameness and joint swelling
- BP measurement, and retinal examination for target organ damage
- Echocardiogram in cases with a suspicion of endocarditis, i.e. pyrexia, novel heart murmur
- Infectious disease screening depending on risk factors
- Test for HAC in dogs with compatible clinical signs
- Renal biopsy
  - Contra-indications
    - Coagulopathy
    - Cystic renal disease
    - Hydronephrosis
    - IRIS stage 4 CKD, i.e severe azotaemia
    - Pregnancy
    - Renal abscess
    - Severe anaemia
    - Uncontrolled hypertension
  - Routine histopathology is not helpful; specialist labs use a combination of:
    - Histopathology
    - Transmission electron microscopy (TEM)
    - Immunofluorescence (IF)
  - Use special fixatives

Treatment

- Considered successful if UPC < 0.5 or a reduction by 50% or more
- Standard therapy for renal proteinuria
  - ACE inhibitor or angiotensin receptor blocker (ARB), or combined therapy used cautiously
  - Omega-3 supplementation
  - Renal diet
  - Prophylactic anti-thrombotics
  - Treatment of any hypertension, e.g. amlodipine

- Immunosuppressive treatment
  - Ideally guided by specialist biopsy interpretation
  - Mycophenolate or chlorambucil are typically the drugs of choice
  - Prednisolone may be used in rapidly progressive cases initially but should be tapered quickly
  - Empirical immunosuppression may be considered, especially in cases with hypoalbuminaemia, progressive azotaemia, or creatinine is >265 mmol/l (3 mg/dl)
    - Pre-renal and post-renal diseases excluded
    - Suspicion of amyloidosis low
    - Triggers (infectious disease, neoplasia) not identified

Monitoring

- Renal parameters should be monitored after each dose adjustment of ACE inhibitor or ARB dosage
- BP, renal parameters, urinalysis including UPC should be monitored at least quarterly

Prognosis

- Azotaemic dogs with nephrotic syndrome are associated with a poor prognosis: survival typically < 60 days)
- Non-azotaemic dogs that do not have nephrotic syndrome may experience extended survival: > 2 years
- Prognosis is improved for ICGN cases that receive immunosuppression

5.12.1D PYELONEPHRITIS

Aetiology

Pyelonephritis describes infection of the renal pelvis and surrounding renal parenchyma; the most common cause is extension of lower urinary tract infections, with haematogenous spread a less commonly documented cause.

Pyelonephritis may present as acute onset disease or, in some circumstances, there may be a chronic insidious onset. In the latter cases an accompanying azotaemia may be due to under-lying CKD predisposing to infection or related to the infection causing renal injury.

As with all UTIs the emphasis is to consider an underlying risk factor in dogs with a diagnosis or high clinical suspicion of pyelonephritis, as addressing this, where possible, is important for successful treatment.

Major signs

- Abdominal or lumbar pain
- Haematuria
- PU/PD
- Pyrexia
- Stranguria
- Urinary incontinence
- Vomiting

Minor signs

- Anorexia, inappetence
- Lethargy
- Weight loss

Potential sequelae

- Anuria due to AKI
- Struvite urolithiasis
- Ureteric obstruction: uroliths composed of blood clot, inflammatory cells and bacteria

Predisposition

- Females and older dogs (> 7 years) may be at increased risk

Historical clues

- Acute pyelonephritis causes sudden or recent onset signs; these dogs are more likely to present with pyrexia
- Chronic pyelonephritis dogs may present with a more insidious onset signs and the diagnosis may be challenging
- Risk factors for development of pyelonephritis
- Altered urine concentration: CKD, diuretics, hepatic dysfunction
  - Immunosuppression
  - Incontinence: neurological disorders, congenital disorders, urethral sphincter mechanism incontinence
  - Urogenital neoplasia
  - Urolithiasis

ORGAN SYSTEMS

Physical examination
- Abdominal or lumbar spinal pain
- Dehydration
- Pyrexia
- Renal pain or asymmetry (renomegaly) on palpation where conformation allows

Laboratory findings
Haematology
- May be mild to moderate poorly regenerative anaemia
- May be leukocytosis, neutrophilia ± left shift

Serum biochemistry
- Azotaemia in ~40% of cases
- Electrolyte disturbances
  - Hyperkalaemia
  - Hyperphosphataemia
  - Hypokalaemia

Urinalysis
- Isosthenuria or hyposthenuria: USG < 1.030 in ~70%
- Sediment examination
  - Bacteriuria
  - Haematuria
  - Pyuria in 70%
  - ± Renal casts, in particular granular
- Urine culture: positive in only ~80% of cases when collected by cystocentesis, and even fewer if recent antimicrobial treatment

Imaging
Plain radiographs
- May detect renomegaly
- Assess for risk factors, in particular urolithiasis

Ultrasound
- Altered renal size: small or large
- Assess for risk factors
- Increased renal hyperechogenicity
- Pyelectasia
- Reduced corticomedullary differentiation
- Ureteral dilatation

Special investigations
- Pyelocentesis for sediment analysis, cytology, and culture

- Tissue biopsy for histopathology and culture (rarely performed)
- Urine cytology (submitted in EDTA) may complement sediment examination in cases with a suspicion of pyelonephritis

Treatment
- Antimicrobial therapy
  - Choice and duration should be guided by culture results and antimicrobial stewardship guidelines
  - Empirical treatment may be commenced pending culture results or in cases with a high clinical suspicion and supportive investigation findings

Monitoring
- Repeat sediment and culture analysis after onset of therapy, and after the end of treatment

Prognosis
- Variable, although generally fair to good
- Those cases with underlying predisposing factors that are not possible to address are likely to have a poorer prognosis

5.12.1E   RENAL TUBULAR DISORDERS

Aetiology
- Abnormal renal tubular function results in diminished reabsorption of water and various constituents with clinical signs related to their loss or the formation of calculi
  - Urinary loss of one or more metabolites: albumin, amino acids, bicarbonate, glucose, sodium, potassium, phosphorus, uric acid
- Tubular defects
  - Genetic: Fanconi syndrome causing a range of tubular dysfunctions
  - Renal glucosuria
    - Selective inability to reabsorb glucose despite euglycaemia
  - Renal tubular acidosis
    - Type I (distal): the ability of the distal tubule to secrete hydrogen ions is defective
    - Type II (proximal): the ability to reabsorb bicarbonate in the proximal tubule is reduced

- Causes hyperchloraemic metabolic acidosis
- Secondary to tubular injury
  - Infection: leptospirosis
  - Part of specific disorder
  - Toxins: gentamicin, heavy metals, jerky treats

Major signs
- PU/PD
- Signs of renal insufficiency may be present
  - Halitosis
  - Oral ulceration
  - Vomiting
- Signs related to urolithiasis: haematuria, pollakiuria, stranguria

Minor signs
- May be incidental finding

Potential sequelae
- Development of CKD in Fanconi syndrome
- Electrolyte disturbances related to losses may result in clinical signs, e.g. muscle weakness if hypokalaemic
- May be at increased risk of urinary tract infection with glucosuria

Predisposition
- Congenital disorders (Fanconi): Basenji, Scottish terrier
- Labrador retrievers with copper-accumulation hepatopathy have been described to display transient glucosuria
- Renal glucosuria: Norwegian Elkhound
- Selective cobalamin deficiency (Imerslund-Gräsbeck syndrome, *q.v.* section 5.7.1.2C) associated with failure of tubules to reabsorb albumin

Historical clues
- Risk factors for leptospirosis: vaccination status, lifestyle
- Ingestion of jerky treats

Physical examination
- Typically unremarkable
- In Labrador retrievers may be evidence of hepatic dysfunction

Laboratory findings
Haematology
- Evidence of systemic inflammation ± thrombocytopenia in leptospirosis

Biochemistry
- Euglycaemia useful to exclude diabetes mellitus as a cause for glucosuria
- May detect electrolyte changes

Urinalysis
- May detect lower USG
- Glucosuria
- Urine culture to assess for pyelonephritis

Imaging
Plain radiographs and ultrasound
- Abdominal imaging may be useful, especially in dogs with underlying hepatopathy

Special investigations
- DNA test for inherited Fanconi syndrome in Basenjis
- Pyelocentesis for cytology and culture in dogs with dilated renal pelvis and suspicion of pyelonephritis
- Tests for copper-accumulation hepatopathy when index of suspicion present, *q.v.* section 5.6.5
- Tests for leptospirosis (blood and/or urine PCR, serology)
- Venous blood gas

Treatment
- Address electrolyte disorders where suitable, e.g. potassium supplementation
- Jerky-treat induced glucosuria typically resolves slowly with no treatment

Prognosis
- Variable, depending on aetiology and clinical course
- Jerky-treat-induced glucosuria typically resolves within weeks

5.12.2 LOWER URINARY TRACT DISEASES

Problems
Presenting complaints
q.v. section 1
1.5 Anorexia/hyporexia/inappetence
1.9 Bleeding
1.11 Constipation
1.19 Dysuria
1.27 Haematuria and discoloured urine
1.48 Urinary incontinence
1.49 Vomiting
1.51 Weakness, collapse and syncope

Physical abnormalities
q.v. section 2
2.1 Abdominal enlargement
2.4 Arrhythmias
2.17.1 Abdominal pain
2.23 Prostatomegaly

Laboratory abnormalities
q.v. section 3
3.4 Azotaemia
3.13 Creatinine
3.23.1 Hyperkalaemia
3.27.1 Hyperproteinaemia
3.29 Urea
3.32.1 Leukocytosis
3.32.2 Leukopenia
3.36 Urine protein:creatinine (UPC) ratio

Diagnostic Approach
1 Distinguish inflammatory from obstructive disease by noting the ability to pass urine and size of bladder post-voiding
2 Dysuria must be distinguished from urinary incontinence and from increased frequency because of PU/PD, *q.v.* sections 1.19, 1.48
3 Urinalysis for sediment examination and cytology to detect inflammatory and neoplastic disease
4 Radiographs and ultrasonography to image the lower urinary tract and detect urolithiasis, neoplasia, and structural abnormalities
5 When a UTI is diagnosed, consider risk factors for development and address these in addition to antimicrobial therapy

Diagnostic Methods
History
- Ability to pass urine
- Duration of current episode
- Number of past episodes and response to treatment
- Pollakiuria suggests inflammation of lower urinary tract
- Presence of gross haematuria
- Presence or absence of urination, tenesmus and haematuria

Clinical signs
- Dysuria
- Haematuria
- Incontinence
- Pollakiuria
- Stranguria

Clinical examination
Visual inspection
- Observe urination pattern in dog
  - Does dog strain to urinate?
  - Does dog actually pass urine and empty bladder?

Physical examination
- Abdominal palpation
  - Empty or distended bladder
    - A full bladder despite attempts to urinate indicates either an obstruction or an atonic bladder
  - Pain on palpation of kidneys or dorsal abdomen
  - Sublumbar area for lymphadenopathy
- Acute/complete urethral obstruction: bladder feels very round, firm and distended
  - If not obstructed, the bladder can be expressed or catheterised
- Pyrexia: pyelonephritis, neoplasia
- Rectal palpation
  - Bladder neck
  - Intrapelvic urethra
  - Prostate size, symmetry, pain, and fluctuance

Laboratory findings
Haematology
- Generally unremarkable

Serum biochemistry
- Azotaemia: post-renal or with concurrent AKI or CKD

Urinalysis
- Full urinalysis including sediment and urine specific gravity

Imaging
Abdominal radiography
- Assess renal size ± shape
- Radiopaque calculi
- Urinary tract rupture: ascites, caudal peritonitis, intrapelvic soft tissue swelling, retroperitoneal space widening
  - Perform positive contrast studies to identify the site of leakage

Thoracic radiography
- If cardiorespiratory signs or checking for metastasis from urinary tract neoplasia
- Uraemic pneumonitis is a very rare finding in advanced disease: patchy alveolar and diffuse interstitial pulmonary infiltrates

Contrast radiography
Lower urinary tract contrast studies to assess for causes of urinary tract obstruction and presence of urethral rupture

Ultrasonography
- Bladder: size, mural lesions or intravesical abnormalities, e.g. calculi
- Prostate: enlargement and echoarchitecture
- Kidneys: size, shape and echoarchitecture
- Sublumbar lymph node size
- Ureteral emptying into bladder neck (ureteral jets): ectopic ureters

Special investigative techniques
- Acid–base status
- Biopsy: catheter suction, FNA, surgical
- Neurological examination
- Passage of urinary catheter
  - Check patency: strictures, urethral calculi, mass lesions
- Prostatic wash
- Urethrocystoscopy
- Urodynamic pressure profile

5.12.2A FUNCTIONAL DISORDERS OF URINATION

Aetiology
Dysuria may manifest as pollakiuria and/or stranguria caused by:
- Primary urinary tract problem
  - Detrusor atony
    - Detrusor atony occurs due to overdistension of the bladder and results in disruption of innervation and stretch of the intercellular tight junctions of the muscle fibres. It may result from any cause of urethral obstruction; certain metabolic disorders may increase the risk, e.g. electrolyte disturbances, glucocorticoids, polymyopathy
  - Reflex dyssynergia
    - Reflex dyssynergia is an idiopathic disorder where there is a failure of coordination of relaxation of the urethral sphincter and contraction of the detrusor muscle
- Secondary problem
  - Neurological disorders, e.g. spinal cord disease, neuropathy, dysautonomia
  - Structural disease, e.g. uroliths, neoplasia, urethritis

Major signs
- Pollakiuria
- Stranguria

Minor signs
- Dyschezia
- Haematuria
- Nocturia
- Signs of systemic illness or neurological disease depending on the cause
- Urinary incontinence

Potential sequelae
- Urinary tract obstruction
- Urinary tract infection
- Urinary tract rupture

Physical examination

- Clinical examination, including assessing for concern of urethral obstruction; in particular, assess for size of bladder and presence of bradycardia suggestive of hyperkalaemia
- Rectal examination to assess for urethra
- Try to pass a urethral catheter to assess for obstruction; can be done conscious in amenable dogs

Laboratory findings

Haematology
- Usually unremarkable

Biochemistry
- Assess for presence of post-renal azotaemia and electrolyte changes if concerns of ureteric or urethral obstruction

Urinalysis
- Sediment examination
- Urine culture

Imaging

Plain radiographs and ultrasound
- Exclude other causes of dysuria with plain radiographs, contrast radiography (retrograde urethrogram) and ultrasound as appropriate

Special investigations

- Exclude other causes, e.g. investigation for neurological disorders, where appropriate

Treatment

- Detrusor atony
  - In some cases of urethral catheterisation, addressing any cause of obstruction and prompt medical management (e.g. bethanechol) may be adequate
  - Bladder rest may be needed in some cases
    - In-dwelling urinary catheter for 5–7 days
    - Cystotomy tube for longer-term management
- Reflex dyssynergia
  - Medical management may be trialled, e.g. diazepam, prazosin, tamsulosin described
  - Some dogs may require cystotomy tube placement

Prognosis

- Prognosis is variable, depending on underlying cause and duration of bladder overdistension if detrusor atony

5.12.2B NEOPLASIA OF THE URINARY SYSTEM

Aetiology

Neoplastic transformation and proliferation of urinary tract cells.
- May affect the kidneys, bladder, urethra or, less commonly, ureter
  - Lymphoma
  - Nephroblastoma
  - Renal carcinoma and cystadenocarcinoma
  - Transitional cell carcinoma (TCC), also termed urothelial carcinoma (UC)
- For prostatic neoplasia, *q.v.* section 2.23

Major signs

- Abdominal pain
- Constipation
- Dysuria
- Haematuria or discoloured urine
- Urinary incontinence

Minor signs

- Anorexia
- Vomiting
- Weakness or collapse

Potential sequelae

- Hydronephrosis and ureteric obstruction
- Urethral obstruction

Predisposition

- Bladder TCC: Scottish terrier, Shetland sheepdog, WHWT
- Renal cystadenocarcinoma and nodular dermatofibrosis (RCND): GSD

Historical clues

- Lawn herbicide exposure in Scottish terriers may increase risk of development of TCC

Physical examination
- Assess thoroughly for mass lesions by abdominal palpation
- Rectal examination to assess urethra and for lymph node enlargement

Laboratory findings
Haematology and biochemistry
- Typically unremarkable
- Azotaemia if urethral or ureteric obstruction

Urinalysis
- Cytology and sediment examination may detect neoplastic cells
- Urinary tract infection may be present in dogs with neoplasia

Imaging
Plain radiographs
Thoracic radiographs to screen for metastasis

Ultrasound
- Assess for presence of mass lesion or suspicion of infiltrative disease, e.g. loss of corticomedullary definition with hyperechoic renal cortices in renal lymphoma
- Assess for metastasis

Special investigations
- Assess for presence of BRAF gene mutation on urinalysis or cytology samples
- DNA test for RCND
- Urinary catheter-guided samples of bladder or urethra
- Renal FNA, in particular in cases with a suspicion renal lymphoma

Treatment
- Dependent on neoplasm type
  - Surgery for unilateral renal carcinoma or nephroblastoma
  - TCC
    - Typically not amenable to surgery due to location
    - Chemotherapy may be appropriate, e.g. mitoxantrone
    - Palliative effect of NSAIDs, e.g. piroxicam, meloxicam

- Palliative urinary diversion (cystotomy tube), or stents may be considered in some cases but are associated with complications

Prognosis
- Typically guarded unless curative surgery possible

5.12.2C URETHRITIS

Aetiology
Inflammation of the urethra often associated with a UTI. Proliferative urethritis is an aberrant immune response resulting in lymphoplasmacytic, suppurative inflammation.
  Urethritis may occur secondary to:
- Infection
- Neoplasia
- Trauma, e.g. repeated urethral catheterization

Major signs
- Dysuria
- Haematuria
- Pollakiuria
- Stranguria

Minor signs
- Inappetence
- Lethargy

Potential sequelae
- Partial or complete urethral tract obstruction may develop

Historical clues
- May be associated with other urinary tract disorders, e.g. neoplasia, previous catheterisation, UTI

Physical examination
- Clinical examination, including assessing for concern of urethral obstruction; in particular, assess for size of bladder and presence of bradycardia suggestive of hyperkalaemia
- Rectal examination to assess urethra
- Try to pass a urethral catheter to assess for obstruction

ORGAN SYSTEMS

Laboratory findings
Haematology
- Usually unremarkable

Biochemistry
- Post-renal azotaemia and hyperkalaemia with urethral obstruction

Urinalysis
- Sediment analysis
  - Crystalluria
  - Haematuria
  - Pyuria and/or bacteriuria if concurrent urinary tract infection

Imaging
Plain radiographs and ultrasound
- Risk factors for development of UTI, e.g. urolith, urinary tract neoplasia
- Contrast study
  - Neoplasia or urolithiasis causing urethral obstruction
  - Proliferative urethritis may be mistaken for neoplasia

Special investigations
- Cystoscopy
- Urethral biopsy for tissue culture and histopathology

Treatment
- Treatment of bacterial infection
- In cases of proliferative urethritis, prednisolone is typically used when infection is resolved (in some cases NSAIDs have been described)

Prognosis
- Generally reasonable prognosis
- Urethritis with complete urethral obstruction may be challenging to manage
- Cases with concurrent neoplasia are associated with a poor prognosis

5.12.2D   URINARY TRACT INFECTION (UTI)

Aetiology
Urinary tract infection (UTI), or bacterial cystitis, occurs due to a failure of host defences and resultant bacterial infection, typically through ascending infection.

   Risk factors for development of UTI
- Diabetes mellitus
- Dilute urine, e.g. CKD, liver disease
- Hyperadrenocorticism
- Immunosuppression
- Neoplasia of the urinary tract
- Urinary catheterisation
- Urinary incontinence

Major signs
- Haematuria
- Pollakiuria
- Stranguria

Minor signs
- Urinary incontinence: urge incontinence

Potential sequelae
- Pyelonephritis
- Urolithiasis (struvite)

Predisposition
- As per for risk factors above
  - Golden retrievers are predisposed to ectopic ureter, therefore at greater risk of UTI
- Females at greater risk due to shorter urethra
- Hooded vulva

Physical examination
- Bladder typically small on examination

Laboratory findings
Haematology
- Usually unremarkable
- Inflammatory leukogram may increase index of suspicion of pyelonephritis

Biochemistry
- Usually unremarkable
- Azotaemia in cases with concerns of pyelonephritis

Urinalysis
- Sediment examination
- Urine pH, alkaline pH may increase index of suspicion of urease-producing bacteria
- Urinary culture, ideally from cystocentesis sample

Imaging
Plain radiographs and ultrasound
Risk factors for development of UTI, e.g. urolith, urinary tract neoplasia

Treatment
- Antimicrobial therapy should be aimed at the shortest course and, ideally, guided by culture and sensitivity results
- Antimicrobial treatment is not typically recommended for subclinical bacteriuria, i.e. where there are no clinical signs
- In cases with recurrent or persistent UTI the emphasis is on addressing the underlying risk factors for the development of UTI rather than pursuing repeated antimicrobial therapy in isolation

Prognosis
- Good for simple infection
- Guarded if underlying predisposition, e.g. chronic pyelonephritis, urolithiasis

5.12.2E   UROLITHIASIS

Aetiology
Urolithiasis is the concretion of minerals within the urinary tract. Nephroliths and ureteral calculi are uncommon: cystic calculi are quite common.
- Calcium oxalate
- Calcium phosphate
- Cystine
- Mixed
- Silica
- Struvite – magnesium ammonium phosphate (triple phosphate)
- Urate
- Xanthine

Major signs
Upper urinary tract uroliths
- Haematuria
- Lumbar pain

Lower urinary tract uroliths
- Dysuria
- Haematuria
- Pollakiuria
- Stranguria

Minor signs
- Anorexia
- Vomiting
- Weakness or collapse

Potential sequela
- Hydronephrosis and ureteric obstruction
- Complete urethral obstruction

Predisposition
- Young: urate urolithiasis in congenital porto-systemic shunt (PSS)
- Breed associations: there are many breed-associated uroliths, e.g. Miniature schnauzers are predisposed to struvite and calcium oxalate uroliths, urate uroliths in Bulldog, Dalmatian, Black Russian terrier
- Struvite calculi associated with UTI by urease-positive bacteria
- Xanthine calculi in dogs treated chronically with allopurinol for leishmaniasis

Historical clues
- Algorithms are available online that help predict urolith based on breed, age, gender, urine pH and stone density and appearance on radiographs, e.g. Minnesota Urolith Centre App

Physical examination
- Clinical examination, including assessing for concern of urethral obstruction; in particular, assess for size of bladder and presence of bradycardia suggestive of hyperkalaemia
- Rectal examination to assess urethra
- Try to pass a urethral catheter to assess for obstruction

Laboratory findings
Haematology
Usually unremarkable

Biochemistry
- Assess for hepatic function (including bile acid stimulation test) in dogs with a clinical suspicion of PSS or diagnosis of urate urolithiasis
- Total and ionised calcium if calcium-based uroliths
- Post-renal azotaemia and electrolyte changes in cases with concerns of ureteric or urethral obstruction

ORGAN SYSTEMS

Urinalysis
- Sediment analysis
  - Crystalluria
    - Does not prove presence of uroliths
    - May suggest composition of confirmed uroliths
  - Haematuria
  - Pyuria and/or bacteriuria if concurrent urinary tract infection
  - Urine pH is important as it influences urolith formation and dissolution

Imaging
Plain radiographs
- Include extra-pelvic urethra in male if obstruction suspected
- Presence of radio-opaque calculi
  NB: Urate and cystine calculi may be radiolucent.
- Lower urinary tract contrast studies to assess causes of urinary tract obstruction and haematuria
  - Pneumocystogram
  - Positive contrast retrograde (vagino)-urethrogram

Ultrasound
- Ureters, bladder and urethra (proximal) for uroliths

Special investigations
- Genetic tests
  - Hyperuricosuria in Bulldog, Dalmatian, Black Russian terrier
- Urine culture where appropriate, e.g. struvite urolithiasis with alkaline urine, radiopaque stone
- Stone analysis

Treatment
- Interventions for any type of urolith aim to decrease urine specific gravity, with modification of urine pH depending on the nature of the stone
- Androgen-dependent cysteinuria may improve following castration
- Cystoliths
  - Hydropulsion for small urocystoliths
  - Medical dissolution can be considered for struvite, urate, and cysteine urocystoliths
  - Non-clinical uroliths unlikely to cause obstruction can be left
  - Surgical removal of cystoliths is advised for stones that are causing clinical signs or present a risk for obstruction
  - Low purine diet for dogs treated chronically with allopurinol
- Nephroliths
  - Do not need to be addressed unless they are causing outflow obstruction, severe renal haemorrhage or urinary infection
  - Dissolution may be attempted in dogs with a suspicion of struvite nephrolith, e.g. struvite urolithiasis with alkaline urine, radiopaque stone, UTI with urease-producing bacteria
- Ureteric uroliths causing complete obstruction require surgery in order to preserve nephron function
  - Stenting
  - Subcutaneous ureteral bypass (SUB)

Prognosis
- Depends on the composition of the stone and whether underlying abnormalities can be addressed

ABBREVIATIONS

A/C	alternating current
ACA	aminocaproic acid
ACE (ACEi)	angiotensin converting enzyme (inhibitor)
ACh	acetylcholine
AChR	acetylcholine receptor
ACT	activated clotting time
ACTH	adrenocorticotrophic hormone
ADH	antidiuretic hormone
AF	atrial fibrillation
AgNOR	argyrophilic nucleolar organiser region
AHDS	acute haemorrhagic diarrhoea syndrome
AIEC	adherent-invasive *E. coli*
AKI	acute kidney injury (formerly acute renal failure, ARF)
AL	alimentary lymphoma
ALL	acute lymphoblastic leukaemia
ALP (SAP)	(serum) alkaline phosphatase
ALT	alanine aminotransferase
AMH	anti-mullerian hormone
AML	acute myeloid leukaemia
ANA	antinuclear antibody
aPTT	activated partial thromboplastin time
ARAS	ascending reticular activating system
ARB	angiotensin receptor blocker
ARD	antibiotic-responsive diarrhoea
ARDS	acute respiratory distress syndrome
ARE	antibiotic responsive enteropathy
ARVC	arrhythmogenic right ventricular cardiomyopathy
ASAC	anal sac adenocarcinoma
ASD	atrial septal defect
AT	antithrombin
ATP	adenosine triphosphate
AV	atrioventricular (valve) or arteriovenous (fistula)
BAER	brainstem-auditory evoked response
BAL	broncho-alveolar lavage
BCS	body condition score
BID	twice daily (q12h)
BMBT	buccal mucosal bleeding time
BOAS	brachycephalic obstructive airway syndrome
BP	blood pressure
BPH	benign prostatic hypertrophy
BPM	beats per minute
BUN	blood urea nitrogen
BW	body weight
CAV	canine adenovirus (ICH)

Notes on Canine Internal Medicine, Fourth Edition. Victoria L. Black, Kathryn F. Murphy, Jessie Rose Payne, and Edward J. Hall.
© 2022 John Wiley & Sons Ltd. Published 2022 by John Wiley & Sons Ltd.

CDI	central diabetes insipidus
CDM	canine degenerative myelopathy
CDRM	canine degenerative radiculomyelopathy
CDV	canine distemper virus
CGL	chronic granulocytic leukaemia
CH	chronic hepatitis
CHF	congestive heart failure
CHOP	cyclophosphamide-doxorubicin-vincristine-prednisolone
CHPG	chronic hypertrophic pylorogastropathy
CIE	chronic inflammatory enteropathy (aka IBD)
CIRD	canine infectious respiratory disease
CKCS	Cavalier King Charles spaniel
CKD	chronic kidney disease (formerly chronic renal failure, CRF)
CLL	chronic lymphocytic leukaemia
CML	chronic myeloid leukaemia
CNS	central nervous system
COP	cyclophosphamide-vincristine-prednisolone
cPL	canine pancreatic lipase
CRGV	cutaneous and renal glomerulovasculopathy
CRP	C-reactive protein
CRT	capillary refill time
C/S	culture/sensitivity
CSF	cerebrospinal fluid
CT	computed tomography
CUPS	chronic ulcerative paradental stomatitis
CVC	caudal vena cava
DAT	direct antiglobulin test
DCM	dilated cardiomyopathy
DDAVP	desmopressin
DDx	differential diagnosis
DFA	direct fluorescent antibody
DGGR	1,2-o-dilauryl-rac-glycero-glutaric acid-(6'-methylresorufin)
DI	diabetes insipidus
DIC	disseminated intravascular coagulation
DJD	degenerative joint disease
DKA	diabetic ketoacidosis
DM	diabetes mellitus
DNA	deoxyribonucleic acid
DV	dorso-ventral (view)
EBP	eosinophilic bronchopneumopathy
ECG	electrocardiogram
EDTA	ethylenediaminetetra-acetic acid
EEG	electroencephalogram
EE/EGE	eosinophilic enteritis/gastroenteritis
EHBDO	extrahepatic bile duct obstruction
EHPSS	extrahepatic portosystemic shunt
ELISA	enzyme-linked immunosorbent assay
EMG	electromyogram
EOD	every other day
EPA	eicosapentaenoic acid

ABBREVIATIONS

EPI	exocrine pancreatic insufficiency
EPO	erythropoietin
ERG	electroretinogram
ETD	every third day
FB	foreign body
FC	flow cytometry
FCE	fibrocartilaginous embolism
FDP	fibrin degradation product
FISH	fluorescent *in-situ* hybridisation
FNA	fine needle aspirate
FRE	food-responsive enteropathy
fT4	free thyroxine
GA	general anaesthesia
GB	gall bladder
GC	granulomatous colitis
G-CSF	granulocyte-stimulating colony factor
GDV	gastric dilatation-volvulus
GFR	glomerular filtration rate
GH	growth hormone
GHRH	growth hormone releasing hormone
GI	gastrointestinal
GIST	gastrointestinal stromal tumour
GME	granulomatous meningoencephalitis
GOLLP	geriatric onset laryngeal paralysis and polyneuropathy
GORD	gastro-oesophageal reflux disease
GSD	German shepherd dog
HAC	hyperadrenocorticism
Hb	haemoglobin
HCT	haematocrit
HDDS	high-dose dexamethasone suppression test
HE	hepatic encephalopathy
HGE	haemorrhagic gastroenteritis (aka AHDS)
HGMS	histology-guided mass spectrometry
HO	hypertrophic osteopathy
HPT	hyperparathyroidism
HUC	histiocytic ulcerative colitis – *q.v.* GC
IBD	inflammatory bowel disease (aka CIE)
IBS	irritable bowel syndrome
ICGN	immune complex glomerulonephritis
ICH	infectious canine hepatitis
IDDM	insulin-dependent diabetes mellitus
IFAT	immunofluorescent antibody test
IgA	immunoglobulin A
IGF	insulin-like growth factor
IHC	immunohistochemistry
IHPSS	intrahepatic portosystemic shunt
IM	intramuscular
IMHA	immune-mediated haemolytic anaemia
IMPA	immune-mediated polyarthritis
IPSID	immunoproliferative small intestinal disease

IMTP	immune-mediated thrombocytopenia
IOP	intraocular pressure
IRE	immunosuppressant-responsive enteropathy
IV	intravenous
IVDD	intervertebral disc disease
IVFT	intravenous fluid therapy
IVIG	intravenous immunoglobulin
IVU	intravenous (excretory) urogram
KCS	keratoconjunctivitis sicca
LDDS	low-dose dexamethasone suppression (screening) test
LE	lupus erythematosus
LI	large intestine
LN	lymph node
LOPP	lomustine-vincristine-procarbazine-prednisolone
LP	laryngeal paralysis
LPC	lymphocytic-plasmacytic colitis
LPE	lymphocytic-plasmacytic enteritis
MCT	mast cell tumour
MCT	medium chain triglyceride
MDS	myelodysplastic syndrome
MG	myasthenia gravis
MGCS	Modified Glasgow Coma Scale
MLK	morphine-lidocaine-ketamine
MO	megaoesophagus
MPS	mucopolysaccharidosis
MRI	magnetic resonance imaging
MUO	meningoencephalitis of unknown origin
MVD	microvascular dysplasia
NDI	nephrogenic diabetes insipidus
NE	necrotising encephalitis
NIDDM	non-insulin-dependent diabetes mellitus
NPO	*nil per os* (nothing by mouth)
NRE	non-responsive enteropathy
NSAID(s)	non-steroidal anti-inflammatory drugs
NTI	non-thyroidal illness
OAVRT	orthodromic atrioventricular reciprocating tachycardia
OESD	Old English sheepdog
OHE	ovariohysterectomy
OSPT	one-stage prothrombin time
Pa	partial pressure
PARR	PCR for antigen receptor rearrangements
PAS	periodic acid schiff
PCNA	proliferating cell nuclear antigen
PCR	polymerase chain reaction
PCV	packed cell volume
PD	polydipsia
PDA	patent ductus arteriosus
PDH	pituitary-dependent hyperadrenocorticism
PFK	phosphofructokinase
PHPT	primary hyperparathyroidism

PIE	pulmonary infiltrate with eosinophils
PIMA	precursor-targeted immune-mediated anaemia
PIVKA	proteins induced by vitamin K antagonism
PLE	protein-losing enteropathy
PLN	protein-losing nephropathy
PLR	pupillary light response
PMI	point of maximal intensity
PO	*per os* (by mouth)
POMC	pro-opiomelanocortin
PPDH	pleuroperitoneal diaphragmatic hernia
PPI	proton pump inhibitor
PRAA	persistent right aortic arch
PRCA	pure red cell aplasia
PS	pulmonic stenosis
PSS	porto-systemic shunt
PT	prothrombin time
PTE	pulmonary thromboembolism
PTH	parathyroid hormone (parathormone)
PTH-rp	PTH-related peptide
PTT	activated partial thromboplastin time
PU	polyuria
PU/PD	polyuria/polydipsia
PVH	portal vein hypoplasia
PVR	peripheral vascular resistance
QID	four times daily (q6h)
q.v.	*quod vide* (see related material)
RAAS	renin-angiotension-aldosterone system
RBC	red blood cell
RCND	renal cystadenocarcinoma and nodular dermatofibrosis
RF	rheumatoid factor
ROTEM	rotational thromboelastometry
SARDS	sudden acquired retinal degeneration syndrome
SAT	slide agglutination test
SC	subcutaneous
SDMA	symmetric dimethylarginine
SG	specific gravity
SI	small intestine
SIBO	small intestinal bacterial overgrowth
SID	once daily (q24h)
SLE	systemic lupus erythematosus
SPE	serum protein electrophoresis
SRE	steroid(immune suppressant)-responsive enteropathy
SRMA	steroid-responsive meningitis-arteritis
SV	stroke volume
SVT	supraventricular tachycardia
T3	triiodothyronine
T4	thyroxine
TAP	trypsinogen activation peptide
TCC	transitional cell carcinoma
TCT	thrombin clot time

ABBREVIATIONS

TECA	total ear canal ablation
TEG	thromboelastography
TEM	transmission electron microscopy
TGAA	thyroglobulin autoantibody
TIBC	total iron binding capacity
TID	three times daily (q8h)
TLI	trypsin-like immunoreactivity
TMJ	temporomandibular joint
TPMT	thiopurine S-methyltransferase
TOD	target organ damage
TP	total protein
TRH	thyroid-releasing hormone
TSH	thyroid-stimulating hormone
TT4	total thyroxine
TVT	transmissible venereal tumour
TXA	tranexamic acid
UCCR	urine cortisol creatinine ratio
UDCA	ursodeoxycholic acid
UK	United Kingdom
UPC	urine protein:creatinine ratio
URT	upper respiratory tract
USG	urine specific gravity
USMI	urinary sphincter mechanism incompetence
UTI	urinary tract infection
VD	ventro-dorsal (view)
VPC	ventricular premature contraction
VSD	ventricular septal defect
vWD	von Willebrand disease
vWf	von Willebrand factor
WBC	white blood cell
WHWT	West Highland White terrier
WNL	within normal limits

ABBREVIATIONS

Page numbers in bold denote pages with the most complete relevant information.
q.v., the information is found at the alternative site
see also, contains related information

Notes on Canine Internal Medicine, Fourth Edition. Victoria L. Black, Kathryn F. Murphy, Jessie Rose Payne,
and Edward J. Hall.
© 2022 John Wiley & Sons Ltd. Published 2022 by John Wiley & Sons Ltd.